# THE TEAM PHYSICIAN'S HANDBOOK

Edited by

**MORRIS B. MELLION, M.D.**
Medical Director, Sports Medicine Center; Associate Professor, Departments of Family Practice and Orthopaedic Surgery (Sports Medicine), University of Nebraska Medical Center; Associate Professor, School of Health, Physical Education and Recreation, and Team Physician, Men's and Women's Sports, University of Nebraska at Omaha, Omaha, Nebraska.

**W. MICHAEL WALSH, M.D.**
Associate Professor of Orthopaedic Surgery and Rehabilitation, and Director, Sports Medicine Program, Department of Orthopaedic Surgery and Rehabilitation, University of Nebraska Medical Center, Omaha, Nebraska.

**GUY L. SHELTON, P.T., A.T.C.**
Lead Sports Physical Therapist and Clinical Instructor, Division of Physical Therapy Education, University of Nebraska; Clinical Instructor, Department of Orthopaedic Surgery and Rehabilitation, University of Nebraska Medical Center; Co-Director, Sports Rehabilitation, Sports Medicine Center, Omaha, Nebraska.

HANLEY & BELFUS, INC./Philadelphia
MOSBY–YEAR BOOK/St. Louis • Baltimore • Boston • Chicago • London
Philadelphia • Sydney • Toronto

Publisher:        HANLEY & BELFUS
                  210 S. 13th Street
                  Philadelphia, PA 19107
                  (215) 546-7293

North American and worldwide sales and distribution:

                  THE C.V. MOSBY COMPANY
                  11830 Westline Industrial Drive
                  St. Louis, MO 63146

In Canada:        THE C.V. MOSBY COMPANY, LTD.
                  5240 Finch Avenue East
                  Unit 1
                  Scarborough, Ontario M1S 5A2
                  Canada

**The Team Physician's Handbook**                    ISBN 1-56053-001-4

Library of Congress Catalog Card Number 90-82905

Last digit is the print number: 9 8 7 6 5 4 3 2

## DEDICATION

Being a team physician is often a family affair, which involves both joy and sacrifice. For the many afternoons, evenings, and weekends we spent on home and away sidelines, rather than with them; for the years they spent sitting on hard, cold bleachers supporting us in our labor . . . we lovingly dedicate *The Team Physician's Handbook* to our families:

Irene, Rosie, and Frank Mellion
Claire, Pat, Ryan, Megan, and Tim Walsh
Beverly, Austin, Franklin, and Wade Shelton

# CONTENTS

## *Part IV:* **SPECIFIC SPORTS**

# CONTRIBUTORS

**ROSEMARY AGOSTINI, M.D.**
Clinical Instructor in Orthopedics, University of Washington; Clinical Teaching Faculty, Department of Family Practice, Swedish Hospital; Staff, Virginia Mason Sports Medicine Clinic; Cleveland High School Team Physician, Seattle, Washington; Chief Medical Officer of Men's Volleyball and Wrestling, 1990 Goodwill Games

**LOREN H. AMUNDSON, M.D.**
Professor of Family Medicine, University of South Dakota School of Medicine, Sioux Falls, South Dakota; Member, American Board of Family Practice Committee to Develop Certificate of Added Qualifications in Sports Medicine

**MARK L. AMUNDSON, M.S., P.T., A.T.C.**
Director, Brookings Sports Medicine Center; Adjunct Faculty, South Dakota State University, Brookings, South Dakota; Vice President, South Dakota Athletic Trainers Association; Member of the Licensure Commission (National Level) of National Athletic Trainers' Association

**THOMAS R. BAECHLE, Ed.D.**
Associate Professor and Chairman, Department of Physical Education/Exercise Science, Creighton University, Omaha, Nebraska; Certified Strength and Conditioning Specialist, National Strength and Conditioning Association; Certified Exercise Test Technologist and Exercise Specialist, American College of Sports Medicine; Level I Weightlifting Coach, U.S. Weightlifting Federation

**DONALD R. BENNETT, M.D.**
Reynolds Professor of Neurology, University of Nebraska College of Medicine, Omaha, Nebraska; Neurological Consultant, Athletic Department, University of Nebraska at Lincoln, Lincoln, Nebraska

**JAMES B. BENNETT, M.D., F.A.C.S.**
Clinical Associate Professor and Chief, Hand and Upper Extremity Surgery Division, Department of Orthopedic Surgery, Baylor College of Medicine, Houston, Texas; Team Consultant, Houston Oilers Professional Football and Houston Astros Professional Baseball

**KRIS E. BERG, Ed.D.**
Professor, School of Health, Physical Education, and Recreation, University of Nebraska at Omaha, Omaha, Nebraska

**T. A. BLACKBURN, JR., R.P.T., A.T.C.**
Staff, Rehabilitation Services of Columbus, Columbus, Ohio

**DANIEL BLANKE, Ph.D.**
Associate Professor, School of Health, Physical Education, and Recreation, University of Nebraska at Omaha, Omaha, Nebraska

**WARREN DANIEL BOWMAN, JR., M.D., F.A.C.P.**
Member, Department of Internal Medicine, Billings Clinic, Billings, Montana; Associate Clinical Professor of Medicine (WAMI), School of Medicine, University of Washington, Seattle; National Medical Advisor, National Ski Patrol System, Inc.; Chairman, Medical Committee, National Association for Search and Rescue

**LARRY E. BRAGG, M.D.**
Assistant Professor of Surgery, Department of Surgery, University of Nebraska and Omaha Veterans Administration Medical Centers, Omaha, Nebraska

**DAVID E. BROWN, M.D.**
Assistant Professor (Orthopaedic Surgery), University of Nebraska Medical Center, Omaha, Nebraska; Team Orthopaedic Surgeon, University of Nebraska—Omaha; Team Orthopaedic Surgeon, Wayne State College

**WILLIAM L. CAPPIELLO, M.D.**
Associate Director, Sports Medicine Fellowship Program, Department of Orthopaedics, Kaiser Permanente Medical Center, Santa Clara, California

**RICHARD L. CARTER, M.D.**
Chief Resident, Department of Neurological Surgery, University of Florida College of Medicine, Gainesville, Florida

**IGNAZIO CARUSO, M.D.**
Sports Orthopedic Surgeon, Rome, Italy

**GUGLIELMO CERULLO, M.D.**
Sports Orthopedic Surgeon, Rome, Italy

**GERALD R. CHRISTENSEN, M.D.**
Associate Professor of Ophthalmology and Pathology, University of Nebraska Medical Center, Omaha, Nebraska

**WILLIAM G. CLANCY, JR., M.D.**
Clinical Professor of Orthopaedics and Sports Medicine, University of Virginia School of Medicine; Staff, Alabama Sports Medicine and Orthopedic Center, Birmingham, Alabama

**PATRICK E. CLARE, M.D.**
Associate Professor Orthopedic Surgery, University of Nebraska Medical Center; Team Physician, University of Nebraska Athletic Department, Lincoln, Nebraska

**LEON F. DAVIS, M.D., D.D.S.**
Associate Professor, Oral and Maxillofacial Surgery, University of Nebraska Medical Center, Omaha, Nebraska

**ARTHUR L. DAY, M.D.**
Professor and James and Newton Eblen Eminent Scholar, Department of Neurosurgery, University of Florida College of Medicine, Gainesville, Florida; Team Neurosurgeon, University of Florida; Chairman of the Sports Medicine Committee of the American Association of Neurological Surgery/Congress of Neurological Surgery Joint Section on Neurotrauma and Critical Care

**PAUL W. ESPOSITO, M.D.**
Assistant Professor of Orthopaedic Surgery, University of Nebraska Medical Center, Omaha, Nebraska

**DENISE M. FANDEL, M.S., A.T.C.**
Instructor and Head Athletic Trainer, University of Nebraska at Omaha, Omaha, Nebraska

**JOHN A. FEAGIN, JR., M.D.**
Associate Professor, Department of Surgery (Orthopaedic Surgery), Duke University Medical Center; Chief of Orthopaedics, Durham VA Hospital; Associate Professor, Biomedical Engineering, Duke University, Durham, North Carolina; Clinical Professor of Orthopaedic Surgery, Uniformed Services University of the Health Sciences, Bethesda, Maryland

**THOMAS P. FERLIC, M.D.**
Clinical Assistant Professor, Director of Hand Surgery, Department of Orthopaedic Surgery and Rehabilitation, University of Nebraska Medical Center, Omaha, Nebraska

**RICHARD B. FLYNN, Ed.D.**
Dean, College of Education, and Professor of Physical Education, University of Nebraska at Omaha, Omaha, Nebraska

**VITTORIO FRANCO, M.D.**
Sports Orthopedic Surgeon, Rome, Italy

**JAMES BOLAN GALLASPY, JR., M.Ed., A.T.C.**
Associate Professor, Athletic Department, The University of Southern Mississippi, Hattiesburg, Mississippi

**JAMES G. GARRICK, M.D.**
Director, Center for Sports Medicine, Saint Francis Memorial Hospital, San Francisco, California; Chairman of Sports Medicine Epidemiology Sub-Committee, Research and Education Committee, American Orthopaedic Society for Sports Medicine

**ANN C. GRANDJEAN, Ed.D.**
Director, International Center for Sports Nutrition, and Assistant Professor, Sports Medicine Program, Department of Orthopaedic Surgery and Rehabilitation, University of Nebraska Medical Center, Omaha, Nebraska

**GARY ALAN GREEN, M.D.**
Clinical Assistant Professor, Division of Family Medicine, UCLA School of Medicine, Los Angeles, California

**WILLIAM D. HAFFEY, M.S.**
Supervisor, Omaha Metro Varsity Football Officials; Assistant Principal, Westside Middle School, Omaha, Nebraska

**RONNIE D. HALD, P.T., A.T.C.**
Sports Physical Therapist, University of Nebraska Medical Center; Co-Director, Sports Rehabilitation, Sports Medicine Center, Omaha, Nebraska

**BRIAN C. HALPERN, M.D.**
Sports Medicine New Jersey, Marlboro, New Jersey

**RICHARD W. HAMMER, M.D., F.A.A.P.**
Clinical Assistant Professor of Pediatrics, University of Nebraska Medical Center, Omaha, Nebraska; Member, Sports Medicine Committee, United States Swimming; Member, Education and Athletic Medicine Committee, Nebraska Medical Association; President, Cornhusker State Games

**JIMMY H. HARA, M.D.**
Associate Clinical Professor, Division of Family Medicine, UCLA School of Medicine; Assistant Chief of Service and Residency Program Director, Department of Family Practice, Kaiser Permanente Los Angeles, Los Angeles, California

**THOMAS M. HEISER, M.D.**
Associate Professor of Orthopaedic Surgery, University of Nebraska Medical Center, Omaha, Nebraska; Co-Team Physician, University of Nebraska at Lincoln, Lincoln Nebraska

**TODD PAUL HENDRICKSON, M.D.**
Assistant Professor, Psychiatry, University of Nebraska Medical Center and Creighton-Nebraska Department of Psychiatry, Omaha, Nebraska; Consultant, Sports Medicine Program

**GREGORY P. HESS, M.D.**
Clinical Instructor, Orlando Regional Medical Center, Florida; Team Physician, Approved and Registered, U.S. Alpine Ski Team

**JEFFREY W. HILL, M.D.**
Assistant Professor of Family Practice, University of Nebraska Medical Center, Omaha, Nebraska; Medical Director, Bike Ride Across Nebraska

**JERRY W. HIZON, M.D.**
Associate Faculty, Department of Family Medicine, University of California, Irvine, Medical Center, Irvine, California; Team Physician, Temecula Valley High School; Medical Director, T.A.C.C. Sports Medicine Center

**DAVID O. HOUGH, M.D.**
Associate Professor of Family Practice and Director of Sports Medicine, Michigan State University College of Human Medicine, East Lansing, Michigan; Director of Sports Medicine and Head Team Physician, Michigan State University

**STEPHEN C. HUNTER, M.D.**
Assistant Clinical Professor, Department of Orthopaedic Surgery—Sports Medicine, Tulane University School of Medicine; Team Physician, Columbus College, Columbus, Georgia; Member American Academy of Orthopaedic Surgeons Committee on Sports Medicine

**WALTER W. HUURMAN, M.D.**
Associate Professor of Orthopaedic Surgery and Rehabilitation, and Assistant Professor of Pediatrics; Director of Children's Orthopaedics, Department of Orthopaedic Surgery and Rehabilitation, and Department of Pediatrics, University of Nebraska Medical Center; Vice-Chief of Staff, University of Nebraska Hospital, Omaha, Nebraska

**DANIEL JOSEPH JOYCE, M.D.**
Primary Care Sports Medicine Physician, Lititz, Pennsylvania; Team Physician, Millerville University, Millerville, Pennsylvania

**MICHELE J. JULIN, PA-C, M.S.**
Physician Assistant, Sports Medicine Center, Omaha, Nebraska

**TIMOTHY F. KELLY, M.A., A.T.C.**
Assistant Athletic Trainer, United States Military Academy, West Point, New York

**ROGER H. KOBAYASHI, M.D.**
Associate Professor of Pediatrics, UCLA School of Medicine, Los Angeles, California

**MARK A. KWIKKEL, M.A., A.T.C., L.A.T.**
Assistant Athletic Trainer/Instructor, School of Health, Physical Education, and Recreation, University of Northern Iowa, Cedar Falls, Iowa

**RICHARD W. LATIN, Ph.D.**
Associate Professor, Exercise Science, School of Health, Physical Education, and Recreation, University of Nebraska at Omaha, Omaha, Nebraska

**NAPOLEON LEE, M.D.**
Senior Research Fellow, UCLA Center for Health Sciences, Los Angeles, California

**WADE LILLEGARD, M.D.**
Sports Medicine Fellow, Michigan State University College of Human Medicine, East Lansing, Michigan

**CHERYL LINDLY, M.A., A.T.C.**
Former Head Athletic Trainer, Papillion-La Vista High School; Physician Assistant Student, University of Nebraska College of Medicine, Omaha, Nebraska

**MONTY SCOTT MATHEWS, M.D.**
Assistant Professor of Family Practice, University of Nebraska Medical Center, Omaha, Nebraska

**JAMES DOUGLAS MAY, M.A., A.T.C.**
Athletic Trainer, The McCallie School, Chattanooga, Tennessee

**CHRIS McGREW, M.D.**
Sports Medicine Fellow, Michigan State University College of Human Medicine, East Lansing, Michigan

**MARK E. McKINNEY, Ph.D.**
Associate Professor, Department of Medicine, Texas College of Osteopathic Medicine, Fort Worth, Texas

**THOMAS L. MEHLHOFF, M.D.**
Clinical Instructor, Division of Orthopedic Surgery, Baylor College of Medicine, Houston, Texas; Team Consultant, Houston Astros Professional Baseball

**MORRIS B. MELLION, M.D.**
Medical Director, Sports Medicine Center, Omaha, Nebraska; Associate Professor, Departments of Family Practice and Orthopaedic Surgery (Sports Medicine), University of Nebraska Medical Center; Associate Professor, School of Health, Physical Education and Recreation, and Team Physician, Men's and Women's Sports, University of Nebraska at Omaha, Omaha, Nebraska

**TERRY L. NICOLA, M.D., M.S.**
Clinical Instructor, Harvard Medical School and Tufts University School of Medicine, Boston, Massachusetts; Director of Sports Medicine, Spaulding Rehabilitation Hospital, Boston, Massachusetts

**THOMAS A. NIQUE, M.D., D.D.S.**
Assistant Professor, Oral and Maxillofacial Surgery, University of Nebraska Medical Center, Omaha, Nebraska

**LAURA E. PETER, M.D.**
Medical Student, University of Nebraska College of Medicine, Omaha, Nebraska

**GIANCARLO PUDDU, M.D.**
Sports Orthopedic Surgeon, Rome, Italy

**JAMES C. PUFFER, M.D.**
Associate Professor and Chief Division of Family Medicine, UCLA School of Medicine, Los Angeles, California

**AMANDA DUFFY RANDALL, M.S.W., A.C.S.W.**
Clinical Psychotherapist/Instructor, Eating Disorders Program, University of Nebraska Medical Center, Omaha, Nebraska

**Wm MacMILLAN RODNEY, M.D.**
Professor and Chairman of Family Medicine, The University of Tennessee, Memphis, College of Medicine, Memphis, Tennessee

**SHARON JANE ROWE, M.A., C.T.R.S.**
Wellness Coordinator, University of Nebraska Medical Center, Omaha, Nebraska; Certified Aerobics Fitness Instructor

**J. RICHARD STEADMAN, M.D.**
Chairman, Medical Group, United States Ski Team; Orthopedic Surgeon, Vail, Colorado

**GUY L. SHELTON, P.T., A.T.C.**
Lead Sports Physical Therapist and Clinical Instructor, Division of Physical Therapy Education, University of Nebraska; Clinical Instructor, Department of Orthopaedic Surgery and Rehabilitation, University of Nebraska Medical Center; Co-Director, Sports Rehabilitation, Sports Medicine Center, Omaha, Nebraska

**MICHAEL A. SITORIUS, M.D.**
Chairman, Department of Family Practice, University of Nebraska Medical Center; Associate Team Physician, University of Nebraska Omaha, Omaha, Nebraska

**HAROLD K. TU, M.D., D.M.D.**
Associate Professor, Oral and Maxillofacial Surgery, University of Nebraska Medical Center, Omaha, Nebraska

**W. MICHAEL WALSH, M.D.**
Associate Professor of Orthopaedic Surgery and Rehabilitation, and Director, Sports Medicine Program, Department of Orthopaedic Surgery and Rehabilitation, University of Nebraska Medical Center, Omaha, Nebraska

**JERRY WEBER, M.S., P.T., A.T.C.**
Assistant Athletic Trainer/Physical Therapist, University of Nebraska at Lincoln, Lincoln, Nebraska

**JOHN M. WILHITE, M.D.**
Group Practice, The Woodlands Sports Medicine Centre, The Woodlands, Texas

# PREFACE

*The Team Physician's Handbook* is written for the many thousands of physicians who are fortunate enough to provide care in a wide variety of team, school, league, and club settings. Being a team physician is both an honor and a challenge. It may be an awesome responsibility for the uninitiated. For the family physician, pediatrician, or internist, there may be unique musculoskeletal problems not seen in daily practice. For the orthopedic surgeon, there will be medical and psychological problems that are alien to the operating room and the cast room. And for physicians from other narrowly defined specialties, the broad knowledge base necessary for care of athletes may pose an even greater challenge.

This book is designed to be both a ready reference and a detailed resource for team physicians, athletic trainers, and other health professionals caring for athletes. It is written in outline format with liberal use of bold type to indicate topic headings and critical points. This approach is designed to provide immediate access to a large volume of well-organized, practical information. The book is divided into four major parts. The first part contains general chapters relating to sports, exercise physiology, and a variety of other general concerns. Part II provides in-depth treatment of important general medical problems. Part III describes specific injury prevention, diagnosis, and treatment. It is organized primarily by body part, but there are also chapters on musculoskeletal injuries in general and on athletic taping. Finally, Part IV deals with the sports medicine issues of most of the popular team sports in the United States. In Part IV a chapter on dance has been included, because caring for a group of dancers is a responsibility very similar to that of being a team physician.

The sport-oriented chapters contain a great deal of overlap with the anatomically oriented injury chapters, as well as with some of the more general chapters in the first two parts of the book. It was decided to permit this overlap in order to provide the reader with sport-specific insights into many of the common injuries.

Morris B. Mellion, M.D.
W. Michael Walsh, M.D.
Guy L. Shelton, P.T., A.T.C.

# Acknowledgments

We would like to express our personal thanks to the many people who helped us make this book possible.

First, thanks go the student-athletes at the University of Nebraska at Omaha. It has been a pleasure to care for you and to be challenged by your wants, desires, and needs. Dr. Robert Gibson and Miss Connie J. Claussen, M.A., athletic directors; Ms. Denise M. Fandel, M.S., A.T.C., and Mr. Thomas A. Frette, M.A., A.T.C., athletic trainers; and the entire coaching staff, training room staff, and equipment manager staff have fostered an ideal setting for us to provide team physician services in a variety of extremely competitive men's and women's sports.

We want to thank Ms. Kathleen Knudsen, as well as several student athletic trainers and a student equipment manager, for posing for photographs. A word of thanks goes to the publishers, Hanley and Belfus, Inc., who once again have provided the highest level of professional support in the creation of this book.

We wish to offer special thanks to Ms. Mary Walsh Jones and Ms. Deborah K. Caddell for their tireless efforts in working and reworking the manuscript. Thanks also to the computer scientists and programmers who designed the word processor.

Finally, we have the deepest appreciation for the opportunity to work with an extremely bright, articulate group of sports medicine and exercise science colleagues, the authors and co-authors of this book. They are the people who support us directly on the campuses of the University of Nebraska Medical Center and the University of Nebraska at Omaha, as well as many others from around the country who devote part or all of their careers to the health and welfare of athletes.

Thank you all very much.

Morris B. Mellion, M.D.
W. Michael Walsh, M.D.
Guy L. Shelton, R.P.T., A.T.C.

Omaha, Nebraska

# Chapter 1: The Team Physician

MORRIS B. MELLION, MD
W. MICHAEL WALSH, MD

I. **Being a Team Physician: A Special Privilege, an Awesome Challenge**

   A. **Special role: Team physicians have a unique responsibility for important decisions.** They are expected by school, community league, or professional team administrators to make major decisions about athletes' health, qualifications to join the team, and ability to participate safely. These decisions are often made in a setting of intense time pressure. They may affect the competitive success of the team as well as the athlete. They often influence the athlete's mental and economic, as well as physical, well-being. Level of performance and scholarships and professional opportunities may depend on timely, high quality medical care.

   B. **The team physician addresses the physical, emotional, and spiritual needs of the athlete in the context of the sport and the needs of the team.** Consequently, family physicians, pediatricians, general internists, and other generalists are best suited by training to function as team physicians. When orthopedists, emergency physicians, general surgeons, gynecologists, and other specialists function as team physicians, their success depends on their individual ability and training to meet the athletes' broad range of medical and psychosocial needs.

      1. **To perform effectively, the team physician must maintain a broad, up-to-date knowledge base that addresses athletics as well as medicine:**
         a. **Medicine**
            i. Musculoskeletal system
            ii. Growth and development
            iii. Cardiorespiratory function
            iv. Gynecology
            v. Dermatology
            vi. Neurology
         b. **Psychology and behavior**
         c. **Pharmacology**
            i. Therapeutics
            ii. Performance aids
            iii. Recreational drugs
         d. **Exercise science**
            i. Exercise physiology
            ii. Biomechanics
            iii. Specific sports

   C. **The team physician has a range of ethical responsibilities that reflect the many relationships involved in the care of the team. Responsibilities to the athlete, the team, and the institution and its representatives must be balanced.**

      1. **Responsibilities to athletes:**
         a. **To allow to participate**—Should not arbitrarily disqualify athletes from participation for reasons that are insignificant or out of line with current thinking. Especially in school-based programs, athletes have a right to participate if there is no valid medical contraindication.
         b. **To protect** from injury, reinjury, permanent disability, and themselves: When there is valid medical contraindication to participation or resumption of participation, athletes must be counseled and thoroughly informed. May be especially difficult to reason with an athlete who has a "participate at any cost" attitude.
         c. **To provide optimal health care.**
         d. **Confidentiality:** Often compromised by relationship to school/professional club. Seldom may information be held in strict doctor-patient confidentiality. However, the team physician must be sensitive as to how widely information is disseminated. For example, if an athlete wishes to resign from the team without having the physician tell others the medical reasons for this decision, that wish should be honored.

1

2. **Responsibility to the team: to facilitate success of the group,** who have all dedicated time and effort to the sport.
3. **Responsibilities to the coach:**
   a. **To facilitate success:** So that the coach does not view the team physician as an impediment to success, but rather as a part of the team striving for success.
   b. **To educate the coach** about improvements in medical and preventive care. Continuing education of the coaching staff is important to eliminate archaic and possibly harmful techniques.
   c. **To protect from possible future liability.**
4. **Responsibilities to the institution:**
   a. **To facilitate success** in light of financial commitment.
      i. To provide optimal health care for the athletes.
      ii. To prescreen scholarship and professional athletes.
   b. **To protect from liability.**

D. **Availability is a cornerstone for success as a team physician.** Personal availability and a well-organized coverage system are essential. Availability is important:
   1. **On the sidelines:** The front lines of sports medicine, especially for contact sports. A physician who covers a team solely from the stands or the office does not truly deserve the title "team physician."
   2. **In the training room:** Important to demonstrate interest in the team by seeing athletes in their own environment, rather than only in the physician's environment.
   3. **In the office:** Team physicians may wish to make special accommodations in their office schedules for athletes with urgent problems.
   4. **Nights and weekends:** Most athletic activity goes on outside the normal work day. Team physicians should always be available to coaches or trainers.
   5. **Unstructured time with the athletic trainer and/or coach.**

E. **Who serves as team physician?**
   1. *The Physician and Sportsmedicine* 1987 survey of 29,000 team physicians presented the following data:
      a. **Specialty**
         i. 23% family physicians
         ii. 17% orthopedists
         iii. 13% general practitioners
         iv. $\geq$ 4% other specialists (osteopaths, internists, general surgeons, pediatricians, and obstetricians/gynecologists)
      b. **Sport**
         i. > 12,000 football
         ii. < 6,000 basketball
   2. **Some physicians share responsibility by pairing a generalist and a specialist;** for example, team physician and team orthopedist. This is probably the ideal situation, since the majority of injury problems are musculoskeletal. Therefore, a generalist (family physician, pediatrician, internist) and orthopedist should be able to deal effectively with most problems that arise. They can then call upon other specialists as necessary.

F. **Team physicians derive a variety of rewards from service in this capacity.**
   1. **Satisfaction:** Immense personal satisfaction
      a. By providing a service to community.
      b. From working with young, motivated patients.
   2. **Credibility:** Undoubtedly, affiliation with teams, from high school to professional, enhances a physician's prestige in the community and may contribute to practice building.
   3. **Remuneration:** Serving as a team physician should be a labor of love. At anything less than a professional team level, most of the time spent will be as a "volunteer." Above the high school level, some compensation may be a part of the agreement. However, this will be extremely variable, ranging from zero to a

considerable retainer with a professional club. Some colleges and universities provide team physician services through Student Health or an affiliated medical school, but most of these arrangements include large amounts of "volunteer" time as well. Surgeons may receive surgical fees for procedures performed, but often these services are provided on a discount basis as well.

G. **Relationship of team physician to institution:**
1. It is important for both physician and institution to establish **an explicit formal relationship between the physician and the school, league, or team.** It should include job description, any fiscal arrangements, and a statement of expectations. Whenever possible, especially if monetary arrangements are involved, it should be in writing. If a formal contract is not appropriate, it is even more critical to discuss these items before the season begins.
   a. **Who hires** or obtains the services of the team physician:
       i. Athletic director
      ii. Athletic trainer
     iii. Business manager or other officer of professional team
   b. **Job description** of team physician
       i. Person to whom team physician reports
      ii. Services provided by team physician
          (a) At home
          (b) Away
              (i) Reimbursement for travel expenses, if any
     iii. Remuneration and benefits
      iv. Any other expectations of the institution or the physician.

II. **The Sports Medicine Team** (Fig. 1).

The team physician cares for an athletic team and also serves as a key player on the sports medicine team, which consists of the athlete, the team physician, and the coach, each of whom has a support system to draw upon, and the athletic trainer, when one is available. The care of the athlete is a team effort in which the members of the sports medicine team support each other for the benefit of the athlete and the athletic team. Like the athletic team itself, sports medicine services are best provided when done so following a team concept of this kind.

A. **The athlete's support system:**
   1. Teammates
   2. Family and significant others
   3. Friends
   4. Teachers
   5. Athletic trainer
B. **The team physician's support system:**
   1. Clinical support
      a. Medical specialists
      b. Physical therapists
      c. Sports psychologists/ psychiatrists
      d. Nutritionists
      e. Dentists
      f. Podiatrists
      g. Equipment managers
      h. Health educators
   2. Research support
      a. Medical researchers
      b. Exercise physiologists
      c. Sports psychologists
      d. Kinesiologists
      e. Nutritionists
      f. Physical educators
      g. Sociologists
      h. Equipment industry
   3. Athletic trainer
C. **The coach's support system:**
   1. School and/or league administration
      a. Athletic director
   2. Coaching staff
   3. Athletic trainer
   4. Equipment manager
D. **The athletic trainer:** He/she occupies a unique position at the center of the athletic health care triangle.
   1. Therapist and counselor for the athlete

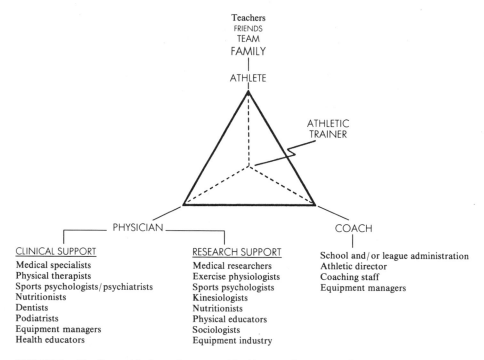

**FIGURE 1.** The Sports Medicine Team. Modified from Mellion MB: **Office Management of Sports** **Injuries & Athletic Problems.** Philadelphia, Hanley & Belfus, Inc., 1988.

      2. Advisor and friend to the coach
      3. Eyes and ears for the team physician
         a. Triage/screening
         b. Supervision of conditioning, care, and rehabilitation
         c. Continuous functional evaluation of the athlete
      4. Every high school and college athletic program should have a certified athletic
         trainer.

   III. **Roles and Functions of the Team Physician: The team physician has a variety of**
      **roles and functions, which include:**
     A. **Medical supervision of athletes:** Herein lies the traditional function of a team
        physician, which has now been greatly expanded.
       1. **Prevention:**
         a. The team physician is responsible for the **preparticipation evaluation:**
            i. Qualification of athletes
              (a) General
              (b) Sport-specific
           ii. Counseling on appropriate sports
          iii. Treatment and rehabilitation of deficits
         b. The team physician is often asked for advice on **proper conditioning**
          **techniques** to prevent or rehabilitate injuries:
           i. Preseason and in-season
           ii. General and sport-specific
         c. The team physician may be asked for advice on **protective equipment:**
           i. Selection
           ii. Fit
           iii. Injury and reinjury prevention

2. **Supervision**
   a. On-site coverage: field, gym, arena, pool
      i. Game and practice coverage
         (a) Physician present for high-risk situations and high-risk sports.
         (b) When a physician is not available for coverage, athletic trainer or other personnel trained in prevention, recognition, and initial evaluation and care of injured athletes should be present.
   b. Tournaments
3. **Evaluation**
   a. Preparticipation evaluation
   b. Illness and injury
      i. On the field
      ii. In the training room
      iii. In the team physician's office
      iv. In the student health clinic
      v. In the emergency room
4. **Management**
   a. Treatment
   b. Consultation and referral when appropriate
B. **Administration: The team physician may be expected to perform a variety of administrative functions.**
   1. **Develop a general system of care for the team.**
   2. Establish **guidelines for consultation** with team physician or referral to consultant.
   3. **Plan and organize preparticipation evaluation:**
      a. Determine content and standards of the evaluation.
      b. Establish guidelines for participation.
      c. Arrange location.
      d. Secure and coordinate personnel.
   4. **Prearrange system of emergency care.**
C. **Logistics:** The team physician should ensure the availability of:
   1. General medical equipment and supplies
   2. Emergency equipment.
   3. Emergency transport.
      a. Ambulance present at high-risk events
   4. Referral to hospital staffed to care for anticipated injuries
   5. Communication
      a. Telephone on sidelines
      b. Radio
D. **Coordination and medical supervision**
   1. Medical personnel
   2. Athletic trainers
   3. Paramedical personnel
E. **Legal and medicolegal**
   1. Contract with school, league, or team
   2. Permission to treat minors
   3. Liability
      a. Institutional liability
      b. Professional liability
   4. Athlete's right to participate
   5. Treatment of athletes on out-of-state trips
      a. Legality
         i. For *major* athletic events the host state or country generally passes legislation granting visiting team physicians temporary licenses.
         ii. For routine competitions and tournaments it is recommended that the traveling team physician work through the host team or tournament physician or local physician in the host town.

     b. "Good Samaritan" laws
         i. No suit has yet been brought against a team physician traveling with a team to another state over the issue of practicing without a license.
     c. Professional liability insurance coverage

F. **Medical insurance**
     1. School, league, or team insurance
     2. Dealing with coverage problems
         a. Capitated medical care systems: HMOs, PPOs
         b. Military dependents
         c. Coverage for preventive services
         d. Coverage for cognitive vs. procedural services

G. **Communication/liaison**
The ideal team physician is a skilled communicator who can often resolve conflicts or enhance cooperation among members of the athletic and sports medicine teams. Certain relationships often require special attention:
     1. Athlete–coach
     2. Athlete–parents
     3. Team physician–parents
     4. Team physician–athlete's family doctor
     5. Athlete–medical colleagues and consultants
     6. Athletic trainer–coach
     7. Injured athlete–press

H. **Education**
The team physician can serve as an educator at many levels and to many audiences in sports medicine.
     1. Audiences:
         a. Athletes
         b. Coaches
         c. Athletic trainers
         d. Administration, especially athletic directors
         e. Medical personnel
             i. Medical students
             ii. House officers
             iii. Colleagues and consultants
         f. Paramedical personnel
         g. Parents
         h. General public
     2. Methods
         a. One-on-one instruction and preception
         b. In-service training
         c. Lectures, workshops, seminars
         d. Formal instructional courses
         e. Newsletters
         f. Audio and video instructional tapes
         g. Written books and articles in sports and professional journals

I. **Student**
     1. Responsibility for remaining current with a body of knowledge that changes rapidly.
     2. Opportunity to learn about life, sport, and medicine from highly motivated athletes, coaches, and other members of the sports medicine team.

J. **Healer**
Even in this highly technical era of medicine, the intangible effect of the "laying on of hands" and the supportive care of the team physician are often the keys to recovery and participation for the athlete.

## RECOMMENDED READING

1. American Academy of Pediatrics: Sports Medicine: Health Care for Young Athletes. Evanston, Illinois, American Academy of Pediatrics, 1983.
2. Howe WB: Primary care sports medicine: A part-timer's perspective. Phys Sportsmed 16(1):103–114, 1988.
3. Lombardo JA: Sports medicine: A team effort. Phys Sportsmed 13(4):72–81, 1985.
4. Samples P: The team physician: No official job description. Phys Sportsmed 16(1):169–175, 1988.

# Chapter 2: The Team Physician, The Athletic Trainer, and the Training Room

CHERYL LINDLY, MA, ATC
DENISE FANDEL, MS, ATC

I. **Roles of the Certified Athletic Trainer**

    A. **Responsible** for prevention, emergency care, first aid, evaluation, and rehabilitation of injuries to athletes under his/her care.

    B. **Liaison** between the team physician, the athlete, the athlete's parents and the coaching staff.

    C. **Consultant** to the coaching staff on conditioning, nutrition, and protective equipment

II. **Education of Certified Athletic Trainer**

    A. **Methods of achieving certification by the National Athletic Trainers' Association (NATA)**

        1. **Internship pathway**

            a. 1500 hours of supervised athletic training experience

                i. 25% in high risk sports

                ii. Supervised by a Certified Athletic Trainer

            b. Coursework

                i. Anatomy

                ii. Physiology

                iii. Exercise physiology

                iv. Kinesiology

                v. Advanced athletic training classes

            c. Bachelor's degree

                i. Usually in a related field

            d. Passing score on certification exam

        2. **Curriculum pathway**

            a. 800 hours of supervised athletic training experience

            b. Graduation from approved curriculum

            c. Passing score on certification exam

    B. **State certification and licensure**

        1. Many, but not all, states certify or license athletic trainers practicing in their states.

        2. May or may not reflect the same competencies measured in the NATA Certification Exam.

III. **Roles and Responsibilities of the Certified Athletic Trainer**

    A. **Prevention of injuries**

        1. Education of athletes and student trainers

        2. Conditioning

            a. Development of conditioning programs

        3. Pre-season screening

            a. Identify factors that put athlete "at risk"

            b. Correct deficiencies

                i. "Prehabilitation"—begin work on deficits before injuries occur

                ii. Referral for further workup

        4. Taping and bracing

            a. Prescribe when needed

    B. **Emergency care and first aid**

        1. Necessary equipment should be available

        2. Communication procedures for emergency situations

            a. Scenarios and procedures should be rehearsed by entire staff.

        3. Provide prompt, accurate triage.

C. **Injury evaluation**
1. Acute injuries
2. Chronic injuries
3. Referral to team physician or specialist where appropriate

D. **Treatment**
1. PRICES (See Chapter 29 on "Musculoskeletal Injuries in Sports")
2. Qualified use of modalities
   a. Cold/heat
   b. Ultrasound
   c. Electrical stimulation

E. **Rehabilitation** (therapeutic exercise)
1. Development of individual exercise prescriptions
2. Supervision of programs
3. Evaluation/modification in program as progress deems necessary
4. Return to competition
   a. Functional testing

IV. **How the Athletic Trainer and Physician Function as a "Team"**

A. **Standard operating procedures should be written whenever possible**
1. Emergency care
2. Transportation
3. Modalities
4. Other treatments and procedures

B. **Coordination of referrals**
1. To physician
2. From physician
3. Between physicians
4. With other health care providers

C. **Game coverage procedures**
1. Establish roles in emergency situations
   a. On-field assessment
   b. Off-field assessment
2. Provide emergency equipment (See Chapter 17, "Injuries and Emergencies on the Field")

D. **Return to play decisions**
1. Define parameters
   a. Range of motion
   b. Strength
   c. Functional ability
   d. Functional taping/bracing?

E. **Open lines of communication**
1. On treatment/rehabilitation
2. On return to competition
3. On emergency care

V. **Training Room Management**

A. **Record keeping**
1. Injury reports
2. Home care instructions
3. Referrals
4. Treatment records
5. Rehabilitation progress notes
6. Insurance

B. **Budgeting**
1. Consult with team physician regarding specific needs

C. **Equipment and supplies**
1. Basic training room supplies and equipment
   a. Taping
   b. Wound care
   c. Rehabilitation devices
      i. Sandbag weights
      ii. Surgical tubing
      iii. Exercise equipment
      iv. Proprioception boards
   d. Modalities
      i. Whirlpool
      ii. Ultrasound
      iii. Ice machine/freezer
      iv. Hydrocollator
      v. Electrical stimulators
2. Emergency equipment and supplies
   a. Spine boards and stretchers
   b. Cervical immobilizer
   c. Splints
      i. Air
      ii. Basswood
      iii. Rapid evacuation form immobilizer
      iv. Knee immobilizer
   d. Slings
   e. Crutches

D. **Equipment available for team physician use only**
   1. Prescription medication samples
   2. Suture kit
   3. Cardiorespiratory emergency medications
E. **Student trainers**
   1. Education
      a. Hands-on experience
      b. Didactic methodology
      c. Preparation for certification examination
   2. Supervision
F. **Professional relationships with support personnel**
   1. Coaches
   2. Administrators
   3. Strength and conditioning coaches
   4. Nutritionists
   5. School nurses
   6. Physical therapists

VI. **Summary**

The athletic trainer is a vital member of the team of allied medical professionals who value and care for the health of interscholastic and intercollegiate athletes. It is important for the team physician to understand the potential for a working relationship with the athletic trainer.

Although often limited by time, space, and budget, the athletic trainer, with guidance from the team physician, can make a vast improvement in the level of care provided for the athletes through timely treatment, rehabilitation, and emergency care.

For the team physician, the athletic training staff acts as a daily liaison with student athletes. As more and more schools hire certified athletic trainers, the effectiveness of the team physician becomes proportionally greater. We hope that in the years to come every educational institution will see fit both to hire a certified athletic trainer and to expand the role of the team physician, thereby allowing the formation of a health care team whose primary concern is the welfare of the student athlete.

# Chapter 3: Coaching and Its Role in Injury Prevention

JAMES B. GALLASPY, JR., ATC
J. DOUGLAS MAY, ATC

I. **Introduction.** The coach is a key member of the sports medicine team. His/her responsibilities include the general care and well-being of athletes through good coaching and leadership, preparticipation screening, and a proper playing environment.

   A. In schools, conferences, and leagues where athletic trainers are not available, the coach's role in prevention and care of injuries in athletes is magnified.

II. **Good coaching and positive leadership are essential for an optimal sports environment.**

   A. **Leadership**
      1. **Based on positive reinforcement:** telling the athlete what he or she is doing right.
      2. **Leadership by example**
      3. **Open, honest communication**
         a. With players
         b. Among coaches
         c. With officials
      4. **Understand and meet the emotional needs** of athletes and fellow coaches.
         a. The most emotionally vulnerable athletes generally respond more positively to good coaching and more negatively to poor coaching than their more stable teammates.

   B. **Administration**
      1. **Recruit only qualified coaches and assistants.**
      2. **Encourage effectiveness training for coaches.**
         a. Hold coaching clinics for assistants.
         b. Use courses and clinics in the community or region. Common sponsoring organizations include:
            i. Local colleges and universities
            ii. American Coaching Effectiveness Program (P.O. Box 5076, Champaign, Illinois 17701)
            iii. Little League Baseball, Inc. (P.O. Box 3485, Williamsport, Pennsylvania 17701)
            iv. National Youth Sports Coaches Association (2611 Okeechobee Road, West Palm Beach, Florida 33409)
      3. Insist on teaching only safe athletic techniques.
      4. Obtain services of a team physician and/or a certified athletic trainer whenever possible.

   C. **Proper and safe fundamentals**
      1. Coach should **know the individual sport thoroughly** in order to:
         a. Teach proper athletic skill techniques.
         b. Correct poor mechanics, which might otherwise lead to overuse injuries.
         c. Teach other coaches and athletes injury prevention by means of
            i. On-field coaching
            ii. Clinics
            iii. Written material
         d. Stress the proper fundamentals that lead to success.

2. **Good coaching guidelines prevent injury and reduce liability risk.**
    a. Advise the athlete (or parents) of inherent dangers of the sport.
    b. Supervise constantly and attentively.
    c. Properly prepare and condition the athlete.
    d. Properly instruct the athlete in the skills of the sport.
    e. Insist on safe techniques
    f. Ensure that safe equipment and facilities are used by the athlete at all times.
    g. Ensure that proper precautions are taken in extremes of heat and cold.
        i. The coach may occasionally even need to cancel practice or competition.
    h. **Recognize physical and emotional injury early and arrange consultation before the problem becomes more severe.**
D. **Officiating and sportsmanship**
    1. The coach should appreciate the role of the rules and the officials in prevention of injuries (Chapter 4).
    2. **The coach should insist that athletes observe the rules and demonstrate proper sportsmanship.**
E. **Conditioning.** The coach is generally responsible for the total conditioning effort, for which the following guidelines are helpful (See also Chapters 6–8):
    1. Teach the athletes the importance of all aspects of conditioning for both maximum performance and injury prevention.
    2. The conditioning program should contain preseason, in-season, and postseason phases.
    3. The conditioning program should contain multiple components, with the emphasis on each determined by the specific sport.
        a. Aerobic power
        b. Strength
            i. Requires special coach training for
                (a) Strength coaching in general        (c) Flexibility
                (b) Specific age/maturity group         (d) Proprioception, agility,
                    coaching                                and coordination
F. **Nutrition** (See Chapter 13)
    1. The coach should understand and teach current valid concepts of nutrition.
    2. The coach should attempt to "debunk" popular nutritional myths that may be harmful to the athlete.
    3. **The coach is obliged to prohibit the use of banned or harmful substances.**
G. **Weight and body composition**
    1. The coach should use and teach **a scientific approach to the issue of weight reduction in athletics.**
        a. **Avoid archaic and/or harmful methods** of body weight manipulation, such as:
            i. Bizarre diets                v. Diuretics
            ii. Fasting                     vi. Rubber suits
            iii. Induced vomiting           vii. Hot boxes
            iv. Purging
    2. The coach should understand and employ valid methods of assessing weight and body composition.

III. **Preparticipation evaluation.** The coach is responsible for ensuring that preparticipation evaluation is performed in compliance with appropriate school, league, or conference regulations.

A. Much of that responsibility may be shared with or assigned to the team physician or athletic trainer; however:
    1. **The coach must ensure that no player practices or competes without proper preseason clearance.**
    2. The coach must ensure **proper follow-up on deficiencies before athletes are permitted to participate:**
        a. Treatment                c. Medical clearance
        b. Rehabilitation

        3. Similarly, the coach is responsible for the same medical evaluation, treatment, rehabilitation, and clearance pattern for the injured athlete during the season.

  B. **Coaches are often major participants in performing the preparticipation evaluation:**
      1. **Conditioning evaluations:**
         a. Aerobic power
         b. Strength
         c. Speed
         d. Agility and coordination
      2. **Musculoskeletal evaluations**
         a. Flexibility
         b. Strength
            i. Manual muscle testing
           ii. Muscle girth measurements
         c. Range of motion
      3. **Body composition measurements**
      4. **Nutrition evaluations**

IV. **Playing Environment**

  A. **Temperature** (See Chapters 11 and 12)
      1. The coach should understand the effects of heat and cold on the safety and performance of the athlete.
      2. **The coach is responsible for measuring temperature and humidity and rescheduling or canceling practices or competitions when conditions are not safe.**
      3. The coach is responsible for **preventive measures,** including but not limited to:
         a. Educating the athlete about safety precautions in hot or cold weather.
         b. Ensuring proper clothing for the weather.
         c. In hot conditions:
            i. Providing adequate fluid replacement
           ii. Providing adequate rest breaks
           iii. Monitoring fluid loss
               (a) Supervising "weigh-in" and "weigh-out" procedures

  B. **Athletic facilities and equipment**
      1. The coach should **set standards for periodic inspection** of athletic facilities and playing surface, particularly prior to practices and competition.
      2. The coach should ensure that safety devices, such as mats and pads, are properly placed and maintained and that dangerous obstacles are eliminated from the playing area.
      3. The coach should ensure that the playing field or facility is properly lighted for the sport.
      4. The coach has responsibilities involving **individual equipment** which include ensuring that protective equipment is:
         a. Properly selected and high quality
         b. Issued by a well-trained individual who can ensure proper fit
         c. Properly maintained and inspected
         d. Properly used by the athlete

  C. **Emergency planning**
      1. The coach is responsible for **developing a plan to evaluate, treat, and transport medical emergencies that occur during practice and competition.**
         a. Plan should be in writing.
         b. Responsibility may be shared with or assigned to the team physician and/or athletic trainer.
         c. Plan should include prior arrangements for transportation of injured athletes and spectators to medical facilities and prior coordination with the referral facility.
      2. **Coaches should have current American Red Cross advanced first aid and cardiopulmonary resuscitation training, or the equivalent, as minimal preparation for handling athletic emergencies.**

# Chapter 4: The Role of Rules and Officials

WILLIAM D. HAFFEY

I. **The Role of Rules**

Rules were developed for the distinct purpose of permitting a congruent transition throughout the length of the contest. **They maintain a consistency in the operation of the mechanics of the contest and a concern for the safety of the participants.** Rules also provide information by which coaches may instruct players and fans may become more enlightened about the sport. They are basic or established criteria by which the officials will work a contest.

A. **Rules.** The rules are divided into several specific areas, each designed to aid in the smooth and normal progress of a contest.

1. **The field of play, the court, the pool.** The rules committee involved with establishing the specifications has set up standards that must be adhered to. The specifications for areas of participation allow consistency between schools and states, and across the country.

2. **Game equipment.** All equipment such as goals, bases, mats, ladders, screens, balls, clocks, yardage chains, etc., used for sports activities must adhere to the standard established by the rules committees.

3. **Player equipment.** The rule books list mandatory equipment that all participants must wear. These items may include helmet, mouth pieces, pads, shoes, jerseys, pants, and uniforms. These items will be professionally manufactured and not altered to decrease protection of the athlete. The mandatory equipment required for all sports is listed in all official rule books.

   a. Game or contest administrators, coaches, and equipment managers must review annually the mandatory equipment that must be worn by participants.

   b. The rule books are reviewed and updated annually.

4. **Illegal equipment.** No player wearing illegal equipment should be permitted to participate. Questions relating to the legality of a player's equipment will be discussed in Section II A.1.d. (below). The list of illegal equipment is for the express purpose of ultimate protection for individuals participating in a contest.

   a. Game or contest administrators, coaches, equipment managers, and officials must know which equipment is illegal for participants to wear during a contest.

   b. The use of illegal equipment should be definitely restricted during practice sessions.

5. **Terminology.** All participants, coaches, fans and officials should be familiar with terms or phrases expressing certain actions involved in an individual sport.

6. **Specific rules. Rules were developed to control the actions of the participants involved with the contest.** As one of the basic fundamentals of the game, coaches should familiarize each player with the rules involved in the sport. Players need not know the technicalities involved with the administration of all the rules, but they should have at least a working knowledge of them.

7. **Violations.** It is a recognized fact that participation in sports activities may result in injury. Some of the sports are more vigorous than others, and physical contact has to be accepted as a consequence. The safety of participants should receive considerable attention. Those responsible for teaching participants of a sport should see that proper techniques are the only methods taught. It is the responsibility of those involved in administering an athletic program to see that coaches teach techniques that are within the rules.

8. **Fouls and penalties.** It is recognized in sports that the basic principle behind the enforcement philosophy is that you are only entitled to advantage gained without the assistance of a foul. The administration of penalties is the responsibility of the official in charge of the contest. Also, coaches should have a basic working knowledge of the fouls and penalties.

## II. The Role of the Official

The official is the essential third party of an athletic contest. The players and coaches make up the other two points of the triangle. The official's primary job is to see that a contest progresses according to the stipulated rules and regulations. He/she must know the rules and mechanics of the sport, have courage to administer the rules, possess tact and poise to insure confidence, be in physical condition to work the sport, and possess the judgment and common sense to execute instinctive reactions to situations that arise during a contest.

### A. Official's duties

The duties can be divided into two areas: pregame duties and game duties.

#### 1. Pregame duties

The general pregame duties for officials follows a similar pattern for contests.

a. The official, regardless of the contest, should have **a precontest meeting to discuss all facets of the contest.** The precontest meeting should follow a well-planned outline. Another objective of this meeting is to get all officials involved mentally to work the contest. The precontest meeting boils down to a "nuts and bolts" meeting.

b. **Inspect the entire area** where the activity will take place. Observe any unusual markings or serious irregularities, and advise the rest of the personnel working the contest. they will take measures to correct or remove any hazardous obstructions within or near the boundary areas of the activity.

c. **Inspect and approve all equipment** and see that all equipment necessary for the proper conduct of a contest is in the proper place and condition.

d. **Check mandatory player equipment.** During pregame, the officials can spot-check player equipment, bandages, tapes, etc. They can have necessary corrections made prior to the contest.

   i. **Football.** Prior to the start of the game, the head coach or his designated representative shall be responsible for verifying to the referee or umpire (depending on whether it is college or high school) that all of the players are in compliance with the rules on mandatory equipment required of all participants. The legality of a player's equipment shall be determined by the umpire.

   (a) NCAA Coaches Certification, in football, implies that all players have been informed what equipment is mandatory by rule and what constitutes illegal equipment, have been provided the equipment mandated by rule, have been instructed to wear and how to wear mandatory equipment during the game, and have been instructed to notify the coaching staff when equipment becomes illegal through play during the game.

   (b) In high school, when any required player equipment is missing or when illegal equipment is found, correction must be made before participation.

   ii. **Wrestling**

   (a) Before a dual meet begins, the referee shall visit each team's dressing room to inspect contestants for presence of oils, improper clothing, all jewelry, long fingernails, and improper grooming. Clarify the rules with coaches and contestants upon request, and review the scorer and timekeeper signals and procedures to be used.

   (b) The legality of all equipment, including mats, markings, uniforms, and supplementary devices, pads and taping, shall be decided by the referee.

   iii. **Basketball**

      (a) The referee shall not permit any player to wear equipment that, in his/her judgment, is dangerous to other players.

      (b) Any equipment that is unnatural and designed to increase a player's height or reach, or to gain an advantage, should not be used.

   iv. **Baseball**

      (a) Prior to the start of the game, the umpire-in-chief shall ascertain legality of all equipment, especially bats and helmets.

      (b) During introduction of umpires and coaches, the coach's acceptance of responsibility for players being properly equipped is part of the pregame duties of officials.

   v. **Soccer**

      (a) The head referee shall inspect and approve the game balls, field of play and nets, inquire about local ground rules, and determine if a fair game may be started.

      (b) Illegal equipment shall not be worn by any player. This applies to any equipment that, in the opinion of the referee, is dangerous and confusing.

   vi. **Volleyball**

      (a) The referee will check players for proper/legal uniforms and equipment.

      (b) The legality of game equipment shall be determined by the referee.

2. **Game duties**

General duties involve knowing the rules and mechanics to officiate the sport within general established guidelines. One of the official's primary concerns, regardless of the sport, is the safety of the participants.

   a. **Whenever game and player equipment can adversely affect the safety of a player, the officials must take precautions to correct the situation.**

   b. **During the contest, whenever damaged or illegal equipment is detected, the officials must take steps to correct the problem,** in accordance with the stipulated rules.

   c. **Injuries.** There are no known steps to prevent all the injuries that can and do occur during athletic contests. Specific procedures do exist when a participant is injured. The following are examples in certain sports.

     i. **Football**

      (a) An injured or apparently injured player who is discovered by an official while the ball is dead and the clock is stopped, and for whom the ready-for-play signal is delayed, or for whom the clock is stopped, shall be replaced for at least one down unless the halftime or overtime intermission occurs.

      (b) In college, the player may remain in the game if his team is charged a timeout in the interval between downs. If the team's charged timeouts have been exhausted, the injured player must leave for one down, whether in college or high school. Any official may stop the clock for an injured player.

     ii. **Wrestling**

      (a) Wrestlers are entitled to injury timeouts and injury recovery time.

      (b) If a competitor is rendered unconscious, he shall not be permitted to continue after regaining consciousness without the approval of a physician. If a physician recommends that an injured wrestler not continue, even though consciousness is not involved, he shall not be overruled.

     iii. **Track**

      (a) A competitor who has been rendered unconscious during a meet shall not be permitted to resume participation in that meet without written authorization from a physician.

      (b) A competitor who scratches from an event because of illness or an injury must have a signed statement from a physician that he/she has permission to participate later in the meet. This statement is required by some state athletic associations.

    iv. **Volleyball**

      (a) In case of injury, the referee may interrupt play and, after sufficient time for replacement of the injured player, direct a replay.

      (b) In case of injury to a starting player during warmups, substitution shall be made without penalty and no entry is charged to the injured player.

    v. **Basketball**

      (a) When a player is injured, the official may suspend play either after the ball is dead or when it is in control of the injured player's team, or when the opponents complete play.

III. **Liability Insurance**

  A. **Sports officials should consider carrying a liability policy.** It has often been said, with much truth, that in America anyone can sue anyone else for almost anything.

  B. **Officials working nonprofessional sports should definitely consider carrying liability insurance.**

  C. Examples of recent legal cases involving sports officials.

    1. *Dailey v. McNeese (Alabama).* This case involves a claim by a high school football player who was injured during the course of the game when an opponent intentionally struck him in the groin, resulting in his testicles being removed. The local officials' association has been sued, based on its failure to supervise the game.

    2. *Rapfogel v. Morris County Industrial Recreation Assn. (New Jersey).* This case involves a claim by a fan who was injured by a foul ball and claims the umpire and the recreational softball league failed to warn her of the danger.

    3. *Thomas v. Board of Education of Hamilton (Ontario, Canada).* This case involves a claim against a local football officials' association arising from a high school football player who was injured when he was tackled during a game. The claim is that the local association failed to insure that there was proper medical supervision in attendance at the game to handle such injuries.

    4. *Heimbaugh v. City and County of San Francisco (California).* This case involves a claim by a recreation baseball player against an umpire claiming he was negligent for allowing the game to proceed with improper bases. The player slid into the base and was injured.

    5. *Uhrigh v. Township of Cranford, et al. (New Jersey).* This is a claim by a recreation wrestler who was injured when his opponent picked him up and slammed him to the mat. The referee is being sued for his failure to properly supervise.

    6. *Frazier v. Rutherford Board of Education (New Jersey).* This is a claim by a high school track man who was injured when he slipped off the take-off board in the long jump competition. There is a claim against the sports official for failure to make sure that the take-off board was in a safe, clean, and dry condition.

    7. *Pichardo v. North Patchogue Medford Youth Athletic Association (New York).* This case involves a claim by a young baseball player who was struck and killed by lightning during a game and his estate is suing the league and umpires.

## RECOMMENDED READING

1. Bunn W: The Art of Officiating Sports. Englewood Cliffs, NJ, Prentice-Hall, 1957.
2. Clegg T, Thompson WA: Modern Sports Officiating. Dubuque, IA, William C. Brown Company, 1979.
3. Goldberger AS: Sports Officiating—A Legal Guide. New York, Leisure Press, 1984.
4. Baseball Rulebook. Mission, KS, National Collegiate Athletic Association, 1988.
5. Basketball Rules and Interpretations Book. Mission, KS, National Collegiate Athletic Association, 1987.
6. Basketball Rules. Kansas City, National Federation of State High School Associations, 1988/89.

7. Football Rules and Interpretation Book. Mission, KS, National Collegiate Athletic Association, 1987.
8. Football Rules. Kansas City, National Federation of State High School Associations, 1988.
9. Football Officials Manual. Kansas City, National Federation of State High School Associations, 1988/89.
10. Football Case Book. Kansas City, National Federation of State High School Associations, 1988.
11. Boys Gymnastics Rules. Kansas City, National Federation of State High School Associations, 1988/89.
12. Girls Gymnastics Rules. Kansas City, National Federation of State High School Associations, 1988/89.
13. Soccer Rules. Kansas City, National Federation of State High School Associations, 1988/89.
14. Volleyball Rules. Kansas City, National Federation of State High School Associations, 1988/89.
15. Swimming, Diving, and Water Polo Rules. Kansas City, National Federation of State High School Associations, 1988/89.
16. Track and Field and Cross Country Rules. Kansas City, National Federation of State High School Associations, 1988.
17. Wrestling Rules. Kansas City, National Federation of State High School Associations, 1988/89.

# Chapter 5: The Preparticipation Physical Examination

JIMMY H. HARA, MD
JAMES C. PUFFER, MD

I. **General Overview**

  A. **Manpower needs and cost efficacy:**
    1. Over 1 million man-hours examining over 6 million youngsters.[28]
    2. Increasing numbers of adults.
    3. Cost efficacy is questioned.[24,29] Study by Risser[24] uncovered only 16 problems in 763 adolescents; one treated and cleared and only 2 of 16 ultimately disqualified. Cost of identifying these three adolescents was $4537 per athlete.

  B. **Likened to elephant being examined by blind men:**[10]
    1. **School administrator:** fulfills legal and insurance needs.
    2. **Coach:** assures health and fit athletes.
    3. **Idealist:** allows mechanism for injury prevention.
    4. **Physician:** uncovers "treatable" conditions.
    5. **Reality:** annual period of frustration, unkept office appointments, and frantic phone calls.

  C. **Potential merits:**
    1. Valuable foundation for provision of care by team physician or primary care physician.
    2. Only if conducted in a rigorous and comprehensive fashion with proper emphasis on format, scope, frequency and content.

II. **Format of Examination**

  A. **Group examination:**
    1. Advocated by Garrick as a high volume, expedient, low cost arrangement.[10,17]
    2. Station-by-station performed by a variety of personnel, including primary care physicians, orthopedists, trainers and physician extenders.[10,21]
    3. According to Garrick, superior to private office examinations in ability to identify abnormalities.[9]
    4. Mustering needed individuals and coordination of schedules not often feasible outside of academic institutions.[12]

  B. **Private office setting:**
    1. Championed by Runyun as an ideal setting.[27]
    2. Family physician, because of longstanding relationship with athlete, thorough knowledge of medical history and prior injuries, and awareness of athlete's physical maturity, is in best position to conduct examination.[21]

III. **Scope of Examination**

  A. Some contend that this represents a rare opportunity to provide comprehensive care.
  B. Rice feels this is not intended to be a substitute for routine periodic comprehensive health screening or a relationship between primary care physician and his patient.[23]

IV. **Objectives of Examination**

  A. Determination of general health.
  B. Assessment of cardiovascular fitness.
  C. Evaluation of pre-existing injuries.
  D. Assessment of size and maturation.

E. Restriction of activity or disqualification from specific activity.
F. Recommendations for appropriate activity when specific participation has been restricted.
G. Establishment of a comprehensive data base.

V. **Frequency of Examination**

A. Ability to achieve objectives dependent upon frequency.
B. Many school districts require annual examination prior to participation in a given sport.
C. NCAA and other governing bodies suggest entry-level comprehensive examination with annual follow-ups.[29]

VI. **Content of Examination**

A. Many school districts and institutions will provide a specific form; if not provided, suggest "Athletic Competition Health Screening Form" developed by Commission on Public Health and Scientific Affairs of the American Academy of Family Physicians (Fig. 1).
B. **Health history** concentrates on prior disease and injuries as well as cardiovascular and musculoskeletal systems, and **in fact most disqualifying conditions show up on the form.**[11]
C. Examination of youngsters should include **assessment of physical maturity** using standard Tanner staging criteria.[32]
D. **Cardiovascular assessment:**
   1. **Outflow tract obstruction is major cause of sudden death in young athletes.**[18]
   2. **Critical question:** "Have you ever felt dizzy, fainted, or actually passed out while exercising?"[12]
   3. Accentuation of systolic murmur with Valsalva suggests asymmetric septal hypertrophy and obstructive hypertrophic cardiomyopathy.[30]
   4. **Ventricular dysrhythmias that disappear with exercise are generally regarded as benign.**
   5. **Unexplained ventricular ectopy should raise possibility of cocaine abuse.**[12]
   6. **Upper limits of blood pressure not requiring evaluation:**[2,33]
      a. 130/75 for children 11 years and younger.
      b. 140/85 for children 12 years and older.
   7. **Systolic hypertension in young athletes usually related to anxiety or inappropriate cuff size in huskier individuals.**[33]
E. Musculoskeletal assessment:
   1. Orthopedic screening assessment should be accomplished in 90–120 seconds.[2]
   2. **Elements of rapid musculoskeletal screen:**
      a. Observe general habitus.
      b. Cervical range of motion (look up, down, over the shoulders, then ear lobes to shoulder tips).
      c. Trapezii, deltoids, and rotator cuffs (shoulder shrug, abduction to 90°, internal-external rotation of shoulders).
      d. Extensor-supinator wad and medial-volar complex (supinate then pronate wrist with elbows at 90°).
      e. Hand function and rotational deformities (spread fingers then make fist).
      f. Duck walk—uncovers hip, knee and ankle disorders.
      g. Quadriceps function (knee extension and thigh tightening, watching vastus lateralis carefully).
      h. Toe touch—checking for scoliosis and tight hamstrings.
      i. Toe walk and heel walk—uncovers leg and foot problems.
   3. More than 90–120 seconds are only necessary if abnormalities are uncovered by history or examination.

VII. **Injury Prevention**

A. An oft-quoted goal, but in reality doubtful if accomplished.

## Athletic Competition Health Screening Form

NAME _____

SCHOOL _____

AGE _____ GRADE _____

DATE OF BIRTH _____ SEX _____

Family Physician _____ Phone _____

Address _____

| HEALTH HISTORY<br>Parent or guardian<br>Answer "yes" or "no" ONLY | YES | NO |
| --- | --- | --- |
| Chronic/Recurrent Illness? | | |
| Hospitalization? | | |
| Surgery Other Than Tonsils? | | |
| Injuries Treated by<br>  Physician? | | |
| Current Medications? | | |
| Organs Missing? | | |
| Heat Exhaustion/Stroke? | | |
| Dizziness, Fainting, Convul-<br>  sions and/or Headaches? | | |
| Knocked Out? | | |
| Concussion? | | |
| Wear Glasses or Contacts? | | |
| Hearing Defects? | | |
| Dental Appliances<br>  Bridge/Brace/Cap/Plate? | | |
| Cough/Pain? | | |
| Problems with Blood Pressure,<br>  Heart or Murmurs? | | |
| Problems with Liver,<br>  Spleen, Kidney? | | |
| Hernia? | | |
| Recurrent Skin Disease? | | |
| Bone/Joint Injury?<br>  Sprain/Dislocation?<br>Injury that Caused a Missed<br>  Practice/Event? | | |
| Allergy to Medications?<br>  Name | | |
| Tetanus Booster in the<br>  Last 10 Years? | | |

The Above Information is Current
and Correct to the Best of My
Knowledge

_____
Signature of
Parent or Guardian

_____
Date

| VITALS | SATISFACTORY YES | SATISFACTORY NO | PHYSICAL EVALUATION COMMENTS | Recommend Follow-up |
| --- | --- | --- | --- | --- |
| Ht | | | | |
| Wt | | | | |
| BP _____ | | | | |
| GENERAL | | | | |
| HEAD | | | | |
| EYES | | | ACUITY  R      L | |
| ENT | | | | |
| DENTAL | | | | |
| CHEST | | | | |
| HEART | | | | |
| ABDOMEN | | | | |
| GENITALIA | | | | |
| SKIN | | | | |
| EXTREMITIES<br>BACK NECK | | | | |
| ALLERGY | | | | |

SUMMARY OF COMMENTS

SPORTS PARTICIPATION APPROVED     Yes _____     No _____

LIMITATIONS

_____
Physician Signature

_____
Date

**FIGURE 1.** Athletic competition health screening form developed by the Commission on Public Health and Scientific Affairs of the American Academy of Family Physicians. The forms are available from the AAFP Order Department at $5 per pad of 50 two-part (self-carbon) forms. A sample copy is available free on request. Reprinted with permission.

1. Marshall suggests use of musculoskeletal flexibility and laxity measures.[19]
2. Jackson and others feel that assessments of flexibility and laxity are not reliable predictors of injury risk.[15]
3. Physician may play important role by assuring preseason conditioning[21] and concentrating on prior injuries:[6]

   a. Moretz and Grana demonstrated lowering of injury rates as season
      progressed.[20]
   b. Reinjury of a previously injured joint is most common clinical scenario.[6]
  B. Sports medicine literature abounds with various **parameters:**
   1. **Body composition**—skin fold calipers, submersion weights
   2. **Strength**—isokinetic devices
   3. **Flexibility**—sit and reach, goniometry
   4. **Power**—vertical leap, Jyvskala test
   5. **Endurance**—12-minute run
   6. **Balance**—stork test, decremental balance beams
  C. Utility of above parameters may be more for physiologic profiling to monitor
     efficacy of training and rehabilitation rather than injury prevention.[22]

VIII. **Classification of Sports**
  A. AMA and American Academy of Pediatrics established guidelines for criteria
     disqualifying athletes based upon level of contact.[2,4]
   1. Hirsch[13] and Birrer[5] modified original AMA/AAP contact/noncontact division:
      a. Hirsch included levels of strenuousness.
      b. Hirsch and Birrer suggested a collision level of contact.
      c. Birrer subdivided noncontact into endurance and leisure.
   2. American Academy of Pediatrics has more recently modified its schema,
      defining contact/collision, limited contact/impact, and noncontact categories
      (Table 1).[3]
  B. **Collision/contact sports**
   1. Football                    6. Soccer
   2. Wrestling                   7. Lacrosse
   3. Hockey                      8. Martial arts
   4. Basketball                  9. Boxing (AMA and AAP have taken official
   5. Baseball                       positions in opposition to boxing as a sport)

IX. **Disqualifying Conditions**
  A. **Caveats in regard to disqualifying conditions:**
   1. Indicate to athlete alternative activities that are permissible and healthier than
      no activity at all.[32]

**TABLE 1.**  Classification of Sports

| | | | Noncontact | |
| Contact/Collision | Limited Contact/Impact | Strenuous | Moderately Strenuous | Nonstrenous |
|---|---|---|---|---|
| Boxing | Baseball | Aerobic dancing | Badminton | Archery |
| Field hockey | Basketball | Crew | Curling | Golf |
| Football | Bicycling | Fencing | Table tennis | Riflery |
| Ice hockey | Diving | Field | | |
| Lacrosse | Field | Discus | | |
| Martial arts | High jump | Javelin | | |
| Rodeo | Pole vault | Shot put | | |
| Soccer | Gymnastics | Running | | |
| Wrestling | Horseback riding | Swimming | | |
| | Skating | Tennis | | |
| | Ice | Track | | |
| | Roller | Weight lifting | | |
| | Skiing | | | |
| | Cross-country | | | |
| | Downhill | | | |
| | Water | | | |
| | Softball | | | |
| | Squash | | | |
| | Volleyball | | | |

From Pediatrics 81:737, 1988, with permission.[3]

2. **Up to the athlete and/or parents to make final decision about participation**[30]— ample **legal precedents** forcing schools and leagues to allow participation.
    a. **In such cases, insist upon legal waiver of responsibility.**
B. Conditions constituting **absolute or relative contraindications** to specific sports activities (Table 2):
    1. **Neurologic**
        a. **Large postsurgical cranial defect:** absolute contraindication for collision/contact.
        b. **Poorly controlled seizures:**
            i. Contraindicate participation in collision/contact and limited contact/impact.
            ii. Contraindicate select noncontact sports:
                (a) High bar and rings
                (b) Swimming and diving
                (c) Weight lifting
                (d) Riflery or archery
        c. **Single concussion**—sidelines for game; **two concussions**—sideline for season; and **three concussions** should require further neurological evaluation prior to decision about participation (but common knowledge that many elite athletes have exceeded this number and still participated).
    2. **Defects in paired organ systems**
        a. Traditionally **absence of vision in one eye and legal blindness in one eye** after correction have been contraindications for collision/contact—but recent advances in protective eye goggles have changed this restriction.
        b. **Retinal detachment** requires consultation with ophthalmologist prior to making decision about advisability of participation.
        c. Recent legal actions[30] have supported participation with **solitary kidney and testicular nondescent;** moreover, protective equipment has improved in this area as well.
    3. **Organ enlargement**
        a. Enlargements of **liver, kidney and spleen** have traditionally constituted contraindications for collision/contact, but this restriction has now been expanded to include limited contact/impact.
        b. Many authorities recommend 3 to 6 months following disappearance of splenomegaly in **Epstein-Barr mononucleosis** before allowing collision/contact.
    4. **Active infection**
        a. **Absolute contraindications for any sport: pyelonephritis, arthritis, osteomyelitis, pulmonary infection (including tuberculosis), and systemic infection.**
        b. **Fever itself should also contraindicate.**
        c. **Active otitis media** contraindicates swimming and diving.
        d. **Boils, impetigo and herpes simplex gladiatorum** disqualify contact/collision and limited contact/impact while contagious.
    5. **Vertebropelvic defects**
        a. Spondylolisthesis with back pain
        b. Legg-Perthes' disease
        c. Slipped capital femoral epiphysis
        d. Spinal epiphysitis
    6. **Cardiopulmonary disorders** (Table 3)
        a. **Asthma**
            i. Only if uncontrolled.
            ii. Exercise-induced bronchospasm often benefited by sports participation.
            iii. Usually benefited by conditioning, particularly aquatic sports.
        b. **Cardiac contraindications**
            i. Mitral and aortic stenosis
            ii. Cyanotic heart disease
            iii. Pulmonary hypertension
            iv. Active myopericarditis

**TABLE 2.**   Recommendations for Participation in Competitive Sports

| | Contact/ Collision | Limited Contact/ Impact | Noncontact Strenuous | Noncontact Moderately Strenuous | Noncontact Nonstrenuous |
|---|---|---|---|---|---|
| Atlantoaxial instability | No | No | Yes* | Yes | Yes |
| * Swimming; no butterfly, breast stroke, or diving starts | | | | | |
| Acute illnesses | * | * | * | * | * |
| * Needs individual assessment, e.g., contagious-ness to others, risk of worsening illness | | | | | |
| Cardiovascular | | | | | |
|   Carditis | No | No | No | No | No |
|   Hypertension | | | | | |
|     Mild | Yes | Yes | Yes | Yes | Yes |
|     Moderate | * | * | * | * | * |
|     Severe | * | * | * | * | * |
|   Congenital heart disease | † | † | † | † | † |
| * Needs individual assessment | | | | | |
| † Patients with mild forms can be allowed a full range of physical activities; patients with moderate or severe forms, or who are postoperative should be evaluated by a cardiologist before athletic participation. | | | | | |
| Eyes | | | | | |
|   Absence or loss of function of one eye | * | * | * | * | * |
|   Detached retina | † | † | † | † | † |
| * Availability of American Society for Testing and Materials (ASTM)-approved eye guards may allow competitor to participate in most sports, but this must be judged on an individual basis. | | | | | |
| † Consult ophthalmologist | | | | | |
| Inguinal hernia | Yes | Yes | Yes | Yes | Yes |
| Kidney: Absence of one | No | Yes | Yes | Yes | Yes |
| Liver: Enlarged | No | No | Yes | Yes | Yes |
| Musculoskeletal disorders | * | * | * | * | * |
| * Needs individual assessment | | | | | |
| Neurologic | | | | | |
|   History of serious head or spine trauma, repeated concussions, or craniotomy | * | * | Yes | Yes | Yes |
|   Convulsive disorder | | | | | |
|     Well controlled | Yes | Yes | Yes | Yes | Yes |
|     Poorly controlled | No | No | Yes† | Yes | Yes‡ |
| * Needs individual assessment | | | | | |
| † No swimming or weight lifting | | | | | |
| ‡ No archery or riflery | | | | | |
| Ovary: Absence of one | Yes | Yes | Yes | Yes | Yes |
| Respiratory | | | | | |
|   Pulmonary insufficiency | * | * | * | * | Yes |
|   Asthma | Yes | Yes | Yes | Yes | Yes |
| * May be allowed to compete if oxygenation remains satisfactory during a graded stress test | | | | | |
| Sickle cell trait | Yes | Yes | Yes | Yes | Yes |
| Skin: Boils, herpes, impetigo, scabies | * | * | Yes | Yes | Yes |
| * No gymnastics with mats, martial arts, wrestling or contact sports until not contagious | | | | | |
| Spleen: Enlarged | No | No | No | Yes | Yes |
| Testicle: Absence or undescended | Yes* | Yes* | Yes | Yes | Yes |
| * Certain sports may require protective cup. | | | | | |

From Pediatrics 81:738, 1988, with permission.[3]

**TABLE 3.**   Cardiac Conditions Contraindicating Participation in Competitive Activities*

| | |
|---|---|
| 1. Obstructive hypertrophic cardiomyopathy | 4. Pulmonic stenosis with RV pressure greater |
| 2. Congenital coronary artery abnormalities | than 75 mm of mercury |
| 3. Cystic medial necrosis of the aorta | 5. Aortic stenosis with a gradient greater than |
| (Marfan's syndrome) | 40 mm of mercury across the valve |

* From Hara JH, Puffer JC. In Mellion MB: Office Management of Sports Injuries & Athletic Problems. Philadelphia, Hanley & Belfus, Inc., 1988, with permission.

      c. **Hypertrophic obstructive cardiomyopathy** (asymmetric septal hypertrophy, idiopathic hypertrophic subaortic stenosis) is a frequent totally unsuspected cause of mortality.[12,18]
          i. Important to listen for systolic murmur accentuated by Valsalva maneuver.[30]
          ii. Some feel echocardiography important.
      d. Other unexpected deaths related to anomalies of coronary circulation.[25]
   C. Important to also be aware of conditions that do not specifically preclude participation (Table 4).

X. **Laboratory Tests**

   A. **Controversial area**[2,12,31]—even role of CBC not settled.[12,31]
      1. Leukocytosis may serve as the only clue of occult infection or dental disease.
      2. Iron deficiency anemia is rare even though iron deficiency is common, particularly in menstruating girls and rapidly growing boys.[2] In spite of poor sensitivity, hematocrit may be most cost-effective and practical screen.
   B. FUA often reveals proteinuria[11] but usually it is benign orthostatic proteinuria.[13,14,30]
   C. EKG generally not warranted, except in suspected Marfan's (Table 5) or other potentially disqualifying cardiac disorder.

XI. **Miscellaneous Considerations**

   A. **Age**
      1. By adulthood most individuals should be aware of their limitations or at least have the potential of exercising good judgment.[23]
      2. Preadolescent youth are a special concern.[16]
         a. William Strong feels younger children tend not to push themselves.[26]
         b. But pushy adults and coaches may be exercising a form of child abuse.[8]
   B. **Gender**
      1. Public Law 92-318 mandates right to participate and equal-quality facilities for women.[12]
      2. Many feel best interests of girls are served by activities exclusively designed for girls.[1,34]
      3. Girls can apparently participate and perform at levels commensurate with boys when differences in height, weight and body composition are considered.[5,7]
   C. **Handicapped**
      1. Special Olympics is an excellent example of the type of program that fosters pride and sense of achievement in dignified manner.
      2. Amputees and limb reduction defects—judged on individual merit.[3,12]

**TABLE 4.**   Cardiac Conditions That Would Not Specifically Contraindicate Participation*

| | |
|---|---|
| 1. Mitral valve prolapse in absence of significant ventricular arrhythmias or severe initial regurgitation | 3. Wolff-Parkinson-White syndrome (WPW) in absence of documented atrial fibrillation with rapid ventricular response |
| 2. Small shunts associated with atrial septal defect (ASD), ventricular septal defect (VSD), or patent ductus arteriosus (PDA) | 4. Primary ventricular arrhythmias in the absence of underlying coronary, myocardial, or valvular disease |

* From Hara JH, Puffer JC. In Mellion MB: Sports Injuries & Athletic Problems. Philadelphia, Hanley & Belfus, Inc., 1988, with permission.

**TABLE 5.**  Suggested Screening Format for Marfan's Syndrome*

Screen all men over 6 feet and all women over 5 feet 10 inches in height with electrocardiogram and slit lamp examination when any two of the following are found:

| | |
|---|---|
| 1. Family history of Marfan's syndrome† | 6. Upper to lower body ratio more than one |
| 2. Cardiac murmur or midsystolic click | standard deviation below the mean |
| 3. Kyphoscoliosis | 7. Myopia |
| 4. Anterior thoracic deformity | 8. Ectopic lens |
| 5. Arm span greater than height | |

\* From Hara JH, Puffer JC. In Mellion MB: Sports Injuries & Athletic Problems. Philadelphia, Hanley & Belfus, Inc., 1988, with permission.
† This finding *alone* should prompt further investigation.

    D. **Drugs**
       1. Cigarette smoking, alcohol, and cocaine are unfortunately seen in athletes as well as society at large.
       2. **Unexplained ventricular ectopy, unexplained seizures, episodic hypertension, and tachycardia may be manifestation of cocaine abuse.**[12]
       3. Anabolic steroids, "blood doping," and other practices engaged in to gain competitive advantage are unfortunately in need of further recognition.

## REFERENCES

1. American Academy of Pediatrics Committee on Pediatric Aspects of Physical Fitness, Recreation, and Sports: Participation in sports by girls. Pediatrics 55:563, 1975.
2. American Academy of Pediatrics Committee on Sports Medicine: Health Care for Young Athletes. Evanston, IL, American Academy of Pediatrics, 1983.
3. American Academy of Pediatrics Committee on Sports Medicine: Recommendations for participation in competitive sports. Pediatrics 81(5):737–738, 1988.
4. American Medical Association: Medical Evaluation of the Athlete. Chicago, American Medical Association, 1971.
5. Birrer RB: Sports Medicine for the Primary Care Physician. East Norwalk, CT, Appleton-Century Crofts, 1984.
6. Birrer RB, Wilkerson LA: Sports Medicine I. Kansas City, MO, American Academy of Family Physicians (Monograph Series), 1985.
7. Carlson KM: Fact vs. fiction: Women in sports. Female Patient 5:48, 1980.
8. Digott RE: Youth in sports: Beware of child abuse. New York Times, Sept. 1, 1977.
9. Du Rant RH, et al: The preparticipation examination of athletes. Am J Dis Child 139:657, 1985.
10. Garrick JG: Sports medicine. Pediatr Clin North Am 24:737, 1977.
11. Goldberg B, et al: Preparticipation sports assessment—an objective evaluation. Pediatrics 66:736, 1980.
12. Hara JH, Puffer JC: The preparticipation physical examination. In Office Management of Sports Injuries & Athletic Problems. Philadelphia, Hanley & Belfus, 1988.
13. Hirsch PJ, et al: Check-out for the would-be athlete. Emerg Med 9(30):65, 1980.
14. Hirsch PJ, et al: Preparticipation evaluation for school athletic programs. J Med Soc NJ 78:585, 1981.
15. Jackson DW, et al: Injury prevention in the young athlete. Am J Sports Med 9:187, 1981.
16. Lendgren CV: Boys in contact sports. Medical Tribune, Nov. 7, 1964.
17. Linder CW, et al: Preparticipation health screening of young athletes. Am J Sports Med 9:187, 1981.
18. Maron BJ, et al: Sudden death in young athletes. Circulation 62:218, 1980.
19. Marshall JL, Tischler HM: Screening for sports. NY State J Med 78:243, 1978.
20. Moretz A, Grana WA: High school injuries. Phys Sportsmed 6:92, 1978.
21. Puffer JC: Sports medicine and the adolescent. Semin Fam Med 2:201, 1981.
22. Puffer JC: Sports medicine: The preparticipation evaluation. West J Med 137:58, 1982.
23. Rice EL: Periodic preparticipation sports examination is advised. Family Practice News 16(12):43, 1986.
24. Risser WL, et al: A cost benefit analysis of preparticipation examinations of adolescent athletes. J School Health 55(7):270, 1985.
25. Roberts WC, et al: Intussusception of a coronary artery associated with sudden death in young college football player. Am J Cardiol 57:179, 1986.
26. Rogers CC: Strong statements on kids and sports. Phys Sportsmed 13(8):32, 1985.

27. Runyan, DK: The preparticipation examination of the young athlete. Clin Pediatr 22:674, 1983.
28. Ryan AJ: Qualifying examinations: A continuing dilemma. Phys Sportsmed 8:10, 1980.
29. Samples P: Preparticipation examinations: Are they worth the trouble? Phys Sportsmed 14(10):180, 1986.
30. Smilkstein G: Health evaluation of high school athletes. Phys Sportsmed 9(8):73, 1981.
31. Smith NJ: Medical issues in sports medicine. Pediatr in Rev 2:229, 1981.
32. Steven MB, Smith GN: The preparticipation sports assessment. Fam Pract Recert 8:68, 1986.
33. Strong WB: Hypertension in sports. Pediatrics 64:693, 1979.
34. Torg BG, Torg JS: Sex and the little league. Phys Sportsmed 2(5):45, 1974.

# Chapter 6: Preseason Conditioning: Aerobic Power

RICHARD W. LATIN, PhD

I. **Introduction**

Cardiovascular fitness is an important physical fitness factor for endurance athletes. Aerobic power is the maximum capability to transport and utilize oxygen and is an index of cardiovascular efficiency. Training programs for aerobic power improvement need to stress the physiological components of the oxygen transport system.

II. **Physiological Components of Oxygen Uptake ($VO_2$)**

Oxygen uptake or $VO_2$ may be mathematically and physiologically defined as:

$$VO_2 = HR \times SV \times a - \bar{v}O_2 \text{ difference}$$

Therefore the system has a central and peripheral component.

A. **Central component**
   1. Heart rate (HR)
   2. Stroke volume (SV)
   3. Cardiac output (Q) = HR × SV
   4. A primary component to oxygen uptake is dictated by the heart's ability to pump large volumes of blood.

B. **Peripheral component**
   1. Arterial – mixed venous oxygen difference ($a - \bar{v}O_2$ difference)
   2. The ability of tissues to extract and utilize oxygen for ATP resynthesis is another primary component of oxygen uptake. This is particularly true for muscles that are being recruited during an activity.

C. **Maximum oxygen uptake ($VO_2$max)**
   1. The measure of $VO_2$max represents the maximum capabilities of the oxygen transport system and aerobic ATP resynthesis.
   2. It is generally expressed in ml of $O_2$ consumed per kg of body weight per minute (ml/kg/min). It may also be expressed in L/min.

III. **Training Principles**

A. **Specificity of training**
   1. Metabolic—This implies stressing the metabolic pathways that would be responsible for the bioenergetics (ATP resynthesis) of a particular exercise task.
   2. Neuromuscular—This implies recruiting the motor units that would be similarly recruited for a given exercise task.
   3. Results are best accomplished by having an individual train using movement patterns and speeds similar to a given exercise task, e.g., a marathoner would train by performing long endurance runs as opposed to short, high-intensity sprints or a cyclist would train by cycling not running (both use leg muscles but different recruitment patterns).

B. **Overload**—In order for adaptive improvement to occur workloads must be imposed that are greater than normally encountered.

C. **Progression**—A gradual systematic increase in training intensity or volume as improvement occurs.

D. **Individuality**—No two individuals will respond or adapt similarly to the same training program. Allowances for initial fitness levels, responses to training, etc. need to be considered.

IV. **Aerobic Training Guidelines**

    A. **Guidelines** proposed by the American College of Sports Medicine[1,3] may be used successfully to train athletes or persons interested in health-related aerobic fitness. These guidelines address intensity, frequency, duration, and mode of aerobic exercise.

    B. **Intensity of exercise training**

       1. Heart rate reserve (HRR) method:

         a. 60–90% of HRR plus the resting heart rate ($HR_{rest}$) may be used to establish appropriate exercise intensities.

         b. Values may be obtained by using the formula developed by Karvonen:[1]

           i. $HR_{max}$ = 220 – age (or other appropriate equations or testing methods).

           ii. $HRR = HR_{max} - HR_{rest}$

           iii. 60–90% of HRR

           iv. Add result to $HR_{rest}$ for exercise target HR.

         c. Example calculation:

           i. Athlete A is 20 years old with $HR_{rest}$ = 60 b/min

           ii. $HR_{max}$ = 220 – 20 = 200 b/min

           iii. HRR = 200 – 60 = 140 b/min

           iv. Selected training intensity = 80%

           v. % HRR = 140 × 0.80 = 112 b/min

           vi. Training intensity = 112 + 60 = 172 b/min.

         d. HR as an indicator of intensity:

           i. Using HR provides a reasonably accurate means of assessing exercise intensity. However, one must use a valid means of quantifying HR such as telemetry, exercise cardiotachometer, or a carefully taught palpation technique.

           ii. Careful consideration should be given to conditions or situations that may affect HR, e.g., medications, heat, altitude, emotional state, overtraining, cardiovascular drift, etc.

       2. Percent $VO_2max$ method:

         a. Workloads that require an oxygen cost of 50–85% of the $VO_2max$ may be used to establish appropriate exercise intensities.

         b. A determination of $VO_2max$ is required.

           i. A maximal exercise test using indirect open circuit calorimetry will provide the most accurate measure of $VO_2max$.

           ii. A field test may be used to estimate $VO_2max$, e.g., Astrand cycle or step test.[4]

         c. Workloads may be established by two methods:

           i. Plot the workload or $HR/VO_2$ relationship obtained during a maximal test (Fig. 1).

           ii. Algebraically determine the oxygen cost of exercise from the equations reported by ACSM[1] (Tables 1, 2).

         d. Example calculation:

           i. Athlete B has a $VO_2max$ = 60 ml/kg/min

           ii. Equation for oxygen cost for running on horizontal surface: $VO_2$ = speed (m/min) × 0.2 + 3.5 ml/kg/min

           iii. Selected training intensity 80% of $VO_2max$: 60 ml/kg/min × 0.80 = 48 ml/kg/min

           iv. Running speed for $VO_2$ = 48 ml/kg/min:

             (a) 48 ml/kg/min = speed (m/min) × 0.2 + 3.5 ml/kg/min

             (b) 44.5 ml/kg/min = speed (m/min) × 0.2

             (c) 222.5 = speed (m/min) or 8.3 mph or 7:14 per mile pace.

           v. Athlete B may run at a 7:14 per mile pace for an appropriate training intensity.

         e. Percent of $VO_2max$ as an indicator of intensity. Using $VO_2$ provides an accurate means of assessing exercise intensity. It is not subject to excessive variation

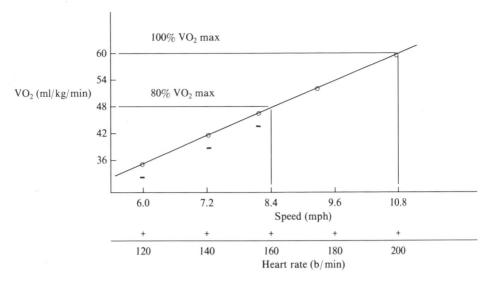

**FIGURE 1.** Relationship between VO₂ and heart rate or workload.

**TABLE 1.** Oxygen Cost of Running*

| Speed (mph) | Pace (min/mi) | VO₂ (ml/kg/min) |
|---|---|---|
| 6.0 | 10:00 | 35.7 |
| 7.0 | 8:35 | 41.0 |
| 8.0 | 7:30 | 46.4 |
| 9.0 | 6:40 | 51.8 |
| 10.0 | 6:00 | 57.2 |
| 11.0 | 5:27 | 62.5 |
| 12.0 | 5:00 | 67.9 |
| 13.0 | 4:37 | 73.3 |

\* Based on the equation:[1] $VO_2$ (ml/kg/min) = Speed (m/min) × 0.2 + 3.5 ml/kg/min.

**TABLE 2.** Oxygen Cost of Cycling*

| Workload (kgm/min) | VO₂ (ml/min) | VO₂ (L/min) |
|---|---|---|
| 450 | 1200 | 1.2 |
| 600 | 1500 | 1.5 |
| 750 | 1800 | 1.8 |
| 900 | 2100 | 2.1 |
| 1050 | 2400 | 2.4 |
| 1200 | 2700 | 2.7 |
| 1350 | 3000 | 3.0 |
| 1500 | 3300 | 3.3 |
| 1650 | 3600 | 3.6 |
| 1800 | 3900 | 3.9 |
| 1950 | 4200 | 4.2 |
| 2050 | 4400 | 4.4 |

\* Based on the equation:[1] $VO_2$ (ml/min) = Workload (kgm/min) × 2 + 300 ml.

**TABLE 3.** Suggested Training Intensities

| Fitness Level | Karvonen Formula | % $VO_2$ max |
|---|---|---|
| Beginner (unconditioned) | 60–70% | 50–65% |
| Intermediate (recreational athlete) | 70–80% | 65–75% |
| Advanced (competitive athlete) | 80–90% + | 75–85% + |

and quantification as is HR and may be the method of choice when $VO_2$max may be accurately determined. However, it would be more difficult to apply this method to some modes of exercise, e.g., swimming, cross-country skiing.
3. Selecting an appropriate intensity.
   a. No exact method exists to establish a starting exercise intensity.
   b. Perceived exertion ratings may allow for an adjustment in initial exercise intensities.
   c. Refer to Table 3 for suggested guidelines.
C. **Frequency of exercise training**
   1. Suggested training frequencies are 3 to 5 days per week.
   2. Endurance athletes may train 5 to 6 days per week; for health-related aerobic fitness or in sports where there is not as great an aerobic demand, 3 days per week is recommended.
D. **Duration of exercise training**
   1. The suggested duration of an individual training session is 15 to 60 minutes.
   2. Fifteen minutes would be the minimal duration required for maintenance or improvement to occur, and 60 minutes or longer may be required in some training sessions for long endurance athletes.
E. **Mode of exercise training**
   1. Exercises that utilize large muscle groups and that are continuous and rhythmic in nature should be used to improve aerobic power.
   2. Exercises that require heavy muscle contractions such as weight training will produce little changes in maximum oxygen uptake.
F. **Effects of exercise mode**
   1. **Central responses** to aerobic exercise modes are relatively nondiscriminatory. Heart rate, stroke volume, and cardiac output adaptations may occur regardless of aerobic exercise mode. Therefore, this component to improving $VO_2$max is nonspecific.
   2. **Peripheral responses** to aerobic exercise modes are highly task-specific. Neuromuscular recruitment of specific motor units and appropriate blood-flow shunts are essential to peripheral physiological and biochemical adaptations that allow for greater tissue utilization of oxygen and improvement of $VO_2$max.
   3. Although a runner may maintain the central component of the oxygen transport system by cycling, the peripheral component is not adequately stimulated, since neuromuscular recruitment is not the same. This would violate one of the tenets of exercise specificity. However, it may be important to consider that many modes of exercise may be used interchangeably if only the health and fitness of the central component (heart) is of concern.
G. **Overload and progression**
   1. Intensity, frequency, and duration may be manipulated to impose a progressive overload.
   2. Intensity of exercise has the greatest influence on improvements of aerobic power.
   3. From the standpoint of progression, frequency should be emphasized first, keeping duration and intensity at a minimum until the desired times per week can be safely (to minimize injury) achieved.
   4. Once the frequency is established, increasing the duration of exercise is emphasized, keeping intensity at a minimum, until a desired length of time is achieved.
   5. Finally intensity is manipulated. As fitness levels improve, gradual increases in the intensity of exercise will stimulate improvement in aerobic power.

**TABLE 4.** Aerobic Fitness Classifications. VO$_2$ max (ml/kg/min)

| | Male Ages | | Female Ages | |
|---|---|---|---|---|
| Category | 13–19 | 20–29 | 13–19 | 20–29 |
| Poor | Below–39 | Below–36 | Below–30 | Below–27 |
| Good | 40–50 | 37–47 | 31–40 | 28–37 |
| Excellent | 51–59 | 48–56 | 41–50 | 38–47 |
| Highly trained | 60–80 | 57–80 | 51–65 | 48–65 |

6. Any abrupt increases in exercise frequency, duration, and especially intensity should be avoided. This only invites introducing the athlete to an underpreparation injury.

H. **Improvement**

1. The amount of improvement in VO$_2$max to expect from training is (1) highly individualized and (2) inversely related to the initial fitness level. An untrained individual may experience a 20–25% increase in VO$_2$max in an 8- to 12-week training period. A trained individual may observe a 5% or less improvement in the same time period (Table 4).

2. A genetically determined peak VO$_2$max may occur in 18 to 24 months of intense training. Up to 70% of this may be achieved in about 3 months.

3. Improvements in endurance performances when VO$_2$max fails to increase are accomplished by the athlete being able to sustain exercise at a higher percent of their VO$_2$max.

4. Percent utilization of VO$_2$max is a powerful predictor of endurance performance among individuals with a similar VO$_2$max.

V. **Methods of Training**

A. **When to begin training?** When to begin training is dictated by the type of sport and the time when a peak level of conditioning is desired. Athletes in sports such as cross country, track, and swimming may use the season itself as a conditioning period, aiming to peak at the season's end for a championship meet. If a season were 10 weeks long, then serious training might start 2 to 4 weeks prior to its beginning. Knowing that it requires 8 to 12 weeks of training to obtain significant levels of improvement, an athlete's training agenda may be planned accordingly.

B. **How much training is needed?** This is also dictated by the sport. A football player requires minimal aerobic fitness and may dedicate three periods per week for 15 minutes to this type of conditioning, whereas a 10 km specialist may train six times per week for about 60 minutes using a variety of high-intensity methods during half of those sessions. Therefore, the amount of aerobic conditioning is influenced by the aerobic metabolic demand of the sport or event.

C. **Long slow duration training.** The emphasis on this type of training is duration rather than intensity. Intensities would typically be about 65% to 75% of HRR + HR$_{rest}$ or 60% to 70% of VO$_2$max. This approach may be used for general conditioning or as a training mode on days following intense workouts. This type of training should not be used exclusively for the competitive athlete, since it lacks the specific neuromuscular and metabolic stress necessary under race conditions. An example of this would be a middle distance runner running 8 miles at a 7:30/mi pace.

D. **Long fast duration training.** This mode of training is typified by higher intensity, moderate duration forms of exercise. Intensities would generally be 80–90% of HRR + HR$_{rest}$ or 80–85% of VO$_2$max. The athlete would maintain a pace just at or below a racing speed. Since the intensity is higher than long slow duration training and the metabolic and neuromuscular components are specific to racing conditions, greater improvements can be made using this training mode. The physical and psychological demands of this type of training are great; therefore, alternating slow and fast workouts or other training variations are recommended. An example of this type of training would be a middle distance runner running 5 miles at a 5:30/mi pace.

E. **Interval training.** This type of training may be used to improve aerobic power by using intervals of intense exercise interspersed with recovery. An athlete may maintain levels of intensity at or above racing conditions for an extended time period. This makes interval training a high-quality conditioning mode that exemplifies the tenants of exercise specificity.

   1. Exercise intervals:
Aerobic training intervals are typically 3 to 5 minutes in duration performed at or above race paces.

   2. Recovery intervals:
Suggested recovery times are from one to one-half the exercise interval time. An example would be 3 minutes of exercise with 3 minutes of recovery. Recovery time may also be judged sufficient when the athlete's HR has returned to about 120 to 130 b/min.

   3. Type of recovery:
Low-level activity (30–50% of $VO_2max$) between exercise intervals will hasten the removal of lactic acid and thus expedite recovery.

   4. Number of intervals:
The suggested number of intervals would be dictated by their length, e.g., shorter intervals like 3 minutes may be repeated 4 to 8 times, longer intervals like 5 minutes may be repeated 3 to 6 times.

F. **Combination programs**
Most successful programs incorporate all three of the previously described methods. Typically, intensive training days or weeks are followed by a corresponding number of easier days or weeks. This is necessary not only for physiological but also psychological standpoints. Refer to Fox et al.[5] for an outstanding treatment of conditioning programs.

VI. **Other Considerations**

A. **Muscle glycogen depletion and restoration.** Many endurance athletes are chronically glycogen-depleted, which causes their performances to suffer. By and large this is due to overtraining and failure to take in an adequate amount of dietary carbohydrates. It takes approximately 48 hours while eating diets high in carbohydrates for complete restoration from a significantly depleted state to occur. No exhaustive training should take place during this time.

B. **Multiple daily training sessions.** Little scientific evidence exists that supports training two or three times per day as being better than a single workout. Although more research in this area is necessary, it is generally recommended that the athlete participate in one high-quality training session on scheduled days.

C. **Quantity vs. quality.** The "more is better" attitude is adopted by many endurance athletes. This type of attitude invites every aspect of overtraining injuries as well as decreased performance. Runners reporting to train 150 miles per week or so are probably spending most of it training by the long slow duration method, which is not as productive for providing improvement. Although no equation exists to establish a "perfect" training regimen, the emphasis should be on quality workouts interspersed with adequate low-intensity recovery days. An excellent example of successful high-quality training is demonstrated by Olympic steeplechase runner Henry Marsh. Marsh reports to train about 35 miles per week for his 3 km event!

## REFERENCES

1. American College of Sports Medicine: Guidelines for Exercise Testing and Prescription. Philadelphia, Lea & Febiger, 1986.
2. American College of Sports Medicine: Position statement on the participation of the female athlete in long distance running. Med Sci Sports Exerc 11(4):ix–xi, 1979.

3. American College of Sports Medicine: Position statement on the recommended quantity and quality of exercise for developing fitness in healthy adults. Med Sci Sports Exerc 19(3):vii–ix, 1978.
4. Astrand P, Rodahl K: Textbook of Work Physiology. New York, McGraw Hill, 1986.
5. Fox E, Bowers R, Foss M: The Physiological Basis for Physical Education and Athletics. Philadelphia, WB Saunders, 1988.
6. Wilmore J, Costill D: Training for Sport and Activity. Dubuque, IA, William C. Brown, 1988.
7. Thomas T, Zebas C: Scientific Exercise Training. Dubuque, IA, Kendall Hunt, 1984.

# Chapter 7: Preseason Strength Training

## THOMAS R. BAECHLE, EdD

I. **Introduction**

This chapter will identify and describe the variables employed in designing safe and effective preseason strength-training programs. These design variables should be carefully manipulated with regard to the demands of the sport, the athlete's capacities and limitations, and the goals of the training program. The following information assumes that the length of the preseason period is 8 weeks.

Strength training is only a part of total athletic conditioning. It is a means to an end, and not an end in itself. Improvement in sports performance, not simply developing superior strength, should be the ultimate goal of strength training. Strength training should be integrated into the total conditioning program to provide an optimal environment also for improvement in agility, power, speed, speed endurance, speed strength, and flexibility, while avoiding over-training. Although not discussed here, sprint training and plyometric exercises for explosive sports are essential if the improved strength levels are to be "converted" to functional sport-specific strength/power.

II. **Strength Training Principles**

A. **Overload and progressive overload principles**
   1. **"Overload"** means imposing a greater stress than that to which the body is accustomed.
   2. **Overload is the stimulus** needed for physiological adaptation and maximum gains.
   3. Introducing overload in a systematic manner is referred to as **progressive overload.** Theoretically, each training session should involve a greater overload than the previous one. In reality, one should recognize the need for variation in training. Well-conceived programs do involve progressively greater overload, but also have time for recovery and adaptation.
      a. The use of variation in training sessions is referred to as **cycling,** and is based upon the concept of **periodization.**
      b. **Periodization** is the systematic organization of the entire training process, e.g., method of training, loads, volumes, and variation needed over an extended period of time.

B. **SAID principle (Specific Adaptation to Imposed Demands)**
   1. Adaptations occurring in response to training are specific to the type of training undertaken. For example, long-distance training is associated with increases in mitochondria number and size, with little or no change in strength levels. Conversely, sprint training has a minimal effect on mitochondria, but produces increased leg strength.
   2. Extent of change is dictated largely by the level of imposed demands and the fitness/training levels of the athlete at the onset of training.

C. **Specificity concept**
   1. **Specificity** is an application of the SAID principle. It refers to training in a specific manner to produce a specific outcome. Its application involves determining the specific or unique demands of the sport, then designing a strength-training program that will stimulate the appropriate adaptation and improved performance in the sport.
   2. In utilizing the specificity concept, the following demands/characteristics of the sport are considered:

a. **Strength:** ability to produce maximum force in a one-time, all-out effort.
b. **Speed strength:** ability to produce high forces at fast velocities.
c. **Muscular endurance:** ability to perform muscular work over an extended period of time without undue fatigue.
d. **Speed endurance:** ability to produce high forces at fast velocities repeatedly over an extended period of time.
e. **Cardiovascular endurance:** ability of the heart and vessels to transport, the lungs to oxygenate, and the muscles to efficiently utilize oxygen.
f. **Power:** ability to exert force rapidly, defined as

$$P = \frac{\text{work}}{\text{time}}$$

g. **Range of movement (flexibility):** ability to move a joint through its entire range of movement.
h. **Metabolic demands:** refers to determining the predominant energy system involved in a particular form or intensity of exercise.
3. Manipulation of the program design variables allows emphasizing or de-emphasizing improvements in the eight characteristics listed above.

III. **Program Design Variables**

A. Choice of exercises for the preseason program
1. Definitions
a. **Core exercises:** exercises that involve two or more joints and large muscle groups.
b. **Secondary exercises:** exercises involving smaller muscle groups.
c. **Power/quick lift exercises:** Core exercises distinguishable by their ballistic nature and recruitment of "power zone" muscles (thighs to rib cage).
2. To select exercises appropriately, apply the specificity concept, i.e., give emphasis to those exercises that work the same muscle groups involved in the sport.
3. Attempt to include at least one exercise for thighs, calf, upper and lower back, shoulders, arms, abdomen, chest, and neck for wrestling and football.
4. Include at least one power exercise (e.g., power clean, hang clean, snatch, push press) to improve neuromuscular coordination and power among "power zone" muscles.
5. For preseason training, include 2 or 3 power movement exercises, 3–4 additional core exercises, and 4–6 secondary exercises.
6. Although the off-season program uses a greater number of core exercises, the end-season program includes more sport-specific or secondary exercises, e.g., wrist curls (baseball, softball), pullovers (volleyball), neck exercises (football, wrestling).
7. Core and secondary exercises commonly included in strength training programs are shown in Table 1.

B. **Order of the exercises**
1. The order in which exercises are performed is important because it may affect the intensity of effort.
a. An appropriate arrangement provides better recovery and, therefore, should enable the athlete to work more intensely.
b. An appropriate arrangement may also help reduce the incidence of injury (e.g., low back exercises before power cleans or squats could predispose the athlete to injury).
2. Exercise order should follow these guidelines:
a. Core exercises first, then secondary exercises
b. Power exercises first, then strength exercises
c. Low back and abdominal exercises last.
3. Once priorities (e.g., power exercises first, strength exercises next) have been established, next consider the order of exercises within both core and secondary exercise categories. Common approaches used include:
a. Alternating push and pull exercises
b. Alternating upper body exercises with lower body exercises.

**TABLE 1.**   Core and Secondary Exercises Commonly Included in Strength Training Programs

I.  Core Exercises

Power movements—quick lifts

| | | |
|---|---|---|
| 1. Power snatch | 4. Hang clean | 7. High pull, from floor |
| 2. Power clean | 5. Push press | and hang |
| 3. Hang snatch | 6. Push jerk | |

Other

| | | |
|---|---|---|
| 1. Squat, front and back | 4. Dead lift, bent-legged | 7. Standing overhead press, in |
| 2. Quarter squat, front and | and straight-legged | front and behind the neck |
| back | 5. Bench press | 8. Bent-over row |
| 3. Leg press, hip sled | 6. Incline press | |

II.  Secondary Exercises

| | | |
|---|---|---|
| Leg extension | Hyperextension | Elbow (bicep) curl |
| Leg curl | "Good morning" | French (tricep) curl |
| Lunge—forward, lateral, and | Pull-over | Reverse curl |
| step-through | Lateral front raise | Dumbbell fly |
| Heel raise | Shoulder shrug | Neck exercises |
| Bent-knee twisting sit-up | | |

Note: *Almost all of the exercises listed above can also be performed with a dumbbell(s).*

4. Table 2 shows how the same 12 exercises might be arranged/ordered into a 3-day-a-week and 4-day-a-week program.
5. Should athletes strength train before or after practice? During the **preseason** and **off-season,** athletes should **strength train first,** then practice the sport. **In season,** athletes should strength train **after practice.**

C.  **Number of repetitions/sets (volume)**
1. Definitions/terms:
   a. **Repetitions:** number of times an exercise is performed before a period of rest.
   b. **Set:** the completion of one series of repetitions, followed by a rest period or a different exercise.
   c. **Volume** = sets × repetitions.
2. Utilizing the specificity concept, volume guidelines for the **core exercises** presented in Table 3 may be summarized as follows:
   a. For **power,** assign 3–6 sets of 1–3 repetitions.
   b. For **muscle strength,** assign 3–5 sets of 3–8 repetitions.
   c. For **muscle hypertrophy,** assign 3–6 sets of 8–12 repetitions.
   d. For **muscular endurance,** assign 2 sets of 15–20 repetitions.
3. Volume guidelines for secondary exercises are 2 sets of 8–12 repetitions, sometimes 15 repetitions when small muscle groups are involved.
4. Table 3 shows that volumes are lowest when training for power and strength, and highest when training for hypertrophy and muscular endurance.
   a. Muscle endurance requirements of certain sports can best be acquired through drills and participation in the sport, rather than through development in the weight room.
   b. For this reason, loads less than 60% are not presented in Table 3.
5. As the season draws nearer, the number of sets typically becomes smaller as loads become heavier. More emphasis and time are given to practicing skills and strategies of the sport.

D.  **Resistance/load assignments**
1. Calculating assignment of resistance/loads typically involves use of a percentage of maximum strength, expressed as either the athlete's 1 repetition max (1 RM) or 10 repetition max (10 RM).
   a. **1 RM:** the maximum amount of weight lifted for 1 repetition.
   b. **10 RM:** the maximum amount of weight lifted for 10 repetitions (with muscular failure occurring during the 11th repetition).

**TABLE 2.** Order of Exercise—3-Day and 4-Day-a-Week Programs

For purposes of comparison, the same 12 exercises are ordered/arranged in 3- and 4-day-a-week programs.

*3-Day-a-Week (Monday, Wednesday, Friday) Program*

| Type of Exercise | Exercise | Muscle Area |
|---|---|---|
| Core, Power | Power clean* | Total body (TB) |
| Core, Power | Power clean from hang* | Total body (TB) |
| Core | Bench press* | Chest (CH) |
| Core | Back squat | Leg (LG) |
| Core | Bent-over row | Upper back (UB) |
| Core | Overhead press | Shoulder (SH) |
| Secondary | Bicep curl | Arm-anterior (A-A) |
| Secondary | French curl | Arm-posterior (A-P) |
| Secondary | Leg extension | Leg-anterior (L-A) |
| Secondary | Leg curl | Leg-posterior (L-P) |
| Secondary | Hyperextensions | Lower back (LB) |
| Secondary | Bent-knee sit-ups | Abdominal (AB) |

The above would be considered a long workout during the preseason for some teams (representing approximately 1½ hours). Should the amount of workout time need to be reduced, the power clean from a hang position and the French curl could be deleted without having a negative effect.

*4-Day-a-Week—Split Program*

| Type† | Monday-Thursday | Muscle Area‡ | Type | Tuesday-Friday | Muscle Area |
|---|---|---|---|---|---|
| C, P | Power clean* | TB, SH | C | Overhead press | TB, SH |
| C, P | Power clean from hang | TB, UB | C | Bent-over row | TB, UB |
| C | Back squat* | LG, CH | C | Bench press | LG, CH |
| S | Leg curl | L-P | S | French curl | L-P, A-P |
| S | Leg extension | L-A | S | Biceps curl | L-A, A-A |
| S | Hyperextension | LB, AB | S | Bent-knee sit-up | LB, AB |

\* Exercises to be cycled.
 For wrestling or football, include neck exercises.
† Type of Exercise: C = Core, P = Power, S = Secondary Exercises
‡ Muscle Area: TB = total body, SH = shoulder, CH = chest, AB = abdominal, A-A = arm-anterior, A-P = arm-posterior, UB = upper back, LB = lower back, LG = leg, L-A = leg-anterior, L-P = leg-posterior.

    2. Utilizing the specificity concept and a 1 RM, resistance/load guidelines presented in Table 3 may be summarized as follows:

        a. For **power,** assign a load that approximates 80% of the 1 RM.

        b. For **muscle strength,** assign a load that approximates 80–90% of the 1 RM.

        c. For **muscle hypertrophy,** assign a load that approximates 70–80% of the 1 RM.

        d. For **muscular endurance,** assign a load that approximates 60–70% of the 1 RM.

  E. **Rest periods**

    1. Table 3 shows application of the specificity concept in determining lengths of rest periods **between sets.**

    2. Longer rest periods (2–4 minutes) are more appropriate for **strength and power** development, whereas rest periods for **muscular endurance** are 30 seconds or less. The rest periods for **hypertrophy** fall somewhere in between.

  F. **Frequency of training:** Once exercises have been selected, decide when they will be performed during the week.

    1. The three common approaches are:

        a. To work out **3 days a week** (Mondays, Wednesdays, Fridays, or Tuesdays, Thursdays, Saturdays) and perform all exercises each day.

**TABLE 3.**   Specificity Concept Applied to Program Design Variables

| Intensity Classification | Outcome of Training | % of 1 RM | Repetition Range | Sets | Rest Between Sets |
|---|---|---|---|---|---|
| Very heavy | Power | 80 | 1–3 | 3–6 | 2–4 minutes |
| Heavy | Strength | 90–80 | 3–8 | 3–5 | 2–4 minutes |
| Moderate | Hypertrophy | 80–70 | 8–12 | 3–6 | 30–90 seconds |
| Light | Muscular endurance | 70–60* | 12–15+ | 2–3 | 30 seconds or less |

* Note: *Although it is common to see percentages of less than 60% recommended for developing muscular endurance, especially in circuit training programs, the author's opinion is that endurance activities associated with the sport, not strength training, should be relied upon to produce the needed changes in sport-specific muscular endurance.*

       b. To work out **4 days a week** (Mondays, Tuesdays, Thursdays, Fridays), splitting up exercises into body "parts," working some on Mondays and Thursdays, others on Tuesdays and Fridays ("split" program).

       c. To work out **6 days a week,** dividing exercises into 3 categories, performing each twice a week, but not 2 days in succession.

   2. Only the 3- and 4-day-a-week programs are discussed here. They are presented in Tables 2, 4, and 5.

F. **Variation**

   1. Varying training loads and volumes is important. By varying loads and/or volumes, there is a greater chance for sufficient recovery, optimal adaptation, and maximum gains. There is less chance that over-training signs and symptoms will occur.

   2. Tables 4 and 5 show variations of load and volume within the week, and from week to week, with increasingly greater intensities as the 8-week cycle of training continues.

       a. The variations of training loads in Tables 4 and 5 use the 1 RM, although the 10 RM could have been used.

       b. Variation of load and volume is typically used only with core exercises.

   3. Training loads and volumes in a **3-day-a-week program** can be varied in the following manner (Table 4):

       a. Monday: heavy loads

       b. Wednesday: light loads

       c. Friday: moderate loads.

   4. The **4-day-a-week (split) program** can be varied in the following manner (Table 5):

       a. Monday—heavy loads; Thursdays—light loads; performing power cleans, power cleans from a hang, back squats, leg curls, leg extensions, and hyperextensions.

       b. Tuesdays—light loads; Friday—heavy loads; performing overhead presses, bent-over rows, bench presses, biceps curls, French curls, and bent-knee sit-ups.

   5. The **8-week cycles** presented in Tables 4 and 5 assume that athletes have been strength training during the off-season.

   6. Should the preseason be longer than 8 weeks, another cycle can be developed, using the guidelines presented.

       a. Succeeding cycles should begin with 2 weeks of high volumes and light loads, then progress, using higher loading percentages than those used during the first 8-week cycle.

       b. The 1 RM determined during the 8th week of the cycle should be used in assigning training loads for the next cycle.

   7. **Be aware that:**

       a. Power movements (e.g., snatches, high pulls from the floor, power snatches) are very stressful exercises.

       b. Repetitions for **power exercises** should not exceed 5 (in a set).

       c. Repetitions for **partial power exercises** (e.g., hang cleans, hang snatches, partial pulls) should not exceed 6 (in a set).

**TABLE 4.** 3-Day-a-Week, 8-Week Training Cycle (For Selected Core Exercises)

| Week | Variables | Monday (Heavy) | Wednesday (Light) | Friday (Moderate) |
|---|---|---|---|---|
| 1 | % 1 RM | 60 | 50 | 55 |
|   | SETS | 3 | 3 | 3 |
|   | REPS | 10 | 10 | 10 |
| 2 | % 1 RM | 70 | 60 | 65 |
|   | SETS | 3 | 3 | 3 |
|   | REPS | 8 | 7 | 7 |
| 3 | % 1 RM | 75 | 68 | 72 |
|   | SETS | 4 | 3 | 3 |
|   | REPS | 6 | 8 | 8 |
| 4 | % 1 RM | 70 | 60 | 65 |
|   | SETS | 3 | 3 | 3 |
|   | REPS | 8 | 8 | 7 |
| 5 | % 1 RM | 80 | 70 | 76 |
|   | SETS | 3 | 3 | 4 |
|   | REPS | 5 | 8 | 6 |
| 6 | % 1 RM | 85 | 72 | 80 |
|   | SETS | 4 | 4 | 4 |
|   | REPS | 4 | 7 | 5 |
| 7 | % 1 RM | 90 | 75 | 83 |
|   | SETS | 4 | 4 | 4 |
|   | REPS | 2 | 5 | 4 |
| 8 | No training on Monday and Friday. Test for 1 RM on Wednesday and recalculate next cycle of loads using the new 1 RM. | | | |

All exercises are performed each day.

The above cycle pertains to loads and volumes for *selected* core exercises. Two sets of 8–12 repetitions are recommended for secondary exercises and other core exercises.

Note: *No more than 5 repetitions in a set should be performed in power movement exercises, such as the power snatch or power clean from the floor position, and no more than 6 repetitions in a set in partial movement exercises, such as the power snatch and clean from a hang position.*

     d. As the training cycle continues, the 1 RM should increase. Therefore, training loads based on a percentage of the original 1 RM may represent a smaller percentage of the new 1 RM. There are methods to anticipate 1 RM increases during the cycle; however, they may overestimate.

     e. The key is to **observe athletes on a daily basis,** being alert to situations requiring modifications in training intensities.

IV. **Over-training Considerations**

  A. **Over-training:**

    1. A condition characterized by a plateau or drop-off in performance.

  B. Characteristics of over-training:

    1. Extremes in **muscle soreness and stiffness.**

    2. **Inability to complete training sessions** that normally would be completed.

    3. **Higher** than normal resting **heart rate.**

    4. **Greater susceptibility** to colds and other illnesses.

    5. Unexplained **loss in body weight.**

    6. **Loss of appetite.**

    7. **Higher** than normal resting **blood pressure.**

  C. Ways to avoid over-training:

    1. Consider stress imposed on the body by the total program (running, agility drills, plyometrics), not just strength training.

    2. Increase training intensity gradually.

**TABLE 5.**  4-Day-a-Week, 8-Week Split Program Training Cycle (For Selected Core Exercises)

| Week | Variables | Monday (Heavy) | Tuesday (Light) | Wednesday | Thurrsday (Light) | Friday (Heavy) |
|------|-----------|----------------|-----------------|-----------|-------------------|----------------|
| 1 | % 1 RM | 60 | 55 | REST | 55 | 60 |
|   | SETS | 3 | 3 |  | 3 | 3 |
|   | REPS | 10 | 8 |  | 8 | 10 |
| 2 | % 1 RM | 65 | 60 | REST | 60 | 65 |
|   | SETS | 3 | 3 |  | 3 | 3 |
|   | REPS | 8 | 7 |  | 7 | 8 |
| 3 | % 1 RM | 75 | 68 | REST | 68 | 75 |
|   | SETS | 4 | 3 |  | 3 | 4 |
|   | REPS | 6 | 8 |  | 8 | 8 |
| 4 | % 1 RM | 70 | 60 | REST | 60 | 70 |
|   | SETS | 3 | 3 |  | 3 | 3 |
|   | REPS | 8 | 7 |  | 7 | 8 |
| 5 | % 1 RM | 80 | 70 | REST | 70 | 80 |
|   | SETS | 3 | 3 |  | 3 | 3 |
|   | REPS | 5 | 8 |  | 8 | 5 |
| 6 | % 1 RM | 85 | 72 | REST | 72 | 85 |
|   | SETS | 4 | 4 |  | 4 | 4 |
|   | REPS | 4 | 7 |  | 7 | 4 |
| 7 | % 1 RM | 90 | 75 | REST | 75 | 90 |
|   | SETS | 4 | 4 |  | 4 | 4 |
|   | REPS | 2 | 5 |  | 5 | 2 |
| 8 | No training on Monday, Tuesday, Thursday, and Friday. Test for 1 RM on Wednesday and recalculate next cycle of loads using the new 1 RM. | | | | | |

Exercises are performed on the following days:
  Mondays, Thursdays:  Shoulder, upper back, chest, arms, abdomen;
  Tuesdays, Fridays:     Power movements, thighs, legs, lower back.

The above cycle pertains to loads and volumes for *selected* core exercises. Two sets of 8–12 repetitions are recommended for secondary exercises and other core exercises.

Note: *No more than 5 repetitions in a set should be performed in power movement exercises, such as the power snatch or power clean from the floor position, and no more than 6 repetitions in a set in partial movement exercises, such as the power snatch and clean from a hang position.*

  3. Provide adequate recovery time.
  4. Assure proper nutrition.
  5. Assure adequate sleep.

V.  **The Total Program**
  A.  Although it is beyond the scope of this chapter, it is important to mention that well-designed programs consider all requirements (running, jumping, agility, speed, speed endurance, speed strength, functional strength, and flexibility) of the sport.
  B.  Designing a total program that will integrate the training for each of these requirements at the right time, at the correct intensity, and within the context of the sport season requires considerable effort and knowledge.
  C.  References at the end of this chapter are ideal sources of information on this topic.

*SUGGESTED READING*

1.  Fleck S, Kraemer W: Resistance Training. Urbana, IL, Human Kinetics, 1987.
2.  Garhammer J: Sports Illustrated Strength Training. New York, Harper & Row, 1986.
3.  State Clinic Association Curriculum: Lincoln, NE, National Strength and Conditioning Association, 1987.
4.  Stone M, O'Bryant H: Weight Training, A Scientific Approach. Minneapolis, Burgess International, 1987.

# Chapter 8: Preseason Conditioning: Flexibility

DANIEL BLANKE, PhD

## I. Introduction

Flexibility is the ability to move the joints of the body through the range of motion (ROM) for which they are intended. Although there is little evidence that excessive flexibility improves performance, there is some indication that lack of flexibility can hamper performance and may lead to injury. It is therefore important that an athlete maintain adequate flexibility. Since changes in the ROM are best developed over a long time, it is important for an athlete to include flexibility training in a preseason conditioning program.

## II. General Principles of Flexibility

### A. Definitions of terms

The following are defined for the purpose of this chapter.

1. **Stretch**—Increasing the length of a tissue.
2. **Stretching**—The process of increasing the length of a tissue.
3. **Elastic stretch**—A temporary increase in the length of a tissue that returns to its original length when the stress is removed.
4. **Plastic stretch**—A more permanent increase in the length of a tissue that remains elongated after the stress is removed.
5. **Flexibility training**—A program of stretching exercises designed to increase the ROM of the targeted joints to a desired level. Once that level is attained, flexibility training can be used to maintain the desired ROM.

### B. Characteristics of connective tissue

1. Connective tissue is one of the most widely varied types of tissue. Although cartilage, bone, blood, and lymph are types of connective tissue, the connective tissue that is found in tendons, ligaments, intramuscular and extramuscular layers of fascia, and joint capsules is the type of connective tissue that we are concerned about as we discuss flexibility training. This type of connective tissue is **primarily collagenous fibers** arranged in a protein-polysaccharide ground substance.[7] It possesses both **elastic and plastic properties.** This type of connective tissue is referred to as dense or collagenous connective tissue.[9] References made to connective tissue in this chapter will imply this dense or collagenous type of connective tissue.
2. Connective tissue exhibits **high tensile strength** and therefore is **difficult to elongate.**
3. Connective tissue is primarily responsible for limiting joint ROM. It is therefore the target of flexibility training. Joint flexibility can be increased through stretching exercises that increase the length of the connective tissue structures.

### C. Plastic versus elastic stretch

1. When connective tissue is stretched, some of the elongation is elastic and some is plastic. Once the force causing the stretch in the connective tissue is removed, the elastic elements return to their resting length whereas the plastic components remain elongated.
2. **Flexibility training should be designed to produce plastic rather than elastic deformation.** Plastic deformation results in a more permanent change in length of the tissue.
3. **Low force loads applied for long periods of time result in a greater incidence of plastic deformation.** Flexibility training should therefore reflect these force and time requirements.

41

D. **Specificity of flexibility training**
   1. The amount of flexibility in any joint is **specific** to that joint and is not a general characteristic.
   2. Increasing flexibility in any joint will not result in an increase in any other joint. To increase flexibility of any joint, stretching exercises that increase the length of the connective tissue surrounding and crossing that joint are necessary.

E. **The effects of temperature on flexibility training**
   1. **Stretching connective tissue under conditions of elevated temperature results in greater plastic deformation.**[7] It is difficult to elevate tissue temperature deep within large muscles with topical application of heat. In a clinical environment, deep heating methods of diathermy or ultrasound may be beneficial, but in the nonclinical environment the **temperature is best elevated through several minutes of muscle activity.**
   2. In order to gain maximum benefit of plastic deformation of connective tissue after stretching, the connective tissue should be allowed to **cool while the stress is applied.** This implies that the most effective flexibility training can be done after the tissue temperature has been elevated by allowing the tissue to cool during the training period. This substantiates the normal practice of training for increased flexibility during the cool-down portion of an exercise bout.

F. **Effects of age on flexibility**
   1. Flexibility tends to **decrease with age.**[6] The effects of aging on flexibility can be reduced by consistently participating in a program designed to maintain or enhance flexibility.

G. **Effects of sex on flexibility**
   1. **Females tend to be more flexible than males of the same age.**[6] The difference in flexibility between males and females of the same age is partly due to the differences in muscle mass and quantity of connective tissue, but also due to the greater tendency for girls and women to participate in activities such as dance, slimnastics, and gymnastics that typically promote flexibility.

H. **Effects of habitual movement patterns on flexibility**
   1. Habitual movement patterns have the greatest effect on flexibility. Moving the joint through a limited range of motion will decrease the flexibility of the joint over time due to **adaptive shortening** of the muscle and connective tissue. The elastic nature of connective tissue causes it to shorten when no load is applied. To reduce the potential for limited ROM, it is important to exercise the joint through full ROM whenever possible.

I. **Retention of flexibility**
   1. The greatest loss of flexibility occurs in the first 2 weeks after termination of flexibility training. After 4 weeks the athlete will continue to lose flexibility but will still be more flexible than prior to starting a flexibility training program.[8] It is therefore important to **train for flexibility on a regular basis.** If training is not possible due to illness or injury, flexibility will deteriorate but the increases on joint ROM gained in flexibility training will not be completely eroded even after 4 weeks of inactivity.

J. **Stretch reflex**
   1. The stretch reflex is a protective reflex due to the action of the muscle spindles. When a muscle is stretched rapidly, especially at its greatest length, the muscle spindle sends a stimulus to the CNS, which in turn sends a stimulus back to the muscle. The muscle responds by contracting. The force of contraction is somewhat related to the speed of the muscle as it is being stretched. The purpose of this reflex is to protect the muscle and associated joints from injury by limiting the ROM of the muscle.
   2. The stretch reflex hampers flexibility training by actively contracting the muscle that is in the process of being elongated. **Slow movements that reduce the intensity of the contraction and delay the activity of the stretch reflex until reaching maximum ROM are more desirable than fast movements that elicit the stretch reflex.** Flexibility training that uses slow movements therefore will reduce the incidence of injury.

K. **Preseason versus in-season flexibility training**
1. **Considerable time is required to develop a significant increase in the flexibility of a joint.** This necessitates that the majority of flexibility training be done **preseason or off-season.**
2. Essentially, it is **important to maintain flexibility during the entire off-season. Preseason workouts can then be used to increase flexibility for the upcoming season.** This pattern will result in a progressive increase in flexibility over an athletic career. An athlete that begins flexibility training with the first practice and stops with the last game will only begin to demonstrate the improvements in flexibility late in the season. This pattern will result in a progressive decrease in flexibility over an athletic career.

III. **Role of Flexibility in Injury Prevention**

A. **Optimal flexibility**
1. **Optimal flexibility** is extremely difficult to define. It is dependent more on the expected activity and **is therefore a relative term rather than an absolute value.** Optimal flexibility for a gymnast may be considerably different than optimal flexibility for a marathon runner. We must also identify optimal flexibility at a specific joint, since flexibility is not a general factor and is joint specific.
2. **Optimal flexibility can be described as the required amount of flexibility or ROM at the joint that will allow for maximum performance of the defined activity while protecting the joint from acute or chronic injury.** This definition will allow for differing amounts of flexibility at any joint dependent upon the activity level of the joint and yet not encourage excessive flexibility, which can result in acute or chronic joint injury.

B. **Flexibility versus stability**
1. **Although lack of flexibility can result in a poor performance, there is little evidence that excessive flexibility can result in outstanding performance.** The amount of flexibility necessary at a joint is dictated by the maximum ROM experienced during the performance of the activity. If this ROM is less than the ROM normally exhibited by a nonathlete of this age and sex, then the athlete should be encouraged to maintain the flexibility expected to match the nonathlete. If the ROM is greater than that normally exhibited by a nonathlete of this age and sex, then the athlete must increase his/her flexibility to meet the demands of the sport or activity in which he/she is participating.
2. **There is a concern over excessive increases of flexibility.**[3] Just because a little bit is good does not imply a lot is better. **There is a trade-off between flexibility and stability.** Increasing flexibility can lead to decreased stability. This is especially evident when the flexibility increases are the result of lengthening the connective tissue structures that stabilize the joint. Athletes should be encouraged to maintain flexibility at the level necessary for maximum performance in their chosen activity, but not in excess of that amount, as excessive flexibility can be associated with a decrease in stability and therefore a greater tendency for injury.
3. **Permanently elongating connective tissue results in some mechanical weakening of the tissue.** Flexibility training with **low stress applied over a long period of time results in less mechanical weakening** than training of a short duration with a large amount of force.

C. **Muscle strain versus joint sprain**
1. When a lack of flexibility is noted in an athlete, that athlete is more prone to muscle strain, whereas an athlete with a large amount of flexibility at a joint may be more prone to joint sprain. Increasing flexibility in the athlete with limited range of motion will help reduce the incidence of muscle strains. **Excessive increase in the flexibility of an athlete increases the likelihood of joint sprains while reducing the tendency for muscle strains.**

IV. **Role of Flexibility in Performance Enhancement**

A. **Effects of limited flexibility**

1. The quality of a performance is affected by many variables. One of the variables that can affect a performance is the lack of flexibility. Swimmers lacking flexibility in the ankles or shoulders will not be able to orient the foot or arm to the water for maximum push, pull, or lift. Divers lacking low back and hamstring flexibility will not be able to achieve the tight pike position necessary to rotate rapidly or secure a high score. The gymnast lacking flexibility, like the diver, will not be able to achieve certain positions, which will definitely affect the athlete's score. These are a few of the examples of the effect of inadequate flexibility on performance. **For any activity, the coach or athlete must evaluate the activity to determine the maximum ROM necessary for optimum performance of the activity then increase the flexibility during the off-season to this required level.**

V. **Techniques for Improving Flexibility**

   A. **Introduction**
      1. There are several techniques that can be used to increase flexibility. All techniques that follow have been shown to increase flexibility if practiced **regularly.** Unlike training to increase strength, flexibility training should be **practiced daily or more than once per day.** Some techniques are more conveniently practiced with a partner, whereas others are easily practiced alone. At least one technique has been shown to increase the chance of muscle and joint injury and therefore is not advocated. Choice of the technique to use should be made by the athlete or coach in light of what will be practiced regularly, as that is the most crucial factor.

   B. **Static stretching**
      1. Static stretching is done by slowly moving the joint to the end of the ROM then holding the position for 5 to 60 seconds. It is important when moving to the end of the ROM to stop at the point of moderate discomfort and prior to pain. As a result of the slow movement, there is a reduced tendency to elicit the stretch reflex. **Static stretch is therefore one of the safest techniques for increasing flexibility.**

   C. **Static stretching with contraction of the antagonist**
      1. Static stretching with contraction of the antagonist is done by slowly moving the joint to the end of the ROM then isometrically contracting the antagonist muscle group for 5 to 30 seconds. This is the muscle group directly opposite the muscle being stretched. It is again important to move the joint just to the point of moderate discomfort and no farther. **This technique enjoys all the benefits of static stretching with the added benefit of further reducing the tendency to elicit the stretch reflex by actively contracting the antagonist muscle group.** By the action of reciprocal inhibition, there is a release of an inhibitory transmitter substance at the spinal cord to reduce the activity of the muscle being stretched.

   D. **Static stretching with contraction of the agonist—proprioceptive neuromuscular facilitation (PNF)**
      1. Static stretching with contraction of the agonist is performed by slowly moving the joint to the end of the ROM, then isometrically contracting the agonist muscle group for 5 to 30 seconds. This is a contraction of the muscle group that is being stretched. No movement should occur in the muscle being stretched. The contraction must therefore be isometric. **It is theorized that the isometric contraction of the muscle being stretched will further relax the muscle after the contraction, possibly through the action of the Golgi tendon organ, and therefore allow additional ROM at the joint.** Minimally, the isometric contraction will put an additional stretch on the connective tissue surrounding the joint and therefore allow greater ROM.

   E. **Static stretching with contraction of the agonist followed by contraction of the antagonist—PNF**
      1. Static stretching with contraction of the agonist followed by contraction of the antagonist is performed by slowly moving the joint to the end of the ROM then isometrically contracting the agonist muscle group for 5 to 30 seconds. As with

the previous PNF method, this is contraction of the muscle group being stretched. This is followed by relaxing the agonist and contracting the antagonist muscle group, the group opposite the group being stretched, for 5 to 30 seconds while attempting to stretch the muscle group even more.

F. **Ballistic stretching**
1. Ballistic stretching is performed by quickly moving the joint to the end of the ROM. It often **uses bouncing, jerking movements or momentum to force the joint beyond its normal ROM.** The movements may be described as pulsing, bobbing, swinging or kicking movements. **Although ballistic stretching has been shown to increase flexibility it is NOT a recommended technique because of the increased potential of injury that is associated with this type of flexibility training.** There is a greater tendency for injury as a result of the additional forces that are present with movement. These forces are in the direction opposite to the direction of the forces incurred in stretching the muscle and therefore can lead to muscle or connective tissue tears or bone avulsion.

VI. **Identifying Flexibility Requirements of Selected Sports**

A. **Evaluating sports for flexibility requirements**
1. The flexibility required for any activity can be determined by identifying the ROM required for each movement of the activity. It therefore becomes **important to analyze the activity carefully** to determine the maximum ROM necessary for performing the activity.
2. As an example, jogging requires little ROM at the hip, knee, ankle, foot, shoulder, elbow, or trunk. When the speed of the jog is increased to running, the ROM of each joint increases. Sprinting demands even greater ROM at the joints with the largest differences occurring at the knee and hip. **The flexibility requirement increases as the ROM requirement of the joint increases.**
3. Sports such as diving, dance, and gymnastics require a large amount of flexibility, especially in the wrists, shoulders, back, and hips, because of the ROM necessary for performance of many of the component activities. Since showing flexibility is part of the scoring system for diving and gymnastics, and part of the aesthetic value of dance, inadequate flexibility results in lower scores whereby optimal flexibility will allow for higher scores.
4. After identifying the flexibility requirements of a sport, the next task is to **develop the appropriate flexibility training program.** A series of flexibility exercises that will increase the flexibility of the joints to the level necessary for optimal performance of the sport must be identified.
5. The **technique of flexibility training** will also need to be identified. The athlete can then begin to increase flexibility with daily training.

B. **Flexibility requirements for selected sports**
1. **Each sport or game, because of its inherent activity, has a certain flexibility requirement.** Sports that require considerable upper body motion will have a greater requirement for the upper body flexibility, whereas those with considerable lower body activity will require more lower body flexibility. Some sports require rotational flexibility, whereas others require only linear flexibility training. Anderson[1] and Beaulieu[2] have identified flexibility training programs for a variety of sport activities as well as detailed descriptions of flexibility exercises for every joint.

VII. **Flexibility Myths and Misconceptions**

A. **Flexibility exercises to avoid**
1. There are several exercises that have been used to increase flexibility that should be **avoided.** These exercises are identified as placing excessive pressure on the spinal discs, the arterial system, knee ligaments, or the sciatic nerve. Beaulieu[3] identified high risk flexibility exercises, whereas Anderson[1] identifies the incorrect and correct position for stretching specific joints.
2. **Yoga plow**—This exercise places excessive strain on the neck and lower back.

3. **Hurdler's stretch**—This exercise applies excessive pressure to the medial collateral ligament of the knee when performed with one hip joint abducted and inwardly rotated, the knee flexed, and the leg outwardly rotated.
4. **Duck walk**—This exercise applies excessive pressure to the ligaments and menisci of the knees.
5. **Toe touching**—This exercise applies excessive pressure to the lumbar discs when performed from a standing position with the knees fully extended.
6. **Straight leg sit-ups or double leg raises**—These exercises apply excessive pressure to the lumbar vertebrae and strengthen the hip flexors when abdominal endurance is the desired goal.

B. **Flexibility Myths**
1. **Pulsing is better than bouncing.** It is a myth that rapid pulsing, which is essentially short bounces at the end of the ROM, is a desirable technique to improve flexibility. This technique is occasionally taught in conjunction with dance exercise. It is still **ballistic** in nature and therefore a less desirable technique for improving flexibility.
2. **Flexibility training should be used for warm-up.** To reduce the chance of muscle injury and increase the effect of flexibility training, the muscle temperature should be elevated prior to stretching. The temperature of the muscle can be most easily elevated by exercise. **Easy, rhythmical exercise should precede easy stretching in the warm-up portion of an exercise bout. Flexibility training is most effective after an exercise bout when the muscle temperature is most elevated.**

VIII. **Summary**

Flexibility training should be a part of the conditioning program for **every athlete. Significant increases in the level of flexibility take from 6 to 12 weeks to develop.** Although flexibility training should take place during the season of competition, it **must be started preseason and should be continued throughout the year.** Flexibility training should take place **daily.** Each session should begin with several minutes of warm-up exercises designed to **increase the temperature of the muscle.** The warm-up exercises should be followed by **specific exercises designed to increase the flexibility of the joints that are used in the activity** for which the athlete is training. The technique used for flexibility training is up to the discretion of the athlete or coach. **Ballistic training should be avoided.**

## REFERENCES AND SUGGESTED READINGS

1. Anderson B: Stretching. Bolinas, CA, Shelter Publications, 1984.
2. Beaulieu J: Stretching for All Sports. Pasadena, Athletic Press, 1980.
3. Beaulieu J: Developing a stretching program. Phys Sportsmed 9(11):59–66, 1981.
4. Etnyre B, Lee E: Comments on proprioceptive neuromuscular facilitation stretching techniques. Res Q Exerc Sport 58(2):184–188, 1987.
5. Etnyre B, Lee E: Chronic and acute flexibility of men and women using three different stretching techniques. Res Q Exerc Sport 59(3):222–228, 1988.
6. Rasch P, Burke R: Kinesiology and Applied Anatomy. Philadelphia, Lea & Febiger, 1978.
7. Sapega A, Quedenfeld T, Moyer R, Butler R: Biophysical factors in range-of-motion exercises. Phys Sportsmed 9(12):57–64, 1981.
8. Thomas T, Zebas C: Scientific Exercise Training. Dubuque, Kendall Hunt, 1984.
9. Tortora G, Anagnostakos N: Principles of Anatomy and Physiology. New York, Harper & Row, 1987.

# Chapter 9: Sports Surfaces

RICHARD B. FLYNN, EdD

## I. Introduction

It is generally accepted that the type of surface upon which an activity or sport is played can affect the quality of performance. Other aspects of the game influenced by the playing surface include speed, costs, player comfort, and player safety.

Unfortunately, there is no one surface that will satisfactorily meet the needs of participants for all indoor and outdoor activities. Each activity has its own unique characteristics requiring a particular type of surface for optimal performance. Economical considerations often dictate a common surface be used to support a variety of activities especially at recreational and amateur levels.

Planners of formal sports facilities are urged to consult with the various governing organizations regarding rules, regulations, and standards that may affect the type of surface necessary for sanctioned participation in a particular sport.

The purpose of this chapter is to outline some of the surfaces used for different sporting activities, relate surface selection to player performance and safety, and identify factors to be considered in the selection of sports surfaces.

A. **Range of surfaces.** There are literally hundreds of surfaces available as possible choices for sporting events. Some of these surfaces are natural and are formed from products found in nature, whereas others are more complex, requiring processing and/or the use of synthetic materials.

1. **Natural surfaces**
   a. Earth—loams, sand, sand-clay, clay-gravel, fuller's earth, stabilized earth, etc.
   b. Turf (grass)—bluegrass mixtures, bent, fescue, Bermuda, etc.
   c. Aggregates—gravel, graded stone, graded slag, shell, cinders, etc.
   d. Masonry—flagstone (sandstone, limestone, granite), brick, etc.
   e. Wood flooring—usually polished hard woods
   f. Miscellaneous—tanbark, sawdust, shavings, cotton-seed hulls, etc.

2. **Non-natural surfaces**
   a. Asphalt—penetration-macadam, asphaltic concrete (cool and hot poured), sheet asphalt, natural asphalt, sawdust asphalt, vermiculite asphalt, cork asphalt, other patented asphalt mixes.
   b. Synthetics—rubber, synthetic resins, rubber asphalt, chlorinated butyl-rubber, mineral fiber, plastics, vinyl, etc.
   c. Concrete—monolithic, terrazzo, pre-cast.

B. **Factors influencing choice of surfaces.** In general, safety, the appropriateness of the surface properties for the specified sport, and the material properties related to wear and maintenance all need to be considered when selecting a surface.[1] Following are additional factors that may influence the choice of surface:

1. Expected multiplicity of use
2. Durability
3. Dustless and stainless
4. Reasonable initial cost and economy
5. Ease and cost of maintenance
6. Pleasing appearance
7. Non abrasiveness
8. Resiliency and consistency of resiliency
9. Year-round usage

      10. Color and color stability
      11. Impact absorption
      12. Effects of temperature and sun (for outdoor surfaces)
      13. Tensile strength
      14. Texture.
  C. **Ideal surface conditions.** There is no one surface that will satisfactorily meet the needs of all activities. Each activity has its own surface requirements that dictate what type of materials can be used. Ideally most sports or activities need the following conditions to be met:
      1. A surface that provides appropriate traction.
      2. A surface that is smooth and even.
      3. A surface that provides consistent hardness.
      4. A surface that has enough spring to prevent injuries.

II. **Surfaces for Outdoor Sporting Events**

  A. **Outdoor field events.** Football, soccer, baseball, field hockey, and lacrosse are all played on outdoor fields. The surface material, whether natural or artificial, is critical to the use and success of the field as a site for practice and games.
    1. **Surface requirements**
      a. Smooth and uniform.
      b. Resilient enough to prevent injuries, but hard enough to facilitate running.
      c. Providing traction.
    2. **Surface options**
      a. **Grass:** blue grass mixtures, bent, fescue, and Bermuda are popular natural fields for athletics.
        i. Advantages of grass
          (a) Attractiveness
          (b) Resiliency
          (c) Nonabrasiveness
          (d) Relatively dust free
          (e) Cool temperature maintained by surface even in hot weather
          (f) Generally regarded as safe.
        ii. Disadvantages of grass
          (a) Difficult to maintain when there is intense usage
          (b) Expense of watering (can be very costly in some parts of the country)
          (c) Field cannot be used, without damage, when wet or frozen
          (d) Field must be given time to recuperate after heavy use
          (e) Requires scheduled aeration, fertilization, deep watering, seeding, and trimming.
      b. **Synthetic turf.** Synthetic turf is a tufted carpet made from polyvinyl chloride or urethane plastic. The composition of the subcarpet base varies in thickness and resiliency. Embedded in, or bonded to, the subcarpet base are plastic fibers resembling grass. The density and height of the blades vary with anticipated use. Recent innovations in synthetic turf include the use of more porous materials that facilitate better drainage, and now with some materials there is no grain, or direction, in the field.
        i. Advantages of synthetic turf
          (a) Consistently smooth and uniform surface.
          (b) Greatly expands the effective use of an area (allows multi-use including recreational activities and instructional classes rather than just formal athletics).
          (c) Provides the opportunity for use under all but the most adverse weather conditions.
          (d) Generally regarded as safe.
          (e) Provides economic benefits through reduced acreage requirements.
          (f) Increased use and decreased maintenance costs.

      (g) Many top regional, state, national, and international events are conducted on synthetic surfaces, providing for greater uniformity in performance.

      (h) Does not cause allergies.

      (i) No bald spots.

  ii. Disadvantages of synthetic turf

      (a) Initial costs are high, sometimes double or triple depending on grading, subsurface, installation process, and selected material.

      (b) Maintenance, although minimal in some cases, is necessary. When required it is both costly and time consuming. Maintenance is reduced if measures are taken to reduce or eliminate vehicular and pedestrian traffic and security measures are taken to reduce vandalism and misuse.

      (c) Aspects of the weather do affect outdoor synthetic surfaces. Extreme temperatures may alter the resiliency of the surface. The character of the composition may also alter over a short period of time either from temperature extremes or ultraviolet exposure.

      (d) Limited research studies have indicated a heat build-up on the surface that may affect the performer.

      (e) Surface is abrasive.

3. **Relationship between turf type and injuries.** There have been many, many studies over the years comparing injury rates on artificial vs. natural turf.

  a. **Sub-factors that affect injury rates**

    i. May be greater frequency of play on synthetic surfaces

    ii. Varying surface pad thicknesses

    iii. Different equipment padding

    iv. Different types of injuries

    v. Varying coaching methods

    vi. Inaccurate recording of injuries

    vii. Varying shoe-turf interactions.[16]

  b. **Recent research highlights.** Although many comparisons of injury rates on artificial versus natural grass have been conducted since artificial turf was first introduced, the results are not entirely conclusive. The research suggests there is a slightly higher injury rate on artificial turf. As developments in artificial turf have taken place over the years, it appears progress is being made toward artificial turf becoming safer. Following are results of several recent major studies:

    i. NCAA Injury Surveillance System data from 1982–1987 found "the injury rate on artificial turf has been consistently higher than on natural turf over the five-year sample. The magnitude of this difference, however, has decreased from an almost 85% higher injury rate on artificial turf in 1982 to only a 14% difference in 1986."[13]

    ii. Another NCAA pilot study on Division I-A football teams found "that more injuries occurred on natural as opposed to artificial surfaces. However, this data must be evaluated with consideration to the small number of schools sampled and the single year of reporting."[6]

    iii. NFL-related representatives have drawn conclusions inconsistent with each other:

      (a) "Virtually all studies indicate that artificial turf is more hazardous, although not all have been statistically significant"—James Garrick, former medical advisor for the NFL Management Council and the NFLPA Joint Safety Committee.[7]

      (b) "Our studies have not shown a significant difference in major injuries (an injury that keeps a player out for at least 21 days) on artificial turf compared with natural turf. . . . Obviously, minor scrapes and abrasions are more prevalent on artificial surfaces"—Jim Miller, Director of Administration Council.[7]

        (c) An NFL study based on games played in NFL stadiums 1980–1985 found "higher rates [of injury] per team-game on the Astro-Turf than on grass surfaces. . . . These data indicate if an NFL team were to play all its regularly scheduled games on Astro-Turf, it could expect to have one additional MAJOR knee injury as compared to a complete season on grass."[17]

      iv. "[A] professional football franchise was studied consecutively from 1960 through 1985 for injuries incurred during regular-season games. . . . Since the team's first games on synthetic surfaces in 1968, there was no difference in the rates of significant injuries per game (0.57 vs 0.67) or major injuries per game (0.22 vs 0.33) between games played on grass or artificial turf, respectively"—James Nicholas, Lenox Hill Hospital, New York.[14]

B. **Outdoor basketball**
  1. **Surface requirements**
    a. Smooth
    b. Hard.
  2. **Recommended options**
    a. Asphaltic concrete
      i. Durable
     ii. Can be used year-round
     iii. Dust-free
     iv. Drains quickly
     v. Marks easily and with a high degree of permanence
     vi. Neat appearance
    vii. Colors easily
    viii. Easy to maintain.
    b. Portland cement concrete
      i. More expensive to install
     ii. May crack when used in an extreme cold climate.
    c. Synthetic surfaces
      i. Same advantages as asphaltic concrete
     ii. Aesthetically pleasing
     iii. More expensive to install.

C. **Outdoor tennis**
  1. **Factors to consider in selecting a surface**
    a. Player preference
    b. Maintenance cost and amount of maintenance required
    c. Initial construction cost
    d. Surface on which player can slide or not slide
    e. Length of time until resurfacing is required
    f. Resurfacing cost
    g. Softness of surface desired for player comfort
    h. Surface adaptability for other uses
    i. Fast or slow surface
    j. Uniformity of ball bounce
    k. Effect of color on glare and heat absorption
    l. Drying time after rain
    m. Availability of service from court builder
    n. Color fastness of surface and its effect on ball discoloration
    o. Effect of abrasive surfaces on ball, rackets, shoes, and falling players
    p. Quality of lines and markings
    q. Hazards, maintenance of lines.[9]
  2. **Classification of tennis court surfaces**
    a. Pervious construction (one that permits water to filter through the surface):
      i. Fast dry (fine crushed aggregate)
     ii. Clay

         iii. Grass

         iv. Others (dirt, grit, etc.).

   b. Impervious construction (one on which water does not penetrate, but runs off the surface):

       i. Non cushioned

         (a) Concrete

         (b) Asphalt

            (i) hot-plant mix

            (ii) emulsified asphalt mix

            (iii) combination of hot-plant and emulsified mix

            (iv) penetration macadam

            (v) asphalt job mix

         (c) Others (wood, etc.).

       ii. Cushioned construction

         (a) Asphalt bound systems

            (i) hot-leveling course and hot-cushion course

            (ii) cold-leveling course and cold-cushion course

         (b) Synthetic

            (i) elastomer

            (ii) textile

         (c) Others.

 D. **Outdoor track**

   1. **Options**

     a. Natural or aggregate materials

     b. Asphalt-bound

     c. Latex or latex-bound

     d. Polyurethane or polyurethane-bound

     e. Pre-manufactured rubber mats.

   2. **Factors for considerations**

     a. Cost for the foundation and drainage

     b. Cost of the surface

     c. Color options

       i. Performance is enhanced on colors other than black.

       ii. Surface temperature is reduced on nonblack surfaces in turn lengthening surface life.

       iii. A color surface change in a nonblack surface indicates need for maintenance.

       iv. A nonblack surface is "treated" better by athletes and spectators.

III. **Surfaces for Indoor Sporting Events**

 A. **Multipurpose use.** The best choice of flooring depends on expected use. Wood is an excellent all-round surface, although it lacks the durability and flexibility that might be demanded by extensive community use of the facility. Synthetic surfaces are excellent for all normal game-type activities and can better accommodate chairs, tables, and booths. Some activities require specialized flooring, such as dance, weight training, and body conditioning.

   1. **Surface options**

     a. Wood

     b. Synthetic

       i. Prefabricated

       ii. Poured-in-place

     c. Carpet

   2. **Life-cycle costs.** Variability in initial costs and maintenance costs will affect choice of a multipurpose activity surface.[19]

   3. **Advantages and disadvantages of various options** (see Section IIIB2, a and b)

 B. **Basketball/volleyball**

   1. **Surface requirements**

      a. Hard, but resilient

      b. Smooth and even.

  2. **Surface options.** The best options for basketball and volleyball are either wood or synthetic flooring of a nonslip nature.

      a. Wood (generally hard northern maple):

          i. Advantages

             (a) Natural resiliency due to organic nature.

             (b) Variability in resilience based upon choice of subflooring (floating systems with foam or rubber underlayment, sleeper systems, and spring systems under plywood).

             (c) Can be sanded to accept a wide variety of finishes.

             (d) Traction is superb for basketball, volleyball, and others.

             (e) Properly maintained wood floor can outlast the building.

         ii. Disadvantages

             (a) High initial cost.

             (b) Maintenance costs can be high (but with new polyurethane finishes, maintenance costs are decreasing).

             (c) Can warp when exposed to moisture.

             (d) Is not as versatile as some synthetics (for example, is too smooth for indoor tennis).[12]

      b. Synthetics (plasticized polyvinyl chlorides or polyurethanes):

          i. Advantages

             (a) Prefabricated floors are uniform in thickness (poured-in-place floors may not be).

             (b) Prefabricated floors are durable (poured-in-place floors may disintegrate, harden, shrink, and crack due to ultraviolet rays and evaporating chemicals).

             (c) Resilient.

             (d) Available in a wide variety of colors, textures, and amount of traction.

             (e) Initial cost usually lower than wood.

             (f) Unaffected by moisture.

             (g) Not slippery when wet.

             (h) Versatile for multiple uses.

         ii. Disadvantages

             (a) Can be difficult to keep clean.

             (b) Ultraviolet rays can cause disintegration in some cases.

             (c) Plasticizers in poured-in-place floors may cause unpleasant odors.

             (d) Poured-in-place floors can be difficult to repair in worn areas.

             (e) Poured-in-place floors may not be uniform thickness.

C. **Dance**

  1. **Surface requirements**

      a. Has shock absorbing qualities.

      b. Will "give" under impact to some degree, and absorb some of the impact energy in doing so.

      c. Will not deform permanently or dent under pressure or impact in normal use.

      d. Should not be "dead" or softly yielding as sand is, but should return some bounce to the shoe.

      e. Should not be absolutely rigid or hard and should not give the impression of being so.

      f. Nonslippery but smooth and permitting of gliding.

      g. Constructed for easy cleaning.[4,18]

  2. **Design options for subflooring.** There are seven major types of subflooring:[18]

      a. **Anchor sleeper construction.** 2 × 3 inch or 2 × 4 inch sleepers of varying lengths leveled and anchored to the concrete substrate with mechanical fasteners.

b. **Resilient rubber padded sleeper with floating floor.** 2 × 3 inch sleepers with resilient rubber or vinyl pads attached to the underside of the sleeper.

c. **Spring-coil.** Spring-coil resembles a miniature coil spring used in the automobile industry but is designed specifically for flooring applications.

d. **Spring-leaf.** Spring-leaf resembles the leaf spring suspension of an automobile, only it is smaller.

e. **Resilient foam underlayment.** Foam underlayment sheets of varying thicknesses and densities deaden sound and absorb shock. Subflooring is laid over foam sheeting.

f. **Multilayered basket-weave sleeper or joist construction.** Stacked layers of 1 × 4 inch or 2 × 3 inch alternating perpendicular to one another.

g. **Mastic set floor.** Mastic set floors of different compositions provide cushioning but very little return of energy. Mastic can be applied under subfloor components at various thicknesses.

3. **Surface materials.** The materials laid over the subfloor systems vary greatly, but all are intended to have the proper surface friction, uniformity of surface, and long-term performance.

   a. Wood products
   - i. Northern hard-strip maple
   - ii. Strip oak
   - iii. Pine
   - iv. Fir
   - v. Birch.

   b. Synthetic products
   - i. Vinyl roll sheet goods
   - ii. Linoleum
   - iii. Portable synthetic flooring mats

   c. Coatings/wood finishes
   - i. Varnish
   - ii. Linseed or tung oil
   - iii. Epoxy ester (preferred when dance involves street shoes)
   - iv. Polyurethane
   - v. Moisture-cure urethane
   - vi. Penetrating oil—modified urethane
   - vii. Natural uncoated wood.

D. **Aerobics**

  1. **Surface requirements**
   - a. Compliance
   - b. Foot stability
   - c. Traction
   - d. Resiliency
   - e. Impact independence (ability to isolate the absorption of impact energy).

  2. **Surface options**

    a. Foam systems with carpet:
   - i. Advantages
     - (a) Low cost
     - (b) Self-installation
     - (c) Generally low maintenance cost
     - (d) Quieter
     - (e) Often can be used for multipurposes
     - (f) Carpeting provides a good surface to lie down on and is perceived aesthetically as softer to dance on
     - (g) Good on compliance characteristics.
   - ii. Disadvantages
     - (a) Limited life expectancy of the foam
     - (b) Hygiene problems related to the carpet covering
     - (c) Some carpet coverings inhibit foot glide and pivot
     - (d) Less resilience.[2]

    b. Hardwood floor systems:
   - i. Advantages of hardwood
     - (a) Ideal for lateral movements
     - (b) Provides considerable shock absorption

        (c) Dependent on underlayment of the subflooring
        (d) Can be beautiful depending on type of wood and finish
        (e) Very long life expectancy (30 years possible)
        (f) Good for foot stability, surface traction, and resilience.
    ii. Disadvantages
        (a) Cost
        (b) Periodic maintenance requirements
        (c) Usually require mats or carpeting over the wood
        (d) More restrictive use (avoid tables, chairs, and street shoes)
        (e) Less compliant.[15]

  c. Carpeting over hardwood flooring
  d. Multi-purpose synthetics (polyurethane or micro-cell foam).
    i. Advantages
        (a) Easy to clean
        (b) Wears well
        (c) Provides good shock absorbency
        (d) Provides good traction
        (e) One-fourth the price of wood flooring
        (f) Micro-cell foam is available in interlocking sections that are movable.[8]

**E. Tennis**

1. **Surface requirements.** Tennis can be played indoors on any firm surface of sufficient size for a tennis court. The composition of a synthetic surface can be altered to offset the bounce of the tennis ball. A surface constructed for playing basketball usually proves to be too fast for tennis competition but will suffice for beginning instruction.

2. **Synthetic options**
  a. Carpet—textile materials that are installed permanently or rolled out as a temporary surface.
    i. Features
        (a) Coated for wearability
        (b) Generally fast playing
        (c) Allows a low bounce
        (d) Allows a quiet game
        (e) Required minimal maintenance.
  b. Modular surfacing—interlocking gridwork of various chemical compositions, the most common being a combination of polypropylene and rubber.
    i. Features
        (a) Usually one square foot in size
        (b) Can form a new surface over an existing court
        (c) Requires minimal maintenance
        (d) Quiet, cushioned effect
        (e) Durable
        (f) Relatively higher in cost
        (g) Not recommended for tournament play since variations in temperature can cause expansion and contraction.
  c. Synthetic sand-filled turf—made of loosely woven polypropylene fibers with a rubber-like backing, filled with graded sand; appearance like a grass court.
    i. Features
        (a) Consistency of bounce
        (b) Easy on the legs
        (c) Minimal maintenance
        (d) Can be laid over deteriorated surfaces
        (e) Sand may shift during the course of play
        (f) Has a tendency to absorb odors.
  d. Removable court surfaces—12-foot-wide strips of various synthetic surfaces.
  e. Asphalt-bound.[20]

F. **Racquetball/handball/squash.** Floors should be hardwood, as in standard gymnasium construction.

G. **Indoor tracks.** Alternative surfaces for indoor tracks include polyurethane or polyurethane-bound, latex or latex-bound, both of which can be either premanufactured or poured-in-place.

IV. **Shoes in Relation to Playing Surfaces**

A. **General information.** Shoe technology is rapidly evolving. Different players need different shoes. College teams have tended to adopt "team" shoes in the past, and high school and younger teams have tried to emulate this pattern. Sports shoes, however, should be selected and fitted for each individual on the basis of their foot, their sport, and the predominant surface.

It should be noted that some shoes that may be suited well for one surface or activity may not be appropriate for another surface or activity, and may lead to not only poorer performance but also an increased chance for injury.

1. **Outdoor field events (football, soccer, etc.)**
   a. "Astro-turf bottoms," or "hard ground cleat shoes" are the currently preferred shoes for use on either synthetic outdoor surfaces or hard natural turf. These shoes typically have between 70–150 smaller studs that are part of the shoe, with approximately 1 to 2 lb of pressure on each stud. These shoes also include some of the cushioning that was first introduced in running shoes. These shoes should have a predominantly carbon-rubber blend base.
   b. Soft-ground situations require molded-bottom, larger, fewer-stud shoes (12–15 studs totally).
   c. Soccer, as opposed to football, has disallowed the anterior toe cleat in shoes—otherwise the shoes are similar to those preferred for football.
   d. The requirements for baseball shoes are similar to those for football and soccer, but baseball shoes are very entrenched in tradition—three studs in front and back in a triangular fashion. The plastic-stud shoes are safer than metal-stud shoes.

2. **Tennis.** With the wide spectrum of surfaces used for tennis, it is difficult to prescribe a single shoe type.
   a. A rubber-blend base is preferred for playing tennis on grass.
   b. Polyurethane is often used in the outsole and midsole of tennis shoes for surfaces more abrasive than grass. However, some people would prefer a lighter shoe on an abrasive surface, even though the shoe would wear more rapidly.

3. **Basketball/volleyball.** Court shoes in general need to have a cupsole. This provides a stable base for feet that move both forward and side-to-side.
   a. Synthetic surfaces. Generally these floors "grab" more, so a shoe that blends polyurethane and rubber is typically preferred.
   b. Hardwood surfaces. A more purely rubberized or higher blend of rubber is usually selected for use on a hardwood floor.
   c. **Typical problems.** A usual difficulty for the basketball team player is the necessity to rotate between synthetic and hardwood floors as he/she plays different teams on varying home courts.

4. **Racquetball/squash/handball.** These sports are almost always played on hardwood, and therefore a higher blend of rubber-based shoe is preferred.

5. **Track.** Running shoes are used for track. If an individual will be running off-road, he/she should select a more studded pattern on the outsole.

6. **Aerobics.** Aerobic shoes need the following features to provide best support:
   a. External heel counters
   b. Forefoot support across the shoe or built into the shoe's lacing pattern
   c. Mid-sole cushioning of compressed EVA (effavinyl acetate)
   d. Full leather upper
   e. Internal heel counters.

## V. Conclusion

The public's increased interest in exercise has raised the level of consciousness concerning sports injury prevention and treatment. Often due to poor or inappropriate surfaces, a large number of individuals have suffered injuries to feet, ankles, knees, hips, and/or backs while attempting to improve the condition of their heart and lungs. Owing in part to publicity and encouragement provided by sports medicine personnel and facility planners, surface manufacturers have become increasingly aware of the relationship between surfaces and safety.

More research and study related to sports surfaces is needed. Expressed concern for safety and injury prevention has prompted a recent increase in the amount of research on sports surfaces and on shoe performance, and some manufacturers have sought a market advantage by making significant improvements in their products. All sports participants, from casual to highly competitive, stand to benefit from an increase in both research and product improvement.

## *REFERENCES*

1. CDDS Seminar: Research Activities Into Synthetic Surfaces. Cologne, Germany, 1988, p 143.
2. Choosing the right aerobics surface. Athletic Business 11(4):78–83, 1987.
3. Court sentences. Athletic Business 10(8):30–36, 1986.
4. Dance Facilities. Washington, D.C., American Alliance for Health, Physical Education and Recreation, 1972.
5. Di Geronimo JW: We've learned the hard way. Athletic Business 9(8):64–75, 1985.
6. Dick R, Assistant Director of Sports Sciences, National Collegiate Athletic Association (personal correspondence, August 1988).
7. Duda M: NFLPA presses for new turf studies. Phys Sportsmed 13(9):29, 1985.
8. Ferguson M: Great strides in flooring. Athletic Business 13(1):November 1989.
9. Flynn RB (ed): Planning Facilities for Athletics, Physical Education and Recreation. Reston, VA, American Alliance for Health, Physical Education, Recreation, and Dance, 1985.
10. Handbook of Sports and Recreational Building Design. London, The Architectural Press, 1981.
11. Hay C: Cushioning, control features mark aerobics shoes' development. Sports Mednotes. Omaha, NE, University of Nebraska Medical Center Sports Medicine Program, February 1989, p 2.
12. Miller DA: Sports surface specs. Athletic Business 12(8):72–78, 1988.
13. National Collegiate Athletic Association Injury Surveillance System, 1982–1987. Mission, KS, National Collegiate Athletic Association, 1988.
14. Nicholas JA, Rosenthal PP, Glime G: A historical perspective of injuries in professional football. JAMA 260:1988.
15. On solid ground: The importance of proper flooring. IRSA Club Business, September 1986, pp 35–37.
16. Penman KA: Planning Physical Education and Athletic Facilities in Schools. New York, John Wiley & Sons, 1977.
17. Powell JW: Incidence of injury associated with playing surfaces in the National Football League, 1980–1985. Athletic Training, Fall 1987.
18. Seals G: A study of dance surfaces. Clin Sports Med 2:557–561, 1983.
19. Sports surface improvements. Athletic Business 13(7):35, 1989.
20. U.S.T.A. Facilities Committee: Tennis Courts 1984–1985. Lynn, MA, H.O. Zimman, Inc. for the United States Tennis Association, 1984.

# Chapter 10: Team Hygiene and Personal Equipment

MARK A. KWIKKEL, MA, ATC, LAT

I. **Importance of Hygiene.** The lack of personal hygiene can lead to a multitude of bacterial, fungal, and even viral infections. Personal hygiene is very important not only for athletes but also for the team physician and other allied health professions as well.

   A. **Dealing with large numbers of athletes.** In dealing with athletic teams, numbers can range from seven or eight on the golf or tennis team to well over 130 on the football team. The larger the squad, the higher the incidence of hygiene problems. The lack of personal hygiene can lead from infection problems to complaints by other team members of the offensive odors generated by an individual. Showering with copious amounts of water and deodorant soap should be stressed.

   1. Showers before examination by the physician or athletic trainer are a common practice in nonemergency situations.

   B. **The locker room environment.** Damp, dark areas are a prime breeding ground for mold, mildew, and bacteria. The shower and drying area as well as sweat-soaked clothing need proper cleaning.

   C. **Cleaning and disinfecting the locker room.** The locker room should be disinfected daily with industrial cleaners. A well-trained custodial staff should know the proper techniques for cleaning and disinfecting a locker room.

   1. Daily damp mopping.
   2. Carpeted areas should be vacuumed daily. Use of antifungal carpets is recommended.
   3. Biweekly high pressure steam cleaning.
   4. Weekly disinfection of lockers.
      a. Germatox (Pioneer Manufacturing, Cleveland, Ohio.)*
      b. Wavicide (Wave Energy Systems, Inc., Cedar Grove, NJ).

II. **Personal Equipment.** All sports have one thing in common, workout and competition clothing. These items need to be properly laundered. Sports such as hockey, football, wrestling, and lacrosse have special protective equipment that need special attention.

   A. **Proper clothing** for each sport is highly recommended. Clothing should be of a nonbinding nature.

   B. **Laundry facilities.** Clothing should be laundered daily. Athletic facilities should be equipped with a commercial washer and dryer designed to handle their laundry.

   1. **Washing.** Clothing should be washed in warm water (100–105°F) using heavy-duty detergents, all-fabric bleach, and fabric softener.
   2. **Drying.** Clothing should be **dried completely.** It is highly recommended that a cooling period be used to avoid shrinkage. Clothing should be folded promptly.
      a. **Home facilities.** Institutions that cannot provide laundry service should provide **written instructions on the care that should be given the athletic clothing.**
   3. **Laundry facilities on road trips.** Many teams find themselves needing laundry facilities while participating away from home.

---

* The companies and products listed in this chapter are for example purposes only. There are many good products on the market to choose from. The author chose these products because of his familiarity with them.

      a. Take clothing items to a coin-operated laundry.

      b. Make arrangements with the host team to have items laundered.

      c. Bring extra items of clothing on road trip.

C. **Cleaning specialized equipment.** Specialized equipment needs to be cleaned periodically with a spray disinfectant/deodorant.

    1. Football equipment. Spraying should include:

      a. Helmets

      b. Shoulder pads

      c. Thigh pads, hip pads, tail pad

      d. Knee pads.

    2. Wrestling equipment. It is extremely important that the wrestling mat be disinfected before and after each practice and competition. A chlorine bleach solution (1 part chlorine bleach; 2 parts water) should be kept in a spray bottle near the mat to clean any blood (see Section IV). (Thor Germicidal Detergent, Huntington Laboratories, Huntington, IN.)

    3. Other sports considerations. It is necessary to disinfect the protective equipment of each individual sport as necessary.

III. **Athletic Training Room and Examination Areas.** Daily cleaning of the athletic training room and examination areas is extremely important.

    A. **Keeping facilities clean.** It is usually the facilities custodial staff that does general cleaning and disinfecting, yet there are certain items that need to be cleaned by the athletic training staff.

      1. Daily cleaning responsibilities.

        a. Disinfection of treatment and taping tables (Iso-Quin; Cramer Chemical Company, Gardner, KS).

        b. Disinfection of whirlpools.

        c. Removal of trash.

        d. Vacuum or sweep floor.

    B. **Hand washing.** It is highly recommended that hand washing with Betadine soap be used before and after examination of athletes. This is especially important following an event or practice when examining a large number of athletes.

IV. **HIV/AIDS Concerns in Athletics.** With the growing problem of human immunosuppressive virus (HIV) and the AIDS epidemic, it is very important that certain precautions be taken when dealing with blood and open wounds.

    A. HIV/AIDS precautions

      1. Use latex gloves when examining and managing open wounds.

      2. Wash hands thoroughly before and after treating an athlete with an open wound.

      3. Use proper eye protection when treating open wounds.

      4. Use chlorine bleach (1 part chlorine bleach; 2 parts water) in spray bottles to clean tables and other surfaces that become contaminated with blood. Paper towels should be discarded in a plastic garbage bag and incinerated as soon as possible.

    B. Prevention of HIV transmissions. It is recommended that the **Centers for Disease Control Recommendations for Prevention of HIV Transmission in Health-Care Settings** be read and followed in the physicians office and in the athletic training room.[1,2]

## REFERENCES

1. Centers for Disease Control: Recommendations for prevention of HIV transmission in health-care settings. MMWR 36(suppl 25):1987.
2. Centers for Disease Control Update: Universal precautions for prevention of transmission of human immunodeficiency virus, hepatitis B virus, and other bloodborne pathogens in health-care settings. MMWR 37:377–388, 1988.

# Chapter 11: Safe Exercise in the Heat and Heat Injuries

MORRIS B. MELLION, MD
GUY L. SHELTON, RPT, ATC

I. **Heat Transfer and Heat Dissipation**

  A. **Increased heat load** of exercise
  1. Muscles can generate $\geq 20$ times as much energy at maximal activity as at rest, leading to huge increases in heat load.
  2. Well-conditioned endurance athletes can generate and dissipate 1033 Kcal heat per hour safely into environment.

  B. **Peripheral mechanisms—minor effect**
  1. Small amount of heat produced by muscle is transferred passively by **conduction** through tissue to overlying skin.
  2. Some of heat from muscle is carried by **convection** via the venous blood in superficial veins en route to the heart.

  C. **Central mechanisms—major effect**
  1. Most of the heat produced in exercise is transported by the blood from the working muscles to the venae cavae and then the heart. The warmed blood from the muscles mixes with the venous return from the rest of the body and enters the heart to form the cardiac output, much of which is pumped to the vessels of the skin for heat dissipation.
     a. Blood has a high **heat capacity.** It can transport a relatively large quantity of heat with only a moderate increase in temperature.
     b. Early in exercise, heat production exceeds heat loss, producing an increase in body core temperature.
     c. The rise in core temperature is sensed by **thermodetectors** in the hypothalamus, the spinal cord, and limb muscles, and provides the stimulus to initiate sweating and increase skin blood flow.
  2. Skin blood flow transfers heat by **convection** to the skin where it is lost by:
     a. **Evaporation** of sweat
     b. **Radiation**
     c. **Convection**
     d. **Conduction**
  3. **Radiation and convection** dissipate most of the heat when the ambient temperature is less than 68°F (20°C), and **evaporation accounts for most of the heat loss when the temperature is above 68°F.**
     a. In heavy exercise, evaporation can account for up to 85% of heat loss.
     b. The **evaporative heat loss** of 1 liter of water at 86°F is 580 Kcal.
     c. 70-kg athlete sweats 1–2 liters/hour during intense exercise in the heat. Larger athletes may sweat considerably more.
  4. After the heat-dissipating mechanisms are brought into play, the core temperature reaches a plateau, where it remains until the exercise's demand is past.
     a. In elite athletes, the equilibrium between heat production and heat dissipation may be as high as 104°F without diminished performance.
  5. If the heat-dissipating mechanisms fail or if there is an overwhelming heat stress, the core temperature may continue to rise, even to dangerous levels.

D. **Conflicting demands for cardiac output and plasma volume during exercise in the heat**
   1. In first 10–20 minutes of exercise, approximately 15% of the intravascular fluid volume is shunted to the working muscles.
   2. Increases of skin blood flow cooling also shunt blood from the central circulation and effectively lower central plasma volume.
      a. Skin blood flow may be 15–25% of cardiac output during intense exercise in a hot environment.
   3. Sweating can easily produce losses of 1–2 liters/hour, thus causing further losses in plasma volume.
   4. As plasma volume (or central blood volume) decreases, there is less blood returning to the heart to be pumped. Therefore, stroke volume and cardiac output decrease.
      a. If this process were to continue, the system would collapse.
   5. The process can be changed favorably by:
      a. Reducing exercise overload (slowing down).
      b. Building plasma volume by drinking water or other specific hypotonic fluids.
      c. Shifting blood flow away from skin.
         i. If this shift is too great, core temperature may rise dangerously.
E. **Dehydration**
   1. Sweat is HYPOTONIC; very little salt is lost. Even less salt is lost in the well-conditioned, heat-acclimatized athlete.
   2. Loss of sweat results in increased electrolyte concentration in the remaining plasma, which is HYPERTONIC.
      a. When the plasma is hypertonic, the thresholds for sweating and vasodilation are elevated.
   3. Taking salt pills or drinking salty (normotonic or hypertonic) salty solutions may make the plasma more hypertonic.
   4. Water reduces the hypertonic state of the plasma back to normal osmolality.
   5. For most exercise situations, **cold water** is the best fluid replacement. Generally, obtaining salt only from normal sodium content of a well-balanced diet is adequate.
   6. **For prolonged or repetitive endurance exercise in the heat,** there is growing evidence that a **hypotonic salt solution** may retard dehydration and speed rehydration.
      a. The addition of carbohydrate in the form of up to 7% glucose polymer may also be helpful.
   7. Thirst is not an adequate guide for fluid consumption in humans.
      a. For optimum hydration, the athlete should drink before, during, and after exercise.
      (See Chapter 13, "Nutrition," for a more detailed discussion of fluid, electrolyte, and carbohydrate replacement.)
F. **Acclimatization and training effect**
   1. **Acclimatization** to exercise in the heat
      a. Adults: 4–7 sessions of exercise in the heat
         i. 1–4 hours/session
      b. Children slightly longer.
      c. **Physiologic effects of acclimatization**
         i. Earlier initiation of sweating
         ii. Increased rate of sweating
         iii. Earlier skin vasodilatation
         iv. Core and skin temperature lower at given workload and heat stress
         v. Increased basal plasma volume
         vi. Heart rate lower at given workload and heat stress
         vii. Sweat sodium concentration lower
         viii. Perceived intensity of exercise reduced
         ix. Thermal comfort increased.

2. The **training effect** related to increased level of physical conditioning also contributes to improved capacity for exercise in the heat, due to:
   a. Increased basal plasma volume
   b. Lower sweat sodium concentration.
G. **Exercise, fever, and antipyretics**
   1. Core temperature elevations caused by **fever** and illness are additive to those caused by exercise.
      a. Therefore, **cardiac output and aerobic capacity are reduced in the febrile athlete.**
         i. **Exercise with a fever may be dangerous, especially in the heat.**
   2. Core temperature elevations caused by exercise cannot be reduced by using aspirin, acetaminophen (Tylenol), or other **antipyretics.**

II. **Exertional Heat Illnesses**
   A. There are four exertional heat syndromes:
      1. **Heat syncope** is a transient hypovolemic syncopal episode.
      2. **Heat cramps, heat exhaustion, and heat stroke** form a progression of increasingly severe heat illnesses caused by dehydration, electrolyte losses, and failure of the body's thermoregulatory mechanism.
   B. **Heat syncope**
      1. Syncope (fainting) or light-headedness usually seen at the end of a race. The athlete is maximally vasodilated; and when activity is stopped, **much of the blood volume "pools" in the lower extremities;** consequently, the heart has too little venous return to pump an adequate supply to the brain.
      2. Predisposing factors:
         a. Ending exercise without cool-down
         b. Dehydration
         c. Lack of acclimatization
         d. The same phenomenon may occur when going from the cold (such as a cold bath) to a hot sauna or whirlpool.
      3. Treatment:
         a. Lie down and elevate legs slightly.
         b. Rest in a cool place.
         c. Drink cold water.
      4. Complications: Rare.
   C. **Heat cramps**
      1. Muscular tightening and spasm seen during or after intense, prolonged exercise in heat.
         a. May be exquisitely painful
         b. Lower extremity muscles most common, but any muscles may be affected, including abdominals and intercostals.
      2. Predisposing factors:
         a. Lack of acclimatization
            i. Also seen in well-conditioned athletes in long or repetitive endurance events.
         b. Ongoing negative sodium balance
            i. The already sodium-depleted athlete loses additional sodium in sweat and replaces the accompanying volume loss with water, producing even further dilutional hyponatremia.
         c. Diuretics, especially first few weeks of therapy.
      3. Treatment:
         a. Rest and cooling down.
         b. Massage (knead) affected muscles.
         c. Oral hypotonic salt solution
            i. 1 teaspoon table salt/1 quart water.
         d. If sodium replenishment fails to resolve heat cramps, evaluate potassium, calcium, and magnesium levels.
      4. **May be warning sign of impending heat exhaustion.**

D. **Heat exhaustion**
1. A serious acute heat injury with hyperthermia due to dehydration, hyponatremia, or both. Sweating mechanisms are generally working, but the amount of sweating may be reduced due to dehydration. Core temperature significantly elevated, but generally < 103° F.
2. Symptoms:
   a. Fatigue
   b. Profound weakness
   c. Lightheadedness
   d. Profuse sweating, unless dramatically dehydrated
   e. Nausea, vomiting
   f. Headache
   g. Myalgias
   h. Mental status generally normal, but may be mildly impaired.
3. Predisposing factors:
   a. Dehydration—acute and chronic
   b. Negative sodium balance over time
   c. Lack of acclimatization to heat.
4. Treatment:
   a. Rest
   b. Rapid cooling
   c. Fluid and electrolyte replacement
      i. Hypotonic oral fluids
      ii. D5/1/2 normal saline intravenously
         (a) Start with 1 liter over 30–60 minutes
         (b) Measure serum sodium
            (i) If markedly elevated, hydrate cautiously to avoid inducing cerebral edema.
E. **Heat stroke—a medical emergency**
1. Extreme hyperthermia with thermoregulatory failure and profound central nervous system dysfunction
   a. **Core temperature ≥ 105° F**
      i. Often as high as 107°–108° F
   b. Patient hot, flushed, dry
      i. **Sweating mechanism frequently has failed.**
2. **Not spontaneously reversible**
   a. **Thermoregulatory failure prevents control of elevated core temperature without external cooling,** even in those few heat stroke patients who retain the ability to sweat.
   b. Progresses to cardiovascular and central nervous system collapse in the absence of prompt intervention.
3. Progressive CNS impairment
   a. Confusion
   b. Disorientation
   c. Agitation
   d. Hysterical behavior
   e. Delirium
   f. Seizures
   g. Coma.
4. **Multiple electrolyte and metabolic abnormalities**
   a. Hyperkalemia or hypokalemia
   b. Hypernatremia or hyponatremia
   c. Hypocalcemia
   d. Hyperphosphatemia
   e. Hypoglycemia
   f. Lactic acidosis
   g. Uremia.

TABLE 1. Severe Complications of Heat Stroke

| | |
|---|---|
| Cardiovascular: | Arrhythmias<br>Myocardial infarction<br>Pulmonary edema |
| Central nervous system: | Cerebral or spinal infarction<br>Coma<br>Seizures |
| Gastrointestinal: | Hepatocellular necrosis<br>Upper gastrointestinal bleeding |
| Hematologic: | Disseminated intravascular coagulation<br>Metabolic lactic acidosis |
| Musculoskeletal: | Rhabdomyolysis<br>Myoglobinemia |
| Pulmonary: | Adult respiratory distress syndrome<br>Pulmonary infarction |
| Renal: | Acute renal failure |

5. **Complications** extend to all major organ systems (see Table 1).
6. **May be part of a continuum with heat exhaustion, but in some individuals the sweating mechanism stops functioning at a relatively low level of heat exposure.**
   a. In these patients, exertional heat stroke **may be a variant of malignant hyperthermia.**
7. Predisposing factors:
   a. Genetic predisposition.
   b. Dehydration—acute and chronic.
   c. Lack of acclimatization to heat
      i. Often seen on an exceptionally hot spring day.
   d. Negative sodium balance over time may be a factor.
   e. Frequently occurs near a race finish line where the already dehydrated athlete increases speed, producing increased muscle blood flow, secondarily decreased skin blood flow, and a resultant rise in core temperature.
8. Treatment:
   a. **Immediate external cooling in the field**
      i. Wet patient down with a tepid or cool spray (or a single layer of wet cheesecloth or thin sheeting) and use a large fan to speed evaporation.
      ii. Remove patient's clothing and pack him/her in ice.
         (a) Less effective, but may be best option in the field.
      iii. **Monitor rectal temperature**
         (a) External cooling may be discontinued when the core temperature drops to 102° F and stabilizes.
         (b) Sophisticated **emergency or intensive care facility** necessary
            (i) Heat stroke patients frequently require:
               - airway management
               - oxygenation ± respirator
               - careful fluid and electrolyte administration
               - circulatory support
               - cardiac, hemodynamic, and laboratory monitoring.
         (c) Dantrolene may be helpful in some subsets of patients:
            (i) Known malignant hyperthermia
            (ii) Patients on neuroleptic agents with exertional heat stroke.
F. **Populations at increased risk**
   1. **Healthy individuals**
      a. Poorly acclimatized
      b. Poorly conditioned
      c. Inexperienced competitor (limited judgment about heat risk)

   d. **Salt or water depleted**
   e. **Large and/or obese**
      i. Generate more heat for same level of activity.
      ii. Dissipate heat less efficiently (due to lower body-surface-to-mass ratio).
      iii. Obese individuals demonstrate higher tissue temperature elevations from the same heat load because adipose tissue has a lower specific heat than lean tissue.
      iv. Obese individuals have fewer heat-activated sweat glands in skin overlying adipose tissue.
   f. **Children**
      i. Sweat less.
      ii. Require greater core temperature increases to trigger sweating.
      iii. Acclimatize more slowly.
      iv. Lower cardiac output at given metabolic rate; therefore, may lack adequate blood flow for both muscle and cooling needs.
      v. High surface-area-to-body-mass ratio
         (a) Works as advantage ordinarily.
         (b) When sun is hot or ambient temperature is high, they absorb relatively more heat from the environment.
   g. **Elderly**
      i. Age-related limitation on full heat acclimatization (probably related to sweating mechanism).
      ii. Decreased maximum heart rate with age leads to decreased maximum cardiac output.
   h. **Previous heat injury**
   i. **Sleep deprivation**
      i. Decreased sweat rate
      ii. Decreased skin blood flow response to heat load
2. Acute illnesses
   a. **Fever**
      i. Reduced cardiac output
      ii. Increased metabolic demand for blood flow throughout body.
   b. **Gastrointestinal illnesses**
      i. Increased blood flow to GI tract competes with skin blood flow for cardiac output.
      ii. Dehydration and electrolyte disturbances.
3. **Chronic illnesses**
   a. Cardiac disease
   b. Cystic fibrosis
   c. Diabetes, uncontrolled
   d. **Eating disorders**
      i. Fluid and electrolyte problem
      ii. Compulsive over-exercising
   e. Hypertension, uncontrolled
   f. Malignant hyperthermia.
4. **Abuse of alcohol and other substances**
   a. Alcohol
   b. Amphetamines
   c. Cocaine
      i. **Acute cocaine intoxication may be difficult to differentiate from heat stroke.**
   d. Hallucinogens
   e. Laxatives
   f. Narcotics.
5. **Medications**
   a. Anticholinergics
   b. Antihistamines

    c. Beta blockers

    d. Diuretics

    e. Neuroleptics, especially tricyclic antidepressants and MAD inhibitors.

III. **Prevention of Heat Illness**

  A. **Medical history and evaluation**—Identify those individuals at increased risk.

    1. **Further workup/treatment**

      a. Acute illness

      b. Chronic illness

      c. Substance abuse.

    2. **Risk factor correction**

      a. Acclimatization

      b. Conditioning

        i. Preseason conditioning (strength, endurance, skills acquisition).

        ii. Increased awareness of heat stress signs and symptoms in workout situations.

        iii. Delay full participation until minimum conditioning level met.

      c. Obesity

        i. Weight loss program is best done in the off season.

        ii. During season, peak performances are often required; this is difficult if calorie restriction is enforced.

        iii. Calorie restriction might make it more difficult to take in proper electrolyte replacement through diet.

      d. Sleep deprivation

        i. Delay participation until adequate rest is achieved.

        ii. Allow time for adequate sleep/rest during season.

    3. **Participant education: athlete, coach, parent**

      a. Inexperienced athlete

      b. Obese athlete

      c. Child athlete

      d. Elderly athlete

      e. Athlete with previous heat illness

      f. Athlete on certain medications

      g. All others with risk factors.

    4. **Activity restriction**

      a. Used in situations specified above where other modifications do not allow safe participation.

      b. Temporary restrictions may be imposed until certain risk factors corrected.

      c. Restrictions may be absolute or relative, depending on each individual situation.

  B. **Atmospheric conditions**

    1. High heat and humidity

      a. Severely limit body's ability to dissipate heat.

      b. Exercising athlete cannot go by "how hot or humid it feels" to judge the environmental heat stress.

    2. Increased awareness of atmospheric conditions needed—**objective measures.**

      a. **Weather reports**

        i. U.S. Weather Service.

        ii. Local radio and television stations.

        iii. Provide approximate temperature and humidity readings.

        iv. Table 2 and Figure 1 show how relative degrees of heat stress can be determined.

        v. Simple and convenient.

        vi. These remote temperature and humidity readings do not allow for variances due to local geography or distance between the weather reporting site and the workout area.

TABLE 2.    Heat Stress (Apparent Temperatures in °F)*

| | | \multicolumn{11}{c|}{Air Temperature (°F)} |
|---|---|---|---|---|---|---|---|---|---|---|---|---|
| | | 70 | 75 | 80 | 85 | 90 | 95 | 100 | 105 | 110 | 115 | 120 |
| | 0% | 64 | 69 | 73 | 78 | 83 | 87 | **91** | **95** | **99** | **103** | **107** |
| | 10% | 65 | 70 | 75 | 80 | 85 | **90** | **95** | **100** | **105** | **111** | **116** |
| | 20% | 66 | 72 | 77 | 82 | 87 | **93** | **99** | **105** | **112** | **120** | **130** |
| | 30% | 67 | 73 | 78 | 84 | **90** | **96** | **104** | **113** | **123** | **135** | **148** |
| Relative | 40% | 68 | 74 | 79 | 86 | **93** | **101** | **110** | **123** | **137** | **151** | |
| humidity | 50% | 69 | 75 | 81 | 88 | **96** | **107** | **120** | **135** | **150** | | |
| (%) | 60% | 70 | 76 | 82 | **90** | **100** | **114** | **132** | **149** | | | |
| | 70% | 70 | 77 | 85 | **93** | **106** | **124** | **144** | | | | |
| | 80% | 71 | 78 | 86 | **97** | **113** | **136** | | | | | |
| | 90% | 71 | 79 | 88 | **102** | **122** | | | | | | |
| | 100% | 72 | 80 | **91** | **108** | | | | | | | |

DANGER ZONE = >90° F (boldface temperatures above).

* Adapted from: "Heat Wave," U. S. Department of Commerce, National Oceanic and Atmospheric Administration, National Weather Service, NOAA/PA 85001, 1985.

   b. **Sling psychrometer** (Fig. 2)
       i. Measures dry-bulb (DB) and wet-bulb (WB) temperature at the activity site.
      ii. Relative humidity then determined from a chart supplied with the instrument.
     iii. Table 2 and Figure 1 show how relative degrees of heat stress can be determined.
     iv. Readily available, reasonably inexpensive, accurate, portable, and easy to learn to use.

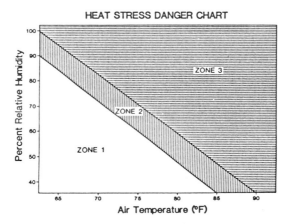

HEAT STRESS DANGER CHART

**FIGURE 1. Heat Stress Danger Chart.** Environmental conditions in **zone 1** are fairly safe for participation. Normal heat stress precautions should be taken. In **zone 2**, moderate heat stress precautions should be taken. Workouts should be less intense, shorter, and with more frequent fluid breaks. More careful observation of individuals at increased risk. In **zone 3**, heat stress danger is at its greatest. Workouts should be rescheduled to a cooler part of the day. Workouts should be relatively easy. Light clothing and a minimum of equipment should be worn. Extra fluids for everyone and close observation for early heat injury symptoms are essential. (Adapted from Fox EL, Mathews DK: *The Physiological Basis of Physical Education and Athletics*, 3rd ed. Philadelphia, Saunders College Publishing, 1981.)

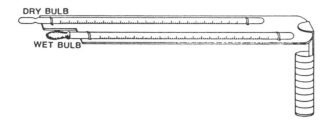

**FIGURE 2. Sling Psychrometer.** Wick on wet bulb is moistened with distilled water and the unit is rotated overhead. Evaporative cooling causes the wet bulb temperature to decrease. The dry bulb and wet bulb readings are used to determine % relative humidity.

    c. **Heat index thermometer** (Fig. 3)
        i. Measures DB, WB, and black bulb (BB) temperatures.
        ii. BB thermometer provides a measure of the radiant heat gained.
        iii. Wet Bulb Global Temperature (WBGT) index calculated using the following formula:
$$WBGT = 0.7 \, (WB) \times 0.1 \, (DB) \times 0.2 \, (BB)$$
        iv. The WBGT index is compared to published guidelines that indicate relative levels of heat stress risk and provide suggestions for activity modification.
C. **Workout schedule**
    1. Identifying adverse environmental conditions has absolutely no benefit unless appropriate steps are taken to **adjust the practice or competition schedule.**
    2. **Reschedule** workouts, practices, and competitions to cooler time of day or **cancel** altogether.
    3. **Alter** practices and workouts:
        a. Decreased intensity
        b. Shorter duration
        c. More frequent breaks.

## HEAT INDEX THERMOMETERS

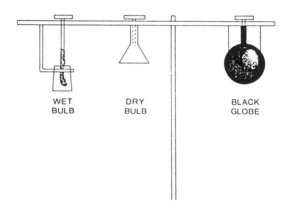

**FIGURE 3. Heat Index Thermometers.** Homemade unit consists of three thermometers mounted on a board. The bulb of the wet thermometer is enclosed in a moistened wick. The bulb of the dry thermometer is in an inverted funnel to shield it from direct sunlight. The bulb of the black globe thermometer is enclosed in a black copper globe to absorb radiant energy. An electronic heat index thermometer is also commercially available (Reuter-Strokes, Cambridge, Ontario).

D. **Clothing**
  1. Restrictive clothing and bulky protective equipment block skin surface area.
     a. **Reduce cooling by**
        i. Radiation
        ii. Convection
        iii. Evaporation.
     b. Examples:
        i. Helmets
        ii. Heavy, long-sleeved uniforms
        iii. Protective pads
        iv. Rubberized workout suits.
  2. **Some oil-based or gel-based sunscreens may block evaporative cooling.**
  3. **Useful strategies:**
     a. Short-sleeved, loose-fitting, open weave or mesh jerseys allow better evaporation.
        i. Short midriff T-shirts, especially under football shoulder pads.
     b. Practice or play in shorts when possible.
     c. Light-colored uniforms reflect sunlight.
     d. Change uniforms so soaked with sweat that they block evaporation from the skin.
     e. Wearing no shirt
        i. Benefit: better heat loss from evaporation and convection
        ii. Risk: more radiant heat gain.
E. **Body weight**
  1. **Acute weight loss = dehydration.**
     a. $> 2\%$ affects performance
     b. $> 3\%$ affects thermoregulatory capacity.
  2. **Nude weight measured and charted before and after practice or competition.**
     a. Supervised and checked by athletic trainer or coach.
     b. **Caution indicated when:**
        i. Workout weight loss $> 3\%$
        ii. Athlete fails to regain previous day's weight loss by workout time the next day.
  3. Athletes with large or persistent acute weight loss should be restricted from activity until rehydrated.
F. **Observe:**
  1. Athletes at increased risk for heat illness.
  2. Overachiever
     a. May be less aware of the early signs of heat illness.
  3. Unacclimatized athletes.
  4. Inexperienced athletes.
  5. Athletes with excessive practice weight loss.
G. **Education**
  1. All involved with athletics and fitness should have a basic understanding of heat illness and its causes, treatment, and prevention.
  2. **Medical personnel:**
     a. Should be able to provide sound advice on the prevention, recognition, and treatment of various types of heat illness.
     b. Good communication among coaches, athletes, and medical staff is essential.
  3. **Coaches:**
     a. Should set aside myths that can contribute to additional heat stress.
     b. Should be trained to recognize early signs of heat illness and apply appropriate first-aid measures.
     c. Responsible to coordinate the prevention program in the absence of an athletic trainer.
  4. **Athletes:**
     a. Should be able to recognize the symptoms of heat illness in themselves.
     b. Should be aware of the initial treatment.

    c. Should understand heat illness prevention principles.

    d. Should understand how to adjust training program to allow for the heat.

    e. Should understand how to consider personal medical conditions and their effect on the ability to adapt to heat stress.

H. **Fluid replacement**

    1. **Most important factor in preventing heat stress syndromes!!**

    2. Indicators of adequate hydration

        a. Post-workout body weight equal to pre-workout body weight

        b. After workout, urine appears clear and unconcentrated.

(See Chapter 13, "Nutrition," for more details on fluid and electrolyte replacement.)

## RECOMMENDED READING

1. American College of Sports Medicine: Position stand on prevention of thermal injuries during distance running. Sports Medicine Bulletin 19(3):8, 1984.
2. Anderson RJ, Reed G, Knochel J: Heatstroke. Adv Intern Med 28:115–140, 1983.
3. Andrews JR, Massey M, Mullins L, et al: Heat illness in athletes. J Med Assoc Alabama 45(2):29, 1975.
4. Bar-Or O: Climate and the exercising child. In Bar-Or O: Pediatric Sports Medicine for the Practitioner: From Physiologic Principles to Clinical Applications. New York, Springer-Verlag, 1983, pp 260–299.
5. Fortney SM, Vroman NB: Exercise, performance, and temperature control: Temperature regulation during exercise and implications for sports performance and training. Sports Med 2:8–20, 1985.
6. Gieck J: Heat and activity. Athletic Training 9(2):78, 1974.
7. Grisolfi CV, Wenger CB: Temperature regulation during exercise: Old concepts, new ideas. In Terjung RL (ed): Exercise and Sports Science Review, Vol. 12. Lexington, MA, D.C. Heath, 1984, pp 339–372.
8. Kenney WL: Physiologic correlates of heat intolerance. Sports Med 2:279–286, 1985.
9. Kobayashi Y, Ando Y, Takeuchi S, et al: Effects of heat acclimatization of distance runners in a moderately hot environment. Eur J Appl Physiol 45:189–198, 1980.
10. Nadel ER: Recent advances in temperature regulation during exercise in humans. Fed Proc 44:2286–2292, 1985.
11. Shapiro Y, Magazanik A, Udassin R, et al: Heat intolerance in former heatstroke patients. Ann Intern Med 90:913–916, 1979.

# Chapter 12: Safe Exercise in the Cold and Cold Injuries

WARREN D. BOWMAN, JR., MD, FACP

I. **Physiologic Changes During Cold Exposure**

  A. **Introduction.** Man has evolved as a tropical animal with only limited ability to adapt to cold through prolonged exposure. Many creatures, such as the arctic fox, adapt well to cold; their mechanisms of adaptation are demonstrable to only a small extent in man. However, in Eskimos and Gaspé Peninsula fishermen, enhancement of peripheral circulation has been shown to occur with exposure, allowing them to work for prolonged times with their hands in cold water. Anecdotal reports, such as John Harlin preparing for the North Face of the Eiger, attest to the value of skiing barehanded and carrying snowballs in the unprotected hands.

  B. **Internal heat production.** Humans, as homeotherms. must control their body temperatures within narrow limits (75–105°F/24–40.5°C) for survival and within even more narrow limits for the level of function needed for optimum performance.

   1. **When exposed to cold, the body behaves as though it were made up of two separate compartments:**
      a. **The core** (central nervous system, heart, lungs, liver, etc.)
      b. **The shell** (skin, muscles and extremities).
   2. **The body guards the core temperature by decreasing circulation to the shell upon exposure to cold.**
      a. **The resultant shell cooling can interfere with the ability to perform well athletically** because it weakens and slows muscle contractions and delays nerve conduction time.
   3. Cold, stiff muscles require a longer, more careful warmup period to prevent injury.
   4. Heat is produced three ways by the body:
      a. **Resting heat production, the byproduct of basal biochemical reactions, amounts to about 50 kcal/m$^2$/hr.**
      b. Basal heat production can be increased up to 6 times by **shivering,** up to 10 times by **vigorous exercise,** and to a minor extent by **semiconscious activity such as foot stamping.**
      c. **Nonshivering thermogenesis** is a weak form of heat production mediated through increased secretion of the hormones thyroxine, epinephrine, and norepinephrine.
   5. **External heat** can be added from the sun, a stove, or a fire.

  C. **Heat loss.** Heat is lost from the body by the four following mechanisms:

   1. **Conduction:** Direct transfer of heat by contact between the body and a colder object.
   2. **Convection:** Transfer of heat when air of a lower temperature moves across the body surface.
   3. **Evaporation:** Loss of heat when water or other volatile liquid on the body surface is transformed into vapor.
   4. **Radiation:** Loss of heat by infrared rays to a cooler object not in contact with the body.
   5. A small amount of heat is also lost when **inspired air** is warmed to body temperature before being expired.
   6. Heat loss can be decreased **involuntarily** by decreasing sweating and reducing shell circulation. The most important and efficient methods, however, are **voluntary** ones such as adding clothing and seeking shelter.

D. **Wind chill.** The athlete must consider not only the actual temperature but also the effect of wind in accelerating heat loss. This refers to both natural wind and the air movement created by a moving body.

    1. The greatest effect of wind is exerted in the first 20 mph—greater wind speeds have little additional effect (Fig. 1).

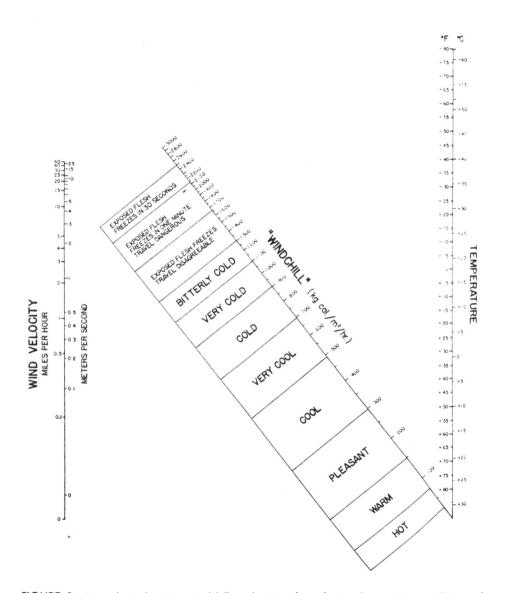

**FIGURE 1.** Line chart showing windchill and state of comfort under varying conditions of temperature and wind velocity. The numbers along the right-hand margin of the diagonal center block refer to the "windchill factor"—the rate of cooling in kilogram-calories per square meter per hour of an unclad, inactive body exposed to specific temperatures and wind velocities. Windchill factors above 1400—the value at which exposed flesh freezes—are very dangerous. (From Consolazio et al: *Metabolic Methods*, St. Louis, The C. V. Mosby Company, 1951, with permission.)

a. The danger point is around $-10°F$ ($-23°C$), a temperature below which the amount of air movement created by such activities as running, bicycling, and skiing can produce rapid frostbite of exposed body parts such as the cheeks, chin, and ears.

E. **Effect of cooling on the organ systems.**
   1. As body temperature falls **below 95°F (35°C),** the rates of essential biochemical reactions slow.
      a. **Regulatory center cooling slows the heart and respiratory rates.** The cardiac output and blood pressure fall.
      b. As the skin and muscles cool, **shivering** begins and increases in violence.
   2. **Below 90°F (32°C), shivering gradually ceases** as the muscles become cooler and stiffer.
      a. **CNS cooling leads to a decrease in cerebral blood flow,** dilation of the pupils, and obtundation of the sensorium, leading to stupor and eventually coma.
      b. **Polyuria (cold diuresis)** occurs as the shell vasoconstriction increases the vascular volume in central vessels.
      c. **Acidosis develops** due to shivering and tissue hypoxia with increased lactate production.
      d. **Insulin activity decreases.**
      e. **The myocardium becomes more irritable, and atrial fibrillation frequently occurs.**
   3. **Ventricular fibrillation is a hazard,** especially below $82°F$ ($28°C$). The EKG may show sinus bradycardia, prolongation of the PR, QRS, and QT intervals, nonspecific ST-T changes, and the J waves of Osborn.
   4. **Oxygen requirements decrease to 50% of normal at 82°F (28°C) and 22% of normal at 64°F (18°C).**

F. **Localized cold injury can occur both at temperatures above and below freezing;** the latter is more of a concern in sports medicine. Subfreezing temperatures can cause injury both from local freezing and from interference with circulation.
   1. Intracellular and extracellular ice crystals appear and, as they increase in size, cause cellular damage by direct injury and through osmotic and biochemical changes.
   2. **Blood vessel damage** causes leakage of plasma through vessel walls, leading to intravascular red cell sludging, circulatory stasis, and edema.
   3. Larger arterioles and arteries show spasm and narrowing.

II. **Prevention of Cold Injury.** This can be accomplished by increasing body heat production and decreasing body heat loss. If these mechanisms fail, heat must be added from the outside.

A. **Increasing heat production** can be achieved be eating and by increasing muscular activity—either involuntarily (shivering) or by exercise.
   1. **Eating** provides both the "specific dynamic action" of the digestive process and calories from the food. **Good nutrition and physical conditioning are necessary if prolonged muscular activity or sustained shivering are required to stay warm.** Regular nutritious meals keep glycogen and fat stores replenished.
      a. During prolonged exercise, provision should be made for **snacks at regular intervals.**

B. **Decreasing heat loss.**
   1. The **"layer principle" of clothing** adapts well to outdoor sports. This means wearing several thin layers of insulation rather than a single thick layer. Clothing can then be adjusted to maintain an optimal microclimate of still, warm air next to the body, preventing overheating with excessive sweating on the one hand and chilling on the other.
      a. Sweating not only causes dehydration and electrolyte loss but wets garments, interfering with their insulating ability.
   2. The **best fabrics** for cold weather sports clothing are those that have high insulating properties that are not diminished significantly by wetting. These

fabrics include **wool, wool/synthetic blends, polypropylene, and treated polyesters such as Capilene.**

   a. **Cotton should not be worn** since it has poor insulating ability, which is markedly decreased by wetness.

   b. Pile garments, and those containing a filler such as down, Dacron, Hollofil and Quallofil, are less useful during exercise because their thickness produces excessive insulation, leading to overheating; they are more useful when worn during the warm-up or the "cooling down" period following exercise.

3. **Wind protection.** This is essential and is provided by wearing **an outer jacket and pants made of windproof fabric** such as Gortex, Nylon, 60/40 cloth, etc. The jacket should have a **hood with a drawstring.**

4. **Protection for special body parts.** Body parts that are normally exposed, such as the face, or that have a large surface-area to volume ratio, such as the ears, fingers, toes, extremities, etc., require special attention.

   a. **Blood supply to the head is not decreased by cold exposure, leading to considerable heat loss from radiation if the head is uncovered.**

      i. **Wear a cap,** preferably the ski-type that can be pulled down over the ears.

      ii. **The exposed face, which can be subject to frostbite at low temperatures, can be covered** with a face mask, balaclava, or a ski-type "neck warmer" that can be pulled up over the lower face.

      iii. Ski goggles can be worn to protect the eyes; they must be well ventilated.

         (a) Athletes who wear glasses may wish to use contact lenses, remembering that at very cold temperatures they may actually freeze to the eyeball.

         (b) Glasses and goggles tend to fog unless well ventilated; this can be prevented to some extent by treating them with antifog preparations.

   b. **Hands** should be protected with polypropylene gloves. At lower temperatures, wool mittens with windproof outer mittens of Gortex or Nylon are advisable.

   c. Athletic shoes should be sized large enough to contain suitable socks. For cold weather running, wear an inner pair of polypropylene socks and an outer pair of heavy wool socks, especially when running in snow where the feet may become wet.

   d. Since trunk cooling leads to vasoconstriction in the skin and extremities, **prevent cold hands and feet by adequate trunk insulation,** thereby providing a greater supply of warm blood to the extremities. Insulate well high heat loss areas where there are large blood vessels close to the skin, such as the groin and sides of the neck, or where there is little natural insulation, such as the sides of the chest.

5. **Avoid wetting** by rain, snow, or perspiration, since heat loss is increased both by evaporation and by decreasing the insulating ability of clothing. A water-repellent jacket and pants of Gortex or similar material should be worn during activities in rain or wet snow.

6. If the conditions are bad enough, it may be better to **cancel the workout and seek shelter.** The combination of wind and cold rain or wet snow, as in a blizzard around 32°F (0°C), is particularly dangerous.

7. **Warming up.** Cold muscles, tendons, and joints are more prone to strains and sprains because they are stiffer and less coordinated. Injury can be prevented by proper warm-ups.

   a. **Since the body should be warm before warm-up exercises begin, they are preferably performed indoors prior to outdoor activity.**

   b. If performed outdoors, protective clothing should be worn to prevent cooling.

   c. If the body shell has already cooled before exercises are started, the activity should start less abruptly and be done slower and for a longer time.

**TABLE 1.** Hypothermia

| F° | C° | Signs and Symptoms |
|---|---|---|
| 99–96 | 37–35.6 | Intense shivering. Impaired ability to perform complex tasks. |
| 95–91 | 35–32.8 | Violent shivering, dysarthria, sluggish thinking, amnesia. |
| 90–86 | 32.4–30 | Shivering ceases, muscular rigidity supervenes. Movements jerky, sensorium dull. |
| 85–81 | 29.8–27 | Coma, areflexia, atrial fibrillation. |
| Below 78 | Below 25.6 | Failure of cardiac and respiratory center control. Pulmonary edema, ventricular fibrillation. Death. |

III. **Types of Cold Injury**

  A. **Hypothermia.**

    1. **Diagnosis.** Hypothermia, or "exposure," exists when the body core temperature falls below 95° F (35° C).

      a. Anticipate hypothermia when suitable climatic conditions exist, and suspect it when an athlete shivers, appears clumsy, apathetic, or confused, or has slurred speech, stumbles, and drops things (Table 1).

      b. Hypothermia is more of a danger to athletes exposed to cold for long periods of time, such as long-distance runners and Nordic ski racers, but any injured or ill athlete who has been exposed to cold weather or cold water is a hypothermia suspect until proven otherwise.

      c. **Low reading thermometers should be available in first aid kits during cold weather athletic events.** They may be purchased from the National Ski Patrol System, Inc., 133 South Van Gordon St., Suite 100, Lakewood, CO 80228.

    2. **Field first aid and prehospital management.**

      a. For purposes of field first aid, **hypothermic patients are divided into those with mild hypothermia (rectal temperature 90° F [32° C]) or above, and those with moderate to severe hypothermia (rectal temperature below 90° F [32° C]).**

      b. In all cases of definite or suspected hypothermia, **get the patient out of the cold and wind** and into a tent or other shelter.

        i. **Replace wet clothing with dry.**

          (a) In severely affected patients, clothing should be cut off to avoid the type of jostling that may precipitate ventricular fibrillation.

          (b) Insulate the patient with dry clothing, blankets, or a sleeping bag; cover the head and do not allow him/her to sit, stand, or walk until rewarmed.

        ii. Make arrangements for speedy transportation to a hospital in all but the mildest cases.

      c. **Field first aid then depends on the patient's core temperature.**

        i. If no thermometer is available, it can be estimated by noting the level of consciousness and whether shivering is present.

          (a) **A patient who is still shivering will likely have a core temperature of 90° F (32° C) or above.**

          (b) **A patient who is not shivering or whose level of consciousness is impaired is likely colder than 90° F (32° C).**

      d. **Mild hypothermia.** Previously healthy athletes with mild hypothermia can almost always be safely rewarmed on the spot by any means available.

        i. Hot water bottles, heating pads, or canteens full of hot water, all wrapped to avoid causing burns, can be used.

        ii. One or two healthy persons can get into a sleeping bag or blanket roll with the patient.

        iii. Hot tubs (around 110° F [43° C]) and electric blankets can be used if available.

iv. Special devices have been developed that deliver heated, humidified air or oxygen (e.g., UVIC Heat Treat, APPLINC Saving Breath).

v. If well insulated, a patient who is shivering vigorously will usually be able to rewarm him/herself without the addition of outside heat.

vi. Hot drinks are useful (mainly for morale purposes) after the patient has been partly rewarmed and is able to swallow.

e. **Moderate to severe hypothermia.** In this case, **the best field results will be obtained by preventing further heat loss** by one of the methods listed above, which can be applied during transportation, **and taking the patient to definitive medical care rather than attempting to rewarm in the field.**

i. Avoid active rewarming methods such as a hot tub or electric blanket. These patients are in "cold storage" and will be relatively stable for a number of hours if treated gently. **Once rewarming starts, serious electrolyte, metabolic, and cardiovascular changes occur that are impossible to diagnose and treat in the field.**

ii. **Since these patients will be dehydrated, start an intravenous infusion of 5% glucose/normal saline if available, warmed at least to body temperature.**

iii. **The usual procedures of basic life support should be followed, except that CPR should not be given unless ventricular fibrillation is likely.**

(a) **In severe hypothermics, the presence of a heart beat may be difficult to document without using a cardiac monitor.**

(b) **Closed chest cardiac massage, however, will very likely precipitate ventricular fibrillation if it does not already exist.**

(c) Since the blood pressure is normally low in hypothermia and will respond to rewarming, do not use the pneumatic anti-shock garment (PASG) without additional indications such as traumatic shock or a pelvic fracture.

iv. Handle the hypothermic gently during transport, avoiding sudden bumps and changes of direction.

3. **In-hospital treatment.** With close attention to hydration, oxygenation, acid/base balance, and pH, mild to moderate hypothermics (rectal temperature 85° F [29°]) or above can be rewarmed externally with an electric blanket or a hypothermia device such as the Blanketrol, with the addition of heated, humidified oxygen. Severe hypothermics are best treated with central core rewarming techniques such as peritoneal dialysis or partial cardio-pulmonary bypass.

B. **Frostbite is actual localized freezing of body tissues to variable depth depending on the temperature, length of exposure, amount of insulation, adequacy of circulation, contact with metal, wetting, and other factors.** The most commonly affected parts are those at the body periphery and/or those that have a large surface area-to-volume ratio or exposed position. Frostbite can be a danger to Alpine and Nordic ski racers, gatekeepers at Alpine races, and cold-weather distance athletes such as speed skaters, bicyclers, and runners. Team sports held outdoors in cold weather, such as football, soccer, field hockey, and bobsledding, can also cause frostbite in poorly dressed participants. Figure skating and ice hockey, which are usually held on indoor rinks, are less of a hazard because the air is warmer and natural wind is absent.

1. **Diagnosis.** Frostbite is generally divided into **superficial** and **deep.**

a. **Superficial frostbite, sometimes called "frostnip," involves the outer layers of the skin.**

i. **Symptoms include a burning feeling followed by numbness.**

ii. **Inspection** shows a greyish or pale area of skin, usually on the face or extremities. The deeper tissues remain soft and pliable. After thawing, the area becomes red, sensitive, and swollen to varying degrees. In the more severe cases, a few small blebs may appear. A few days later, the skin is shed by flaking or peeling.

b. **Deep frostbite** is a much more serious and less common injury, and should be seen rarely, if at all, during well-managed athletic events. It is most common in the ears, nose, fingers, toes, and extremities.
   i. **The affected part typically becomes painfully cold, then stops hurting and becomes numb.**
   ii. **Inspection** shows a cold, firm, rigid, pale, or waxy member resembling a piece of chicken removed from the freezer. After thawing, blisters develop within hours to days and may have a startling appearance.

2. **First aid and prehospital management.**
   a. **Superficial frostbite can be thawed on the spot** by direct body heat such as a warm hand on a frozen cheek or a frozen finger held inside a jacket in the patient's armpit.
      i. **Attention should then be paid as to why the frostbite occurred.**
         (a) The patient should put on protective clothing and in many cases be taken to a shelter where general body warming can be performed. As mentioned before, additional trunk insulation is desirable since an increase in core temperature causes peripheral vasodilation, increasing the amount of warm blood available to the shell.
   b. **Deep frostbite is best rewarmed under controlled conditions in a hospital.**
      i. Experience has shown that the least tissue damage results if rewarming is rapid and is performed in a water bath at a temperature of 104°F to 108°F (39°C–42°C).
      ii. During transport, keep the part frozen, although the patient's body should be prevented from cooling further.
      iii. Refreezing should be avoided since it inevitably leads to tissue loss.

IV. **Miscellaneous Cold-related Illnesses**
   A. **Raynaud's syndrome.** This syndrome is not rare in young athletes, especially women. It is characterized by bilateral episodic spasms of digital blood vessels caused by emotion or cold exposure. It can be due to an underlying disease or anatomic abnormality but is usually idiopathic. The fingers are most commonly affected.
      1. **Signs and symptoms.** During the ischemic phase, the affected fingers are cold, pale, and numb; this phase is followed by hyperemia with redness, throbbing pain, and swelling.
      2. **Treatment and prevention.**
         a. **Attacks can be terminated by warming the hands.**
         b. The patient should have a **thorough medical evaluation to rule out an underlying condition,** such as collagen-vascular disease, thoracic outlet compression syndromes and other neurologic conditions, cryoglobulinemia, and cold agglutinin disease.
         c. Smoking should be avoided.
         d. Hands should be protected properly during cold weather.
         e. Attacks can be prevented to some extent by prophylactic use of reserpine, vasodilators such as prazosin or tolazoline, or calcium channel blockers.
   B. **Cold-induced asthma.** In many asthmatics, attacks are precipitated by breathing cold air or by exercise. In some, attacks occur only in the cold. Attacks can frequently be prevented by the prophylactic use of standard oral bronchodilators such as long-acting theophylline preparations and/or inhalation bronchodilators such as metaproterenol or albuterol.
   C. **Cold-agglutinin disease.** Cold-agglutinin disease may be idiopathic or occur as a complication of a *Mycoplasma* infection.
      1. **Signs and symptoms,** which are caused by intravascular agglutination of RBC due to an antibody that is activated by cold exposure, include cyanosis and pain or numbness of exposed body parts, such as the ears and fingers.
      2. **Treatment:** warming.
      3. It is differentiated from Raynaud's syndrome by the lack of blanching followed by hyperemia. In the mycoplasmal variety, which is self-limited, there is

frequently a history of a recent upper respiratory infection, particularly bronchitis.

4. **Prevention** consists of avoidance of cold exposure or the use of protective clothing.

## RELATED READING

1. Lloyd EL: Cold stress in sport. In Hypothermia and Cold Stress. Rockville, MD, Aspen Publishers, 1986.
2. Lereim I: Sports at Low Temperatures. Federation Internationale de Ski, Worbstrasse 210, Postfach, CH-3073 Gumligen, Switzerland.
3. Bowman WD: Cold injuries. In Current Emergency Therapy 1985. Rockville, MD, Aspen Publishers, 1985.
4. Bowman WD: Outdoor Emergency Care. Denver, National Ski Patrol, 1988.
5. Pozos RS, Wittmers LE Jr (eds): The Nature and Treatment of Hypothermia. Minneapolis, MN, University of Minnesota Press, 1983.
6. Wilkerson JD, Bangs CC, Hayward JS: Hypothermia, Frostbite, and Other Cold Injuries. Seattle, The Mountaineers, 1986.

# Chapter 13: Sports Nutrition

## ANN C. GRANDJEAN, EdD

Good nutrition is basic to athletic performance. The well-nourished athlete has more energy and stamina than the under-nourished athlete and therefore is able to train harder. Generally, the same basic dietary principles that promote good health for the general public will maximize performance for most athletes. In certain conditions, however, such as heavy weight training and endurance sports, the requirements may vary. To provide sound nutritional information to athletes, physicians should be aware of the current sports nutrition recommendations.

I.  **Basic Nutrition**
   A.  **The diet**
      1.  The best diet for any athlete is based upon physical, sociological, and psychological factors, as well as the type and intensity of the sport and training program.
      2.  The diet should consist of a wide variety of foods—breads and cereals, fruits and vegetables, dairy products, and protein sources—to ensure that nutrient requirements are met.
      3.  There is no such thing as a "good" or "bad" food. This label mistakenly places focus on the quality of individual foods and de-emphasizes the importance of the quality of the athlete's diet as a whole. As long as a variety of different foods are consumed in moderation, extra energy needs can be met with any foods or beverages the athlete likes.
      4.  **A person must consume approximately 1800 calories from a variety of foods to meet nutritional requirements. Foods and beverages consumed beyond that level are needed solely to meet energy needs.**
         a.  **Athletes at risk**
            i.  Athletes who "make weight," e.g., wrestlers, boxers.
            ii.  Athletes of small body size, e.g., gymnasts, ballet dancers, figure skaters.
   B.  **Energy requirements**
      1.  Depend on body size, demands of sport, age, sex, and nontraining activity level, with **body size being the primary determinant.**
      2.  Table 1 compares approximate caloric expenditures per hour of various activities.
   C.  **Sources of calories.**
      1.  **General recommendations**
         a.  Carbohydrates      50–60%
         b.  Protein      10–15%
         c.  Fats      30–35%
         d.  Alcohol      No more than 2%
      2.  **Athletes with special needs.** There is evidence that some forms of heavy training increase the requirements for certain nutrients.
         a.  **Endurance athletes**
            i.  Increased carbohydrate intake
            ii.  Increased protein intake.
         b.  **Heavy weight training**
            i.  Increased protein intake
            ii.  Calorie intake to support development.
   D.  **Carbohydrate**
      Adequate carbohydrate intake plays a role in long-term health. Carbohydrate foods contribute essential vitamins and minerals and fiber.

**TABLE 1.** Approximate Calories Used Per Hour*

| Activity | 205 lb person | 125 lb person |
|---|---|---|
| Archery | 420 | 268 |
| Baseball—infield or outfield | 382 | 234 |
| —pitching | 488 | 299 |
| Basketball—moderate | 575 | 352 |
| —vigorous | 807 | 495 |
| Bicycling—on level ground,  5.5mph | 409 | 251 |
| 13.0 mph | 877 | 537 |
| Canoeing—4 mph | 565 | 352 |
| Dancing—moderate | 341 | 209 |
| —vigorous | 464 | 284 |
| Fencing—moderate | 409 | 251 |
| —vigorous | 837 | 513 |
| Football | 678 | 416 |
| Golf—twosome | 443 | 271 |
| —foursome | 332 | 203 |
| Handball or hardball—vigorous | 797 | 488 |
| Horseback riding—walk | 270 | 165 |
| —trot | 551 | 338 |
| Motorcycling | 297 | 182 |
| Mountain climbing | 820 | 503 |
| Rowing—pleasure | 409 | 251 |
| —rowing machine or sculling 20 strokes/min | 1116 | 684 |
| Running—  5.5 mph | 887 | 537 |
| —  7 mph | 1141 | 669 |
| —  9 mph level | 1269 | 777 |
| —  9 mph, 2.5% grade | 1480 | 907 |
| —  9 mph, 4% grade | 1564 | 959 |
| —  12 mph | 1606 | 984 |
| —  in place, 140 count/min | 1993 | 1222 |
| Skating—moderate | 465 | 285 |
| —vigorous | 837 | 513 |
| Skiing—downhill | 789 | 483 |
| —level, 5 mph | 956 | 586 |
| Soccer | 730 | 447 |
| Squash | 849 | 520 |
| Swimming—backstroke—20 yds/min | 316 | 194 |
| —40 yds/min | 682 | 418 |
| —breaststroke—20 yds/min | 392 | 241 |
| —40 yds/min | 786 | 482 |
| —butterfly | 956 | 586 |
| —crawl—20 yds/min | 392 | 241 |
| —50 yds/min | 869 | 532 |
| —sidestroke | 682 | 418 |
| Tennis—moderate | 565 | 347 |
| —vigorous | 797 | 489 |
| Volleyball—moderate | 465 | 285 |
| —vigorous | 797 | 489 |
| Walking—2 mph | 286 | 176 |
| —110–120 paces/min | 425 | 260 |
| —4.5 mph | 540 | 331 |
| —downstairs | 544 | 333 |
| —upstairs | 1417 | 869 |
| Water skiing | 638 | 391 |
| Wrestling, judo, or karate | 1049 | 643 |

* From Grandjean AC: Nutrition for Sport Success. Reston, VA, The American Alliance for Health, Physical Education, Recreation and Dance, 1984, p 6, with permission.

1. **Role in exercise**
    a. Primary energy source
    b. Protein sparing
    c. Carbohydrate is the substrate used to form glycogen.
        i. **Muscle glycogen**
            (a) Important in endurance exercise.
            (b) Low levels are associated with exhaustion and fatigue during heavy exercise.
            (c) Research shows that consuming adequate carbohydrate before and during exercise will delay the onset of fatigue and allow the athlete to compete for a longer period of time.
2. **Recommended intakes**
    a. 5 g of carbohydrate per kilogram body weight should more than adequately replace glycogen depleted during **day-to-day** training.
    b. 500–600 g of carbohydrate (2500–3000 kcal) eaten during the 24 hours **following strenuous exercise** will replenish muscle glycogen.
E. **Protein**
Needed for building and repairing tissue.
1. **Role of exercise**
    a. Research shows that changes in protein metabolism occur with exercise.
        i. Protein synthesis is decreased.
        ii. Leucine, an essential amino acid, is used directly as oxidizable fuel during exercise. The rate of oxidation increases as the intensity of exercise increases.
2. **Protein requirements**
    a. Protein requirements depend on:
        i. Body size
        ii. Type, intensity, and duration of sport
        iii. Age
        iv. Calorie intake.
    b. An important factor affecting protein requirements of athletes is the interrelationship of protein and energy (calories).
        i. Increasing energy intake will improve nitrogen balance. Thus, protein requirements decrease as energy intake increases. In turn, **the lower the athlete's calorie intake, the higher the protein requirement.**
    c. **Consuming adequate carbohydrate during heavy training provides protein-sparing effect.**
3. **Recommended intakes**
    a. The recommended dietary allowance for the nonexercising adult is 0.8 g/kg/bw.
    b. An athlete's normal protein intake (10 to 15% of total calories) is generally adequate as long as energy intake is sufficient to maintain competitive weight.
        i. **Athletes who may require a more protein-dense diet.**
            (a) Low-energy consumers, e.g., wrestlers, figure skaters, gymnasts.
            (b) Athletes consuming vegan diets (all-vegetable diet without any meat, milk products, or eggs).
    c. A well-balanced diet will most likely provide 80–100 g of good quality dietary protein.
    d. Research shows that **endurance- and weight-training athletes may require 1.0–1.5 g protein/kg/d.**
F. **Fat**
Fat is a concentrated source of energy. It functions as a carrier of fat-soluble vitamins, adds palatability to the diet, and has protein-sparing action.
1. **Role in exercise**
    a. Fat is a major source of energy during exercise.
        i. Chief advantage—role of fatty acid oxidation in sparing glycogen stores.
    b. Trained subjects oxidize more fat and less carbohydrate than untrained subjects.
    c. Exercise performed under aerobic conditions promotes fat oxidation.

2. **Recommended intakes**
   a. High-fat diets are not recommended.
      i. Increased risk of heart disease, some cancers, and obesity.
   b. Dietary fat should not exceed 30 to 35% of total calories.
   c. High-fat diets compromise carbohydrate intake.
G. **Vitamins**
   Nutrients required in small amounts for normal metabolism, growth, and development (Table 2).
   1. **Role in exercise**
      a. Function as co-enzymes—important in metabolism of carbohydrate, protein, and fat.
      b. **Intakes greater than the Recommended Dietary Allowance (RDA) will not provide more energy or enhance performance.**
   2. **Recommended intakes**
      a. The RDA can usually be obtained by eating a varied diet, assuming calorie intake > 1800 calories.
      b. Taken in excess, vitamins provide no advantage, can be toxic, and can interfere with the absorption and metabolism of other nutrients.
H. **Minerals**
   1. Essential constituents of all cells.
      a. Macronutrients—minerals present in relatively large amounts in the body > 100 mg/day, e.g., calcium, phosphorus, magnesium.
      b. Micronutrients—"trace minerals" present in small amounts < 100 mg/day, e.g., iron, zinc, copper, iodine, and manganese.

**TABLE 2.**  Recommended Daily Dietary Allowances*

| Age (Years) | Children 7–10 | Males 11–14 | 15–18 | 19–24 | 25–50 | 51+ | Females 11–14 | 15–18 | 19–24 | 25–50 | 51+ |
|---|---|---|---|---|---|---|---|---|---|---|---|
| **Weight** | | | | | | | | | | | |
| (kg) | 28 | 45 | 66 | 72 | 79 | 77 | 46 | 55 | 58 | 63 | 65 |
| (lb) | 62 | 99 | 145 | 160 | 174 | 170 | 101 | 120 | 128 | 138 | 143 |
| **Height** | | | | | | | | | | | |
| (cm) | 132 | 157 | 176 | 177 | 176 | 173 | 157 | 163 | 164 | 163 | 160 |
| (in) | 52 | 62 | 69 | 70 | 70 | 68 | 62 | 64 | 65 | 64 | 63 |
| Protein (g) | 28 | 45 | 59 | 58 | 63 | 63 | 46 | 44 | 46 | 50 | 50 |
| **Fat-soluble vitamins** | | | | | | | | | | | |
| Vitamin A ($\mu$g RE) | 700 | 1000 | 1000 | 1000 | 1000 | 1000 | 800 | 800 | 800 | 800 | 800 |
| Vitamin D ($\mu$g) | 10 | 10 | 10 | 10 | 5 | 5 | 10 | 10 | 10 | 5 | 5 |
| Vitamin E (mgd–TE) | 7 | 10 | 10 | 10 | 10 | 10 | 8 | 8 | 8 | 8 | 8 |
| **Water-soluble vitamins** | | | | | | | | | | | |
| Vitamin C (mg) | 45 | 50 | 60 | 60 | 60 | 60 | 50 | 60 | 60 | 60 | 60 |
| Thiamin (mg) | 1.0 | 1.3 | 1.5 | 1.5 | 1.5 | 1.2 | 1.1 | 1.1 | 1.1 | 1.1 | 1.0 |
| Riboflavin (mg) | 1.2 | 1.5 | 1.8 | 1.7 | 1.7 | 1.4 | 1.3 | 1.3 | 1.3 | 1.3 | 1.2 |
| Niacin (mg NE) | 13 | 17 | 20 | 19 | 19 | 15 | 15 | 15 | 15 | 15 | 13 |
| Vitamin B-6 (mg) | 1.4 | 1.7 | 2.0 | 2.0 | 2.0 | 2.0 | 1.4 | 1.5 | 1.6 | 1.6 | 1.6 |
| Folacin ($\mu$g) | 100 | 150 | 200 | 200 | 200 | 200 | 150 | 180 | 180 | 180 | 180 |
| Vitamin B-12 ($\mu$g) | 1.4 | 2.0 | 2.0 | 2.0 | 2.0 | 2.0 | 2.0 | 2.0 | 2.0 | 2.0 | 2.0 |
| **Minerals** | | | | | | | | | | | |
| Calcium (mg) | 800 | 1200 | 1200 | 1200 | 800 | 800 | 1200 | 1200 | 1200 | 800 | 800 |
| Phosphorus (mg) | 800 | 1200 | 1200 | 1200 | 800 | 800 | 1200 | 1200 | 1200 | 800 | 800 |
| Magnesium (mg) | 170 | 270 | 400 | 350 | 350 | 350 | 280 | 300 | 280 | 280 | 280 |
| Iron (mg) | 10 | 12 | 12 | 10 | 10 | 10 | 15 | 15 | 15 | 15 | 10 |
| Zinc (mg) | 10 | 15 | 15 | 15 | 15 | 15 | 12 | 12 | 12 | 12 | 12 |
| Iodine ($\mu$g) | 120 | 150 | 150 | 150 | 150 | 150 | 150 | 150 | 150 | 150 | 150 |

* Adapted from Food and Nutrition Board, National Academy of Sciences, National Research Council, Revised 1989.

2. **Role in exercise**
   a. Important regulators of physiological processes involved in athletic performance.
      i. Maintenance of body fluid balance
      ii. Muscle contraction
      iii. Blood clotting.
3. **Recommended intakes**
   a. For the RDA of minerals, see Table 2.
   b. A balanced diet, sufficient in calories, will provide adequate levels of minerals.
      **NOTE:** A nutrient-by-nutrient review is not practical here. Iron and calcium, however, warrant special attention because of the interest in these two minerals shown by many coaches and athletes, and the fact that American diets are often inadequate for these minerals.
4. **Iron**
   a. Mineral frequently deficient in the American diet.
   b. Functions of iron:
      i. Oxygen transport
         (a) Hemoglobin
         (b) Myoglobin.
      ii. Oxidative metabolism
         (a) Cytochrome C.
   c. **Recommended Dietary Allowance:**
      i. Males:　　11–18 years　　　　　　18 mg
      　　　　　　　19 years and up　　　　10 mg
      ii. Females:　11–50 years　　　　　　18 mg
      　　　　　　　Pregnant or lactating　　18 mg
      　　　　　　　51 years and up　　　　10 mg
   d. Absorption of iron:
      i. Iron is absorbed in two forms by the body—heme and nonheme:
         (a) Heme iron is better absorbed of the two and is found exclusively in animal tissues, especially red meats.
         (b) Nonheme iron is the iron found in plant sources such as cereals and grains. It is poorly absorbed.
      ii. The body regulates absorption according to its needs.
   e. **Foods that increase iron absorption:**
      i. Meat, fish, and poultry (heme iron sources).
      ii. Vitamin C-rich foods, such as orange juice or tomatoes, increase absorption of nonheme iron.
   f. **Factors that decrease iron absorption:**
      i. Tea　　　　　　　　v. Bran
      ii. Coffee　　　　　　vi. Antacids
      iii. Soy products　　　vii. Fiber.
      iv. Eggs
   g. **Those at risk of becoming iron deficient:**
      i. Females—increased losses through menstruation, pregnancy.
      ii. Children and adolescents undergoing their growth spurt.
      iii. Vegetarians—due to poor absorption of nonheme iron food sources.
      iv. Low-calorie diets (<1800 kcal).
      v. Endurance athletes, especially runners.
         (a) Research has shown lower serum ferritin and hemoglobin levels.
   h. **Stages of iron deficiency:**
      i. Stage 0. Measurements are normal
      ii. Stage 1. Iron stores become depleted and serum ferritin decreases to < 20 ng/ml. Free erythrocyte protoporphyrin (Fep), hemoglobin (Hgb), and transferrin saturation levels are normal.
      iii. Stage 2. Decreased transferrin saturation; increased Fep.
      iv. Stage 3. Hemoglobin decreased <12 g/dl.

    i. **Factors contributing to poor iron status in athletes.**
       i. **Heavy training**
         (a) With heavy training, there is an increase in plasma blood volume that dilutes the red blood cells and lowers hemoglobin levels. "Dilutional pseudoanemia":
           (i) Does not appear to affect performance
           (ii) Does not require medical supervision.
       ii. **Footstrike hemolysis**
         (a) Impact of hard foot strikes can destroy normal red blood cells.
         (b) May contribute to true anemia in distance runners.
         (c) Research shows that modern running shoes may reduce footstrike impact in runners.
         (d) Does not appear to affect performance.
       iii. **Increased iron losses** as a result of:
         (a) Sweating
         (b) Gastrointestinal blood loss.
       iv. **Inadequate dietary intake**
         (a) Female athletes often fall below recommended levels of 18 mg iron/day.
         (b) Contributing factors:
           (i) Low calorie intakes
           (ii) Poor absorption of nonheme iron.
  j. **Effects of iron status on performance**
       i. Well documented that iron deficiency anemia affects performance.
         (a) Decreases the capacity of skeletal muscle to consume oxygen and produce ATP.
       ii. Iron deficiency without anemia has been shown to diminish oxidative metabolism in humans.
  k. **Diagnosis of iron deficiency in athletes**
       i. Hemoglobin levels $< 12$ g/dl in males and 11 g/dl in females.
       ii. Serum ferritin below 20 or 25 ng/ml.
       iii. Transferrin saturation levels $< 15\%$.
       iv. Mean Corpuscular Volume (MCV) of 85 fl or below.
  l. **Recommendations**
       i. Routine screening tests should be performed on prospective athletes.
         (a) Hemoglobin and hematocrit levels drawn one or two times per year. NOTE: Hemoglobin concentration varies greatly in normal subjects, and lesser degrees of iron deficiency can go undetected if it is the only measurement used. For a complete assessment of iron status, a battery of tests is indicated.
       ii. If levels are abnormal, 300 mg of ferrous sulfate one time per day, gradually increasing to three times per day, is recommended. If ferrous sulfate is not well tolerated, ferrous fumarate or ferrous gluconate should be prescribed. Treatment may also include 250 mg of ascorbic acid three times per day.
        **Caution:** Overuse and abuse of dietary supplements is not uncommon among athletes. Self-treatment should be discouraged.
       iii. If the athlete does not respond to therapy after 3–6 months, further workup is recommended.
       iv. Athletes need to be aware of food sources of dietary iron (Table 3).
         (a) Daily diet should contain 1–2 servings of meat, green leafy vegetables, and fresh fruit.
         (b) Use of enriched cereals and breads provides additional iron.
         (c) Avoid drinking coffee or tea with meals. They inhibit iron absorption.
5. **Calcium**
Calcium deserves brief mention because of the incidence of amenorrhea in female athletes and the role of calcium in bone density and therefore stress fractures and healing.

**TABLE 3.**  Food Sources of Iron

| Food | Portion Size | Iron (mg) |
|------|-------------|-----------|
| *Liver—pork | 3 oz | 17.7 |
| *Liver—lamb | 3 oz | 12.6 |
| *Liver—chicken | 3 oz | 8.4 |
| *Oysters, fried | 3 oz | 6.9 |
| *Liver—beef | 3 oz | 6.6 |
| Apricots, dried | ½ cup (12 halves) | 5.5 |
| *Turkey, roasted | 3 oz | 5.1 |
| Prune juice | ½ cup | 4.9 |
| Dates, dried | ½ cup (9 dates) | 4.8 |
| *Pork chop, cooked | 3 oz | 4.5 |
| *Beef | 3 oz | 4.2 |
| Prunes, dried | ½ cup (10 prunes) | 3.9 |
| Tostada, bean | 1 | 3.2 |
| Kidney beans, cooked | ½ cup | 3.0 |
| Baked beans with pork & molasses | ½ cup | 3.0 |
| *Hamburger | 3 oz | 3.0 |
| Soybeans, cooked | ½ cup | 2.7 |
| *Enchilada, beef | 1 | 2.6 |
| Raisins | ½ cup | 2.5 |
| Lima beans, canned or fresh cooked | ½ cup | 2.5 |
| Refried beans | ½ cup | 2.3 |
| Figs, dried | ½ cup (4 figs) | 2.2 |
| Spinach, cooked | ½ cup | 2.0 |
| *Taco, beef | 1 | 2.0 |
| Mustard greens, cooked | ½ cup | 1.8 |
| Corn tortilla, lime treated | 8″ diameter | 1.6 |
| Peas, fresh cooked | ½ cup | 1.4 |
| Enchilada, cheese & sour cream | 1 | 1.4 |
| *Egg | 1 large | 1.2 |
| *Chicken, roasted, dark meat | 3 oz | 1.2 |
| *Chicken, roasted | 3.5 oz (½ breast) | 1.0 |
| *Sardines | 1 oz (2 medium) | 1.0 |
| *Shrimp, deep fat fried | 3 oz (5 large) | 1.0 |
| *Haddock fillet | 3 oz | 0.9 |

* Foods of animal origin. Iron in foods of animal origin (except milk and milk products, which have little iron) is absorbed more efficiently than iron in foods of plant origin.

   a. **Functions of calcium:**
      i. Structural support of teeth and bones
      ii. Normal blood clotting
      iii. Muscle contraction and relaxation
      iv. Nerve transmission.
   b. **Requirements**
      i. Greatest during adolescence
      ii. Recommended Dietary Allowance: 800 mg—children and adults; 1200 mg—adolescents, pregnant and lactating women.
      iii. Some experts recommend that postmenopausal and amenorrheic females increase intake to 1000–1500 mg/day.
   c. **Inadequate dietary intake**
      i. May increase risk of osteoporosis in susceptible individuals.
      ii. Inadequate intakes of dietary calcium have been reported in some female athletes, particularly those participating in gymnastics, ballet, and figure skating.

d. **Absorption of calcium**
   i. The body's ability to absorb dietary calcium is affected by the presence of other nutrients and dietary substances as well as by physiological factors.
      (a) **Factors that increase calcium absorption:**
         (i) Increased need
         (ii) Vitamin D
         (iii) Lactose
         (iv) Weight-bearing exercise
         (v) Estrogen.
      (b) **Factors that decrease calcium absorption:**
         (i) Fiber
         (ii) Oxalic acid (contained in spinach, beet tops, collard greens, chocolate, and rhubarb)
         (iii) Phytic acid (found in the outer layers of cereal grains and thus in whole-grain products)
         (iv) Alcohol
         (v) Inactivity
         (vi) High protein intakes.
   ii. **Exercise** plays an important role in minimizing bone loss in females.
      (a) Studies show that bone mineral content is significantly higher in athletes versus nonathletes.
   iii. **Athletic amenorrhea**
      (a) Reports suggest that young women who exercise strenuously to the point of amenorrhea may be at risk for bone demineralization.
   iv. **Recommendations**
      (a) Athletes should be aware of food sources of calcium (Table 4).
      (b) Athletes who ingest less than 2000 kcal per day may require a calcium supplement.
      (c) Amenorrheic women should be evaluated, i.e., patient history, including:
         (i) Menstrual cycle history
         (ii) Level of physical activity
         (iii) Nutritional history
         (iv) Weight control practices.

## II. Fluids and Electrolytes

### A. Water

1. **The athlete's most important nutrient.**
   a. Must be consumed regularly and in sufficient amounts to ensure normal functioning of the body and thermal regulation.
   b. Failure to replace water loss results in dehydration, which has been shown to cause decrements in performance.
2. **Effects of exercise on water balance.**
   a. **Sweating—primary method of thermoregulation.**
      i. The greater the intensity and duration of the sport, the greater the heat production and sweat loss.
      ii. **Sweat loss equal to 2 to 3% of body weight can cause measurable impairments in thermal regulation, cardiovascular performance, and performance.**
3. **Dehydration**
   a. **Symptoms**
      i. **0.5% body weight loss**—thirst
      ii. **2% body weight loss**—stronger thirst, general discomfort, loss of appetite, decrement in performance.
      iii. **3% body weight loss**—dry mouth, decrease in urine.
      iv. **4% body weight loss**—apathy, increased effort for exercise, flushed skin, impatience.
4. **Rehydration**
   a. **Goals**
      i. Replace water that is lost and prevent hypohydration.
         (a) **Thirst is not a sensitive indicator of water need.**

**TABLE 4.** Food Sources of Calcium

| Food | Portion Size | Calcium (mg) |
|------|--------------|--------------|
| **Dairy Products** | | |
| Yogurt, plain | 1 cup | 415 |
| Skim milk | 1 cup | 296 |
| Whole milk | 1 cup | 288 |
| Cottage cheese | 1 cup | 282 |
| Swiss cheese | 1 oz | 248 |
| Mozzarella cheese | 1 oz | 207 |
| Cheddar cheese | 1 oz | 204 |
| Ice cream | 1 cup | 175 |
| **Meats** | | |
| Oysters | 1 cup | 343 |
| Salmon (with bones) | 1 oz | 86 |
| Sardines (with bones) | 1 oz | 74 |
| **Vegetables** | | |
| Turnip greens | ½ cup | 184 |
| Mustard greens | ½ cup | 183 |
| Collard greens | ½ cup | 152 |
| Spinach | ½ cup | 83 |
| Broccoli | ½ cup | 67 |
| White beans | ½ cup | 50 |
| Cabbage | ½ cup | 49 |
| Kidney beans | ½ cup | 48 |
| Lima beans | ½ cup | 38 |
| Carrots | ½ cup | 37 |
| **Fruits** | | |
| Prunes | 8 large | 90 |
| Orange | 1 medium | 62 |
| Tangerine | 1 large | 40 |
| **Nuts** | | |
| Almonds | ½ cup | 152 |
| Walnuts | ½ cup | 60 |
| Peanuts | ½ cup | 54 |
| Pecans | ½ cup | 43 |

     ii. **Drink water before, during, and after an event or practice session**
         (a) 2 cups water 2 hours prior to exercise.
         (b) 2 cups water 15–20 minutes prior to exercise.
         (c) 4–6 oz water every 10–15 minutes during exercise.
     iii. **The most accurate method of monitoring hydration is for athletes to weigh nude before and after practice sessions or competitions.**
         (a) One half-quart (16 oz) of water equals 1 pound of body weight.
   5. **Fluid replacement**
     a. Cold fluids increase gastric emptying and stabilize body core temperature.
     b. Water or hypotonic saline, 200–400 ml every 15–20 minutes.
     c. Simple sugar concentration should be ≤ 2.5 g of sugar/100 ml of water. Glucose polymers ≤ 7.5%.
     d. Research shows that athletes involved in endurance events benefit from polymer-containing drinks with concentrations of 5.0 to 7.5% carbohydrate.
     e. Research also shows that rehydration during and after exercise in hot weather will occur quicker when sodium is taken in with fluids. However, more research is needed.
  B. **Electrolytes**
   1. **Role in exercise**
     a. Regulation of body water distribution between various fluid compartments.
     b. Muscle and nerve contraction.
     c. Enzymatic control of cellular reactions.

2 Although sweat is hypotonic, it contains some **electrolytes.**
  a. **Sodium**
    i. Sodium is the mineral most affected by physical exercise. A deficiency can impair performance.
    ii. **The best method of maintaining salt balance is by salting food during meals.**
    iii. Under extreme conditions, athletes who sweat profusely, who are not acclimated to the heat, or who have low sodium intakes may experience heat cramps or exhaustion due to sodium depletion.
      (a) Treatment:
        (i) A typical diet should provide adequate amounts of sodium.
        (ii) May need to increase intake of foods higher in sodium (pizza, ham, salted snack foods, etc.) and/or salt foods.
        (iii) The daily requirement for the active normal adult in a temperate climate is 1100–3300 mg (47.8–143.4 mEq).
      (b **Cautions**
        (i) **Avoid salt tablets,** which are irritating to the stomach and can increase the danger of dehydration.
        (ii) **Overloading with salt** has been associated with body potassium depletion, which may increase the risk of heat stroke.
  b **Potassium**
    i. Plays an essential role in muscular contraction and nerve conduction. Potassium is lost in sweat; however, **losses can generally be replaced with a balanced diet** providing approximately 1875–5625 mg/day (47.9–143.8 mEq).
    ii. There is no substantial evidence to support the use of supplements or potassium-rich beverages or electrolyte beverages containing potassium.
    iii. **Ingestion of potassium in chemical forms is discouraged** because of the possibility of gastric distress, sharp elevation of plasma potassium, and risk of cardiac toxicity.
    iv. Potassium needs can be met by increasing potassium-rich foods, such as citrus fruits and juice, tomatoes and tomato juice, potatoes, bananas, peaches, milk, and peanuts, in the diet.
  c **Renal conservation**
    i. **Exercise causes a reduction in renal blood flow,** the extent of which varies with the intensity of exercise.
    ii. Moderate exercise has been shown to reduce blood flow nearly 30%, whereas strenuous exercise may cause it to drop as much as 75%.
      (a) Changes appear within 10 minutes of the onset of exercise.
    iii Intense exercise can reduce glomerular filtration rate by up to 50% of resting value and increase circulating levels of plasma antidiuretic hormone.
      (a) **Urine flow is decreased and plasma volume conserved.**
    iv. **Cautions**
      (a) These alterations in renal function coupled with *extremely* high water intake may contribute to hyponatremia.
      (b) In cases of extremely high water intake, high sodium-chloride intake and/or low potassium intake, hypokalemia should also be considered.
C. **Sport drinks**
  1. Sport drinks are commercial preparations that are often promoted (1) as a source of sodium, potassium, and sugar; (2) to be superior to water for fluid replacement; and, (3) to have anti-fatigue properties due to carbohydrate and electrolyte content.
    a. **Cautions:** the use of sport drinks is controversial, and research is inconclusive as to their effect.
  2. **Major benefits**
    a. Prevention of hypohydration due to an increase in *voluntary* intake of fluids.

3. Practical application
   a. Beverage should empty from the stomach as quickly as plain water.
   b. Simple sugar drinks (glucose, fructose, sucrose) should be diluted with water to decrease concentration to a level of 2.5% or less.
   c. Glucose polymer solutions of 7% (or 7.5%) empty readily and provide a greater carbohydrate load. This is of greatest value to endurance athletes.
   d. Use of sport drinks should be tested during training and not consumed for the first time during competition.

III. **Achieving Competitive Weight**

A. **Body composition**
   1. **Desirable competitive body weight and composition should be achieved during the off-season and maintained throughout competitive season.**
   2. Body composition will vary according to sport.
   3. Great individual variation due to factors such as genetics, etc.
   4. It is impossible and irresponsible to establish fixed body weight or percent body fat for sports and/or athletes.

B. **Weight loss**
   1. Reducing weight to compete in a lower weight classification is a common practice in sports such as wrestling, judo, boxing, and weightlifting.
   2. Techniques used to produce rapid weight loss (fasting, crash diets, dehydration, induced vomiting, laxatives, and diuretics) can endanger an athlete's health and impair performance.
   3. Starvation or extremely low-calorie diets (semistarvation) are not recommended for athletes, *ever*.
      a. **Health concerns:** nutritional deficiencies, dehydration, loss of lean body mass, electrolyte imbalance, increased risk of infection.
      b. **Effect on performance:** decreases in aerobic power and capacity, speed, strength, coordination, and judgment.
      c. **Growth and development:** growth retardation in children.
   4. Recommendations for weight loss:
      a. Decrease caloric intake, increase energy expenditure.
      b. The recommended rate of weight loss is 1–2 pounds per week (caloric deficit of 500–1000 kcal/day).
      c. The safe level of restriction depends on the athlete's normal dietary intake.
         i. Not < 2000 kcal for males.
         ii. Not < 1800 kcal for females.
      d. Maintain best competitive weight throughout the year.

C. **Weight gain**
   1. Goals
      a. To gain lean body mass, not fat. (Muscle mass increases only after a significant period of weight training.)
      b. Consume a diet that meets nutrient needs as well as the increased caloric requirement.
   2. Potential problems
      a. Increasing caloric intake may be difficult. Increasing size of meals is often undesirable, causing discomfort.
      b. Busy schedules, e.g., school, work, training, and travel, may make it difficult for the athlete to take time out to eat.
   3. Recommendations
      a. Gradually increase intake at meals and include 2–4 snacks a day.
      b. Increase intake of high-calorie food.
      c. Monitoring weight gains with skinfold measurements will indicate type of body weight being added.
      d. Rate of gain and location of added muscle will depend on training program, sex, and somatotype as well as genetic factors.

IV. **Food as a Ergogenic Aid**
   A. **Definition:** an ergogenic aid is any substance that helps to increase work output.
      1. In athletics, this term is used to describe drugs, medicines, and dietary regimens believed by some to:
         a. Increase strength and endurance
         b. Increase concentration
         c. Decrease pain
         d. Delay onset of fatigue.
   B. Ergogenic aids can be divided into five categories: (1) pharmacological, (2) *nutritional, (3) mechanical, (4) psychological, and (5) physiological.
   C. **Nutritional aids**
      1. Proposed to increase performance by:
         a. Increasing energy stores in the body (carbohydrate, protein, fat)
         b. Facilitating the biochemical reactions that produce energy.
         c. Modifying the biochemical changes contributing to fatigue.
      2. Examples of nutritional ergogenic aids include:
         a. Dietary regimens used to alter glycogen levels.
         b. Supplements, both nutritive and non-nutritive.
   D. Dietary regimens used to alter glycogen levels
      1. **Carbohydrate loading** is the process of manipulating the diet and amount of exercise in an effort to increase glycogen stores in the muscles.
         a. Several techniques for increasing glycogen levels in the muscle have been reported. Knowing which method is most effective and least harmful to athletes is important.
         b. **The most universally accepted dietary regimen currently recommended is as follows:**
            i. Phase 1—One week prior to competition, gradually reduce activity, with complete rest the day before an event.
            ii. Phase 2—During the first 3 days of this gradual tapering of exercise, consume a normal mixed diet of 50% carbohydrate.
            iii. Phase 3—During the final 3 days, a diet of 525 g of carbohydrate is consumed. NOTE: Total grams of carbohydrate is more important than the percentage from total calories.
         c. **Carbohydrate loading is recommended for:**
            i. Endurance athletes, e.g., long-distance runners, cross-country skiers, road cyclists, endurance swimmers (activities requiring 1.5 hours or more of intense effort at a high percentage of $VO_2$ max).
         d. **Carbohydrate loading is not recommended for:**
            i. Athletes participating in short-term events, such as sprints, or in sports in which the activity may last for a long period of time, but the physical effort is characterized by brief periods of high-energy activity with alternate rest periods, such as football, baseball, wrestling.
            ii. Young children.
         e. **Possible side effects**—Athletes should be informed about potential negative effects of carbohydrate loading.
            i. Repeated glycogen loading can cause:
               (a) Increased water retention and subsequent weight gain.
               (b) Stiffness.
               (c) Cramps.
               (d) Chest pain, electrocardiogram changes, and alterations in blood lipid profiles have been reported, albeit only a few cases.
               (e) Depression, lethargy, and loss of muscle tissue may also occur.
               (f) Some athletes may experience digestive problems on very high-carbohydrate diets.

---

* For purpose of this section, the focus of discussion will be on nutritional ergogenic aids.

(i) Possible solutions:
- Experiment early in the season, not before a big event.
- Liquid carbohydrate source may be used to supplement the loading diet; however, exclusive use of liquid carbohydrate sources is not recommended.

2. **Supplements**
   a. **Nutritive:** Supplements commonly used by athletes include vitamin and mineral combinations, vitamins (both oral and injectable), minerals, protein and amino acids, brewers yeast, and bee pollen. Use of any herbal, vitamin/ mineral, protein/amino acid, and/or other supplement is at the athlete's own risk. *Some dietary supplements have resulted in positive drug tests.*

   i. **Vitamin and mineral supplements**
      (a) All vitamins and minerals needed by the body can be obtained in adequate amounts by consuming an adequate diet—there is no benefit to taking more.
      (b) Research has shown that vitamin and mineral supplementation above the RDA does not improve work output, muscle strength, resistance to fatigue, recovery, cardiovascular function, endurance capacity, or oxygen consumption.
      (c) Potential problems: the fat-soluble vitamins A, D, E, and K can be toxic when taken in high doses.
      (d) Because many athletes have high-energy intakes, they are already consuming 200% or more of the RDA for many nutrients **from food alone.**
      (e) In some cases, the use of a daily multivitamin supplement may benefit the athlete who limits calorie intake, restricts the use of some food groups, or has unusual eating habits.

   ii. **Protein and amino acid supplements**
      (a) There is no evidence that excessive protein (protein powders, pills, etc.) improves athletic ability, supplies extra energy, or increases muscle mass.
      (b) Many athletes consume more than twice the RDA for protein from food alone.
      (c) Athletes consuming adequate dietary protein are consuming adequate amounts of essential amino acids. There is no benefit to taking more.
      (d) Excessive intakes of protein may result in:
         (i) Renal and hepatic stress
         (ii) Gout
         (iii) Dehydration.

   iii. **Bee pollen**—a mixture of bee saliva, plant nectar, and pollen.
      (a) Sold in powder or capsule form.
      (b) Promoted as an energy supplement.
      (c) Potential problems: if taken in large amounts, can cause severe allergic reactions in some individuals.
      (d) Has not been shown to be ergogenic.

   iv. **Brewers yeast**
      (a) Promoted as natural source of protein, B vitamins, minerals, and nucleic acids.
      (b) Is not the same as nutritional yeast, which is fortified with vitamin $B_{12}$.
      (c) Has not been shown to be ergogenic.

   v. **Sodium bicarbonate ($NaHCO_3$) loading**
      (a) Considered as a potential aid to enhance performance.
      (b) Theory: neutralizes the buildup of lactic acid in the muscles and reduces fatigue.
      (c) Studies on the effect of bicarbonates on performance are conflicting.

(d) Not recommended.
(e) Concerns:
    (i) Ethical considerations of taking substance to enhance performance.
    (ii) Large quantities of $NaHCO_3$ may result in diarrhea and/or gastric distress.
    (iii) Disturbances in body sodium and water balance.

vi. **Herbals**
  (a) Common forms supplied to athletes include: teas, capsules, liquids, and tablets.
  (b) Examples of herbs: ginseng, suma, mate
  (c) Cautions:
    (i) Herbs may contain toxic chemicals.
    (ii) No control over substances used in herbs.
    (iii) Some herbs have resulted in positive drug tests.

b. **Non-nutritive**
  i. **Pangamic acid** ("vitamin $B_{15}$")
    (a) Promoted as a dietary supplement to cure fatigue.
    (b) Advocates claim pangamic acid increases oxygen content of the blood.
    (c) Cautions: pangamic acid is *not* a vitamin and some of the compounds being sold under this name are potentially toxic.
  ii. **Bioflavinoids** ("vitamin P")
    (a) Not a vitamin.
    (b) Hesperidin, rutin, and citrin (citrus bioflavinoids) are frequently found in supplements promoted for athletes.
    (c) Have *no* nutritional value.
    (d) Do not enhance athletic performance.

# Chapter 14: Eating Disorders

AMANDA DUFFY RANDALL, MSW, ACSW

I. **Anorexia Nervosa**

A. **Essential features and diagnostic criteria**
1. Refusal to maintain body weight over a minimal normal weight for age and height, e.g., weight loss leading to maintenance of body weight 15% below that of expected normal range.
2. Intense fear of gaining weight or becoming fat, even though underweight.
3. Disturbance in the way in which one's body weight, size, or shape is experienced; the person claims to "feel fat" even when emaciated, or believes that one or several areas of the body are "too fat" even when obviously underweight.
4. In females, absence of at least three (3) consecutive menstrual cycles when otherwise expected to occur (primary or secondary amenorrhea).

B. **Medical symptoms**
1. Hypothermia
2. Bradycardia
3. Hypotension
4. Edema
5. Lanugo (neonatal-like hair on face and/or body)
6. Metabolic changes
7. Amenorrhea.

C. **Associated features**
1. Preoccupation with food; prepare elaborate meals for others yet limit themselves to a narrow selection of low-calorie foods.
2. May hide, conceal, crumble, or throw away food to avoid eating it.
3. Minimization of the severity of the illness or body condition.
4. Delayed psychosexual development of adolescents and/or adults; markedly decreased interest in sex.
5. Compulsive behavior may be present.

D. **Age at onset: early to late adolescence; can range from prepuberty to early 30s (rare).**

E. **Sex ratio: predominantly in females (95%).**

F. **Prevalence: ranges from 1 in 800 to 1 in 100; reported in studies of females between ages 12–18.**

G. **Course: may be unremitting until death, episodic, or consist of a single episode.**

H. **Impairment: severe weight loss often necessitates hospitalization to prevent death by starvation.**

I. **Mortality rates range between 5–18%.**

II. **Bulimia Nervosa**

A. **Diagnostic criteria and essential features**
1. Recurrent episodes of binge eating (rapid consumption of a large amount of food in a discrete period of time).
2. A feeling of lack of control over eating behavior during the eating binges.
3. Regular engagement in either self-induced vomiting, use of laxatives or diuretics, strict dieting or fasting, or vigorous exercise in order to prevent weight gain.
4. Minimum average of two binge eating episodes a week for at least 3 months.
5. Persistent overconcern with body shape and weight.
6. Eating binges may be planned; food consumed often has high caloric content, a sweet taste, and a texture that facilitates rapid eating. The food is usually eaten as inconspicuously as possible or secretly. Food is usually eaten rapidly with

little chewing. Once the eating has begun, additional food is often sought to continue the binge. A binge is usually terminated by abdominal discomfort, sleep, social interruption, or induced vomiting. Vomiting decreases the physical pain of abdominal distention, allowing either continued eating or termination of the binge, and often reduces post-binge anguish. Vomiting may be desired; food is sometimes eaten to vomit, or vomiting will occur after eating a small amount of food. Although eating binges may be pleasurable, disparaging self-criticism with a depressed mood often follow.

    7. Frequent weight fluctuations are common due to alternating binges and fasts.

    8. Patients often feel that life is dominated by conflicts about eating.

B. **Associated features:**

    1. Normal weight range; some individuals overweight or underweight.

    2. Depressed mood is common.

    3. Some subject to psychoactive substance abuse or dependence, most frequently involving sedatives, amphetamines, cocaine, or alcohol.

C. **Age at onset: adolescence or early adult life.**

D. **Course: chronic and intermittent over a period of many years; usually binges alternate with periods of normal eating or fasting.**

E. **Impairment and complications**

    1. Seldom incapacitating except in rare cases.

    2. Dental erosion is common.

    3. Electrolyte imbalance with dehydration can occur, which can lead to severe physical complications (cardiac arrhythmia, sudden death).

      a. Rare complications include esophageal tears and gastric rupture.

III. **Complications of Eating Disorders for Athletes**

A. **Anorexia nervosa and bulimia cause the body to feel the effects of dehydration and starvation, with the following conditions possible:**

    1. Loss of muscle strength and endurance

    2. Decreased aerobic power with decreased oxygen utilization

    3. Loss of speed and coordination

    4. Impaired judgment

    5. Reduced blood volume (and, consequently, less blood flow to the kidneys)

    6. Loss of muscle glycogen

    7. Electrolyte loss

    8. Inability to regulate body temperature

    9. Reduced heart function

    10. Increased heart rate

    11. Amenorrhea

    12. Loss of bone mass during adolescence

    13. Increased susceptibility to injury

    14. Impaired brain function with irritability, depression, and withdrawal.

IV. **Common Behaviors Associated with Anorexia Nervosa or Bulimia**

A. Many athletes engage in weight maintenence or reducing behaviors that are time-limited and appropriate to their performance; not all thin athletes have an eating disorder, just as being at ideal body weight does not indicate that they are necessarily healthy. However, **certain behaviors do merit attention and are often associated with an eating disorder.**

    1. Constant preoccupation with and discussion of weight and dieting (repetitive comments about "feeling fat").

    2. Weight loss below the ideal competitive weight set for that athlete and which continues even off-season.

    3. Purposeless, excessive physical activity that is not a part of the training program.

    4. Extreme weight fluctuations.

    5. Secretive eating or evidence of secretive eating (candy or food wrappers in inappropriate places—food sneaking or stealing).

6.  Vomitus or odor of vomit in restroom, shower, or wastebasket areas.
7.  Bloodshot or watery eyes, especially after using the restroom or areas where vomiting could have occurred.
8.  Complaints or evidence of bloating or edema not explained by medical cause or premenstrual water retention.
9.  Frequent constipation.
10. Lightheadedness, disequilibrium (loss of balance), and mood swings not attributed to any medical cause.
11. Avoidance of situations where the athlete would be observed eating, or refusal to eat with or around others.
12. Intense concern with nutrition information or the eating patterns of others.

V.  **Treatment for Eating Disorders**
    A.  **An eating disorder is a complex psychological and physiological problem that should be diagnosed and treated by a physician, psychologist, and nutritionist trained in the field.** However, coaches and trainers need to be aware of the behaviors that suggest the athlete has an eating disorder, and be informed of resources for treatment. Athletes who exhibit behaviors associated with an eating disorder need to be confronted with the specific observations relating to their behaviors. REFERRAL TO AN APPROPRIATE TREATMENT PROGRAM IS ESSENTIAL FOR RECOVERY OF THE ATHLETE.
    B.  **Treatment generally will consist of a thorough physical, psychological, and nutritional assessment process. Individual, group, and family psychotherapy and nutritional education therapy are required for effective treatment of an eating disorder.** Treatment is often provided on an outpatient basis.
    C.  **For athletes in serious physical condition (severe symptoms of chemical imbalances, dangerously low body weight, or a severe binging/purging cycle), inpatient hospitalization and treatment may be necessary.** Hospitalization is frequently long-term (6 to 10 weeks) and is followed by outpatient aftercare treatment.

VI. **Prevention**

An eating disorder is associated with underlying emotional distress and is not caused by athletic training or participation. Young athletes with an intense desire to succeed and please the coach or trainer can be strongly influenced by comments or behaviors directed toward weight or dieting. Eating disorders in athletes can be reduced by using the following general guidelines:
    A.  Emphasize the role of overall, long-term good nutrition and weight control in optimizing athletic performance.
    B.  Do not overly focus on the effect of lower body weight on athletic performance.
    C.  Set realistic goals that address methods of dieting, rate of weight change, and a *reasonable* target weight for the athlete.
    D.  Never suggest or encourage the use of laxatives, diuretics, or purging behavior to reduce or maintain weight.
    E.  Be aware of the behaviors associated with eating disorders and refer athletes for professional help when appropriate.

# Chapter 15: The Role of Sports Psychology/Psychiatry

TODD P. HENDRICKSON, MD
SHARON J. ROWE, MA, CTRS

*I never hit a shot, not even in practice, without having a very sharp in-focus picture of it in my head.*
                                                    -Jack Nicklaus, Professional Golfer

*If you are relaxing and subconsciously thinking about your coming race, you are going to perform at just about 100% efficiency.*
                                                    -Mark Spitz, Swimmer

*The committed athlete of the future will be able to achieve peak performance ONLY through the use of a comprehensive mental AND physical training program.*

                                                    -Marilyn King, Olympic Pentathlete

Everyone can vividly remember a special time in their athletic lives when everything they did was perfect, effortless, and focused, with an overwhelming rush of excitement and power that accompanied a task that was extraordinarily well done.

Most athletes, whether competitive or recreational, will acknowledge that mental factors and psychological mastery account for 60 to 90% of any given athletic performance. Understanding the role of sports psychology/psychiatry as a major influence on sport behavior and sport performance must be a priority in any sport training program that is designed to maximize both physical and mental preparation. By understanding the effects of psychological factors on behavior or the psychological effects that participation has on the performer, we can evaluate, assess, and assist the athlete in his/her environment.

Understanding the psychological aspects of sport and sport behavior can help us identify strengths and weaknesses, solve performance problems, improve self-esteem, provide a framework for the appropriate use of intervention techniques, and ultimately enhance the performance of the athlete through the facilitation of personal growth.

## I. Historical Background

The study of sport psychology is not new; it has only been within the past 25 to 30 years that it has been scientifically linked to excellence in performance. Much of this progress can be attributed to experts in the U.S. and Soviet Union:

1895—George W. Fritz' investigation of reaction time raises the questions of why physical education needs an understanding of psychology and what psychological benefits can be derived from participating in physical education.

1925—Coleman R. Griffith is hired by the University of Illinois to help coaches improve players' performance. He is intrigued by the psychological effects of Knute Rockne's "pep talks," and the "mental toughness" of football player Red Grange.

1930–1940s—Soviet and American experts study the profound psychological ramifications of the Nazi Holocaust and its survivors; specifically their ability to tap into hidden reserves to find the strength to go on in spite of heinous, abusive treatment.

1950s—Soviet Alexander Romen's basic research using ancient yogic techniques to teach Soviet cosmonauts to control psychophysiological processes while in space leads to programs for teaching optimal sports performance. This field of inquiry comes to be known as "self-regulation training."

American John Lawther's research in motor learning stimulates interest about motivation, team cohesion, interpersonal relationships, and motor control.

1960s—Bruce Ogilvie pioneers clinical work with athletes in their environment(s) focusing on motivation, motives of participation, performance decrements, and the integration of intervention strategies to enhance performance in athletes.

Nov., 1976—*Track and Field News* reports that mental training sessions were being employed by Soviet weight lifters. This report was filed after unprecedented success by Soviet and East German athletes in the 1976 Olympic Games.

1980s—Comprehensive mental training programs begin to flourish and are accepted as legitimate forms of sport training. Performance enhancement programs become more widespread.

II. **Evaluation and Assessment of the Athlete**

For the most effective care, thorough evaluation of the athlete and assessment of the clinical problem are necessary before formulating a management program and selecting therapeutic techniques.

A. **The clinician's qualifications**
   1. Emphasis should be placed on the qualifications of the clinician providing services (i.e., educational background, specialized training, and clinical experience in the field of sports psychology).
      a. Sport psychologist (now a recognized field)
      b. Clinical psychologist
      c. Psychiatrist
      d. Therapists, counsellors.

B. **The scope of clinical problems encountered: the client**
   1. Clients seen may exhibit a range of behaviors, thoughts, and feelings that can either complicate or facilitate personal growth through various mental training programs or interventions.
   2. Clinically, the impression via the evaluation of an athlete may range from mental healthiness (most athletes) to mental illness (i.e., depression, substance abuse, personality disorder, anorexia nervosa, etc.)
   3. Ethical principles of complete confidentiality must be maintained.
   4. The client is the consumer.

C. **The role of the clinician**
   1. **Service**—Provision of services for crisis intervention, stress management, psychological skills training, group and individual psychotherapy, pharmacotherapy, etc.
   2. **Educational**—Care must be taken to provide information to clients regarding theoretical principles being used (i.e., intervention techniques, therapy, expectations of treatment, etc.) so that the client may be able to function independently and with autonomy (i.e., without you). Didactics and group teaching can be extremely helpful when working with athletes.
   3. **Research**—One must be able to validate principles being applied through reproducibility and consistency.

D. **Goals of the evaluation and assessment**
   1. **Diagnosis** is a major goal. Categorization according to the *DSM-III R* (if applicable) multiaxial system should be done with each case.
   2. **Treatment planning** is based on the patient's needs and capacity for responding to various types of treatment.
   3. **Psychological understanding of the patient** is critical regardless of diagnosis or treatment. This allows for greater empathetic communication and affords insight into the patient's likely response to treatment.
   4. **A working alliance** or rapport with the patient is fostered by a thorough evaluation by the treating clinician.

E. **Use of the biological-psychological-sociological model**
   1. **Biological:** medical history, medical status, familial history, current physical skill level/development, and overall physiology of the athlete.
   2. **Psychological assessment** should include:
      a. **Mental Status Examination** (a measure of psychological fitness)

      i. General attitude and behavior (i.e., appearance)

      ii. Speaking style and form

      iii. Affect (emotional tone)

      iv. Mood

      v. Thought content (what the patient thinks about)

      vi. Cognitive function (ability to calculate, concentrate, reason, and abstractly think)

      vii. Insight (into self and/or problems)

      viii. Judgment (right versus wrong).

    b. **Problem-solving skills**

    c. **General reaction to stress**

    d. **Athlete's overall perception of SELF**

  3. **Sociological assessment** should include analysis of the patient's athletic and nonathletic environment. This includes social support systems, family dynamics, interpersonal relationships, substance abuse history, educational background, cultural background, childhood development, and sport-performance experiences (successful and unsuccessful).

F. **Evaluation and assessment procedure**

  1. **The clinical interview with a biopsychosocial orientation.**

  2. **Direct observation of the athlete** (i.e., field study) is a prerequisite for complete evaluation, as one must see the athlete in action to develop a "feel" for how the athlete responds to various internal and environmental stimuli. This can be facilitated through the use of videography (videotape).

  3. **Data gathering,** with the permission of the athlete, can be helpful to comprehend how others see the athlete (i.e., reports from coaches, parents, friends, other athletes).

  4. **Psychological testing** may be helpful in organizing an overall picture of the athlete, although it may not be indicated in all clinical cases. This testing can be extremely beneficial when diagnostic issues are confusing, or when treatment is meeting with resistance (i.e., refractoriness to treatment).

    a. **Personality** can be assessed through the use of the Minnesota Multiphasic Personality Inventory (MMPI), which helps to establish longstanding behavioral patterns and adaptation to life stressors. There are also numerous new tools being tested that give us information about personality traits and their interaction with sport-specific situations.

    b. **Mood assessment** may give valuable feedback regarding an athlete's subjective feeling about himself/herself.

      i. POMS (Profile of Mood States)

      ii. HDRS (Hamilton Depression Rating Scale).

    c. **Anxiety,** which can be crippling to the athlete and may deter performance capabilities, can be identified as well. In most cases, behavior is believed to be determined by the reciprocal interaction of personal traits and the characteristics of different situations. This can be especially helpful in understanding the anxiety-performance relationship.

      i. State/Trait Anxiety Inventory

      ii. Sport Competition Anxiety Test (SCAT)

      iii. Competitive State Anxiety Inventory (CSAI).

    d. **Stress** may be evaluated through the use of the Holmes-Rahe Scale, which helps to identify causes of stress.

    e. **Motivational assessment** can be accomplished through goal analysis and behavioral assessment.

    f. **Thought disorders** may be assessed via the

      i. MMPI

      ii. SCL–90 (Symptom Checklist–90)

G. **Conclusion**

Evaluation and assessment of the athlete can be complex yet challenging. If done appropriately and comprehensively, it can serve as the foundation on which to build individualized programs for performance enhancement and personal growth of the athlete. Once again it should be pointed out that there are numerous intervention techniques available today that profess to enhance performance in athletes. However, care should be taken to evaluate and assess *each* athlete appropriately so that any intervention techniques used will reap maximum benefits for the athlete.

III. **Psychiatric Disorders Seen in Athletic Populations**

    A. **Major depression** (principal disorder of affect and mood)

        1. **Clinical features:** usually of insidious onset; may see symptoms of subjective depression, loss of pleasure, suicidal thoughts, loss of appetite, sleep disturbance, self-reproach, lack of energy, dysphoric (depressed) mood, and feelings of guilt.

          a. In children, one tends to see more somatic symptoms and psychomotor agitation.

          b. In adolescents, one sees more frequent anorexia, weight loss, hypersomnia, and hopelessness.

        2. **Differential diagnosis:** Substance abuse (especially cocaine withdrawal, sedative-hypnotic usage, and anabolic steroid use), anxiety disorders, eating disorders. This type of depression is usually *not* related to specific psychosocial stressors as seen in adjustment disorders.

        3. **Treatment**

          a. Referral to mental health professionals is often appropriate.

          b. Psychosocial therapy (i.e., individual, group, family).

          c. Pharmacotherapy may be indicated, especially if significant disturbance in ability to function on a daily basis is noted. A combination approach of pharmacotherapy and psychotherapy is usually very effective and may be the quickest resolution to symptoms.

    B. **Adjustment disorder** may be considered if the psychiatric symptoms (including symptoms of depression and/or anxiety) seem to be related to a recent (within 3 months) psychosocial stressor(s) and will usually remit when the stress is over. This syndrome is commonly seen in sport-related situations.

        1. Injury, career termination, death of a loved one, loss of a relationship, change in playing status (i.e., demotion of status), change of a coach, change of academic status (i.e., high school to college), loss of a "big game," situational anxiety (i.e., "preperformance anxiety").

        2. Chronic adjustment disorders may be seen in overuse/overtraining syndromes, burnout, and failed physical rehabilitation (i.e., knee injuries).

        3. **Treatment**

          a. Psychosocial therapy (individual or group) can be extremely helpful with this "reactive" depression through a supportive and nurturing approach. Allow time for transition as this clinical situation usually abates.

          b. Pharmacotherapy is rarely indicated here.

    C. **Anxiety disorders**

        1. **Description:** Anxiety is characterized by subjective feelings of anticipation, dread, or apprehension or a sense of impending disaster associated with varying degrees of autonomic arousal and reactivity. Anxiety can lead to changes in behavior, playing an important role in learning and adaptation.

        2. **Generalized anxiety**

          a. Unrealistic or excessive anxiety and worry about various life circumstances

          b. Symptoms of motor tension (trembling, restlessness, easy fatiguability)

          c. Symptoms of autonomic hyperactivity (shortness of breath, dry mouth, sweating, etc.)

          d. Symptoms of vigilance and scanning ("on edge")

          e. **Differential diagnosis:**

             i. Hyperthyroidism, hypertension, caffeinism, unstable angina, substance abuse—stimulants, alcohol withdrawal, major depression, adjustment disorder.

    f. **Treatment:**

       i. **Pharmacologic:** Benzodiazepines are the treatment of choice. Tolerance develops to the sedative effects but not to their anxiolytic properties. These medications do have addictive properties. Combined treatment with antidepressant medication has also been useful.

      ii. **Psychosocial:**

         (a) Behavioral therapy (i.e., systematic desensitization, relaxation training, biofeedback) can be especially helpful

         (b) Individual psychotherapy

            (i) Psychoanalytical

            (ii) Cognitive (identification of irrational beliefs/thoughts).

3. **Obsessive compulsive disorder (OCD) is characterized by the presence of recurrent obsessions and compulsions with near magical thinking.**

    a. **Obsessions: thoughts or images that are involuntary, intrusive, and anxiety provoking. They often have sexual, violent, or derogatory connotations, provoke severe anxiety and may be described as ego-alien.**

    b. **Compulsions:** impulses to perform a variety of stereotyped behaviors or rituals that serve to reduce anxiety or get rid of obsessions (usually the patient experiences a sense of relief upon completing the act). The diagnosis of OCD should be made when these symptoms cause marked distress to the individual or interfere with social or occupational functioning. OCD is often chronic, beginning in childhood to young adulthood with marked variability in dysfunction. In athletes, it is common to see obsessive-compulsive personality traits/characteristics, but less common to see the full-blown disorder.

    c. **Differential diagnosis:** schizophrenia, major depression, exercise addiction, compulsive gambling, substance abuse (esp. alcohol abuse), obsessive-compulsive personality disorder.

    d. **Treatment:**

       i. **Psychosocial:**

         (a) Behavioral therapy: exposure, modelling, response prevention, thought stopping

         (b) Supportive psychotherapy, psychoanalytic psychotherapy.

      ii. **Pharmacotherapy:**

         (a) Antidepressants (imipramine, clomipramine, fluoxetine)

         (b) Monoamine oxidase inhibitors (i.e., Nardil, Parnate)

         (c) Anxiolytics may be used as adjuncts if anxiety is excessive.

D. **Panic disorders**

1. **Panic vs anxiety.** Panic is beyond normal experience, has a sudden onset without a clear precipitant, and is usually associated with physical symptoms (notably activation of the autonomic nervous system). Panic has a catastrophic quality that is not present in anxiety. These individuals have a sense of "impending doom" and may think they are going to die. Disorientation may be seen. Symptoms may last from a few minutes to a few hours.

2. **Panic disorder with agoraphobia**

    a. Panic symptoms *with* a fear of being in places or situations from which escape might be difficult (or embarrassing), or in which help might not be available in the event of a panic attack.

    b. **Common situations:** outside home alone, being in a crowd, travel in a bus/train/car. May be seen in the athlete who is fearful to travel away from his home environment.

    c. **Differential diagnosis:** cardiac arrhythmias, hypoglycemia (seen in athletes who have used dietary restriction), vertigo, drug/alcohol intoxication/withdrawal, hypochondriasis, generalized anxiety disorder, performance anxiety (adjustment disorder), hyperthyroidism.

   d. **Laboratory tests:**
      i. Provocative—lactate infusion induces panic.
      ii. Echocardiography—mitral valve prolapse syndrome may be seen in 8–20% of patients with panic disorder.
   e. **Pharmacotherapy:** Based on severity of attack, frequency, and amount of dysfunction (i.e., progressive) noted. May be especially useful for those who also have prominent depressive symptoms (along with psychotherapy).
      i. Antidepressants (MAOIs, imipramine).
      ii. Benzodiazepines (especially alprazolam [Xanax]) are most helpful because of their rapid onset and can be useful in early treatment at a time when psychosocial dysfunction is at its greatest.
      iii. Beta-blockers (propranolol [Inderal]): contraindicated in athletes with asthma; relative contraindication with heart disease (conduction abnormalities) and diabetes (masks hypoglycemia).
   f. **Psychosocial therapy**
      i. Supportive and insight-oriented approach can be helpful to deal with the psychosocial complications of the panic attacks.
E. **Phobias:** Seen more commonly in athletes than one might think. When panic attacks are present, they generally precede and are more troublesome than phobic symptoms—this combined disorder is now seen as primarily a panic disorder.
   1. **Agoraphobia** without history of panic disorder (as mentioned above):
      a. **Pharmacotherapy:** if panic occurs, same as above.
      b. **Psychosocial therapy:**
         i. Behavioral therapy
            (a) Relaxation response (progressive muscle relaxation, hypnosis, meditation, self-hypnosis, biofeedback, massage).
            (b) Exposure treatment (systematic desensitization, flooding).
         ii. Cognitive therapy
         iii. Psychodynamic psychotherapy
         iv. Support groups, family therapy
   2. **Social phobia:** Some individuals may have specific fears (fear of speaking in public), whereas others may have more general fears of being embarrassed, humiliated, scrutinized, or unable to perform while in public or at social functions (fear of being judged in competition). Key to diagnosis is that anxiety increases as the individual approaches the situation, which may be avoided or be endured with extreme anxiety. In sport situations, the anxiety is usually represented as tremulousness, or saying inappropriate things while in the competitive, feared environment.
      a. **Pharmacotherapy** (usually used only if refractory to psychotherapy)
         i. Benzodiazepines, i.e., anxiolytics.
         ii. Propranolol (has been on the list of "banned" substances in international competition(s) if used for enhancement of performance).
      b. **Psychosocial therapy**
         i. Desensitization through gradual exposure to the anxiety-provoking situation/stimuli. Use of the anxiety hierarchy is essential.
         ii. Psychotherapy if underlying emotional issues are a contributing factor
   3. **Simple phobia:** Usually starts in childhood. A persistent fear of a circumscribed stimulus (object or situation) other than the fear of having a panic attack (as in panic disorder), or of humiliation in social situations (as in social phobia). Exposure to the stimulus produces an immediate anxiety response. The object or situation is usually avoided and this avoidant behavior becomes more and more disruptive to the person's normal routine.
      a. **Pharmacotherapy is usually ineffective** unless panic symptoms are present.
      b. **Psychosocial:** as above, desensitization (progressive exposure) is vital, and insight-oriented approaches may be helpful as adjuncts.
   4. **General considerations of anxiety-related phenomena**
      a. Generalized anxiety—anxiety is chronic.
      b. Obsessive-compulsive—anxiety occurs when behaviors/thoughts resisted.

    c. Panic disorder—anxiety of sudden onset, without clear precipitants.

    d. Phobias—anxiety when confronting stimuli.

    e. Post-traumatic stress disorder—anxiety when trauma recalled.

F. **Post-traumatic stress disorder** is defined by the temporal relationship between a recognizable traumatic event and the development of symptoms that result in impairment of psychological, social, and physical function. Stressors involved are generally outside the range of normal experience (rape, sexual abuse, assault, traffic accidents, natural disasters, extraordinary athletic injury, etc.) and are not frequently seen in athletic populations.

    1. **Clinically one would see disturbances in these three areas:**

        a. The traumatic event is re-experienced.

        b. Numbing of general responsiveness.

        c. Persistent symptoms of increased arousal.

    2. In the athlete, it is not unusual to see **symptoms of physiologic reactivity (increased arousal)** upon exposure to events that symbolize an aspect of the traumatic event (i.e., a gymnast is "paralyzed" on the balance beam after having been previously abducted by a motorcyclist). Exaggerated startle responses are common as well as irritable, oppositional behavior, and difficulty concentrating.

    3. **Normal response to moderate trauma** (not necessarily out of range of human experience).

        a. Anxiety . . . depression . . psychosomatic reactions.

    4. **Common phases of response to severe trauma**

        a. Outcry (ranges from acute alarm to stunned ability to take in the meaning).

        b. Denial (weeks-months): see withdrawal, sleep disturbances, somatic symptoms.

        c. Intrusive (fear, anxiety): startle responses, increase reactivity.

        d. Working through (mourning of the loss or injury): examination of the meaning of the trauma; consideration of plans for coping in the future.

        e. Completion: recognize the impact of the trauma, hopeful about the future, resumption of normal activities.

        f. This process may take up to 2 years to work through. Delayed forms have a worse prognosis.

    5. **Differential diagnosis:** adjustment disorder (some overlap), substance abuse, brief reactive psychosis, panic disorder.

    6. **Prevention/treatment:**

        a. Assistance immediately following the trauma . . . supportive role.

        b. Support groups.

        c. Psychotherapy with an empathetic approach aimed at helping individual recognize connection between the trauma and other conflicts in their lives are generally successful.

        d. Pharmacotherapy may be needed in severe cases, especially if depression or anxiety is prominent.

G. **Personality disorders**

    1. **General considerations:** Everyone has a personality style or certain personality traits that distinguish them from others. This is of course not to say that everyone has a personality disorder. Personality traits are enduring patterns of perceiving, relating to, and thinking about the environment and oneself, and are exhibited in a wide range of important social and personal contexts. Personality disorders become evident when these traits become inflexible and maladaptive, and cause either significant impairment in social or occupational functioning or subjective distress. Usually this maladaptive behavior is evident by adolescence or young adulthood. **Most personality disorders can be grouped into these areas:**

        a. **Odd, eccentric behavior**

            i. Paranoid, schizoid, schizotypal (rarely seen in healthy athletes)

        b. **Dramatic, emotional, or erratic behavior**

            i. Histrionic (hysterical), narcissistic, antisocial, borderline (more common)

        c. **Anxiety, fear as manifestations**

            i. Avoidant, dependent, compulsive, passive-aggressive (more common).

2. **Clinical considerations in athletes**
   a. Manifestations of a personality disorder often develop under extreme or persistently stressful situations that are perceived as harmful to the athlete's self.
      i. **Injury** (i.e., patient sabotages his/her rehabilitation by overworking or missing appointments).
      ii. **Consistently poor performances with resultant worry** (i.e., acting out behavior at practice . . . not obeying rules, getting into fights, back-stabbing, not listening, being consistently late for practice, etc.).
      iii. **Demotion in playing status** due to objective drop off in actual performance (i.e., may have grandiose ideas of his/her playing abilities/ competence . . . narcissistic . . . with claims that the coach is off track or that others are out to get him/her . . . i.e., blaming of others).
   b. Frequently, one of the first and earliest signs that a personality disorder may be affecting an athlete is the subjective feeling in the *coaches* or *sports physician* of anger, frustration, and lack of being in control in dealing with the athlete's needs. This can be a very important insight to be aware of, and its recognition may be the difference between treatment success and failure.
3. **Specific disorders**
   a. **Borderline.** The clinical picture here is dramatic, with a pervasive pattern of mood instability, stormy interpersonal relationships, and disturbed self-image. Impulsivity, inappropriate anger, identity disturbance, chronic feelings of emptiness, and self-abusive behavior (drug use, suicidal gestures, rehabilitative abuse) may be seen. These are extremely challenging patients that probably need to be referred to a mental health specialist as part of the overall treatment plan.
      i. **Helpful hints:** Be consistent with your treatment plan, keep all scheduled appointments, use a "team" approach, explain all procedures, and try to be an empathetic listener without guaranteeing promises that you cannot keep (i.e., false hope).
   b. **Narcissistic.** Tendency to display rage, hypersensitivity to slights, boredom, and exploitive behavior are common. The narcissistic patient is usually aloof and arrogant, accompanied by a sense of entitlement (being special—"I get something for nothing in return"), with brooding preoccupations with issues of self-esteem.
      i. **Helpful hints:** Remember that the patient is in psychological "pain," a straightforward approach is necessary here, as one wants to avoid excessive "joking around" with the person in order to insure treatment compliance. Be "up-front" with behaviors that seem exploitive.
   c. **Histrionic.** Behavioral features of self-dramatization, emotional expressiveness, drawing attention to oneself, craving activity and stimulation, overreacting to minor events, and irrational outbursts—all occurring against a background of dependence and manipulation.
      i. **Helpful hints:** Avoid seductive interactions but encourage the patient to express "real" feelings about his/her treatment.
   d. **Passive-aggressive:** Characteristically, this person procrastinates, resists demands for adequate performance, finds excuses for delays, and finds fault with those he/she depends on, yet refuses to separate him/herself from dependent relationships. Passive, self-detrimental behavior may be an expression of personal conflicts through retroflexed anger. Lack of assertiveness and indirectness of need are common. Frequently, the clinician becomes enmeshed in trying to support the patient's many claims of unjust treatment.
      i. **Helpful hints:** fulfilling the demands of such patients is often to support their disorder, but refusing their demands is to reject them; try to point out consistently the probable consequences of passive-aggressive behaviors as they occur, and try not to get enmeshed in issues outside the treatment plan.

    e. **Other personality disorders seen in athletes:**
       i. **Antisocial**
       ii. **Obsessive compulsive disorder**
       iii. **Dependent**
       iv. **Avoidant.**
  4. **Management:**
    a. **Psychotherapeutic modalities are the primary intervention needed**
       i. **Individual psychotherapy** attempts to overcome resistance to establish a more healthy self.
       ii. **Family therapy** is especially helpful for adolescents and young adults when the family situation is enmeshed.
       iii. **Group therapy** is especially helpful when control is needed for acting-out or impulsive behavior.
    b. **Pharmacotherapy has limited usefulness** here unless there are symptoms of psychosis or major depression (i.e., borderline PD).
H. **Eating disorders** (see also Chapter 14)
  1. Anorexia nervosa
  2. Bulimia nervosa.
I. **Psychoactive substance abuse**
  1. **Alcohol**
  2. **CNS stimulants**
    a. Cocaine
    b. Amphetamine.
  3. **CNS depressants**
    a. Benzodiazepines, barbiturates, meprobamate (Miltown), ethchlorvynol (Placidyl), glutethimide (Doriden).
  4. **Anabolic steroids** (see Chapter 16)
  5. **Opioids** (heroin, morphine, methadone)
    a. Meperidine (Demerol), propoxyphene (Darvon), hydromorphone (Dilaudid), oxycodone (Percocet, Percodan), pentazocine (Talwin).
  6. **Hallucinogens**
    a. LSD, mescaline, psilocybin.
  7. **Arylcyclohexylamines**
    a. Phencyclidine (PCP).
  8. **Cannabinoids** (marijuana, hashish).
J. **Disorders of childhood and adolescence**
In addition to the disorders of adulthood previously discussed (which also apply to children and adolescents), there are a few clinical syndromes that one may see specifically in the child or adolescent who is also a competitive athlete. **Interestingly, because of the time and energy commitment to sport performance by young athletes, it is often in their sport performance and behavior that we see hints that may suggest underlying psychopathology.**
  1. **Symptoms and behaviors that may be indicative of underlying conflict:**
    a. Persistent oppositional behavior: defiant, devious (breaking rules, talking back, etc.).
    b. **Excessive fear:** One may see anxiety and extreme resistance to participate (especially with new skill acquisition).
    c. **Excessive anxiety:** May show up as a need for constant reassurance, lots of self doubt, somatic concerns—stomach problems, sickness, absence from practice, inability to relax.
    d. **Persistent irritability, defensiveness, mood changes:** One may see verbal and physical fights with coaches, teammates, parents. May be indicative of depression, anxiety, substance abuse, etc.
    e. **Lying, cheating behavior:** May be indicative of low self-esteem, personal problems, family problems, etc.
    f. **Frequent, seemingly hard-to-understand injuries:** May be indicative of confusion or dissatisfaction in the athlete owing to conflicts of interest,

interpersonal problems, unmanageable stress, or true questions regarding the motives for participation in sport (i.e., "Am I doing this for myself or someone/something else?").

2. **Evaluation of the child/adolescent: special considerations**
    a. **Care must be taken to consider the physiological and psychological development of the athlete** (i.e., developmental ages) in order to gain a true idea of what the problem is and the appropriateness of intervention strategies.
    b. **Family and social context(s)** are extremely important variables in these age groups.
        i. Example: **"the vicarious athlete":** parents and/or coaches who influence the young athlete in various ways (through pushing, discipline, manipulation) in an attempt, usually unconscious, to fulfill their own unmet needs.
    c. **Sources of information** must include the client, family, coaches, and school representatives.
    d. **Always include a substance abuse history as well as history of sexual and/or physical abuse** (as deemed appropriate).
3. **Clinical syndromes**
    a. **Attention deficit hyperactivity disorder**
        i. **Clinically manifested as:**
            (a) Attention deficits (high distractibility, can't concentrate)
            (b) Hyperactivity (high motor activity, "on the move constantly")
            (c) Coordination problems (in both fine and gross motor systems)
            (d) Impulsivity (sudden change in interest, stealing, substance abuse)
            (e) Perceptual problems (poor school performance in youngster with normal IQ)
            (f) Immature and domineering behavior.
        ii. **Evaluation:** careful listing of symptoms and conditions under their occurrence, pediatric evaluation, testing of motor skills and attention span, IQ testing, school and parent reports.
        iii. **Sports context.** Disorder may be seen in a young athlete who can't seem to sit still or follow instructions, or in an athlete that appears to have a disproportionate problem with learning and developing certain motor skills (i.e., beam routines in gymnastics, baseball swing, shooting baskets, etc.).
        iv. **Treatment:**
            (a) **General:** individual may need special education programs, special activities to enhance coordination and sensory organization, or supportive and directive psychotherapy if child views self as abnormal or worthless.
            (b) **Pharmacotherapy** (methlyphenidate [Ritalin], dextroamphetamine [Cylert]) **after psychiatric consultation.**
    b. **Oppositional defiant disorder**
        i. **General:** Not uncommonly seen in young athlete populations. Typically, one will see temper outbursts, frequent challenging/arguing of authority (i.e., the coach), easily annoyed by others, angry outbursts, use of obscenity, blaming of others for own mistakes, "bossy stubborness." Chronic oppositional behavior almost always interferes with interpersonal relationships and school and athletic performance.
        ii. **Differential diagnosis:** Rule out major depression and conduct disorder
        iii. This behavior can be both normal and adaptive at specific developmental stages and in response to situational crises. If related to a significant stressor, this is an adjustment disorder. However, in the disorder the symptoms are usually prolonged and not transient in nature.
        iv. **Treatment:**
            (a) Individual therapy and counseling with parents/coaches—emphasis is to help understand self-destructive nature of behavior, and one must work on self-esteem (which is typically low).

(b) Family therapy can be helpful for identification of stressors and patterns of behavior.

(c) **Helpful hint:** It is easy to be angry and turned off by this type of problem because this athlete/person threatens *your* authority. Remember, the youngster is telling *you* something, and a more understanding and empathetic approach is desirable. A one-to-one approach may help the youngster open up to you.

c. **Conduct disorder**

The essential feature is a "persistent pattern of conduct in which the basic rights of others and major age-appropriate societal norms or rules are violated." This disorder is one of the disruptive behavior disorders (along with *a* and *b* above).

   i. **Clinically, behavior patterns are repetitive, persistent,** and include stealing (with confrontation of the victim), lying, running away overnight, fire-setting, forced entry, destruction of other's property, cruelty to animals, sexual abuse, substance abuse, use of weapons in fights, frequent physical fights, and lack of regard for other people's sense of autonomy.

   ii. **Treatment approach:** referral to mental health system for evaluation and treatment . . . this person may need more acute care (i.e., hospitalization).

d. **Specific developmental disorders** (reading, arithmetic, language, etc.).

IV. **Intervention Strategies**

A. **General concepts:** It is important to note that there are numerous intervention strategies available for athletes to use in their attempts to solve problems, change or examine certain behaviors, relax, and enhance/maximize their overall performance both on and off the field. Care must be taken to individualize each athlete's program to maximize its effectiveness and to allow the athlete to take as active a part in the program as possible. An educational approach in which one carefully teaches the athlete the concepts of the various intervention techniques has been shown to be very helpful, in that it allows the athlete or team to take a dynamic, active part in his/her own growth and development through the use of these techniques. In order for the techniques to work, the athlete must believe in your ability to give him/her accurate information and he/she must be able to develop a trusting, nurturing, and empathetic relationship with you. Feedback from the sports medicine professional and the athlete is critical; **listen to the athlete.**

B. **Relaxation training**

1. **Concept:** One must realize that increased anxiety levels may hamper sport-related performance by causing muscular tension, nausea, inappropriate focus attention (i.e., easy distractibility), autonomic hyperarousal, and decreased psychological flexibility (i.e., resistance to change). Relaxation techniques can be helpful skills (i.e., they take practice just as do physical skills) in an attempt to decrease anxiety-arousal levels, and to minimize the stress-related anxiety that is common to nearly all sport behaviors.

2. **Types of relaxation training:**

a. **Deep breathing** is the most natural technique to use. When an athlete is tense or nervous, breathing typically will involve the upper chest and the accessory muscles of respiration. When relaxed, the athlete will use more diaphragmatic (i.e., stomach) breathing. The athlete should breathe at his/her own rate, deeply and slowly. As breathing becomes deeper and slower, the athlete will notice that he/she will become more and more relaxed.

b. **Progressive muscle relaxation (Jacobsen)** is usually used with deep breathing exercises and is based on understanding high and low muscle tension, the relative differences between the two, and the subsequent control over muscle relaxation that one can obtain with practice. It is helpful to move slowly through each muscle group until the desired relaxation response is obtained (tense toes, relax toes . . . tense quadriceps, relax quadriceps . . . etc.). Initially, this exercise is best done in a comfortable position and quiet location, but with practice the technique can be used even during competition. Background music without lyrics may be a helpful adjunct for the relaxation process (soothing). It is also helpful to practice this technique at least once or twice each day (especially before and after workouts, prior to bedtime, before competition, etc.) when learning the process. One must be patient!

    c. **Biofeedback** is a type of training that involves necessary physiological feedback (i.e., blood pressure, skin temperature, etc.) via a visual or auditory signal that indicates the athlete's present state of tension. Biofeedback can promote self-awareness by helping athletes become more aware of what causes tension, anxiety, and pain. This awareness can then help to give the athlete alternative ways of responding to particular stressors through the practice of new responses outside biofeedback sessions.

    d. **Autogenic training (Johannes Schultz)**
        i. The word autogenic comes from the Greek words meaning "self-create," implying that one should be able to have control over oneself with the help of one's own concentration. The starting point for autogenic training is the learned ability to exert control over mind and body through thought.
        ii. The process is twofold:
        (a) The first phase involves the use of self-suggestions or self-statements that are implemented to help with self-development (i.e., change behavior, improve attitude/mood, intensify motivation, etc.):
            Examples: "My mind is crystal clear"; "I feel secure"; "I feel strong, active, on the offensive." The self-suggestions can come in several forms: verbal (from oneself), verbal in the form of an imagined thought, auditory (i.e., audiotape), and visual (words as symbols). Once again, it is easier to achieve success with this technique while in a relaxed state, as described above.

    e. **Other techniques:**
        i. **Yoga**
        ii. **Meditation**
        iii. **Massage.**
        iv. **Exercise**

3. **Uses of relaxation training techniques**
    a. **Especially helpful for anxiety and stress-related phenomena** (i.e., anxiety, mood-depression, irritability, distractibility).
    b. Helpful in **pain management** and its relationship to injury and subsequent rehabilitation.
    c. Athlete should confer with his/her physician prior to initiation of a regular relaxation training program.
    d. Relaxation is a helpful preliminary exercise to learn if the athlete is planning to use visualization (visual imagery) as a part of a regular training program.
    e. Once again, if there are any questions regarding the implementation of these techniques, athlete should consult with his/her sport psychologist/psychiatrist/therapist.

C. **Visual/mental imagery (i.e., visualization)**
1. **Concept.** Many athletes have reported that just prior to performance they try to mentally picture themselves going through the forthcoming activity in their mind. Most athletes have an ability to picture in their minds certain aspects (either mechanical-technical or emotional) of their performance without even trying very hard to do so. Visualization can involve creating mental images of oneself, a particular idea, or a desired/experienced emotional response/feeling. The "visualization," in other words, can be used to produce mechanical and technical images of one's performance (past, present, future), *or* it can be used in a kinesthetic fashion to produce images of control, comfort, and relaxation (i.e., emotional).

This conceptual technique can be used with or without relaxation techniques, but relaxation often increases its effectiveness and adds to the learning effect of the training.

The use of visual imagery and its effectiveness remains controversial with regard to its direct effect on performance. Controlled studies are difficult to reproduce, and there are few observable data (i.e., reliance primarily on self-reports) to interpret when one is talking about the images we create in our minds. However, there is a growing body of athletes at all levels that personally attest to its effectiveness in their own training program(s). This technique will continue to stimulate research and development as a viable intervention tool in helping athletes maximize their performance.

2. **Visual-motor-behavioral rehearsal (Suinn) . . . VMBR**
   a. This technique combines deep breathing, muscle relaxation, and visualization in a step-by-step process of gaining control over arousal, stress-related anxiety, negative thoughts/disruptive thoughts, and energy levels (i.e., directing one's energy). It is designed to allow flexibility of thought processes in a relaxed state within each athlete so that he/she may maximize sport performance by learning how to appropriately direct thoughts and emotional energy with regard to performance.

D. **Hypnosis** is a form of attentive, receptive focal concentration with a sense of parallel awareness and a constriction in peripheral awareness. During this focused attention, the athlete is relatively open to receiving information and exploring the mind-body relationship. This approach can help facilitate the evaluation of an athlete's psychological resources for change and also help to adjust therapeutic strategies to the athlete's personal style and abilities. More, specifically, hypnosis has proven effective in the reduction of stress-related anxiety, a phenomenon encountered by nearly all competitive athletes.

E. **Cognitive training/self-regulation**

Most, if not all, athletes have specific vulnerabilities, particular stressors impinging on these vulnerabilities, and habitual patterns of reacting to various situations. Cognitive training can help identify, test the reality of, and correct distorted perceptual conceptualizations of certain beliefs. Cognitive training is based on the underlying theoretical rationale that the way individuals structure their experiences determines how they feel and behave.

The sports therapist plays a vital role in the training, as the proximal goal is to modify the athlete's bias in interpreting personal life experiences and making future predictions. This is attempted through a series of techniques including the **identification of automatic thoughts** (rapid thoughts usually preceding some affect such as anger, anxiety, etc.), **identification of cognitive errors** (i.e., arbitrary inferences, over-generalizations, etc.), **reality testing,** and **monitoring anxiety,** all of which are intended to give the athlete a healthier set of self-referring statements and beliefs (i.e., improve self-esteem/self-concept).

1. **A model of self-regulation (Kirschenbaum)**
   a. **Problem identification** (verbally noted, expressively written down).
   b. **Commitment to change** (to self and others).
   c. **Implementation/execution.** Specific plans are set up and carried out systematically, i.e., change in training routine, use of relaxation training, regular use of positive self-statements, etc.
   d. **Self-monitoring of progress,** including progression and setback . . . i.e., use of feedback for constant reevaluation (videotape, verbal feedback, performance diaries, etc.).
   e. **Generalization.** The hope that improvement and success in certain, specific areas will "generalize" to other areas of performance and/or life skills management.

2. **Uses:**
   a. Stress management, anxiety reduction
   b. Correcting performance flaws (technical or emotional)

       c. Breaking bad habits or undesired patterns of behavior

       d. Performance enhancement, personal growth (life skills management)

       e. Communication problems

       f. Negative attitudes, thoughts.

    3. **Other cognitive models**

       a. Covert conditioning/modeling

F. **Desensitization training**

    1. Desensitization is the gradual ability to tolerate or become insensitive to negative disturbances/situations that typically create a sense of heightened arousal that is uncomfortable (anxiety, fear, panic, etc.).

    2. It is helpful to **analyze performance behavior** and identify which situation(s) stimulate the exaggerated arousal that is uncomfortable. Examples might include:

       a. Balance beam series in front of judges.

       b. A technical free-throw in front of a hostile crowd during a basketball game.

       c. Teeing off at the first hole of the last round of a match-play golf tournament.

       d. Wrestling an opponent one has never been able to beat.

    3. A hierarchy of situations can then be identified and arranged by the athlete along a continuum of least anxious (bottom of the list) to most anxious (top of the list).

    4. With the use of relaxation techniques, the athlete then "desensitizes" him/herself to each situation, starting on the bottom of the list, until the situation can be tolerated with little/no anxiety. Interestingly, this process can be done either via de novo exposure (i.e., actual performance) or through the use of imagery (i.e., imagined situations), or a combination of both.

    5. Once the anxiety-provoking situation is tolerated, the athlete moves "up" the list systematically until the desired performance is obtained.

    6. **Uses:** The training is especially helpful for situational anxiety (i.e., free throws in basketball, hitting with two strikes in baseball, etc.) and phobias (i.e., fear of being judged harshly, fear of heights, etc.). This technique is used in various sport contexts to acclimate athletes to potentially stressful situations. For example:

       a. A professional football team practices with loudspeakers that bring in sound similar to that to be experienced in the upcoming game, which will be in a noisy, domed stadium.

       b. A gymnast practices her backhand spring series on a lower-set balance beam (with padding and with a spotter) before moving up to the competition balance beam (without padding, without a spotter).

       c. A baseball team plays intrasquad games with real-game situations prior to the start of the season.

G. **Motivational goal setting** is the systematic use of short/intermediate/long-term goals that are identifiable and realistic. The goals should be directed toward desired behavior(s) intended to enhance performance, facilitate personal growth, and feel good. It is important to set goals that have emotional or affective significance (i.e., "It feels good," "I want to do this badly," "I need to do this to improve my performance," etc.) in order to facilitate compliance with goal-setting programs.

    In addition, goal-setting programs will lose their effectiveness if they are not periodically re-evaluated and if there is no feedback mechanism put into place (i.e., contact with coaching staff regarding updates on goal-directed behavior).

    It can be helpful to conceptualize goals and/or behavior into four major areas.

    1. Before goals are set, one should **identify areas of strength and weakness (i.e., a "needs" assessment).** This can be done on an individual or team basis.

       a. Athletic/physical . . . athletic, physical skills

       b. Academic/professional/vocational . . . school, sport, work

       c. Social . . . self, friends, family, coaches, significant others, etc.

       d. Spiritual . . . faith, religion.

    2. **Set goals that are performance-related** (i.e., increased strength, increased speed, improved form, a particular score/time, etc.) rather than *strictly* outcome-

related (i.e., win-lose, national championship, etc.). Although general outcome goals can be important in a motivational setting, they are often difficult to put into objective form and can be difficult to apply to the daily setting of practice (physical and mental).

3. **Set goals that are realistic but allow athletes to be a little bit grandiose about what they think they are capable of doing.** Confer with teammates and/or coaches to make sure that they objectively concur with what the athlete thinks he/she is capable of. This process can be extremely helpful and allow the athlete to take risks that will not automatically result in failure.

4. **Be creative with goal-setting.** Make it challenging but fun and enjoyable.

5. Structure the environment for motivational training:
   a. Provide opportunity for skill development and fitness development.
   b. Create practices/games that are fun/exciting.
   c. Allow for socialization needs (i.e., friendship).
   d. Provide a realistic view of success and personal growth.
   e. Allow for athlete's feedback and ventilation.
   f. Provide constructive/specific criticism and positive reinforcement.
   g. Put a premium on open communication.
   h. Promote the use of self-evaluation.

H. **Psychological skills training** (PST) consists of techniques and strategies designed to teach and develop mental skills that facilitate high quality performance, a positive approach to sport competition, and personal growth. The premise is that athletes are generally mentally healthy, but they may benefit from learning cognitive skills that help them cope with the demands of sport and its competitive environment.

This process takes practice and patience. It requires receptiveness from the group/individual being worked with (i.e., players, coaches, trainers, etc.).

The process typically requires several years for players and teams to reach maximum effectiveness and for its acceptance into a regular practice/competition routine.

PST is based on an educational model that attempts to identify the key psychological skills that are usually needed to facilitate personal growth. Many of these skills may be sport-specific. The program then helps individuals develop these skills through the implementation of training methods (i.e., visual imagery, goal-setting, arousal control, etc.).

1. **Typical PST program (adapted from Vealey) for a sports team:**
   a. Overview, presentation of concepts, format
   b. Psychological skills assessment
      i. **Volition:** Why this is important to me.
      ii. **Awareness of self:** use of self-monitoring, self-inventories in major life skills areas (i.e., strengths, weaknesses): academic, athletic, social, spiritual.
      iii. **Self-esteem (Riedler):** understanding of oneself × adaptability to change.
      iv. **Arousal**—anxiety.
      v. **Attentional focus**—concentration.
      vi. **Stress management:** learning to anticipate stressful events.
      vii. **Communication skills/interpersonal skills.**
      viii. **Motivation,** i.e., concepts of goal-setting.
      ix. **Leadership:** personal challenge.
      x. **Lifestyle management.**
   c. **Methods of development**
      i. **Physical practice** (no substitute).
      ii. **Education.**
      iii. **Intervention strategies** (imagery, relaxation, thought control, cognitive-behavioral problem-solving, etc.).
   d. **Application to the sport setting** as well as life skills management.
      i. **Sport-specific** vs. general.

    e. **Constant use of feedback regarding effectiveness of program** (i.e., during and after the season).

      i. Adjustments for competition, variations in performance, problem areas that need more emphasis, injury, etc.

      ii. Use of videotape, self-report evaluations

    f. **Allowance for individual sessions as needed** (coaches, players) . . . i.e., crisis intervention.

    g. **Use of coaching staff to help implement program.**

    h. **Collection of data for evaluation, research.**

V. **Future Directions in Sport Psychology/Psychiatry**

    A. A shift to more community service-based programs.

    B. Premiums placed on certification and training for sports therapists.

    C. Integration into Sports Medicine.

    D. Acceptance at all competitive levels. Programs will become commonplace for the individual athlete and sports team.

    E. Work with athletes at all levels, not just the elite athlete, with special focus on youth development.

    F. Increased competition for services rendered.

    G. Practical application of knowledge through research.

    H. Educational development with coaches, athletes, and parents.

    I. More research with the "non"-athlete.

    J. Expansion of tools available to assess and assist athletes (e.g., psychometric testing, computer-assisted programs).

# Chapter 16: Drugs and Doping in Athletes

JAMES C. PUFFER, MD
GARY A. GREEN, MD

I. **Introduction**

A. **Definition:** Doping is the administration to, or the use by, a competing athlete of any substance foreign to the body or any physiological substance taken in abnormal quantity or by an abnormal route of entry into the body, with the sole intention of increasing in an artificial and unfair manner his performance in competition.[1]

B. **Historical perspective**
1. 1960—Danish cyclist Kurt Enemar Jensen dies during Summer Olympics in Rome from amphetamines and Roniacol.
2. 1964—International Olympic Committee (IOC) adopts definition of "doping."[2]
3. 1964—Tokyo becomes the first Olympiad to perform drug testing. Testing is on a spot basis only and nonpunitive. Several athletes found to be utilizing foreign substances. This led to the establishment of a banned substance list that has been modified and expanded repeatedly (Table 1).
4. 1968—Formal drug testing adopted for the Summer and Winter Olympics. Drug testing has been present at every Olympiad since then and the results are listed in Table 2.
5. 1972—U.S. swimmer Rick DeMont is stripped of gold medal for using ephedrine to treat underlying asthma.
6. 1986—Cocaine-related deaths of Maryland basketball player Len Bias and Cleveland Browns football player Don Rogers give impetus to expand drug testing for intercollegiate athletes.
7. 1988—Canadian Olympian Ben Johnson is stripped of his gold medal following a positive drug test for stanazolol. Engenders public support for investigating the use of anabolic steroids in all sports.

II. **Prevalence of Drugs in Athletics**

A. The scope of the problem has been investigated using self-reporting surveys at a variety of institutions. Purpose is to determine if athletes' drug use differs from the general population.
1. 1981—National Collegiate Athletic Association (NCAA) sanctioned study of the Big Ten Conference surveyed 1140 male athletes competing in four sports as compared to the general student population. Alcohol and marijuana use were similar, 80% and 20%, respectively, for both groups. However, 2% of the athletes, as compared to none of the nonathletes, admitted to using anabolic steroids.[3]
2. 1983—Clement surveyed 1687 Canadian Olympic athletes[4]:
   a. 5% used anabolic steroids.
   b. 21% considered using anabolic steroids.
   c. 10% used psychomotor stimulants.
   d. 57% used alcohol.
   e. 23% used marijuana.
   f. 4% used cocaine.
3. 1985—Anderson and McKeag from Michigan State evaluated 2,048 intercollegiate athletes from 11 schools[5] (Table 3). Drug use can be divided into four basic categories based on this study: anabolic steroids, stimulants, nonsteroidal anti-inflammatory drugs, and recreational drugs.

B. Based on these studies, various types of substances and doping methods will be explored as they relate to their use and abuse by athletes.

**TABLE 1.**   Restricted and Banned Substances and Methods

I. Doping classes
   A. Stimulants
      1. Psychomotor substances
      2. Sympathomimetic amines
      3. Miscellaneous CNS stimulants (including caffeine)
   B. Narcotics
   C. Anabolic steroids
   D. Beta-blockers
   E. Diuretics
   F. Growth hormone

II. Doping methods
   A. Blood doping
   B. Pharmacological, chemical and physical manipulation of the urine.

III. Classes of drugs subject to certain restrictions
   A. Alcohol*
   B. Local anesthetics[†]
   C. Corticosteroids[‡]
   D. Beta 2 agonists[§]

* Not prohibited, but levels (breath or blood) may be requested by an international federation.
† Permitted when medically indicated and documented in writing to IOC Medical Commission.
‡ Banned, except when used topically, via inhalation, locally, or intra-articularly and documented in writing to IOC Medical Commission (oral, intravenous, and intramuscular use banned).
§ Permitted in the aerosol or inhalant form for the treatment of asthma.

**TABLE 2.**   Olympic Game Doping Results

| Site/Year | Positive | No. Athletes Tested |
|-----------|----------|---------------------|
| Grenoble, 1968 | 0 | 86 |
| Mexico City, 1968 | 1 | 668 |
| Sapporo, 1972 | 1 | 211 |
| Munich, 1972 | 7 | 2079 |
| Montreal, 1976 | 11* | 2061 |
| Lake Placid, 1980 | 0 | N/A |
| Moscow, 1980 | 0 | 2200 |
| Sarajevo, 1984 | 1[†] | 408 |
| Los Angeles, 1984 | 11[‡] | 1520 |

* Eight samples positive for anabolic steroids.
† Positive for anabolic steroids.
‡ Ten samples positive for anabolic steroids.

**TABLE 3.**   Drug Use by Intercollegiate Athletes

| Drug | Percent of Athletes |
|------|---------------------|
| Alcohol | 88% |
| Amphetamines | 8% |
| Anabolic steroids | 6.5% |
| Anti-inflammatories | 31% |
| Caffeine | 68% |
| Cocaine | 17% |
| Marijuana | 36% |

III. **Anabolic Steroids**
  A. **Definition:** Testosterone or testosterone-like synthetic drugs that result in both anabolic and androgenic effects, e.g., increased protein synthesis (anabolism) and enhanced development of male secondary sexual characteristics (androgenic).
  B. **History:** Originally developed in the 1930s and used in World War II to help restore positive nitrogen balance to starvation victims.[6] Also, reportedly used by German troops to increase aggressiveness.[7] Introduced to world class athletics in the 1950s.[8]
  C. **Prevalence of use:** It is difficult to assess the number of athletes who use anabolic steroids due to the secretive nature of the practice.
    1. 1988—Buckley et al.[9] surveyed 12th grade male students from 150 high schools across the U.S. and received 3,403 responses, which corresponded to a 50% response rate.
      a. 6.6% used or had used anabolic steroids.
      b. 21% had obtained the drugs from a health professional.
      c. 35% of the users of anabolic steroids were not involved in a school-sponsored sport.
      d. The data from Buckley's study indicate that anabolic steroid use is prevalent in high schools and has broken out beyond traditional "power sports." Further data from Buckley's study are provided in Tables 4 and 5.
    2. There are probably today at least 1 million anabolic steroids users in the U.S. involved in a $100 million black market industry.[10]
  D. **Mechanism of action.**
    1. Anabolic steroids are bound by cytoplasmic proteins and transported to the nucleus. This activates DNA-dependent RNA polymerase and results in the production of messenger RNA for protein synthesis.[11]
    2. There have been numerous studies with anabolic steroids and male athletes that support both improvement in strength,[12–16] as well as no significant improvement in strength.[17–20] A review of these studies in 1984 by the American College of Sports Medicine led to the following conclusions[21]:
      a. In the presence of an adequate diet, anabolic steroids can contribute to increases in body weight and lean mass.
      b. The gains in muscular strength achieved through high-intensity exercise and proper diet can be increased by use of anabolic steroids in some individuals.
      c. Anabolic steroids do not increase aerobic power.
  E. **Potential therapeutic uses:** These uses include the treatment of refractory anemias, replacement therapy in hypogonadal males, and in the management of burn victims.

**TABLE 4.**  Age of High School Senior Respondents at First Use of Anabolic Steroids[9]

| Age | Percent |
| --- | --- |
| <15 | 38% |
| 16 | 33% |
| 17 | 26% |
| >18 | 3% |

**TABLE 5.**  Main Reasons for Using Anabolic Steroids[5]

| Reason | Percent |
| --- | --- |
| Improve performance | 47% |
| Appearance | 27% |
| Prevent or treat sports injury | 11% |
| Social | 7% |
| Other | 8% |

**TABLE 6.**  Two-month history of Anabolic Steroid Use by a Body-Builder[23]

| Drug | Dose | Therapeutic Dose |
|---|---|---|
| Methandrostenolone (Dianabol) | 75 mg subcutaneously every other day | 5 mg daily |
| Methenolone (Primabolin) | 150 mg subcutaneously every other day | |
| Oxandrolone (Anavar) | 20 mg orally daily | 2.5–10 mg daily |
| Oxymetholone (Anadrol) | 100 mg orally daily | 5–10 mg daily |

F. **Dosage**
  1. **When utilized by athletes, doses may be taken in amounts that are 10 to 40 times the therapeutic dose.**
  2. **Athletes frequently use combinations of anabolic steroids ("stacking") or cycling in a pyramidal fashion to achieve maximum effect.**[22] Table 6 describes the 2-month drug history of a body builder.[23]
G. **Adverse reactions:** The side-effects that are experienced in general depend on the amount of testosterone naturally secreted and the stage of development.
  1. **GI**—hepatocellular dysfunction, peliosis hepatis, case reports of hepatocellular carcinoma.[24] Hepatic effects are increased with the 17 alpha-alkylated compounds that are consumed orally.
  2. **Cardiovascular**—increase in total cholesterol, LDL cholesterol, decrease in HDL-cholesterol, hypertension,[21] and reported cases of myocardial infarction[25] and cerebrovascular accident.[26]
  3. **Psychologic effects**—changes in libido, mood swings, aggressive behavior.[21] A **dependence pattern** with opioid-type features has been reported.[23,27] Pope and Katz interviewed 41 body-builders and football players who had used anabolic steroids and, according to *DSM III-R* criteria, found that[28]:
     a. 9 subjects (22%) displayed a full affective syndrome.
     b. 5 subjects (12%) demonstrated psychotic symptoms in association with anabolic steroid use.
     c. The data suggested that major psychiatric symptoms are commonly associated with anabolic steroid use.
  4. **Male reproductive effects**—oligospermia, azospermia, decreased testicular size,[21] gynecomastia.[29] A case of adenocarcinoma of the prostrate has also been reported.[30]
  5. **Female effects**—reduced LH, FSH, estrogens, and progesterone; menstrual irregularities; male pattern alopecia; hirsutism; clitoromegaly; and deepening of the voice.[21] These last three are likely irreversible.
  6. **Youths—irreversible, premature closure of the epiphyses.**[21]
  7. **Miscellaneous**—spontaneous tendon rupture,[31,32] increase in sebaceous glands, and acne.[33] Infectious complications, including AIDS, resulting from the sharing of contaminated needles used with injectable anabolic steroids.
H. **Detection:** As the use of steroids has increased, so have the types of athletes who utilize them. No longer confined to the "power" sports, anabolic steroid use has been detected among many other sports. Clinical suspicion should be aroused by the presence of the above adverse affects. Drug testing, which is discussed later in this chapter, can detect anabolic steroids with a high degree of accuracy.

IV. **Human Growth Hormone**

  A. **Definition:** Human growth hormone (hGH) is a polypeptide hormone composed of 191 amino acids with a molecular weight of 21,500. Normally, 5–10 mg are stored in the anterior pituitary, and adult males have a production rate of 0.4–1.0 mg/day.[34]
  B. **History:** Animal breeders in the 1930s discovered that animals given crude extract of species-specific pituitary glands developed increased muscle mass, decreased body fat, and an accelerated growth rate. Researchers in the 1950s realized that hGH stimulated the production of somatomedins, which increased growth. With

the development of radioimmunoassay in 1961, hGH concentrations were first measured in the plasma. In 1985, the first of two synthetic hGH preparations were sold in the U.S.

C. **Prevalence:** With the growing effectiveness of gas chromatography and mass spectrometry in detecting anabolic steroids and testosterone, many athletes have turned to growth hormone. The prevalence of use is difficult to estimate, since there is no reliable method currently available for detecting exogenous hGH. However, the Food and Drug Administration (FDA) has become concerned due to an increasing number of complaints from endocrinologists and anecdotal reports from team physicians.[35] Evidence of hGH was reportedly found in urine specimens tested at the World Track and Field Championships in Helsinki in 1983, and it is thought to be widely used in football players and body-builders.[34]

D. **Mechanism:** Most of the work on the mechanism of action of hGH has been done on children with hypopituitarism. The scientific literature contains no documented reports of its use or effects on athletes.[34]
   1. **Function:** Administration of hGH to growth hormone-deficient children results in a positive nitrogen balance and a stimulation of skeletal and soft-tissue growth.[34]
   2. **Metabolic effects:** Growth hormone reduces glucose and protein metabolism and has a net anti-insulin effect by inhibiting the cellular uptake of glucose.[34] hGH also stimulates the mobilization of lipids from adipose tissue, and protein synthesis is greatly increased in hypophysectomized animals.[34]
   3. **Effects on muscle:** Several studies have been done that lead to conflicting data on the effect of hGH on muscle.[36–38] A series of animal experiments by Goldberg concluded that growth hormone increased the basal metabolic rate of protein synthesis, but that protein synthesis was also determined by the amount of muscular work.[39] It is difficult to predict the ability of growth hormone to increase contractile elements and improve the performance of normal muscle in normal humans.[34]

E. **Therapeutic uses:** It is clear that hGH is effective in increasing the stature of growth hormone-deficient children[40] and can also increase the rate of growth in some short-statured children who are not hGH deficient.[41,42] It is estimated that in the U.S. the maximum number of people who fit these criteria is approximately 9,000.[35]

F. **Dosage:** Although little information exists concerning athletes' usage of hGH, there have been reports of athletes consuming 20 times the dosage recommended for therapeutic purposes.[35] The therapeutic dose in deficiency states is 0.06 mg/kg three time a week by the intramuscular route,[43] or 1 mg/day in a 50 kg individual. There have been estimates that an 8-week supply would cost between $1,000 and $1,500.[35] Cost alone may discourage athletes from abusing hGH.

G. **Adverse reactions**
   1. **Acromegaly** is a potential serious side effect in those abusing megadoses of hGH. It is estimated that acromegalic patients with hGH concentrations of 5–30 ng/ml have production rates of 1.5–9 mg/day.[44] As little as a twofold increase in the recommended dose may result in acromegaly, leaving a narrow therapeutic window. With athletes consuming up to 20 mg per day, the risk of acromegaly is significant. Complications of acromegaly include diabetes, arthritis, myopathies, and the characteristic coarsening of the bones of the face, hands, and feet.[34]
   2. Formation of **antibodies to hGH** is common and **hypothyroidism** has occurred.
   3. **Creutzfeldt-Jakob disease** has occurred from the use of growth hormone derived from cadaveric pituitary glands.[45] While the use of synthetic hGH will eliminate this problem, athletes often obtain substances from black market sources, thereby increasing their risk for this catastrophic neurologic disorder.

H. **Detection:** hGH has recently been banned by the IOC. However, there currently exists no reliable method of detecting hGH. Team physicians should rely on their clinical suspicion based on the various potential adverse effects.

### V. Amphetamines

A. **Definition:** Amphetamines are stimulants that can be classified as indirect-acting sympathomimetic amines, which have central and peripheral effects.[46]

B. **History:** Amphetamines were first utilized in the 1930s in the treatment of nasal congestion, narcolepsy, and obesity.[46] Experiments describing the effects on human performance were conducted in the 1950s, and the popularity of the drug increased. As previously noted, the Danish cyclist Jensen died during the 1960 Summer Olympics from an overdose of amphetamine.

C. **Prevalence:** Anderson and McKeag found in 1985 that 8% of intercollegiate athletes had utilized amphetamines in the previous year.[5] During that time period, one-third of that group had used amphetamines at least 6 times. Mandell described the "Sunday syndrome" in professional football players who abuse these drugs.[47]

D. **Mechanism of action: Several theories have been proposed** to explain the central and peripheral effects of amphetamines.[46]
   1. Increased liberation of endogenous catecholamines.
   2. Displacement of bound catecholamines.
   3. Inhibition of monamine oxidase.
   4. Interference with catecholamine reuptake.
   5. Production of false neurotransmitters.
      All probably contribute to observed physiologic responses, including increases in blood pressure and heart rate, bronchodilation, increased metabolic rate, and increased free fatty acid production.

E. As amphetamines relate to **athletic performance,** the literature contains contradicting data.
   1. Smith and Beecher reported that 75% of trained swimmers, weight throwers, and runners had improved performance after taking amphetamines.[48]
   2. Chandler demonstrated no substantial improvement in athletic performance.[49]
   3. The explanation for this contradiction may be that tasks that were simple and repetitive resulted in enhanced performance with amphetamines, whereas more complicated maneuvers did not.

F. **Therapeutic uses:** Amphetamines have been used legitimately to treat many conditions. Some of these include refractory obesity, narcolepsy, attention deficit disorder, and severe depression.[46] The high abuse potential of these drugs has limited their utility in these conditions.

G. **Dosage:** When taken orally, amphetamines exert their effects within 30 minutes of ingestion; however, their actions can last for 12 to 24 hours.[46] Dosages are variable, depending on the athlete and type of preparation.

H. **Adverse reactions**
   1. **Central nervous system**—restlessness, insomnia, psychological addiction, psychosis, tremor, anxiety, dizziness, and cerebral hemorrhage.
   2. **Cardiovascular**—lowered threshold for arrhythmias and provocation of angina.
   3. **Miscellaneous**—disruptions in thermoregulation and predisposition to heat illness.

I. **Detection:** Amphetamines are readily detected by urine drug testing, as both unchanged amphetamines and metabolites appear in the urine.[46]

### VI. Cocaine

A. **Definition:** Cocaine is a naturally occurring alkaloid that is derived from the leaves of the *Erythroxylon coca* plant.[50] Although it is a topical anesthetic, it also acts as a CNS stimulant. This has led to its use by athletes as an ergogenic aid.

B. **History:** Cocaine was referred to as the "divine plant of the Incas"[51] and many scientific treatises were written on the subject in the late 19th century. Cocaine use has followed cyclical peaks since that time, with the current epidemic one further episode. National attention was captured by the deaths of athletes Len Bias and Don Rogers and the revelations of cocaine use by basketball player Gary McClain.

C. **Prevalence**
   1. 30 million Americans have tried cocaine, and there are 5 million regular users.[52]
   2. Anderson and McKeag found that 17% of the athletes in their survey had used cocaine in the previous 12 months.[5]
   3. *The New York Times* in 1987 stated, "Cocaine has probably joined rotator-cuff injuries, torn ligaments, and broken bones as a potential occupational hazard for athletes."[53]
D. **Mechanism**
   1. Cocaine acts by increasing the release and blocking the re-uptake of norepinephrine from neurons in the nervous system.
   2. Increased availability of epinephrine causes euphoria, increased blood pressure, tachycardia, and lowered threshold for seizures and ventricular arrhythmias.
   3. Cocaine may cause hyperglycemia, hyperthermia, and an increased peripheral reflex speed.[54]
   4. Cocaine stabilizes axonal membranes and blocks nerve impulse initiation and conduction.[55] Combined with its properties as a vascoconstrictor, cocaine is an excellent topical anesthetic.
E. **Therapeutic uses:** Although scientists of the 19th century hailed cocaine as a cure for a variety of ailments from hemorrhoids to broken bones, its legitimate use is now limited to its properties as a topical anesthetic.
F. **Dosage:** Cocaine is readily absorbed by the intravenous, intranasal, and pulmonary routes. Recreational users of intranasal cocaine can use 1 to 3 g per week.[54] In order to mimic the intense high associated with intravenous use, but without the complications of needles, cocaine users have turned to smoking the substance. This began with the smoking of the free alkaloid form, known as "free base." Recently, the use of ready-to-smoke, low-priced, free base ("crack") cocaine has led to epidemic smoking in urban areas.[56] The effect of crack is rapid and lasts only 5 to 10 minutes. The half-life of cocaine is 2 to 6 hours and can be detected in the urine for 3 to 5 days.
G. **Adverse reactions**
   1. **Cardiovascular:** The increased levels of catecholamines that are associated with cocaine use can directly induce ventricular dysrhythmia, coronary vasospasm with thrombosis, and myocardial infarctions,[54,57] all of which can lead to sudden death, even in those patients without underlying heart disease. Aortic rupture has also been reported, as well as cerebrovascular accidents.[54]
   2. **Central nervous system:** Chronic use can result in agitation, insomnia, and tremulousness. Toxic psychosis, severe depression, paranoia, and dysphorias have been reported,[54] as well as **rapid addiction.**
   3. **Respiratory system:** When taken intranasally, cocaine can cause swelling of the nasal mucosa, rhinitis, sinusitis, epistaxis, and nasal septal necrosis. Bronchitis and bronchiolitis obliterans with organizing pneumonia has been reported.[58]
   4. **Considerations in athletes:** Cocaine has direct effects on central thermoregulation, and an athlete exercising in the heat would be susceptible to hyperthermia. It has recently been proposed that the elite sprint-trained athlete may be at greater risk for severe lactic acidosis and cocaine-induced seizures due to the higher percentage of glycolytic muscle fibers.[59]
H. **Detection:** Cocaine is readily detectable by most drug testing. According to the data from Anderson and McKeag, most cocaine users do not participate in drug use with teammates.[5] It may be difficult for coaches, trainers, or team physicians to detect patterns of cocaine usage.

VII. **Caffeine**

A. **Definition:** Caffeine is a naturally occurring plant alkaloid derived from aqueous extracts of *Coffea arabica* and *Cola acuminata*.[46] It is classified as a CNS stimulant and is found in coffee, tea, and cola drinks. Caffeine is a xanthine and chemically related to theobromine and theophylline. It has been used by athletes for its stimulant properties and potential for increased work and power.

B. **History:** The discovery of caffeine-containing plants that could be made into beverages was probably by paleolithic man.[60] Caffeine has been touted throughout history for its stimulant and antisoporific effects.

C. **Prevalence**
1. Coffee is consumed in 98% of American homes, and the average annual consumption is 16 pounds per person.[46]
2. Although 68% of athletes in Anderson and McKeag's study used caffeine, 82% of the users consumed caffeine three times or fewer per day.[5]
3. Significant amounts of caffeine were found in large numbers of athletes competing in the 1976 Summer Olympic Games in Montreal.[61]

D. **Mechanism of action:** Caffeine is rapidly absorbed and peak levels are achieved in 30 to 60 minutes with a half life of 3.5 hours.[46] General effects include:
1. **GI**—increased gastric acid, pepsin, and small intestine secretion.
2. **Cardiovascular**—tachycardia, tachyarrhythmias, increased stroke volume, cardiac output, and resting blood pressure.
3. **Miscellaneous**—increased diuresis.[46]

E. **Performance:** The increased work and power probably result from:
1. Increased mobilization of free fatty acids.
2. Increased rate of lipid metabolism.[62]
3. Direct effects on muscle contraction secondary to increases in calcium permeability of the sarcoplasmic reticulum.[63]
   Overall, there has been controversy about the ability of caffeine to enhance or prolong work output, and recent studies cast doubts on its effectiveness.[64,65] If there is a benefit in athletic performance, it is limited to endurance activities.[46]

F. **Therapeutic uses:** Caffeine has been utilized as a stimulant in fatigue states, in combination with analgesic compounds, and in diet pills.[46] Table 7 provides information concerning the caffeine content of certain over-the-counter medications.

G. **Dosage:** The IOC has recently set the maximum urinary concentration of caffeine at 12 $\mu$g/ml. A recent study found that in order to exceed that threshold, an individual needed to consume almost 1000 mg of caffeine within 3 hours of testing.[66] The average daily consumption of caffeine per day is approximately 200 mg.[60] It can therefore be assumed that if an athlete has a level above 12 $\mu$g/ml, it is not the result of mere social imbibing of caffeine. Caffeine concentration as it relates to urinary levels is provided in Table 7.

H. **Adverse reactions**
1. **Central nervous system**—anxiety, hypochondriasis, insomnia, headache, tremors, depression, scotomata, and addiction with withdrawal states.[46]
2. **Cardiovascular**—tachyarrhythmias, especially paroxysmal atrial tachycardia, tachycardia.[46]
3. **Renal**—diuretic effect that is of significance in athletes at risk of dehydration.

I. **Detection:** Caffeine can be detected by drug screening and is banned by the IOC at concentrations above 12 $\mu$g/ml. The NCAA allows a maximum level of 15 $\mu$g/ml.

**TABLE 7.**  Caffeine Content of Commonly Used Substances

| Substance | Caffeine Concentration (mg/ml) | Caffeine Level* ($\mu$g/ml) |
|---|---|---|
| Coffee | 55–85 | 1.5–3 (1 cup) |
| Tea | 55–85 | 1.5–3 (1 cup) |
| Cola | 10–15 | 0.75–1.5 (1 cup) |
| Medications | | |
| Cafergot | 100 mg/tablet | 3–6 |
| NoDoz | 100 mg/tablet | 3–6 |
| Anacin | 32 mg/tablet | 2–3 |
| Midol | 32 mg/tablet | 2–3 |

\* Level dependent on size of athlete and rate of metabolism. These figures represent general estimates based on average size and rate of metabolism.

**TABLE 8.** Some of the Many Common Drugs Containing Sympathomimetic Amines

| | | |
|---|---|---|
| Actifed | Dristan | Primatene |
| Contac | Drixoral | Sinu-tab |
| Co-Tylenol | Entex | Sudafed |
| Dexatrim | Phenergan | |

VIII. **Sympathomimetic Amines**

A. **Definition:** Sympathomimetic amines are synthetic congeners of naturally occurring catecholamines.[67] In addition to amphetamines, there are several other weaker sympathomimetic amines that have the potential to be abused by athletes. Examples include phenylpropanolamine, phenylephrine, ephedrine, and pseudoephedrine. Table 8 lists some over-the-counter medications that contain sympathomimetic amines.

B. **History:** The discovery of epinephrine in 1899 led Barger and Dale to the study of synthetic amines in 1910, which were termed "sympathomimetic."[60] Their research suggested that these compounds had an indirect effect on nerve endings.

C. **Prevalence:** Sympathomimetic amines appear in a variety of cold remedies, common nasal and ophthalmologic decongestants, and most asthma preparations. The previously mentioned case of Rick DeMont's disqualification for ephedrine focused attention on the potential use of sympathomimetic amines by athletes.

D. **Mechanism of action:** The response of sympathomimetic amines depends on the relative selectivity of the drug, e.g., alpha, beta 1, or beta 2 agonists.
   1. Alpha effects—smooth muscle contraction, primarily vasoconstriction.
   2. Beta 1 effects—production of intracellular cAMP, and increased heart rate and strength of contraction.
   3. Beta 2 effects—smooth muscle relaxation, bronchodilation, stimulation of skeletal muscle.[67]
      Although earlier scientific studies demonstrated that the use of ephedrine resulted in improved athletic performance, three recent studies have shown no significant increases in performance.[62,68,69]

E. **Therapeutic uses:** The many uses of sympathomimetic amines include the treatment of allergic reactions, asthma, hypotension during spinal anesthesia, atrioventricular block, and nasal congestion.[46]

F. **Dosage:** The many types of drugs in this category have varying potencies and duration of actions.

G. **Adverse reactions:** With increasing doses, anxiety, epigastric distress, palpitations, tremulousness, and both insomnia and drowsiness have been shown to occur.[43]

H. **Detection:** Sympathomimetic amines are banned by the IOC and can be detected by drug testing. The IOC allows the use of inhaled selective beta 2 agonists, terbutaline, albuterol, bitolterol, orciprenaline, and rimiterol. These subtances are not banned by the NCAA.

IX. **Nonsteroidal Anti-inflammatory Drugs**

A. **Definition:** Nonsteroidal anti-inflammatory drugs (NSAIDs) are a class of drugs that have analgesic and anti-inflammatory properties by virtue of their inhibition of prostaglandin synthesis.[70]

B. **History:** NSAIDs are synthetic derivatives of salicylates, which were first isolated from the willow bark in 1829.[60] Although salicylates possess antipyretic properties, the introduction of indomethacin in the 1960s was the first drug of its class to be marketed for anti-inflammatory effects.

C. **Prevalence:** In 1984, more than 26 billion tablets of NSAIDs were consumed in the U.S., including aspirin and over-the-counter ibuprofen.[71] Given their use in soft-tissue injuries, it is not surprising that Anderson and McKeag found that 31% of their sample used these drugs.[5]

D. **Mechanism of action:** Although the exact mechanism is uncertain, inhibition by NSAIDs of the synthesis of prostaglandins has several effects.[70]

1. Inhibition of superoxide generation.
2. Competition with prostaglandins for binding at receptor sites.
3. Inhibition of leukocyte migration.
4. Inhibition of the release of lysosomal enzymes from leukocytes.
5. Interactions with the adenylate cyclase system.
    The effects of these actions is to ameliorate soft-tissue inflammation. In addition, NSAIDs have been shown to uncouple oxidative phosphorylation in skeletal muscle.[72]

E. **Therapeutic uses:** NSAIDs are useful as an adjunct to the treatment of tendinitis, sprains, strains, and other soft-tissue derangements. In addition, they are used in the treatment of rheumatoid arthritis, other rheumatologic conditions, degenerative joint disease, acute and chronic pain, and dysmenorrhea.[70]

F. **Dosage:** A variety of NSAIDs exist today, including the over-the-counter medications aspirin and ibuprofen. Variable half-lives can allow for once-daily dosing.

G. **Adverse reactions**
1. **Gastrointestinal:** GI upset that causes the discontinuation of NSAIDs has been reported in 2-10% of patients with rheumatoid arthritis.[73] Effects include nausea, dyspepsia, gastritis, ulceration, bleeding, and hepatotoxicity.
2. **Renal**—increased serum creatinine, sodium and water retention, hyperkalemia, papillary necrosis, interstitial nephritis, proteinuria, and acute renal failure. Of note is that renal disease appears more frequently in those patients who take NSAIDs while they are hypovolemic.
3. **Hematologic**—bone marrow suppression, reversible inhibition of platelet aggregation, and possible decreased coagulation.
4. **Central nervous system**—headache, tinnitus, dizziness, sedation.[70]
5. **Considerations in athletes:** Uncoupling oxidative phosphorylation can affect oxygen consumption and directly stimulate ventilation, promote sweating and dehydration, and lead to heat illness.[72]

H. **Detection:** All NSAIDs are allowed by both the NCAA and IOC.

X. **Alcohol**

A. **Definition:** Ethanol is the most abused recreational drug in the U.S. and is classified as a depressant.

B. **History:** The fermenting and imbibing of alcohol has been known since ancient times and in the Middle Ages alcohol was thought to be the elixir of life.[60]

C. **Prevalence:** Approximately 70% of adult Americans drink alcohol and the per capita consumption is estimated to be 2.7 gallons per year. Perhaps 5-10% of these drinkers are, or will become, alcoholics, and there are 200,000 annual alcohol-related deaths.[74] The Michigan State study demonstrated that alcohol was far and away the most used drug among intercollegiate athletes.[5]

D. **Mechanism of action:** The physiologic effects of alcohol are well known and will not be reviewed here.

E. **Therapeutic uses:** There are currently no therapeutic uses indicated for ethanol.

F. **Dosage:** The American Medical Association defines alcoholism as "an illness characterized by significant impairment that is directly associated with persistent and excessive use of alcohol. Impairment may involve physiological, psychological or social dysfunction."[74]

G. **Adverse reactions:** Physicians are familiar with the many adverse consequences of alcohol abuse. Following a review of the literature, the American College of Sports Medicine issued a statement regarding the use of alcohol as it relates to athletic performance.[75]
1. The acute ingestion of alcohol has a deleterious effect on many psychomotor skills, including reaction times, hand-eye coordination, accuracy, balance, and complex coordination.
2. Alcohol consumption does not substantially influence physiologic functions crucial to physical performance ($VO_2$ max, respiratory dynamics, cardiac function).

3. Alcohol ingestion will not improve muscular work capacity and may decrease performance levels.

4. Alcohol may impair temperature regulation during prolonged exercise in a cold environment.

   A recent study has also concluded that alcohol is toxic to striated muscle in a dose-dependent manner.[76]

H. **Detection:** Except for shooting events (including the modern pentathlon), neither the NCAA nor the IOC specifically tests for the presence of alcohol. However, breath or blood levels may be determined at the request of an International Federation. Since the effects of alcoholism may take 5 to 20 years to develop and usually occur after age 30, early identification of those athletes with alcohol problems is imperative. Given the negative effects on performance, education is a key role in helping to prevent this problem in athletes.

## XI. Marijuana

A. **Definition:** Marijuana is a naturally occurring cannabinoid containing the active ingredient delta-9-tetrahydrocannabinol (THC). It is currently an illegal drug that is used recreationally as a euphoriant.

B. **History:** Marijuana has been utilized by many cultures for centuries for its mind-altering properties.[77] In the U.S., marijuana has enjoyed popularity over the past 25 years.

C. **Prevalence:** It is estimated that 43 million Americans have tried marijuana and at least 17 million are regular users.[78] Of the 36% of athletes who had used marijuana in the study by Anderson and McKeag, 83% had first tried the drug in junior high or high school.[5]

D. **Mechanism of action:** THC exerts its effects on a variety of tissues, with the CNS and cardiovascular system being most prominent. Effects are dependent on the route, dose, setting, and prior experience of the user.

   1. **Cardiovascular:** Tachycardia is dose-related and can be blocked by propranolol. In addition, increased systolic blood pressure while supine and decreased standing blood pressure are seen.[60]

   2. **Central nervous system**—impaired motor coordination, decreased short-term memory, difficulty concentrating, and a decline in work performance.

   3. **Male reproductive system**—decreased plasma testosterone, gynecomastia, and oligospermia.[79]

E. **Therapeutic uses:** THC has been utilized as an antiemetic agent in conjunction with chemotherapy for cancer patients and for lowering the intraocular pressure in glaucoma.[60]

F. **Dosage:** The THC content of marijuana in the United States can range from 0.5–11%, and the serum concentration is dependent on the smoking technique employed by the user.[60]

G. **Adverse reactions:** There have been well-publicized studies on the side-effects associated with marijuana use. Renaud and Cormier studied the effects on exercise performance.[80]

   1. Reduction of maximal exercise performance, with premature achievement of $VO_2$ max.

   2. No effects on tidal volume, arterial blood pressure, or carboxyhemoglobin as compared to controls.

   3. In addition, marijuana causes inhibition of sweating that can lead to an increase in core body temperature.[60]

H. **Detection:** Marijuana is not banned by the IOC, but it is considered a street drug by the NCAA and is banned. Because of its high lipid solubility, marijuana can be detected for as long as 2–4 weeks by drug testing. Depending upon the concentration sensitivity, passive inhalation could result in a positive test.

## XII. Blood Doping

A. **Definition:** Blood is removed from an athlete and stored in a frozen state, and the individual's red cell mass is allowed to re-equilibrate. Following this, the donated red cells are reinfused, with a resultant increase in red cell mass. Also known as **blood boosting** or **blood packing.**

B. **History:** The earliest report in the medical literature described the infusion of 2000 ml of freshly transfused blood from matched donors to armed forces personnel in 1947.[81] Although a 34% increase in endurance over controls was demonstrated, subsequent studies using refrigerated blood failed to reproduce the results. Later researchers were able to show more impressive results when the blood was frozen at minus 80 degrees C.

C. **Prevalence:** The actual extent of blood doping is unknown; however, there have been widespread rumors of this practice for the past 20 years. The admission by the United States Olympic Committee that 7 U.S. cyclists had engaged in this practice at the 1984 Summer Olympic Games led to widespread publicity.

D. **Mechanism of action:** Transfusion increases the oxygen delivery to exercising muscle, and studies confirm that red cell mass and $VO_2$ max are well correlated.[82] Studies of blood doping in elite runners as compared to controls demonstrated[83]:
   1. Improvement in maximal oxygen consumption.
   2. Increased total exercise time.
   3. Increased hemoglobin concentration.

E. **Therapeutic uses:** Red cell transfusions are limited to those patients with symptomatic anemia.

F. **Dose:** Most studies have utilized 2000 ml of homologous blood or 900 to 1800 ml of cryopreserved autologous blood.[84]

G. **Adverse reactions:** Improperly matched donor blood can result in transfusion reactions that can be fatal. Immune side-effects are reported in 3% of all transfusions.[83] Using donor blood has the attendant risks of infectious complications. There is substantially lower risk with the use of autologous blood.

H. **Detection:** The IOC banned blood doping, but enforcement of this policy is limited by the lack of an effective technique for its detection. Although blood doping is not a "foreign substance," it is a "physiologic substance taken in abnormal quantity an by an abnormal route . . . with the sole intention of increasing in an unfair and artificial manner . . . performance," and therefore violates the IOC definition of doping.

XIII. **Bicarbonate or Phosphate Loading**

A. **Definition:** The ingestion of bicarbonate or phosphate to favorably alter physiologic parameters to improve performance.

B. **History:** These two substances have been recent arrivals within the spectrum of ergogenic aids.

C. **Prevalence:** The extent that these compounds are used is not currently known.

D. **Mechanism of action**
   1. **Bicarbonate loading:** Lactic acid produced during anaerobic metabolism is buffered by bicarbonate. A decrease in intramuscular pH restricts glycolysis and lipolysis, resulting in a decrease in energy production. Studies using endurance athletes given 0.3 g/kg of oral bicarbonate (as compared to placebo) demonstrated:[85]
      a. Increased serum pH before, after, and 3 minutes after exhaustive treadmill exercise.
      b. Run time to exhaustion was significantly increased.
   2. **Phosphate loading:** Increasing serum phosphate causes an increase in red blood cell 2,3 diphosphoglycerate (2,3 DPG) levels, with a resultant shift in the oxygen-hemoglobin curve to the right, and increases oxygen to the tissues. In order to raise serum phosphate, Cade loaded highly trained athletes with 1 g of sodium phosphate four times a day over 3 consecutive days and compared this with placebo. He found[86]:
      a. Significantly increased serum phosphate and red cell 2,3 DPG.
      b. Increased maximum oxygen uptake correlating with the rise in 2,3 DPG.

F. **Dosage:** Studies have utilized 0.3 g/kg of bicarbonate and 1 g of sodium phosphate qid, respectively.

G. **Adverse reactions:** Overdosage of these substances can lead to acid-base disturbances and electrolyte imbalances, depending on the salt utilized.

H. **Detection:** Although neither of these substances is specifically banned, their use violates the IOC definition of doping.

XIV. **Drug Testing**

A. **Purpose:** Drug testing has been the major means of attempting to enforce compliance with a banned substance list. Public awareness has been heightened by positive tests in elite athletes. To date, most drug testing has been of the "announced" variety at championship or Olympic events.

B. **Cost:** Organized athletics has devoted great expense towards the testing of athletes.
   1. $3 million was spent on equipping the drug-testing laboratory in Montreal in 1976.
   2. $1.8 million was spent to fund the UCLA Olympic Analytic Laboratory in Los Angeles for the 1984 Games.
   3. $1 million is spent annually for the NCAA to test athletes.

C. **Reliability:** Several types of tests are available that vary regarding specificity, sensitivity, and expense.
   1. **Thin-layer chromatography (TLC):** This is the least-expensive screening test, but also has less specificity and cannot provide positive identification of a substance. The Centers for Disease Control reviewed 13 laboratories using TLC and found that the laboratories were often unable to detect drugs at concentrations called for by their contracts.[87]
   2. **Radioimmunoassay (RIA) and enzyme-multiplied immunoassay (EMIT):** These are the two most commonly used screening methods. During the 1984 Olympic Games, RIA was used as a screening test for amphetamines, morphine, and benzoylecgonine.[88] Although manufacturers claim a 97–99% accuracy rate, such is not usually the case. In order to avoid false-positive tests when an athlete's career may be at stake, a second, highly sensitive, and highly specific test is required.
   3. **Gas chromatography/mass spectroscopy (GC/MS):** Provides the "gold standard" and is the only drug test that is legally admissible in court. All state-of-the-art laboratories must use GC/MS as a confirmatory test, since it provides a "fingerprint" of the detected substance. At the 1984 Olympics, GC alone was used as a screen for volatile and nonvolatile agents, GC/MS screened for anabolic steroids, and all positives underwent a confirmatory GC/MS.[88] Unfortunately, the high cost of both the equipment and the test prohibits most smaller laboratories from using GC/MS.

D. **Testing for anabolic steroids/testosterone:** In order to combat the use of exogenous testosterone, the ratio of testosterone to epitestosterone has been quantified. The normal ratio of testosterone to its isomer epitestosterone is one-to-one. However, when exogenous testosterone is administered, serum testosterone is elevated out of proportion to epitestosterone. A positive test is considered to be a ratio of greater than 6:1. A recent Swedish study found that ethanol ingestion may increase the testosterone level and urged caution in interpreting these ratios.[89] Diuretics and probenecid have been used by athletes as "masking" agents for anabolic steroids. For this reason, probenecid and diuretics have been added to the banned drug list.

E. **Circumvention by athletes:** Although the GC/MS may approach 100% accuracy, athletes have attempted numerous methods of avoiding detection.
   1. **Masking agents:** Diuretics and tubular blocking agents such as probenecid have been used in order to mask the presence of banned substances in the urine. Most drug tests utilize a minimum urinary specific gravity to combat this, and probenecid and the diuretics have been specifically banned by the IOC.
   2. **Determination of drug half-life:** With announced drug testing, athletes can determine how long a drug can be detected in the urine. Table 9 lists some elimination times.[90] This problem can be addressed with random, unannounced testing.

**TABLE 9.** Drug Clearance Times

| Drug | Approximate Elimination Time |
|---|---|
| Stimulants (e.g., amphetamines) | 1 to 7 days |
| Cocaine: Occasional use | 6 to 12 hours |
|       Repeated use | 3 to 5 days |
| Codeine and narcotics in cough medicine | 24 to 48 hours |
| Tranquilizers | 4 to 8 days |
| Marijuana | 3 to 5 weeks |
| Anabolic steroids | |
|       Fat-soluble injectable | 6 to 12 months |
|       Water-soluble oral | 1 to 6 weeks |
| Over-the-counter cold preparations | |
|       containing ephedrine, etc. | 48 to 72 hours |

      3. **Substitution of urine:** Athletes have developed numerous methods to substitute "clean" urine, including self-catheterization and innovative "delivery systems." In order to eliminate this problem, collection of the urine sample is conducted under constant supervision and close observation.

  F. **Extent of testing**[91]

      1. **Olympic level:** The IOC and the USOC conduct formal drug testing at sanctioned events, such as the Olympics, Olympic Trials, and Olympic Festivals.

      2. **Collegiate level:** The NCAA began testing in 1986 at postseason football games and championship events at the Division I, II, and III levels. A 1986 survey of 257 NCAA affiliated schools found that 28% had a drug-screening program for athletes, and 52% of those schools without such a program were considering one. Drugs most commonly screened were cocaine (99%), amphetamines (97%), and cannabinoids (96%), with steroids being tested by 60%.[92] Testing methods included EIA (56%), TLC (30%), GC (25%), and GC/MS (72%).

      3. **Major League Baseball:** Random tests for cocaine, marijuana, heroin, and morphine are administered among players with specified drug-testing clauses and owners, managers, executives, and umpires.

      4. **National Basketball Association:** Individual players can be tested with "reasonable cause" for cocaine and heroin without prior notice.

      5. **National Football League:** Currently tests are given at all preseason camps and scouting sessions in an announced fashion for "street drugs," anabolic steroids, and amphetamines; may also test with "reasonable cause."

  G. **Effectiveness:** The effectiveness of drug testing in preventing drug abuse by athletes is difficult to evaluate. A 1987 NCAA survey of 407 football players from Division I schools revealed that 63% felt that drug testing was a deterrent to drug use.[93] It is difficult to reconcile the disparity between positive drug tests (0.72% at the 1984 Olympics and 2.5% by the NCAA) and the presumed larger prevalence of drug use by athletes. It is clear that random, unannounced testing provides a greater deterrent.

  H. **Legality**

      1. **Cases allowing testing**

         a. New York court ruled that testing jockeys was allowable.

         b. Louisiana upholds the disqualification of an intercollegiate football player prior to the Sugar Bowl.

      2. **Cases disallowing testing**

         a. 1987—As a result of suit by Stanford athletes, it is ruled that drug testing violates student athletes' right to privacy.

      2. University of California at Berkeley suspends drug testing rather than contest a suit by the American Civil Liberties Union.

         The legal issues surrounding drug testing have yet to be fully resolved, and it is prudent to consult local legal experts before embarking on a testing program.

## XV. Drug Education

The education of athletes is certainly one additional tool that can be utilized to deter drug abuse. To be effective, however, education needs to be started at a young age. This was emphasized by Anderson and McKeag's data, which demonstrated that **most patterns of drug use are established in junior high and high school.**[5] Education begun at the collegiate level is probably too late. In a recent study, 34% of college football players felt that special seminars and courses would discourage drug use.[93] Educational intervention is probably best suited for deterring recreational drug use, since the substances usually impact negatively on performance. Although education may be useful in alerting athletes to the risks involved with the use of performance-enhancing drugs and methods, the positive reinforcement of improved performance makes drug testing a necessary component of deterrence.

## *REFERENCES*

1. Memorandum of Agreement between the United States Olympic Committee and the National Governing Boards, 1985, p 1.
2. Barnes L: Olympic drug testing: Improvements without progress. Phys Sportsmed 8:21–24, 1980.
3. Duda M: Drug testing challenges: College and pro athletes. Phys Sportsmed 11(6):64–67, 1983.
4. Clement DB: Drug use survey: Results and conclusions. Phys Sportsmed 11(9):64–67, 1983.
5. Anderson WA, McKeag DB: The substance use and abuse habit of college student athletes. Mission, KS, National Collegiate Athletic Association, June 1985.
6. Loughton SV, Ruhline RO: Human strength an endurance responses to anabolic steroids and training. J Sports Med Phys Fitness 17:285–296, 1977.
7. Cowart V: Steroids in sports: After four decades, time to return these genies to bottle? JAMA 257(4):421–427, 1987.
8. Wilson JD: Androgen abuse by athletes. Endocr Rev 9:181–199, 1988.
9. Buckley WE, et al: Estimated prevalence of anabolic steroid use among male high school seniors. JAMA 260(23):3441–3445, 1988.
10. Marshall E: The drug of champions. Science 242:183–184, 1988.
11. Windsor RE, Dumitru D: Anabolic steroid use by athletes. Postgrad Med 84(4):37–49, 1988.
12. Ariel G: The effect of anabolic steroid upon skeletal muscle contractile force. J Sports Med Phys Fitness 13:187–190, 1973.
13. Berg A, Keul J: Der Einfluss von anabolen Substanzen auf das Verhalten der freien Serumanimosauren von Normalperson und Scwerathleten in Rule and bei Korperarbeit. Oester Z Sportsmed 4:11–18, 1974.
14. Hervey GR, Knibbs AV, Burkinshaw L, et al: Effects of methandienone on the performance and body composition of men undergoing athletic training. Clin Sci 60:457–461, 1981.
15. Stamford BA, Moffatt R: Anabolic steroid effectiveness as an ergogenic aid to experienced weight trainers. J Sports Med Phys Fitness 14:191–197, 1974.
16. Ward P: The effect of an anabolic steroid on strength and lean body mass. Med Sci Sports Exerc 5:227–282, 1973.
17. Hervey GR: Are athletes wrong about anabolic steroids? Br J Sports Med 9:74–77, 1975.
18. Johnson LD, et al: Effects of anabolic steroid treatment on endurance. Med Sci Sports Exerc 7:287–289, 1975.
19. Loughton SV, Ruhline RO: Human strength and endurance responses to anabolic steroids and training. J Sports Med Phys Fitness 17:285–296, 1977.
20. Stromme SB, Meen HD, Aakvaag A: Effects of an androgenicanabolic steroid on strength development and plasma testosterone levels in normal males. Med Sci Sports Exerc 6:203–208, 1974.
21. American College of Sports Medicine: Stand on the use of anabolic-androgenic steroids in sports. Indianapolis, IN, American College of Sports Medicine, 1984.
22. Burkett LN, Falduto MT: Steroid use by athletes in a metropolitan area. Phys Sportsmed 12(8):69–74, 1984.
23. Tennant F, Black DL, Voy RO: Anabolic steroid dependence with opioid-type features. N Engl J Med 319:578, 1988.
24. Overly WL, et al: Androgens and hepatocellular carcinoma in an athlete. Ann Intern Med 100:158, 1984.
25. McNutt RA, et al: Acute myocardial infarction in a 22 year old world class weight lifter using anabolic steroids. Am J Cardiol 62:164, 1988.
26. Frankle MA, et al: Anabolic androgenic steroids and a stroke in an athlete: Case report. Arch Phys Med Rehabil 69:632–633, 1988.

27. Brower KJ, et al: Anabolic-androgenic steroid dependence. Journal of Clinical Psychiatry 50:31–33, 1989.
28. Pope HG, Katz DL: Affective and psychotic symptoms associated with anabolic steroid use. Am J Psychiatry 145:487–490, 1988.
29. Aiache AE: Surgical treatment of gynecomastia in the body builder. Plast Reconstr Surg 83:61–66, 1989.
30. Roberts JT, Essenhigh DM: Adenocarcinoma of prostate in a 40 year old body-builder. Lancet ii:742, 1986.
31. Kramhoft M, Solgaard S: Spontaneous rupture of the extensor pollicis longus tendon after anabolic steroids. J Hand Surg 11:87, 1986.
32. Back BR, et al: Triceps rupture: A case report and literature review. Am J Sports Med 15:285–289, 1987.
33. Kiraly CL, et al: Effect of testosterone and anabolic steroids on the size of sebaceous glands in power athletes. Am J Dermatopath 96:515–519, 1987.
34. Macintyre JG: Growth hormone and athletes. Sports Med 4:129–142, 1987.
35. Cowart VS: Human growth hormone: The latest ergogenic aid? Phys Sportsmed 16(3):175–185, 1988.
36. Ahren K, et al: Cellular mechanisms of the acute stimulatory effect of growth hormone. In Pecile & Muller (eds): Growth Hormone and Related Polypeptides. Proceedings of the 3rd International Symposium, Milan, September 17–20, 1975. Amsterdam, Excerpta Medica, 1975.
37. Goldberg AL: Work induced growth of skeletal muscle in normal and hypophysectomized rats. Am J Physiol 213(5):1193–1198, 1967.
38. Kostyo JL, Reagan CR: The biology of growth hormone. Pharmacol Ther 2:591–604, 1976.
39. Goldberg AL: Relationship between growth hormone and muscle work in determining muscle size. J Physiol 216(5):655–666, 1969b.
40. Underwood LE: Report of the conference on uses and possible abuses of biosynthetic human growth hormone. N Engl J Med 311:606–608, 1984.
41. Spilotis BE, et al: Growth hormone neurosecretory dysfunction: A treatable cause of short stature. JAMA 251:2223–2330, 1984.
42. VanVliet G, et al: Growth hormone treatment for short stature. N Engl J Med 309:1016–1022, 1983.
43. Physician's Desk Reference, 43rd ed. Oradell, NJ, Medical Economics, 1989, p 1180.
44. AdHoc Committee on Growth Hormone Usage, the Lawson Wilkins Pediatric Endocrine Society, and the Committee on Drugs: Growth hormone in the treatment of children with short stature. Pediatrics 72:891–894, 1983.
45. Koch TK, et al: Cruetzfeldt-Jakob disease in a young adult with idiopathic hypopituitarism: Possible relation to the administration of cadaveric human growth hormone. N Engl J Med 313:731–733, 1985.
46. Lombardo JA: Stimulants and athletic performance: Amphetamines and caffeine. Phys Sportsmed 14(11):128–139, 1986.
47. Mandell AJ: The Sunday syndrome: A unique pattern of amphetamine use indigenous to American professional football. Clin Toxicol 15(2):225–232, 1979.
48. Smith GM, Beecher HK: Amphetamine sulfate and athletic performance. JAMA 170:542–557, 1959.
49. Chandler JV, Blair SN: The effects of amphetamines on selected physiological components related to athletic success. Med Sci Sports Exerc 12:65–69, 1980.
50. Cantwell JD, Rose FD: Cocaine and cardiovascular events. Phys Sports Med 14(11):77–82, 1986.
51. Kunkel DB: Cocaine then and now, Part 1. Emerg Med June 15:125–138, 1986.
52. Roth D, et al: Acute rhabdomyolysis associated with cocaine intoxication. N Engl J Med 319:673–677, 1988.
53. Goodwin M: In sport, cocaine's here to stay. New York Times, May 3, 1987.
54. Cregler L, Mark H: Special report: Medical complications of cocaine abuse. N Engl J Med 315:1495–1500, 1986.
55. Kunkel DB: Cocaine then and now, Part II. Emerg Med July 15:168–173, 1986.
56. Gawin FH, Ellinwood EH: Cocaine and other stimulants. N Engl J Med 318:1173–1182, 1988.
57. Isner JM, et al: Acute cardiac events temporally related to cocaine abuse. N Engl J Med 315:1438–1443, 1986.
58. Patel RC, et al: Free-base cocaine use associated with bronchiolitis obliterans organizing pneumonia. Ann Intern Med 107:186–187, 1987.
59. Giammarco RA: The athlete, cocaine, and lactic acidosis: A hypothesis. Am J Med Sci 294:412–414, 1987.
60. Gilman AG, Goodman LS, Rall TW, Murad F (eds): Goodman and Gilman's The Pharmacologic Basis of Therapeutics, 7th ed. New York, Macmillan, 1985.
61. Laurin CA, Letorneau G: Medical report on the Montreal Olympic Games. Am J Sports Med 6:54–61, 1978.

62. Ivy JL, et al: Role of caffeine and glucose ingestion on metabolism during exercise. Med Sci Sports Exerc 10:66, 1978.
63. Welch JM, et al: Effect of caffeine on skeletal muscle function before and after fatigue. J Appl Physiol 54:1303–1305, 1983.
64. Butts NK, Crowell D: Effects of caffeine ingestion on cardiorespiratory endurance in men and women. Res Q Exerc Sport 56:301–305, 1985.
65. Casal DC, Leon AS: Failure of caffeine to affect substrate utilization during prolonged running. Med Sci Sports Exerc 17:174–179, 1985.
66. Van Der Merwe PJ, et al: Caffeine in sport: Urinary excretion of caffeine in healthy volunteers after intake of common caffeine-containing beverages. South African Med J 74:163–164, 1988.
67. De Meersman R, et al: The effects of a sympathomimetic drug on maximal aerobic activity. J Sports Med 26:251–257, 1986.
68. Sidney KH, Lefoe NM: The effects of Tedral upon athletic performance: A double-blind cross-over study. Quebec City, Quebec, Canada, Quebec City International Congress of Physical Activity Sciences, 1976.
69. DeMeersman R, Getty D, Schaefer DC: Sympathomimetics and exercise enhancement: All in the mind? Pharmacol Biochem Behav 28:361–365, 1987.
70. Amadio P, Cummings DM: Nonsteroidal anti-inflammatory agents: An update. Am Fam Phys 34:147–154, 1986.
71. Sedor JR, Davidson EW, Dunn MJ: Effects of nonsteroidal anti-inflammatory drugs in healthy subjects. Am J Med 81(suppl 2B):58–83, 1986.
72. Day RO: Effects of exercise performance on drugs used in musculoskeletal disorders. Med Sci Sports Exerc 13:272–275, 1981.
73. Butt JH, Barthel JS, Moore RA: Clinical spectrum of upper gastrointestinal effects of nonsteroidal anti-inflammatory drugs. Am J Med 84(suppl 2A):5–14, 1988.
74. Millhorn HT: The diagnosis of alcoholism. Am Fam Phys 37(6):175–183, 1988.
75. American College of Sports Medicine: Position statement on the use of alcohol in sports. Med Sci Sports Exerc 14:ix–x, 1982.
76. Urbano-Marquez A, et al: The effects of alcoholism on skeletal and cardiac muscle. N Engl J Med 320:409–415, 1989.
77. Tashkin DP, Gong H, Fligiel SEG: How the lungs are affected by marijuana smoke. J Respir Dis 8:87–107, 1987.
78. Powell DR: Does marijuana smoke cause lung cancer? Primary Care and Cancer October 1987, p 15.
79. Biron S, Wells J: Marijuana and its effects on the athlete. Athletic Training 18:295–303, 1983.
80. Renaud AM, Cormier Y: Acute effects of marihuana smoking on maximal exercise performance. Med Sci Sports Exerc 18:685–689, 1986.
81. Pace N, Lozner EL, Consolazio WV, et al: The increase in hypoxia tolerance of normal men accompanying the polycythemia induced by transfusion of erythrocytes. Am J Physiol 148:152–163, 1947.
82. Klein HG: Sound Board: Blood transfusion and athletics. N Engl J Med 312:854–856, 1985.
83. Buick FJ, et al: Effect of induced erythrocythemia on aerobic work capacity. J Appl Physiol 48:636–642, 1980.
84. American College of Sports Medicine Position Stand: Blood doping as an ergogenic aid. Phys Sportsmed 16(1):131–134, 1988.
85. Pate RR, et al: Effect of orally administered sodium bicarbonate on performance of high intensity exercise. Med Sci Sports Exerc 17:200–201, 1985.
86. Cade R, Conte M, Zauner C, et al: Effects of phosphate loading on 2,3 diphosphoglycerate and maximal oxygen uptake. Med Sci Sports Exerc 16:263–268, 1984.
87. Hansen HJ, et al: Crisis in drug testing: Results of CDC blind study. JAMA 253(16):2382–2387, 1985.
88. Catlin DH, Kammerer RC, Hatton CK, et al: Analytical chemistry at the games of the XXIIIrd Olympiad in Los Angeles, 1984. Clin Chem 33(2):319–327, 1987.
89. Falk O, et al: Effect of ethanol on the ratio between testosterone and epitestosterone in urine. Clin Chem 34(7):1482–1484, 1988.
90. USOC Drug Education Program: Questions and Answers. Committee on substance abuse research and education, USOC, 1988.
91. Gall SL, Duda M, Giel D, Rogers CC: Who tests which athletes for what drugs? Phys Sportsmed 16(2):155–161, 1988.
92. Summary Report of Drug Screening Questionnaire, December 1986.
93. Abdenour TE, Miner MJ, Weir N: Attitudes of intercollegiate football players toward drug testing. Athletic Training 22(3):199–201, 1987.

# Chapter 17: Injuries and Emergencies on the Field

BRIAN C. HALPERN, MD

I. **Basic Principles of Emergency Treatment**

In any traumatic incident, especially one that occurs on the playing field, **rapid evaluation and management are imperative for a good prognosis. Often, the initial evaluation and treatment determine the ultimate outcome. Good medical care is possible in the emergency setting if trained personnel, who are familiar with athletic injuries, are on the field.**

A. **Adequate preparation**

1. **A team leader** should be designated as the person responsible for supervising on-the-field management of an injury. This position is usually filled by the team physician or trainer. He/she designates responsibilities, prearranges a network of referrals and emergency care, and directs the treatment of injury.

2. **Appropriate health care personnel** should be on or readily accessible to the field to assist the team leader. Their training and expertise should include, at least, basic CPR and life support, as well as how to transport an injured athlete. The medical care provider should not perform procedures or provide treatment that are beyond his/her training.

3. **All necessary emergency equipment** should be at the site of the potential injury (Table 1). It must be in good operating condition, and all personnel must be trained to use it properly in advance.

4. **Ambulance transportation** to a hospital and/or neurosurgical center must be immediately available for high-risk sports and "on call" for other sports.

5. **Telephone link-up** to the emergency room, ambulance, and trauma center is necessary for communication between the medical facility and the team leader. Information on the athlete's condition and the estimated time of arrival is vital so that adequate preparation can be made.

6. **Various injury scenarios** should be worked through prior to their actual occurrence. Once instituted, these strategies promote faster, safer, and more effective care for the injured athlete.

B. **Step-by-step assessment (A,B,C,D,E)**

A careful but swift initial assessment can save the patient's life and prevent further injury. Maintain close and continued observation by **looking, listening, and feeling.** Take all the time necessary for the evaluation and use the letters **"ABCDE"** as a mnemonic for a step-by-step assessment of the patient. Begin with the query "Are you okay?" Touch an arm or leg to see if the patient responds.

1. **A = airway and cervical spine**

    a. **Airway**

      i. Look and listen for spontaneous breathing. If the athlete is in the face-down position and the airway cannot be accessed, he must be brought into the face-up position by **the log roll.** The leader of the team controls the head and gives commands while three members roll (one at the shoulders, one at the hips, and one at the knees). The body must be maintained in line with the head and spine during the roll (Fig. 1).

**TABLE 1.** Equipment List

| *Mandatory for head, neck and other neurologic and orthopedic trauma:* | | |
|---|---|---|
| Spine board | Bolt cutters | Sand bags |
| Stretcher | Rigid cervical collar | |

| *Mandatory for cardiac basic CPR and ACLS (usually supplied by the ambulance):* | | |
|---|---|---|
| Oral and nasal airway | Intravenous D5/Ringer's lactate | BP cuff |
| Oxygen w/mask | MAST | 18-and 14-gauge catheter |
| Suction | Cardiac monitor/defibrillator | Crash cart with cardiac and |
| Esophageal obturator airway | Stethoscope | anaphylactic medications |

| *For general care:* | | |
|---|---|---|
| Scissors | Splints | Suture kit |
| Foil | Crutches | Alcohol and Betadine swabs |
| Tape | Slings | Eye kit with eye chart |
| Bandages | Ice | Irrigation kit |
| Penlight | Tongue depressors | Scalpel |
| Otoscope/ophthalmoscope | Gauze | Syringes and needles |
| Blankets | Band aids | Thermometer |
| Ace bandages | Hemostats | Sterile gloves |

   ii. Establish airway access.

      (a) Remove the face mask using bolt cutters or snap-offs to gain airway access.

      (b) Institute chin or jaw lift with someone always maintaining in-line traction.

      (c) Clear the airway of any material with the finger sweep or with suction. Consider that the tongue has fallen back or that there is a foreign body, such as the player's mouth piece, obstructing the airway.

      (d) Insert an oral or nasal airway to maintain air exchange. **Use the oral airway only in an unconscious person.** It can stimulate vomiting in the responsive patient.

      (e) Use supplemental oxygen with or without the airway in place.

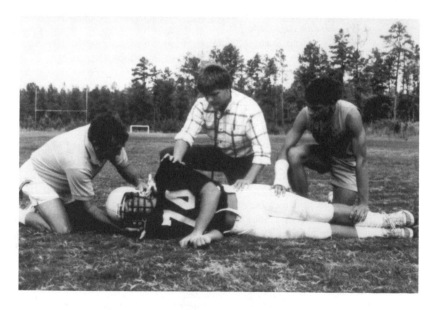

**FIGURE 1.** The log roll.

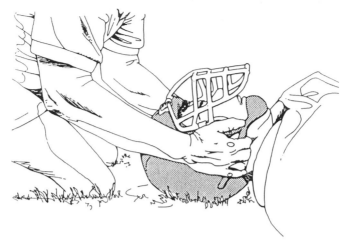

**FIGURE 2.**  In-line traction to maintain head and neck in the neutral position.

   b.  **Cervical spine**
      i.  When a player sustains an injury above the clavicle or a head injury that results in an unconscious state, an associated cervical spine injury should be suspected.
     ii.  The head and neck must be maintained in the neutral position with in-line traction (Fig. 2).
    iii.  Do not remove the helmet when cervical spine injury is suspected.
    iv.  In the unconscious athlete, where cervical spine injury is suspected, do not use ammonia capsules. The athlete should not be made to awaken and suddenly move.

2.  **B = breathing**
   a.  If there is no respiration after the airway is established, proceed with:
      i.  **Artificial ventilation**
        (a)  Mouth-to-mouth
        (b)  Mouth-to-mask ⎫ Safer than mouth-to-mouth for resuscitation
        (c)  Bag-valve-mask: ⎰ with regard to infectious diseases
        During artificial ventilation, the athlete may spontaneously vomit. Suction the airway or do the finger sweep simultaneously with the log roll. Remember, do not extend the neck.
   b.  If spontaneous respiration still does not return:
      i.  Insert an **esophageal obturator airway,** making sure not to flex the neck because of suspected cervical spine injury (contraindicated in a child less than 16 years old).
     ii.  **Endotracheal intubation** is another option, but is **difficult to perform on the field.**
   c.  Continue with artificial ventilation and supplemental oxygen.
   d.  **If stridor, hoarseness, anterior neck pain, bony crepitus, and/or subcutaneous emphysema occurs, then suspect laryngeal fracture or marked laryngeal edema.** If there is laryngeal edema or if ventilation cannot be established with mouth-to-mouth, esophageal obturator airway, or endotracheal tube, consider **needle cricothyroidotomy.**
      i.  Palpate the cricothyroid membrane.
     ii.  Puncture the skin with a 14-gauge catheter over the needle directing it at a 45-degree angle caudad (Fig. 3).

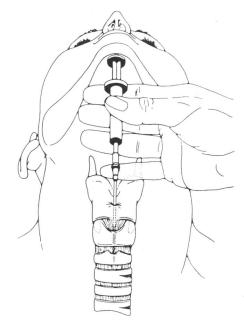

**FIGURE 3.** Needle cricothyroidotomy.

    iii. Aspiration of air signifies entry into tracheal lumen.

    iv. Ventilate through the catheter.

e. Once spontaneous ventilation occurs, or once artificial ventilation has been adequately established:

    i. **Look and listen for asymmetry of the chest wall during respiration** (must remove the chest equipment, including jersey and pads).

    ii. **If asymmetry, tachypnea, or labored respiration occur, consider:**

        (a) **Tension pneumothorax**

           (i) Diagnosis:

- Tracheal deviation
- Unilateral absence of breath sounds
- Distended neck veins
- Cyanosis.

           ii) Treatment:

- Ventilate. Place a large bore needle into the second intercostal space along the midclavicular line on the involved side.
- Ultimately, a chest tube is indicated, but this is done in the hospital setting.

        (b) **Open pneumothorax (sucking chest wound)**

           (i) Diagnosis:

- Decreased breath sounds
- Open chest wound.

           (ii) Treatment

- Ventilate. Place a piece of foil, cloth or other item over the wound. Secure it on three sides, leaving the fourth side open (if all sides are taped down, it can cause a tension pneumothorax).
- Chest tube.

        (d) **Flail chest**

           (i) Diagnosis:

- Asymmetry of chest to wall movement (usually secondary to multiple rib fractures).
(ii). Treatment:
  - Ventilate. Place patient on the involved side, or place sandbags on the involved side. Intubation and a respirator can be used in a hospital setting.
(d) **Massive hemothorax**
  (i) Diagnosis:
    - Decreased breath sounds
    - Shock
    - Dullness to percussion.
  (ii) Treatment:
    - Ventilate.
    - Chest tube.
(e) **Cardiac tamponade**
  (i) Diagnosis:
    - Shock
    - Distended neck veins
    - Decreased heart sounds.
  (ii) Treatment:
    - Ventilate
    - Massive volume infusion intravenously
    - Perform pericardiocentesis in the hospital setting.

3. **C = circulation**
   a. Check the carotid pulse for quality, rate and regularity. **In the emergency setting, do not bother with the blood pressure cuff. Use the pulse as an estimate of the blood pressure.**
      i. **When a carotid pulse is palpable, systolic BP is approximately 60.**
      ii. **When radial pulse is palpable, systolic BP is approximately 80.**
   b. **If the pulse is absent, begin CPR.**
   c. **If the pulse is present, but weak, do the capillary blanch test.** (If the capillary bed stays white for longer than 2 seconds after release, then there is some type of shock.)
      i. Check for areas of hemorrhage and apply pressure.
      ii. Rapidly infuse Ringer's lactate.
      iii. Place EKG leads on the chest and monitor cardiac rate and rhythm.
      iv. Oxygen.
      v. MAST (contraindication in acute pulmonary edema).

4. **D = disability**
   Perform a **limited neurological exam,** assessing the level of consciousness, pupillary size and reaction, extraocular movements, and motor response (Fig. 4). You must record the initial assessment and compare it with subsequent examinations.
   a. **Minimum Grading System:**
      A = alert
      V = responds to vocal stimuli
      P = responds to painful stimuli
      U = unresponsive.
   b. **Moderate Grading System (Glasgow Coma Scale, Table 2).** This system is based on eye opening, verbal, and motor responses. Responsiveness of the patient is expressed by summation of the figures. Lowest score is 3, highest is 15. Score of 7 or less indicates coma:

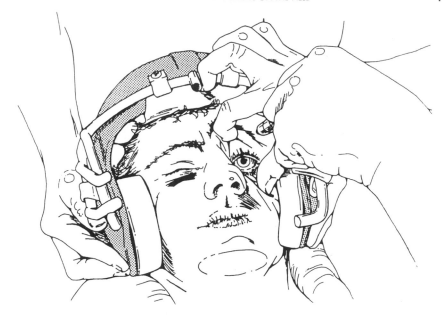

**FIGURE 4.** Assessing pupillary size and reaction.

5. **E =exposure**
   a. Inspect extremities and other body parts for bleeding, fractures and contusions.
   b. Take blood pressure with blood pressure cuff.

II. **Specific Life and Limb Emergencies**

A. **Cardiovascular emergencies** (hypovolemia, myocardial infarction, dysrhythmias):
   Cardiovascular instability is commonly secondary to hypovolemia, but may also be

**TABLE 2.** Glasgow Coma Scale[12]

| EYES: | Open | Spontaneously | 4 |
|---|---|---|---|
| | | To verbal command | 3 |
| | | To pain | 2 |
| | No response | | 1 |
| **BEST MOTOR RESPONSE:** | | | |
| To verbal command: | | Obeys | 6 |
| To painful stimulus | | Localizes pain | 5 |
| | | Flexion-withdraws | 4 |
| | | Flexion-abnormal (decorticate rigidity) | 3 |
| | | Extension (decerebrate rigidity) | 2 |
| | | No response | 1 |
| **BEST VERBAL RESPONSE:** | | | |
| Arouse patient with painful stimulus if necessary | | Oriented and converses | 5 |
| | | Disoriented and converses | 4 |
| | | Inappropriate words | 3 |
| | | Incomprehensible sounds | 2 |
| | | No response | 1 |
| **TOTAL:** | | | 3–15 |

cardiogenic in nature. The initial evaluation and treatment for cardiovascular instability should follow the same method as for circulation (p. 132). The immediate goals are to maintain vascular expansion, optimum cardiac filling, and adequate oxygenation. Packed red blood cells should be given early in the course of shock to provide optimum oxygen carrying capacity. **The initial hemoglobin/ hematocrit may not be low with blood loss, because the diminished red cell mass has not had time to equilibrate with the interstitial fluid that has moved into the vascular tree.** Adequate vascular lines are the priority and, if necessary, early surgical intervention. **The cause of shock must be identified and reversed.**

1. Hypovolemia develops as a result of decreased intravascular volume, secondary to external and/or concealed blood loss. Blood loss leads to decreased preload, which causes decreased cardiac output. The body's response is vasoconstriction to maintain blood pressure. When $1/4$ to $1/3$ of the intravascular volume is lost, the result is hypotension.

   a. Manifestations:
      i. Pallor
      ii. Cool extremities
      iii. Tachycardia
      iv. Hypotension
      v. Diaphoresis
      vi. Oliguria
      vii. Decreased sensorium
      viii. Decreased capillary refill
      ix. Metabolic acidosis
      x. Hyperpnea.

   b. Treatment:
      i. Oxygenation should be used at all times.
      ii. Use intravenous fluids to restore intravascular volume.
         (a) Rapidly infuse 1 or 2 liters of Ringer's lactate/plasmanate or a similar product.
         (b) Maintain hemoglobin at 12 gm% through blood replacement.
            (i) **Estimates, in liters, of localized blood loss from adult fractures:**

| | |
|---|---|
| **Humerus** | **1.0–2.0 liters** |
| Elbow | 0.5–1.5 liters |
| Forearm | 0.5–1.0 liters |
| **Pelvis** | **1.5–4.5 liters** |
| **Hip** | **1.5–2.5 liters** |
| **Femur** | **1.0–2.0 liters** |
| Knee | 1.0–1.5 liters |
| Tibia | 0.5–1.5 liters |
| Ankle | 0.5–1.5 liters |

      iii. Control external and internal hemorrhage.
      iv. Monitor blood pressure, central venous pressure, urine output, electrocardiogram, hemoglobin/hematocrit, arterial blood gases, coagulation profile, electrolytes, etc.

2. **Cardiogenic emergencies** develop as a result of myocardial infarction, dysrhythmia, tamponade, contusion, etc.

   a. Manifestations:
      i. Same as hypovolemia.

   b. Treatment:
      i. Oxygenation.
      ii. Decrease myocardial oxygen demand with a cardioselective beta blocker.
      iii. Improve myocardial contractility with epinephrine, dopamine or dobutamine IV.
      iv. Improve coronary blood flow and decrease left ventricular afterload with IV or sublingual nitroglycerin.
      v. Control pain with morphine sulfate 2–4 mg IV.

      vi. Manage life-threatening dysrhythmia appropriately:
- (a) Ventricular fibrillation: lidocaine IV/cardioversion
- (b) Ventricular tachycardia: lidocaine IV/cardioversion
- (c) Asystole: epinephrine IV/atropine IV
- (d) Electromechanical dissociation: epinephrine IV
- (e) Bradyarrhythmia with symptoms: atropine IV/pacemaker

     vii. Monitor blood pressure, central venous pressure, wedge pressure, vascular resistance (systemic and pulmonary), urine output, electrocardiogram, hemoglobin/hematocrit, arterial blood gases, coagulation profile, electrolytes, oxygen consumption, left ventricular stroke work index, isoenzymes, etc.

B. **Anaphylaxis** is the immediate shock-like, and frequently fatal, hypersensitivity reaction that occurs within minutes of administration of foreign sera or drugs. It may occur after an insect sting.

  1. Manifestations:

| | |
|---|---|
| a. Apprehension | h. Incontinence |
| b. Paresthesia | i. Shock |
| c. Generalized urticaria or edema | j. Fever |
| d. Choking | k. Pupillary dilation |
| e. Cyanosis | l. Loss of consciousness |
| f. Wheezing | m. Seizures. |
| g. Cough | |

  2. Treatment: Follow the algorithm in Figure 5.

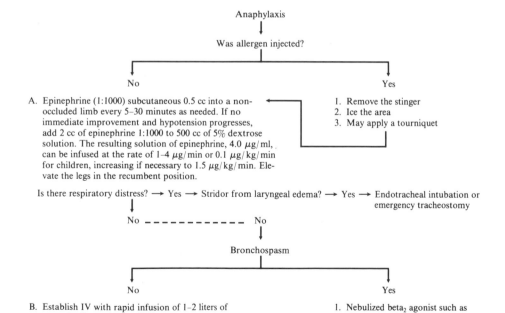

**FIGURE 5.** Treatment of anaphylaxis.

3. Prevention:
   a. Deaths from anaphylaxis can be avoided if correct treatment is provided quickly.
   b. After an episode of anaphylaxis, the cause should be identified and thereafter avoided.
   c. When the cause cannot be identified or avoided, the patient should carry some form of medical identification tag and be equipped with a self-administered epinephrine device.
C. **Central nervous system injuries:**
   1. **Head injury**
      **The leading cause of death on the football field is head injuries. These injuries can be characterized as either diffuse brain injuries (concussive syndromes) or more focal brain syndromes (epidural, subdural, or intracerebral hematomas).** You need to be able to evaluate and treat them quickly.
      a. Diagnosis and treatment:
         The key elements to assess are loss of consciousness, an abnormal neurologic examination, and retrograde and post-traumatic amnesia. **Memory loss is a more sensitive marker than the level of consciousness.** Usually the patient begins with retrograde memory loss and, if the injury is severe, may also develop post-traumatic amnesia. Begin treatment with the ABCDE method that was outlined in the step-by-step assessment and continue appropriate treatment when a specific diagnosis has been made. For easy reference use flow diagram in Table 3.

**TABLE 3.**   Assessment of a Head Injury

| Diagnosis | Mild | | | Moderate | Severe |
|---|---|---|---|---|---|
| | *I* | *II* | *III* | | |
| Loss of consciousness | − | − | − | < 5 min | > 5 min |
| Amnesia | − | + retrograde and post-traumatic | + retrograde and post-traumatic | + retrograde and post-traumatic | + retrograde and post-traumatic |
| Confusion | Slight | Increased | More pronounced | Obvious | For 5 or more min |
| **TREATMENT** | | | | | |
| ABCDE | + | + | + | + | + |
| Immobilize cervical spine and transport to hospital for x-rays and further evaluation | −/+ if also has neck pain or abnormal neurologic or cervical examination | | | + | + |
| Observation out of hospital | + | + | + | − | − |
| Transportation to the hospital for neurosurgical consultation and CT scan/MRI visualization and close observation | − | − | − | + | + |
| Hyperventilate to PCO 22–33 mm mercury, dexamethasone 1 mg/kg and maintain serum osmol. to less than 320 osmol/liter | − | − | − | − | + |
| Return to play the same day if: <br>• Appropriate evaluation on sidelines is negative <br>• No headache, irritability, inability to concentrate or obvious changes in functions (as in normal dexterity, strength and speed) <br>• No photophobia; is first concussion | + | − | − | − | − |

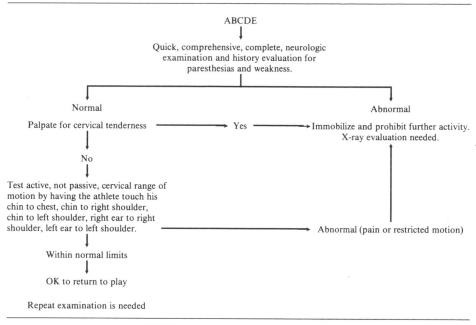

**FIGURE 6.** Assessment of a neck injury.

2. **Neck injury**
   **Usually results in greater morbidity than mortality.** A small fraction of sports-incurred neck injuries result in permanent neurologic injury. **If handled improperly, an unstable lesion without a neurologic deficit can be converted to one with a neurologic deficit and permanent disability.** For diagnosis and treatment see Figure 6.

3. **Back injury**
   For diagnosis and treatment see Figure 7.

D. **Abdominal and pelvic (GI and GU) injuries:**
   With trauma to the abdomen and pelvis, anticipate possible injury to the spleen, pancreas, liver, bowel, kidney, bladder, urethra, testicles, aorta, vena cava, etc. **The key to successful management is rapid detection of a vascular or visceral injury and control of hemorrhage and abdominal contamination.**

   1. Diagnosis:
      a. **General. Signs of significant injury are:**
         i. Decreased bowel sounds
         ii. Tender abdomen
         iii. Hard or rigid abdomen
         iv. Distended abdomen
         v. Flank pain or guarding
         vi. Hematuria
         vii. Inability to void
         viii. Signs and symptoms of shock: hypotension and tachycardia.

   2. Evaluation and treatment:
      a. Conservative
         i. NPO (nothing by mouth)
         ii. Minimal pain medication
         iii. Serial hematocrit and WBC count determinations
         iv. Urinary catheterization
         v. Serial amylase values
         vi. Repeat physical examinations
         vii. If patient develops evidence of blood loss or abdominal tenderness, then a peritoneal lavage should be performed.

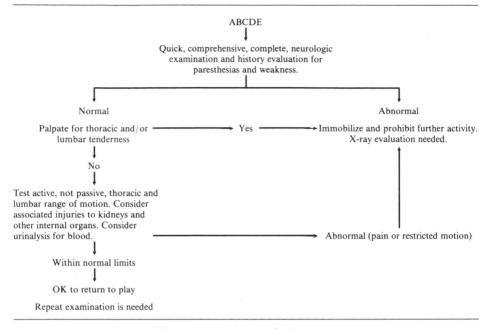

**FIGURE 7.** Assessment of a back injury.

3. Specific examples:
   a. **Spleen**
      i. **Signs and symptoms**
         (a) Abdominal pain in left upper quadrant
         (b) Left shoulder or neck pain
         (c) Frequently associated with left lower rib fractures.
      ii. **Diagnostic work-up**
         (a) Ultrasound
         (b) Spleen scan to detect hemorrhage or intrasplenic hematoma
         (c) CT or arteriography to detect occult hemorrhage or intrasplenic hematoma.
   b. **Liver**
      i. **Signs and symptoms**
         (a) Abdominal pain in right upper quadrant
         (b) Right shoulder or neck pain
         (c) Possible right lower rib fractures.
      ii. **Diagnostic work-up**
         (a) Ultrasound
         (b) Liver scan
         (c) CT or arteriography to detect occult hemorrhage or intrahepatic hematoma.
   c. **Kidney, bladder, urethra**
      i. **Signs and symptoms**
         (a) Hematuria
         (b) Bloody meatal discharge or inability to void
         (c) Flank pain
         (d) Associated pelvic fracture.

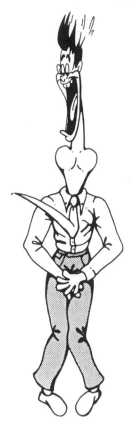

**FIGURE 8.**   Testicular trauma.

   ii. **Diagnostic work-up**
     (a) IVP should be done first because extravasation from cystogram may obscure a lower urethral injury.
     (b) Urethrogram/cystogram.
  d. **Testicles** (Fig. 8)
    i. **Signs and symptoms**
     (a) Inability to void
     (b) Swelling so excessive that the epididymis is indistinguishable from the testes.
     (c) If the testicle cannot be trans-illuminated, there may be testicular rupture.
    ii. **Diagnostic work-up**
     (a) Ultrasound of scrotum
     (b) Doppler study of testicles
     (c) Testicular scan.
    iii. **Treatment**
     (a) For a simple contusion use: ice, scrotal support, analgesics.
     (b) Ambulate when pain and swelling stabilize.
  e. **Rectus abdominis muscle contusion/strain**
    i. **Signs and symptoms**
     (a) Positive bowel sounds
     (b) Superficial, but not deep tenderness to palpation
       (i) Palpate the abdominal wall during Valsalva maneuver
     (c) No distension
     (d) No rigidity
     (e) No signs or symptoms of shock.

        ii. **Treatment**
           (a) Ice
           (b) Rest
           (c) Abdominal support.
    f. **Rectus abdominis muscle hematoma**
      i. **Signs and symptoms**
          (a) Muscle guarding and tenderness
          (b) Increased abdominal pain with straight leg raising and hyperextension of the back
          (c) Nausea and vomiting
          (d) Palpable mass in the abdominal wall.
      ii. **Diagnostic work-up**
          (a) CT scan.
      iii. **Treatment**
          (a) Ice
          (b) Rest
          (c) Abdominal support
          (d) Surgery is necessary only if bleeding continues into the muscle and the hematoma expands.
E. **Eye/ENT injuries**
  1. **Eye**
    **Care for ocular trauma or sudden loss of vision begins with a differentiation between potentially blinding problems and a less serious situation.**
    a. **Signs and symptoms of serious injury**
      i. Blurred vision or abnormal visual acuity that does not clear with blinking
      ii. Loss of all or part of the visual field of the eye
      iii. Sharp stabbing or deep throbbing pain
      iv. Double vision after injury
      v. Black or red eye
      vi. Object in the cornea
      vii. An eye that does not move as completely as the opposite eye
     viii. One eye protruding when compared with the opposite eye
      ix. Abnormal pupil size or shape compared to the opposite eye
      x. Layer of blood between the cornea and iris
      xi. Laceration or penetration of eyelid or eyeball
     xii. A dark subconjunctival mass that may indicate scleral rupture.
    b. **Treatment for abnormal eye exam**
      i. Ask patient to shut eye lightly as if sleeping, tape a sterile eye pad in place, and tape a hard shield over the eye pad.
      ii. Transport to eye facility and make sure that the patient does not squeeze eye tightly shut.
  2. **Ear**
    a. **Signs and symptoms of cauliflower ear**
      i. Throbbing, painful, swollen ear
      ii. Organized hematoma.
    b. **Treatment**
      i. Aspirate the hematoma under sterile technique.
      ii. Compress to area of the hematoma using a collodion pack, plaster of Paris cast, or a silicone mold.
  3. **Nose**
    a. **Signs and symptoms of epistaxis**
      i. Bleeding from the nose.

    b. **Treatment**

      i. Nasal area should be covered with cold cloths or ice and compression.

      ii. If the bleeding is profuse and not easily stopped, careful packing of the anterior nares may reach the area of bleeding and control it. A regular size tampon works well for this purpose.

F. **Extremity injuries**

  1. **The following systems must be evaluated in the affected extremity:**

    a. Vascular

    b. Neural

    c. Osseous

    d. Ligamentous

    e. Muscular

    f. Tendinous

    g. Skin and subcutaneous tissue.

  2. **Management**

    a. **Initial evaluation to detect the following:**

      i. Absent or decreased pulse

      ii. Pallor

      iii. Generalized extremity edema

      iv. Deformity

      v. Local swelling

      vi. Ecchymosis

      vii. Joint laxity

      viii. Obvious soft tissue lacerations or defects

      ix. Decreased motion to command or to painful stimulation

      x. Hypesthesia or anesthesia.

    b. **Initial treatment**

      i. Splint injury

      ii. Cover wound with moist dressing

      iii. Early reduction of dislocation after neurovascular check

      iv. Early transport, especially after neurovascular injury

      v. Rest, ice, compression, elevation.

    c. **Specific injuries**

      i. **Open fractures**

        (a) Wounds should be covered with sterile dressing that has been soaked in saline or Betadine.

        (b) The fracture should be splinted without pulling the exposed bone back into the soft tissue. Do not probe the wound. Do not push extruded soft tissue or bone back into the wound.

        (c) Transport the patient to the hospital to begin antibiotics, tetanus, and repair.

      ii. **Traumatic amputation**

        (a) The proximal stump should first be irrigated with lactated Ringer's injection and a pressure dressing applied with sterile gauze.

        (b) The amputated part should be irrigated in lactated Ringer's injection, wrapped in sterile gauze, and then placed in a plastic bag or aluminum foil. It should then be cooled, not frozen, by placing it into a container of ice.

      iii. **Dislocations**

        (a) Neurovascular assessment

        (b) Reduction on the field before marked muscle spasm occurs

        (c) Splint the injury and do a neurovascular re-check.

      iv. **Vascular injury. Peripheral arterial injury should be suspected in any patient sustaining the following extremity injuries: knee or elbow dislocation, any long-bone fracture (particularly if there is a supracondylar humeral or femoral fracture), or crush injury. Check for** external hemorrhage, pulse deficit, ischemic changes, including pallor or cyanosis, coolness, hypesthesia, and partial or complete paralysis, bruit or thrill, and hematoma.

    (a) Control bleeding by applying direct pressure.

    (b) Immediate revascularization of ischemic extremity.

  v. **Peripheral nerve injury**

    (a) Primary nerve repair only if the laceration is clean, especially with digital nerves of the hand.

    (b) Traction nerve injury usually has continuity of the nerve and function gradually returns.

## *RECOMMENDED READING*

1. Bruno LA, Gennarelli TA, Torg JS: Head and neck injuries. Clin Sports Med 6: 1987.
2. Cantu RC: Guidelines for return to contact sports after a cerebral concussion. Phys Sportsmed 14(10):75–83, 1986.
3. Cloward RB: Acute cervical spine injuries. CIBA Clinical Symposia 32:1–32, 1980.
4. Cowley RA, Dunham CM: Shock Trauma/Critical Care Manual Initial Assessment and Management. Baltimore, University Park Press, 1982.
5. Deshazo WF: Hematoma of the rectus abdominis in football. Phys Sportsmed 12:(9)73–75, 1984.
6. Friedman WA: Head injuries. CIBA Clinical Symposia 35:1–32, 1983.
7. Graver K: A review of the new guidelines for advanced cardiac life support. Fam Pract Recert 10:55–68, 1988.
8. Haycock CE: How I manage abdominal injuries. Phys Sportsmed 14(6):86–99, 1986.
9. Hoover DL: How I manage testicular injury. Phys Sportsmed 14(4):127–129, 1986.
10. Hugenholtz H, Richard MT: The on-site management of athletes with head injuries. Phys Sportsmed 11(6):71–80, 1983.
11. Iverson LD, Clawson DK: Manual of Acute Orthopaedic Therapeutics, 2nd ed. Boston, Little, Brown, 1982.
12. Jennett B, Teasdale G: Predicting outcome in individuals after severe head injury. Lancet 1:1031–1034, 1976.
13. Lehman LB: Nervous system sports-related injuries. Am J Sports Med 15:494–499, 1987.
14. McIntyre KM, Lewis AJ: Textbook of Advanced Cardiac Life Support. Dallas, American Heart Association, 1981.
15. Nelson WE, Gieck JH, Jane JA, Hawthorne P: Athletic head injuries. Athletic Training 19:95–100, 1984.
16. Ormerod AD: Emergency management of anaphylaxis: Treatment and clues to diagnosis. Emergency Decisions. March:31–40, 1988.

# Chapter 18: Youth Sports Leagues

KRIS BERG, EdD

I. **Fitness and Health Status of American Youth**

  A. **National Children and Youth Fitness Study**
   1. A random sample of 8800 boys and girls, grades 5–12, in 19 states.
   2. Students participating in physical education classes outperformed those who were not on a battery of physical fitness tests.
   3. Students participating in community physical activity/sports programs were more fit than those who did not.

  B. **Other national fitness tests**
   1. Lower fitness levels of American youth in the 1980s than previous decades.
   2. Increased body fatness in boys and girls is one of the most consistent findings.

  C. **Physical activity levels of American youth**
   1. A study using Holter monitoring indicated that American youth in a typical day do not exercise vigorously enough to meet criteria for achieving aerobic fitness.

  D. **Cardiovascular disease**
   1. A number of studies indicate that elementary school age children are at risk for coronary heart disease.
      a. American youth have significantly higher levels of total cholesterol and body fatness than youth in Third World nations and Japan.
   2. Fatty streaks are evident in prepubescents.

  E. **Role of youth sports programs**
   1. Critical role in youth fitness.
   2. Physical education programs have been eliminated in some areas and often are poorly funded.

II. **Traits of Sound Youth Sports Leagues**

  A. **Sound coaching**
   1. **American Coaching Effectiveness Program (ACEP)**
      a. Training program for youth coaches
      b. Offered by many colleges, universities, YMCAs, etc.
      c. Content
         i. First aid
         ii. Safety
         iii. Philosophy of developing all children and deemphasizing winning
         iv. Conditioning
         v. Strategy and skill development.
   2. **Handbook for Youth Sports Coaches**
      a. Available from American Alliance Publications, P.O. Box 704, Waldorf, MD 20601
      b. Topics
         i. Goalsetting
         ii. Injury prevention
         iii. Teaching sportsmanship
         iv. Organizing practice.

   3. **"The Winning Trap: Sports and Our Kids"**
      a. A videotape available from National Association for Sport and Physical Education, 1900 Association Drive, Reston, VA 22091.

B. **Sound philosophy**
   1. **The Bill of Rights for Young Athletes**
      a. Formulated by the American Alliance for Health, Physical Education, Recreation and Dance (1979) (Table 1).
      b. Sound criteria for developing, modifying, and assessing youth sports leagues.

C. **Modification of rules to suit developmental level of participants**
   1. Use smaller balls, fields, and courts.
   2. Shorten the duration of games and practices.
   3. Reduce the number of participants playing at one time (e.g., three instead of five basketball players, six instead of 11 soccer players).
   4. Stop play when a rules violation is made and allow the player who normally would be penalized to continue to play without penalty after a brief explanation or demonstration (e.g., a player double-dribbling in basketball is stopped, given a brief explanation, and given the ball again to continue play).
   5. Do not keep score or won-loss records.
   6. Rotate players to different positions each game.
   7. In baseball and softball, use a batting tee or have a coach pitch to his/her own players.

D. **Constructive role of parents**
   1. Parents play a critical role in encouraging children to participate in sport. Constructive parental support should lead to a happy and voluntary involvement of the child in sport. If, however, a child is driven beyond his or her own wishes by a parent playing the role of a "vicarious athlete," then the effects can be destructive.
   2. Parents who coach must be especially aware not to favor or disfavor their own children. This requires considerable sensitivity.
   3. Classic poor examples of a parent coach are illustrated by a son or daughter who pitches or plays quarterback while other equally skilled children are given secondary roles, and a parent who screams at his or her players or at referees.
   4. ACEP training can greatly assist the parent coach, but the individual's own value system is still likely to be openly expressed in a moment of duress on the playing field. Most coaches need to continually remind themselves of the important duties they have assumed in being a volunteer coach.

**TABLE 1.** The Bill of Rights for Young Athletes

| |
|---|
| Right to participate in sports |
| Right to participate at a level commensurate with each child's maturity and ability |
| Right to have qualified adult leadership |
| Right to play as a child and not as an adult |
| Right of children to share in the leadership and decision-making of their sport participation |
| Right to participate in safe and healthy environments |
| Right to proper preparation for participation in sports |
| Right to an equal opportunity to strive for success |
| Right to be treated with dignity |
| Right to have fun in sports |

Reprinted with permission of the American Alliance for Health, Physical Education, Recreation and Dance, 1900 Association Drive, Reston, Virginia 22091.

E. **Assessing the effect on youth**

The following questions provide a simple but effective means of assessing a program:

1. Do children look like they are having fun during games or while at practice?
2. Do they like the coaches?
3. Do they speak of playing the sport again? Do they actually play again?
4. Are their skills noticeably better at the end of the season?
5. Are they bothered by losing?
6. Does everyone play at least half the game?
7. Do skilled performers dominate key positions?
   a. Pitcher
   b. First base
   c. Point guard.
8. Do skilled performers dominate play?
   a. Score most of the goals or baskets
   b. Dribbling the ball
   c. Passing the ball.

III. **Trainability of Youth**

A. **Aerobic power**

1. A number of studies have indicated no change in maximum oxygen uptake due to training in children, or a reduction in trainability due to training.
2. Some suggest that a critical maturational threshold may exist or that children possess an initially high aerobic power not readily improved with training.
3. In most studies not indicating significant gain scores, the exercise was below the intensity, duration, and frequency guidelines used for adults.
4. In most studies demonstrating significant change, adult guidelines were followed.
5. It appears that unless exercise is relatively prolonged and intense, and based on standards recommended for adults, improvement is not likely to occur.

B. **Strength and muscular development**

1. A maturational threshold has been proposed as a requisite for strength and muscle development.
   a. However, several studies indicate that prepubescents and pubescents (i.e., stages 1 and 2 of Tanner's or Greulich's scale) can significantly increase strength.
   b. Because gains in body weight did not occur in these studies, it is suggested that strength gains in children are induced neurologically as typifies the response by women and the elderly.
2. For decades many physical educators and physicians have warned that weight training was not only ineffective in prepubescents and early adolescents, but that it would damage the epiphyseal plate and soft tissues.
   a. The validity of the injury issue was addressed in a recent investigation. Only one training injury occurred in 14 weeks to 32 boys and scintigraphy revealed no bone, epiphysis, or muscle damage.
3. It appears that prepubescents are not only strength trainable but when closely supervised, injury is infrequent.
4. The importance of close supervision is supported by the observation that roughly half of some 35,000 weight training injuries requiring visits to an emergency room occurred in 10–19 year olds, most of whom were training at home.

C. **Recommendations**

1. If wishing to elicit gains in aerobic fitness, adult standards should be used, i.e., 15–20 min duration three or more times weekly at or above 50% of $VO_2max$.

**TABLE 2.**   Strength-training Recommendations for Prepubescent Boys and Girls*

**Equipment**

1. Strength-training equipment should be of appropriate design to accommodate the size and degree of maturity of the prepubescent.
2. It should be cost effective.
3. It should be safe, free of defects, and inspected frequently.
4. It should be located in an uncrowded area free of obstructions with adequate lighting and ventilation.

**Prescribed Program**

1. Training is recommended two or three times a week for 20- to 30-minute periods.
2. No resistance should be applied until proper form is demonstrated. Six to fifteen repetitions equal one set; one to three sets per exercise should be done.
3. Weight or resistance is increased in 1- to 3-lb increments after the prepubescent does 15 repetitions in good form.

**Program Considerations**

1. A preparticipation physical exam is mandatory.
2. The child must have the emotional maturity to accept coaching and instructions.
3. There must be adequate supervision by coaches who are knowledgeable about strength training and the special problems of prepubescents.
4. Strength training should be a part of an overall comprehensive program designed to increase motor skills and level of fitness.

5. Strength training should be preceded by a warm-up period and followed by a cool-down.
6. Emphasis should be on dynamic concentric contractions.
7. All exercises should be carried through a full range of motion.
8. Competition is prohibited.
9. No maximum lift should ever be attempted.

* American Orthopaedic Society for Sports Medicine: Strength-training Workshop. Indianapolis, IN, August, 1985.

    2. Recommendations for safe development of strength in youth have been made recently by the American Orthopaedic Society for Sports Medicine (summarized in Table 2).
        a. Elimination of overhead lifts while standing should be added to their recommendations because of the undue pressure placed on the lumbar spine.
            i. Sitting presses, for example, develop the same upper body muscles as the standing press, but are much safer because of reduced spinal hyperextension.

IV. **Sex Differences**

  A. **Body composition**
    1. Throughout childhood, girls have slightly more body fat than boys.
    2. At puberty, boys rapidly gain muscle mass and lose about 3–5% of body fat between ages 12 and 17, whereas girls gain some lean body mass as well as fat.
    3. Typical body fatness for older teenage girls is about 20–25%, whereas athletic girls will often have less than 16–18%.
    4. Body fatness greatly affects athletic performance. Consequently, exercise is valuable, because by facilitating weight control, other factors are also positively affected:
      a. Aerobic power
      b. Heat tolerance
      c. Ability to handle body parts
        i. Agility
        ii. Power
        iii. Speed.
    5. Body fatness probably influences a person's overall like or dislike for physical activity.

  B. **Physique and performance**
    1. Boys and girls are similar in height and weight until puberty.

2. By maturation, men are considerably heavier and taller, and possess more muscle mass than women.
3. The onset of these changes is so rapid that boys and girls are usually separated in competition well before even the early maturers reach puberty. Third grade is a commonly cited time for this separation.
4. Adolescent growth differs in early and late maturers.
   a. Growth rate (e.g., peak height velocity) is greater the earlier the spurt occurs, but growth also ceases earlier, leading to a reduction in adult height.
   b. Early maturing boys are typically more muscular with shorter legs, whereas early maturing girls have shorter legs and narrower shoulders.
5. The adolescent growth spurt provides the average male with major athletic advantages in comparison to women.
   a. Strength
   b. Speed
   c. Power
   d. Aerobic power
   e. Recent world records in track and swimming place the woman's performance at about 6 to 14% below that of the male's.

C. **Aerobic power**
1. After puberty, endurance performance of girls typically decreases, whereas it increases in boys.
2. In boys, increased androgen secretion leads to increased protein synthesis.
   a. Greater hypertrophy of skeletal and cardiac muscle.
   b. Greater red blood cell and hemoglobin production.
   c. Adolescent and adult males consequently have greater heart size and weight than girls, even when expressed relative to body size.
   d. Net result is an aerobic power and endurance typically about 20–25% greater in males than females.
   e. Group data usually exaggerate the difference, whereas comparison of elite females who are lean, highly trained, and genetically endowed with elite males results in much smaller differences.

D. **Cultural expectations**
1. Most physical activity surveys of children and adolescents show males to be more active in organized sports as well as in recreational physical activity than girls.
2. American culture seems to promote sports and exercise as basic to the male's general development.
3. Only in the last decade or so have girls been widely encouraged to participate in sport.
4. Societal norms regarding females and exercise seem to have changed dramatically.
5. The increased participation of girls coupled with appropriate coaching and facilities will likely continue to increase the need for sound sports programs for girls.

## V. **Differences Between Youth and Adults**

A. **Children should not be treated as miniature adults.**
1. They are remarkably different physically, emotionally, socially, and psychologically.
2. Although the physical differences are obvious, the others may be less so.
   a. For example, it is a common error of many youth coaches to presume that all the participants on a team have winning as their primary goal. However, surveys indicate that most children would rather play a lot on a losing team rather than minimally on a winning team.

    b. Similarly, children do not typically wish to strive for optimal physical conditioning. Spending excessive time on intense and elaborately designed conditioning would not seemingly suit the needs and interests of most children below age 13.

B. **Heat tolerance is less in children.**
  1. Reduced sweating capacity.
  2. Greater body surface area to weight ratio.
    a. Particularly detrimental when ambient temperature exceeds body temperature.

C. **Walking and running eficiency is considerably lower.**
  1. From age 8 to 18, efficiency of locomotion increases about 1% per year.

D. **Effect of maturation rate on sports performance**
  1. Most female athletes tend to initiate menarche later than nonathletes.
  2. Prepubertal sex characteristics such as leanness seem to be advantageous in many sports.
  3. Early maturing boys seem to prevail in team sports where height, weight, and strength are requisites for success.
    a. Several classic studies show that boys competing in the Little League World Series were above average in skeletal growth, and the more mature boys tended to play the critical positions, including pitcher.
  4. Grouping of youngsters to promote equality of competition.
    a. Age and grade level are the predominant modus operandi.
    b. Maturation should be taken into consideration.

E. **Recommendations**
  1. Emphasize fun and skill development. Lacking this, further participation in sports is hampered, as may be the physical activity pattern in adulthood.
  2. Begin specific conditioning work only when youth are old enough to understand its purpose and are willing to subject themselves to vigorous, demanding exercise.
    a. Err on the side of too little rather than too much to reduce the incidence of injury and reduced enjoyment.
    b. Consider conditioning below age 13 to be primarily for the sake of exposure to conditioning.

## RECOMMENDED READING

1. American Academy of Pediatrics: Fitness in the preschool child. Pediatrics 58:88–89, 1976.
2. American College of Sports Medicine: Position statement on the recommended quantity and quality of exercise for developing and maintaining fitness in healthy adults. Med Sci Sports Exerc 10:vii–x, 1978.
3. Berg K, LaVoie J, Latin R: Physiological training effects of playing youth soccer. Med Sci Sports Exerc 17:656–660, 1985.
4. Berg K, Sady S, Beal D, et al: Developing an elementary school CHD prevention program. Phys Sportsmed 11(10):99–105, 1983.
5. Brooks G, Fahey T: Fundamentals of Human Performance. New York, Macmillan, 1987.
6. Consumer Product Safety Commission National Electronic Injury Surveillance System: Report for January 1 through December 21, 1979.
7. Duda M: Prepubescent strenght training gains support. Phys Sportsmed 14(2):157–161, 1986.
8. Gilliam TB, Freedson PS, Geenen DL, Shahraray B: Physical activity patterns determined by heart rate monitoring in 6–7 year-old children. Med Sci Sports Exerc 13:65–67, 1981.
9. Gilliam TB, Katch VL, Thorland W: Prevalence of coronary heart disease risk factors in active children, 7 to 12 years of age. Med Sci Sports Exerc 9:21–25, 1977.
10. Greene L, Osness WL: Health education: Sunflower style. Health Education 10(November-December):34–35, 1979.
11. Hale C: Physiological maturity of little league baseball players. Res Q 27:276–282, 1956.

12. Hamilton P, Andrew GM: Influence of growth and athletic training on heart and lung functions. Eur J Appl Physiol 36:27–38, 1976.
13. Kobayashi K, Kiamura K, Miura M, et al: Aerobic power as related to body growth and training in Japanese boys: A longitudinal study. J Appl Physiol 44:666–672, 1978.
14. Krogman W: Maturation age of 55 boys in the Little League World Series. Res Q 30:54–59, 1959.
15. Martens R: The uniqueness of the young athlete: Psychological considerations. Am J Sports Med 8:382–385.
16. Martens R, Christina RW, Harvey JS, Sharkey BJ: Coaching Young Athletes. Champaign, IL, Human Kinetics Publishers, 1981.
17. Moritani I, deVries H: Neural factors versus hypertrophy in the time course of muscle strength gain. Am J Phys Med 58:115–124, 1979.
18. Pate RR, Blair SN: Exercise and the prevention of atherosclerosis: Pediatric implications. In Strong WB (ed): Atherosclerosis: Its Pediatric Aspect. New York, Grune & Stratton, 1978, Ch 13.
19. Ross J, Gilbert G: The National Children and Youth Fitness Study: A summary of findings. J Phys Educ, Rec Dance January, 3–8, 1985.
20. Sailors M, Berg K: Comparison of responses to weight training in pubescent boys and men. J Sports Med Phys Fit 27:30–37, 1987.
21. Weltman A, Janney C, Clark R, et al: The effects of hydraulic resistance training in pre-pubertal males. Med Sci Sports Exerc 18:629–638, 1986.

# Chapter 19: The Mature Athlete

DAVID O. HOUGH, MD
WADE LILLEGARD, MD
CHRIS McGREW, MD

I. **Introduction***

The number of older adults in America has markedly increased over the past 15 years. Currently, more than 10% of the U.S. population is 65 years of age and older, compared with less than 5% at the turn of the century. The U.S. Census Bureau predicts that approximately 20–21% of the population will be aged 65 and older by the year 2030.

The aging process represents a gradual decline in the ability of the individual to adapt to changes in the environment. As the U.S. population ages, health care providers increasingly will be challenged to meet the special needs of the elderly, especially in helping them to remain more functional. A program of regular exercise is one way this goal may be met. Mature athletes participate in a wide variety of sports, competing in community regional and national levels of competition, including the Senior Olympics, at the highest level.

Physicians often inappropriately tell their older patients with exercised-induced problems to stop their activity altogether. This chapter will look at the importance and benefits of exercise in older people and evaluate the types of injuries seen in this population. There is little evidence that the elderly are less physically active than younger people, and in fact, **exercise may increase longevity in men and women.** The growing importance of the aged and their role in society makes it imperative that the health professional understands their needs and problems.

II. **Principles of Exercise Prescription for the Mature Athlete**

A. Prior to instituting an exercise program in the elderly, consider the following:
   1. The exercise goals of the patient.
   2. The availability of equipment and facilities.
   3. Cost of the program.
   4. Performing a thorough assessment of the patient's health, reviewing:
      a. Appropriate history and physical.
      b. Assessment of nutritional status, present activity level, smoking habits, alcohol use and weight problems.
      c. Diseases that lead to decreased exercise tolerance.
      d. Orthopedic problems and disabilities that produce physical limitations.
      e. Any history of prior injury and rehabilitation.
      f. Present status of the patient's physical condition and training status.
      g. Medications that may interfere with or alter the exercise response.
   5. Laboratory testing—urinalysis, EKG.

* *Editor's note:* This chapter is written from a slightly different perspective than the rest of the book. As group or "team" activities and competitions have become popular for older adults, many of the physicians who care for younger athletes are asked by older patients for advice about safe exercise. "The Mature Athlete" provides insights and guidelines for exercise prescription and participation in a more senior population.

**TABLE 1.** Age-Related Decreases in Functional Status

| | | |
|---|---|---|
| **Cardiovascular system** | ↓ Maximum heart rate | 10 beats/minute/decade |
| | ↓ Resting stroke volume | 30% by 85 years of age |
| | ↓ Maximum cardiac output | 20–30% by 65 years of age |
| | ↓ Vessel compliance | ↑ blood pressure 10–40 mmHg |
| **Respiratory system** | ↑ Residual volume | 30–50% by 70 years of age |
| | ↓ Vital capacity | 40–50% by 70 years of age |
| **Nervous system** | ↓ Nerve conduction | 1–15% by 60 years of age |
| | ↓ Proprioception and balance | 35–40% ↑ in falls by 60 years of age |
| **Metabolism** | ↓ Maximum $O_2$ uptake | 9%/decade |
| **Musculoskeletal system** | ↑ Bone loss—> 35 y.o. | 1%/year |
| | > 55 y.o. | 3–5%/year |
| | ↓ Muscle strength | 20% by 65 years of age |
| | ↓ Flexibility | Degenerative disease or inactivity |

6. Graded exercise test (GXT) in patients with multiple risk factors, or symptoms of coronary artery disease in sedentary males aged 40–59.
   a. The risk of GXT in the elderly may be higher than that in the young population due to the increased incidence of coronary artery disease. After age 65, 30% of patients develop myocardial ischemia during exercise, and the use of a modified GXT protocol is warranted.[3–7]
B. **Physical changes of aging**[1]: The physical changes that occur in aging include (Table 1):
   1. Decreased cardiac output (decreased stroke volume, decreased heart rate).
   2. Decreased ventilatory capacity, pulmonary blood flow, aerobic power, and physical work capacity.
   3. Decreased body muscle mass, nerve conduction, time, and elasticity of tissue and an increased absorption of bone.
   4. Increased incidence of hypertension (BP > 150/95) in 50% of patients over age 80.
   5. Increased potential for developing heat stress.
C. **Benefits of regular exercise in the mature athlete**[3]: The benefits of exercise for older adults include:
   1. Improved muscle tone, range of motion, posture, coordination, and physical work capacity.
   2. Increased $VO_2max$ and decreased blood pressure.
   3. Improved weight control, body image, and a decreased incidence of depression.
   4. Reduction in the incidence of low back pain.
   5. An improvement in the prevention of accidents.
   6. Improved social contacts and sleep patterns.
   7. Improved functional ability and more independence.
D. **Purpose of exercise evaluation:** The purpose of the exercise evaluation is to:
   1. Determine the appropriate exercise (type, frequency, intensity, and duration) for the patient.
      a. The importance of graded exercise testing for patients in this age group should be noted.
   2. Evaluate any chronic health problem that may compromise the patient's physical capacity.
   3. Acknowledge medical conditions that preclude vigorous physical activity, and understand absolute contraindications for exercise participation.
   4. Instruct the patient to start all exercise programs gradually and increase activity levels based on the exercise evaluation.

E. **Guidelines for patient education**[8,9]: Patient education regarding exercise for the mature athlete should include:
   1. Specificity about the exercise prescribed.
   2. Exercise three to four times a week with a proper warmup and cool-down period; avoid hot/humid weather.
   3. A gradual increase in activity from week to week.
   4. Acquainting the patient with the significance of muscle/joint pain and the importance of fatigue.
F. **Goals of the exercise program:** The goals of the mature athlete's exercise program include:
   1. Increased cardiovascular fitness, endurance, flexibility, balance, and strength through walking, jogging, swimming, or biking.
   2. Minimize deconditioning and disuse changes previously attributable to aging.
   3. Increase self-esteem.
G. **Special concern—to avoid unnecessary injury:**
   1. Avoidance of running, jumping rope, and weight lifting in selected patients.
   2. Avoidance of isometric exercise if the patient is hypertensive.
   3. Exercising within the aerobic limits established by the GXT.
   4. Establishing a target heart rate of 60–75% of maximum heart rate.
   5. Informing patients with decreased visual or hearing acuity about the dangers of exercising without special precautions (traffic, etc.).

III. **Common Musculoskeletal Problems of the Mature Athlete**

A. **Common injuries**
   1. The following problems account for the largest number of visits to physicians: low back injuries, acute cervical strains, bursitis/tendonitis of the shoulder, patellofemoral dysfunction, and chronic ankle injuries. Treatment of these injuries is discussed elsewhere.
   2. **Possible contributing factors and disease processes contributing to musculoskeletal complaints include:**
      a. **Decreasing flexibility with aging—primary cause is disuse.** Regular stretching and exercises involving full range of joint motion may retard process.
      b. **Decreased nerve conduction and reaction time**—15% decrease between age 30–70. The patient should progress slowly to allow for neuromuscular adaptation.
      c. **Decreased hearing and/or vision associated with unsteady gait**—use of a stationary bicycle may be useful for those with balance problems.
      d. **Degenerative joint disease**—Increased incidence with aging, almost ubiquitous over age 65. Studies show that jogging is not a causal factor of DJD.[10] If symptomatic, may need to use non-weight-bearing form of exercise such as cycling or water exercises.
      e. **Rheumatoid arthritis**—increased incidence with aging; females > males. Similar recommendations for non-weight-bearing exercises as for DJD.
      f. **Gout**—increased incidence over age 60; males > females, should curtail activity during acute attack, utilizing adequate rest periods, appropriate splinting and medications.
      g. **Decreased muscle mass**—results in decreased strength and shock absorption. Regular exercise helps maintain lean muscle mass.
      h. **Osteoporosis**—more significant for females, may predispose older individuals to increased fractures, especially to the hip, vertebral column, and forearm. Regular weight-bearing exercise may play an important role in prevention.

B. **Principles of injury treatment**
1. Proper analysis of contributing factors with **appropriate modification or correction** is required in the following:
    a. **Specific movements and/or activities;** e.g., a tennis player with tennis elbow requires instruction in proper back-hand technique.
    b. **Training patterns;** e.g., a runner with an overuse injury such as posterior tibialis stress syndrome (shin splints) should reduce mileage and increase strength work and stretching.
    c. **Biomechanical factors;** e.g., a runner with excessive subtalar joint pronation may benefit from a properly designed orthotic.
    d. **Equipment;** e.g., a bicyclist with a knee pain may need an adjustment in seat height and use of lower resistance gears.
2. **Appropriate use of rest (either relative or absolute).**
    a. For a prescribed period of time or related to symptom relief (nonaggravating activities are allowed).
    b. May be expressed in terms of % decrease in activity—often reduced by increments of 15–25% of usual activities until symptoms disappear.
    c. Followed by a gradual return to activity (increase activity by increments of 15–25% over the course of 3–6 weeks).
    d. With increased age of patient, probably need to increase recovery time.
3. **Provision of an appropriate and aggressive rehabilitation program.**
    a. Use of simple, inexpensive equipment (such as free weights or elastic tubing) that can be used at home along with printed material showing rehabilitation methods may increase compliance and recovery.
    b. Rehabilitation should also include range-of-motion and flexibility exercises.

IV. **Exercise Prescription for the Sedentary Adult**

A. **Introduction**

Over the last 30 years, more than 40 published studies have examined the effect of regular physical activity in order to learn whether people who are more active have a healthier life than less active or sedentary people.[11,12] Not all of these studies support the hypothesis that active people are healthier, but most demonstrate that active individuals do better, particularly in relation to chronic disease.

Coronary artery disease is the major disease for which we have evidence that active people are healthier. They have substantially lower mortality rates. Disorders such as obesity, osteoporosis, and hypertension were also less prevalent in this active group. The amount and type of activity that are beneficial seem to be well within the capacity of most adults. Exercise that contributes to lowering the risk for these diseases consists mostly of activities such as walking, stair climbing, hiking, and routine activities of everyday life.

Reduction of other risk factors for heart disease also should be employed. Lowering dietary cholesterol, avoiding cigarettes, and treating hypertension when present should be routine advice for the patient prone to develop heart disease. A comprehensive approach that includes these behavioral modifications, treatment techniques, and a regular exercise program can significantly change the long-term health of the active individual.[13]

B. **Contraindications for exercise training and testing**
1. Exercise testing is useful in patients when the physician must decide whether closer monitoring of the exercise program is indicated. Patients in this category should undergo a medically supervised test for functional capacity.
2. Patients with the following conditions require supervised stress testing[15]:
    a. Recent myocardial infarction or post-coronary artery bypass surgery.

**TABLE 2.**  Conditions Requiring Caution in Exercise Prescription

1. Viral infection or cold
2. Chest pain
3. Irregular heart beat
4. Exercise-induced asthma
5. Prolonged, unaccustomed physical activity
6. Conduction disturbances (LBBB, complete AV block, or bifascicular block with or without first degree block)

     b. Presence of a pacemaker-fixed rate or demand.
     c. Use of chronotropic or inotropic cardiac medications.
     d. Presence of morbid obesity combined with multiple coronary risk factors.
     e. Occurrence of ST-segment depression at rest.
     f. Severe hypertension.
     g. Intermittent claudication.
3. Conditions, both medical and environmental, that require moderation of activity or caution in prescribing exercise are listed in Tables 2 and 3.
4. In general, many patients in the mature athlete age group will require some form of exercise testing prior to instituting an exercise program.

C. **Intensity of exercise**
1. The most important variable in any exercise prescription is **intensity,** but it also is the most difficult factor to determine.
2. Intensity is expressed as a percentage of maximum heart rate (MHR), heart rate reserve (maximum HR minus resting HR), or functional capacity ($VO_2$max or METs).
3. **The intensity rate for proper training depends on the initial fitness level of the adult.**
     a. Unconditioned individuals have a low threshold for improving functional capacity, whereas conditioned patients require a greater intensity level to increase aerobic fitness.
     b. Determining intensity by heart rate.
        i. MHR is determined through a linear relationship between the heart rate and $VO_2$max. Intensity is expressed as a percentage of maximum heart rate ($HR_{max}$), where $HR_{max} = (220 - age) \pm 15$.
        ii. Intensity levels of 60–85% of MHR can induce training. These values correspond to approximately 60–80% of functional capacity.
        iii. The Karvonen method is the preferred method of determining intensity and is based on the maximum heart rate formula of $220 - age \pm 15$ beats.
           (a) Calculate the training heart rate (THR) as follows: $THR = [(0.60$ to $0.85) \times (HR_{max} - HR_{rest})] + HR_{rest}$, where (0.60 to 0.85) represents a potential range of training intensities from 60–85% of MHR.
           (b) The mature athlete should begin exercise at low intensity levels and gradually increase as fitness improves.

**TABLE 3.**  Conditions Requiring Moderation of Activity

1. Extreme heat and high relative humidity
2. Extreme cold, especially when strong winds are present
3. Following heavy meals
4. Exposure to high altitudes (greater than 1700 meters)
5. Significant musculoskeletal injuries

**TABLE 4.**  Average Maximum Heart Rates by Age and Recommended Target Heart Rates (THR) for Normal Asymptomatic Participants During Exercise*

| Age (Yrs) | 20–29 | 30–39 | 40–49 | 50–59 | 60–69 |
|---|---|---|---|---|---|
| $HR_{max}$ | 190 | 185 | 180 | 170 | 160 |
| Peak THR<br>0.9 $(HR_{max}-75) + 75$ | 179 | 174 | 170 | 161 | 152 |
| Lowest THR<br>0.6 $(HR_{max}-75) + 75$ | 144 | 141 | 138 | 132 | 126 |
| Average THR<br>0.7 $(HR_{max}-75) + 75$ | 155 | 152 | 149 | 141 | 135 |

* Modified from the American College of Sports Medicine: *Guidelines for Graded Exercise Testing and Exercise Prescription*, 2nd ed. Philadelphia, Lea & Febiger, 1980. Reprinted from Fox E: *The Physiological Basis of Physical Education and Athletics*, 3rd ed. Philadelphia, Saunders College Publishing, 1981, p 412.

  (c) The Karvonen method is advantageous over simple measures of MHR, since variability in the athlete's resting heart rate is accounted for in the formula.[37] Table 4 shows average maximum heart rates and THR for various age groups.

 D. **Exercise prescription using METs:** Use of METs to prescribe exercise is generally reserved for mature patients with some form of disability, where calculation by percent of MHR is not adequate for defining an exercise level.

  1. A MET is a unit used to describe exercise intensity.

   a. One MET is equivalent to $O_2$ consumption at rest in a sitting position.

   b. One MET = 3.5 ml/kg/min

  2. Maximum MET (MMET) = $\dfrac{VO_2max\ (ml/kg/min)}{3.5\ ml/kg/min}$

  3. Training intensity (TMET) should be between 0.6 and 0.85 MMET.

   a. Low intensity = 0.6 MMET

   b. High intensity = 0.85 MMET

  4. Metabolic cost (in METs) of various activities is readily available (Table 5). This is useful when prescribing exercise prognosis in this patient group.

  5. Energy expenditure can be calculated per session as follows (since 1 MET = 1 kcal/kg/hr): energy expenditure (kcal) = METs × time in activity (in hours) × body WT (in kg). Use this formula to determine how many kcal are burned in each exercise session.

 E. **Cycle ergometry**

  1. Cycle ergometry is used as an alternative to treadmill testing to determine $O_2$ uptake at given workloads.

   a. Calculations are based on the linear relationship of heart rate and $O_2$ uptake ($VO_2$) at varying workloads.

   b. The ergometer is used when the patient has problems with walking or jogging on the treadmill. It is a good alternative when proper protocols are followed.

  2. Maximum oxygen consumption ($VO_2max$) is calculated based on a projected workload at the predicted or known MHR of the mature athlete.

   a. You must have at least two submaximal $VO_2$ determinations, and

   b. The heart rate at submaximal workloads should be between 125–170 beats/minute for the best prediction of $VO_2$.

  3. **Bicycle ergometry protocol principles:**

   a. Multistage tests are more valid than single-stage tests.

   b. Adjust the workload for the mature athlete's age, sex, and level of conditioning.

**TABLE 5.** Average Work Intensities for Activities Suitable for Exercise Prescription*

| Activity | Average Work Intensity | |
|---|---|---|
| | *METs* | *Kcal/hr (75 kg)* |
| Walking, 0% grade | | |
| 2.5 mph | 3.0 | 225 |
| 3.0 mph | 3.3 | 240 |
| 3.5 mph | 3.5 | 262 |
| 4.0 mph | 4.6 | 345 |
| Jogging | | |
| 4.5 mph | 5.7** | 375–490 |
| 5.0 mph | 8.4 | 630 |
| 6.0 mph | 10.0 | 750 |
| 7.0 mph | 11.4 | 855 |
| 8.0 mph | 12.8 | 960 |
| Cycling (ergometer) | | |
| 300 kpm | 3.7 | 278 |
| 450 kpm | 5.0 | 375 |
| 600 kpm | 6.0 | 450 |
| 750 kpm | 7.0 | 525 |
| 900 kpm | 8.5 | 630 |
| 1050 kpm | 10.0 | 750 |
| 1200 kpm | 11.0 | 825 |
| 1500 kpm | 11.3 | 1010 |
| Swimming, crawl*** | | |
| 20 yd/min | 6.0 | 420 |
| 30 yd/min | 9.0 | 675 |
| 40 yd/min | 12.0 | 900 |
| Games (average intensity) | | |
| Basketball | 7–15 | 525–1125 |
| Volleyball | 5–12 | 375–900 |
| Soccer | 7–15 | 525–1125 |
| Handball | 8–12 | 600–900 |
| Tennis | 6–10 | 450–750 |

  * From Hanson PG, Giese MD, Corliss RJ: Clinical guidelines for exercise training. Postgrad Med 67:120, 1980.
  ** Metabolic cost of jogging at 4–5 mph is variable owing to the transition between fast walk and jog.
*** Metabolic cost of swimming is highly variable owing to efficiency, buoyancy, and technique; values may vary by 25%.

    c. Complete at least two stages with the heart rate between 125–170, depending on predicted MHR.
    d. Each stage should last 3 minutes or longer if the heart rate is not stable (within 5 beats/min).
    e. Calculations of $VO_2$ are made from simple graphs.
  F. **Duration of exercise**
    1. Ideal duration of exercise for most mature athletes is 20–60 minutes of continuous aerobic activity at a moderate intensity.
    2. Exercise sessions should be gradually extended from an initial 15–20 minutes as cardiovascular endurance improves. In this age group, instruct the patient to start with walking before jogging and gradually work the patient into a "walk-jog" program.
    3. Once initial fitness programs are underway, you should instruct the patient to extend the exercise session up to 60 minutes.
    4. Fat utilization increases significantly after approximately 20 minutes of light-to-moderate exercise, enhancing body fat reduction during longer periods of aerobic exercise.

5. The mature athlete should avoid high intensity exercise of short duration, as this may lead to increased musculoskeletal injury and the possibility of adverse cardiovascular events.

G. **Frequency of exercise**
   1. A minimum of three exercise sessions per week is necessary to achieve an aerobic effect.
      a. Allows sufficient rest to prevent musculoskeletal overuse syndromes.
   2. In the obese and in adults with low functional capability ($<$ 3 METs), prescribe repeated exercise sessions of 5 minutes each, several times per day.
      a. As functional capacity improves, one or two longer daily sessions should be undertaken.
   3. As functional capacity improves, increase to three or more sessions per week.
   4. Easier days must then be included during which the duration and intensity of exercise are reduced.
   5. Exercise sessions should not exceed 5 days per week.
      a. Progression from 3 to 5 days per week should occur gradually over a 4-week period.
      b. No more than three intense sessions should occur per week.
   6. Exercising 7 days per week does not further improve aerobic power and may serve to initiate overuse problems.
      a. **One exception**—the obese adult who needs daily low-intensity exercise to reduce body fat.

H. **Exercise mode**
   1. Exercise activities that utilize large muscle groups in a rhythmic and continuous manner are the preferred type of aerobic exercise.
      a. Jogging/running, swimming, bicycling or cross-country skiing programs.
      b. Less intense activities such as golf, bowling, and archery offer little training stimulus, as heart rates rarely exceed 100 beats/min.
      c. Rope skipping may produce excessively high heart rates and should be avoided in patients with restricted to moderate exercise intensity levels.
      d. Tennis and squash are adequate training stimuli if the skill level is sufficiently high. Squash, however, involves rapid starting and stopping, increases systolic blood pressure and myocardial oxygen demands, and should be prescribed only in healthy, risk-free patients.
   2. Weight-training programs should be of sufficient intensity to elicit a strength-training effect while minimizing musculoskeletal injury and an elevated blood pressure response.
      a. Avoid sustained isometric activities against heavy resistance, as they are strongly discouraged in unconditioned, hypertensive, and coronary-prone patients.

I. **Monitoring exercise**
   1. The mature athlete should be instructed to stop after 3–5 minutes of exercise. Measure the radial pulse for 6 seconds; then add a zero to yield the heart rate.
      a. Wrist palpation avoids the possibility of reflex hypotension that may occur with overly vigorous carotid massage.
      b. The pulse should be counted immediately after stopping because heart rate decreases rapidly after exercise has stopped.

J. **Progression of the exercise program**
   1. As cardiovascular and musculoskeletal fitness improves, increase the intensity, frequency and duration of exercise.

    a. Increase only one variable in any one session.
2. The rate of progression depends on the athlete's age (in general the older the patient, the slower the progression), functional capacity, overall health status, and exercise goals.
3. Typically, an exercise program is divided into three stages:
    a. Initial conditioning phase
    b. Improvement phase
    c. Maintenance phase.
       i. **Initial conditioning phase:** 2–10 weeks range of duration; average length of approximately 6 weeks.
          (a) **Purpose**—transition from sedentary to active lifestyle; if patient is already fairly active, duration of this phase may be short.
          (b) **Emphasis**—avoiding undue discomfort, which is discouraging to the new athlete.
          (c) **Content**—stretching and light calisthentics for warm-up and cool-down, with low level aerobic activities sandwiched in between. The aerobic phase should initially be 5–10 minutes in duration. The total workout in this phase should progress by 2–3 minutes every 1–2 weeks up to 20 minutes. Training intensity is usually low, approximately 50–60% of functional capacity.
          (d) **Basis for progression**
             (i) **Objective:** decrease in steady-state heart rate at a given intensity (3–8 BPM); voluntary adaption of a slightly faster pace by the patient and improvement in functional capacity.
             (ii) **Subjective:** decrease in fatigue and perceived exertion; improved movement patterns, more relaxed facial expression.
      ii. **Improvement phase:** up to 6 months or more after initial conditioning phase.
          (a) **Purpose**—major physical adaptation.
          (b) **Emphasis**—gradual increase in intensity and duration of exercise.
          (c) **Content**—Intensity and duration alternately increased. Intensity gradually increased from 50–60% to 70–85% of $VO_2max$ for a given duration. When tolerance of the new intensity is achieved, duration can increase, usually in increments of 2–5 minutes per workout. The duration is increased gradually to 30–45 minutes, depending on the intensity level.
          (d) Instruct the patient that further improvements in fitness occur more slowly than during initial conditioning phase.
     iii. **Maintenance phase:** next 6 months.
          (a) **Purpose**—Sustaining the gains made through prior conditioning program
          (b) **Emphasis**—Long term adherence to the exercise program and avoiding injury
          (c) **Content**
             (i) Review of exercise goals—weight control, cardiovascular fitness, competition, etc.
             (ii) Introduction of a variety of other aerobic activities in order to maintain interest and avoid overuse injuries.
             (iii) The patient exercises at 70–85% of functional capacity ($VO_2max$) for 30–45 minutes 3–5 sessions per week.
             (iv) Monitor progress with a training diary and follow-up exercise testing if appropriate.

    (d) Emphasize the fact that musculoskeletal overuse injuries are common **with rapid progression of exercise programs.**

    (e) Adequate rest periods between exercise periods are very important to avoid overuse problems.

## REFERENCES

1. Clarke HH (ed): Exercise and aging. President's Council on Physical Fitness and Sports. Physical Fitness Research Digest 7:1–27, 1977.
2. Williams RS: How beneficial is regular exercise? J Cardiovasc Med 119:1112–1120, 1982.
3. American College of Sports Medicine: Guidelines for Graded Exercise Testing and Exercise Prescription, 2nd ed. Philadelphia, Lea & Febiger, 1980.
4. Barry HC: Exercise prescriptions for the elderly. Am Fam Phys 34(3):155–162, 1986.
5. Elkowitz EB, Elkowitz A: Prescribing exercise for the elderly. J Fam Prac Recert 8:117–130, 1986.
6. Laslett LJ, Amsterdam EA, Mason DT: Exercise testing in the geriatric patient. Ann Intern Med 112:56, 1980.
7. Mean WF, Hartwig R: Fitness evaluation and exercise prescription. J Fam Pract 13:1039–1050, 1981.
8. Smith EL, Gilligan C: Physical activity prescription for the older adult. Phys Sportsmed 11(8):91, 1983.
9. Hanson PG, Giese MD, Corliss RJ: Clinical guidelines for exercise training. Postgrad Med 67:120–138, 1980.
10. Lane N, et al: Long distance running, bone density, and osteoarthritis. JAMA 255:1147–1151, 1986.
11. Laporte RE, Blair SN: Physical activity or cardiovascular fitness: Which is more important for health? A pro and con. Phys Sportsmed 13(3):145–157, 1985.
12. Paffenbarger RS, Hyde RT, Wing AL, et al: Physical activity—all causes of mortality and longevity of college alumni. N Engl J Med 314:605–613, 1986.
13. Simons-Morton BG, Pate RR, Simons-Morton DS: Prescribing physical activity to prevent disease. Postgrad Med 83(1):165, 1988.
14. Goodman JM, Goodman LS: Exercise prescription for the sedentary adult. In Welsh RP, Shephard RJ (eds): Current Therapy in Sports Medicine. Toronto, BC Decker, 1985, pp 17–24.
15. Smith LK: Medical clearance for vigorous exercise. Postgrad Med 83(1):146, 1988.

# PART II

# GENERAL MEDICAL PROBLEMS

## Chapter 20: General Medical Problems in Athletes

MICHAEL A. SITORIUS, MD
MORRIS B. MELLION, MD

I. **General Issues**
   A. **Exercise and the immune system**
      1. Athletes' lore—"Physical exercise will promote resistance to infection."
         a. Anecdotal evidence only that conditioning reduces respiratory illness.
            i. Not verified by epidemiologic study.
         b. Respiratory infections may increase in winter.
            i. May be due to close daily indoor contact.
            ii. No evidence that cold exposure increases viral transmission.
         c. Overtraining increases susceptibility to infection.
      2. **Laboratory studies** support potentially important alterations in the immune system with strenuous exercise.
         a. **Lymphocytes**—increase in total number and enhanced function.
            i. T cells > B cells
            ii. Clinical significance unknown.
         b. **Antibodies**
            i. Decreased IgA level found in saliva in a study of Nordic ski racers.
               (a) Possible etiologies: cold exposure, exercise level, overtraining.
            ii. No change in circulating levels in a study of runners.
         c. **Complement**—not affected in two small studies (N = 26).
         d. **Granulocytes**
            i. Increased transiently (1–2 hours).
            ii. Varied mechanisms—fluid shift to intracellular, ↑ catecholamine levels, ↑ cortisol levels.
            iii. No significant change in total granulocyte count in highly trained athletes vs sedentary individuals.
         e. **Interleukin-1**
            i. An immunostimulant.
            ii. Increased acutely with exercise.
            iii. Increased T cell/B cell activity.
         f. **Interferon**
            i. Transient increase in level 2 hours post-exercise (8 treadmill subjects).
            ii. Increase modest compared to increase with viral infection.
      3. **Can the immune system be damaged?**
         a. Exhaustive exercise acutely lowers helper T-cell/suppressor T-cell ratio—increased risk of infection.

b. Exhaustive exercise may produce antibody decrease in respiratory, salivary secretions—? sign of decreased circulatory immunity
c. Difference in granulocyte response in conditioned vs. unconditioned athlete.[2]
   i. No significant leukocytosis in marathoners following a 13 km run.
   ii. ↑ leukocytes in unconditioned athletes post treadmill test.
   iii. Questionable clinical significance: What does the alteration of leukocyte response to exercise mean? Is it a positive response to conditioning? Does it represent decreases in immune response?

4. **Conclusions:**
   a. Clinical significance of laboratory abnormalities unclear.
   b. Results of clinical trials varied.
   c. Increased risk of infection in overtrained athlete may be result of exercise and immune system responses.
   d. Acute exercise effects different from chronic exercise effects.

B. **Effects of fever on exercise capacity and performance**
   1. **Effects**
      a. Decreased strength
      b. Decreased aerobic power ($VO_2$max)
      c. Decreased endurance
      d. Decreased coordination
      e. Decreased concentration
      f. All can lead to injury.
   2. **Physiologic effects of fever**
      a. **Cardiovascular**—increased cardiopulmonary effort with reduced peak exercise capacity.
         i. Cardiac output ↑ at submaximal levels of activity
            (a) Heart rate ↑
            (b) $O_2$ consumption ↑ at low levels of activity
            (c) Ventilation ↑.
         ii. Maximal cardiac output is reduced
            (a) Maximal workload is reduced
            (b) Blood pressure ↓
            (c) Peripheral resistance ↓
      b. **Temperature regulation abnormal**
         i. Increased set point in hypothalamus.
         ii. Danger may be magnified by dehydration.
      c. **Pulmonary function** abnormal in all but mildest acute respiratory infection
         i. Increased airway resistance
         ii. Decreased diffusion capacity
         iii. Decreased alveolar ventilation to pulmonary capillary gas exchange ratio
         iv. All magnified by increased demands of exercise.
      d. **Musculoskeletal**
         i. Isometric muscle strength ↓
         ii. Early fatigue.
      e. **Psychological**
         i. Desire to complete exercise (conditioning) decreased.
   3. **Recommendations**
      a. **Avoid strenuous conditioning and competition during febrile state.**
         i. Flushing occurs with fever > 38°C (100.4°F) and may be a helpful guide.
      b. Level of exercise on return to participation varies with time away and severity of illness.

C. **Overtraining** ("staleness")
   1. The athlete's training and competition program exceeds the physiological and psychological limits of the body, resulting in multisystem failure.
      a. Results from increase in exercise intensity or exercise volume (of short or medium duration).
         i. **Often a massive increase in exercise.**
      b. **Inadequate nutrition may contribute.**
         i. Differential diagnosis includes eating disorders.
      c. Minor forms of syndrome do exist.
   2. **Symptoms**
      a. Fatigue
      b. Loss of appetite
      c. Sleep difficulty
      d. Apathy (loss of motivation)
      e. Irritability and restlessness
      f. Depressed mood
      g. Heaviness in legs
      h. Chronic muscle soreness
      i. Increased evening fluid intake.
   3. **Signs**
      a. **Increased basal heart rate: most consistent and generally earliest sign.**
         i. **5–10 beat rise is diagnostic.**
         ii. As little as a 2 beat rise in athletes with previously stable basal heart rate may be a clue to an impending problem.
      b. **Weight loss**
         i. Decreased body fat
         ii. Acute and chronic dehydration.
      c. Exaggerated postural blood pressure drop
      d. Decreased muscle size
      e. Lymphadenopathy.
   4. **Laboratory findings**
      a. Increase in serum creatinine kinase
      b. Decrease in cardiac output.
   5. **Associated conditions (may be sequelae)**
      a. **Frequent illnesses and infection**
      b. **Gastrointestinal disturbances**
      c. **Frequent overuse injuries**
      d. **Poor healing of overuse injuries**
      e. **Depression**
      f. **Eating disorders.**
   6. **Performance sequelae**
      a. Decreased speed
      b. Decreased endurance
      c. Increased heart rate recovery time after exercise
      d. Decreased coordination.
   7. **Treatment: Reduce training volume and intensity.**
      a. Minor overtraining problems may respond to training reduction and brief "training holidays" without loss of aerobic power.
      b. **Major overtraining syndromes characterized by multisystem involvement may require several weeks to months break from serious training.**
D. **Runner's high**
   1. **Euphoria often experienced by well-conditioned runners late in a long slow distance run.**
      a. Generally occurs after > 45 minutes of exercise.
      b. Reported in cross country skiing and bicycling, as well.
         i. Probably present in other forms of rhythmical endurance exercise.

2. **Mechanism unknown**
   a. **Prevalent hypothesis is that it results from the release of endorphins associated with endurance exercise.**
      i. Endorphins are endogenously produced peptides that act as mediators at central nervous system morphine receptor sites.

E. **Exercise addiction**
   1. **Defined as addiction because of symptoms that occur after stopping long-term, intense, regular exercise program.**
      a. Occurs in athletes exercising:
         i. Frequently, generally daily
         ii. Intensely
         iii. Long duration.
   2. **Symptoms**
      a. Anxiety
      b. Restlessness
      c. Irritability
      d. Nervousness
      e. Feelings of guilt
      f. Muscle twitching
      g. Bloated feeling
      h. Constipation
      i. Sleep disturbance.
   3. **Controversy: positive vs. negative aspects of exercise addiction**
      a. **Positive addiction**[11]: "That may strengthen us and make our lives more satisfying."
         i. Exercise addiction as **extension of normal behavior.**
         ii. Addiction to exercise and/or meditation replaces other dysfunctional or self-defeating behaviors.
      b. **Negative addiction**[18]
         i. **Compulsion to exercise becomes a distortion of normal behavior.**
            (a) As difficult to treat as any other addiction.
         ii. **Indications of negative addiction:**
            (a) **Less attention to family and other close personal relationships.**
            (b) **Less concern with other external issues such as work performance.**
            (c) "Feeling good becomes more important than anything else."
   4. **Proposed etiology: endorphins**
      a. Unproven.
   5. **Differential diagnosis:**
      a. Eating disorders
      b. Overtraining.
   6. **Therapy: behavioral interventions similar to those used in alcoholics and substance abusers.**
      a. Prognosis similar.

II. **Respiratory Illnesses**

A. **Acute**
   1. **Upper respiratory infections**
      a. Symptoms
         i. Fever
         ii. Chills
         iii. Myalgias
         iv. Nasal congestion
         v. Sore throat
         vi. Fatigue
         vii. Cough
      b. Etiology—viral
      c. Treatment:
         i. Supportive
            (a) Fluids

      (b) Rest

      (c) Antipyretic—aspirin or acetaminophen.

   ii. Medical

      (a) Decongestants

      (b) Antihistamines

      (c) Cough suppressants (e.g., 15 mg dextromethorphan/5 cc, 5–10 cc every 4–6 hours)

      (d) Caution about using prescribed or over-the-counter banned substances (see Chapter 16).

   iii. Prevention—good hand washing to decrease spread since transmission is person to person.

  d. **Factors for return to athletics**

    i. Afebrile

    ii. Myalgias improved

    iii. Gradual re-conditioning.

  e. **Complete re-conditioning may take longer than expected**

    i. Occasionally, seemingly mild viral respiratory illnesses may cause a 4–6 week delay in return to normal performance.

      (a) Possibly due to occult pulmonary damage.

2. **Streptococcal pharyngitis**

  a. Symptoms and signs

    i. Fever

    ii. Sore throat

    iii. Swollen, exudative tonsils

    iv. Anterior cervical lymphadenopathy—tender.

  b. Etiology: **group A beta-hemolytic streptococcus**

  c. Diagnosis

    i. Signs and symptoms

    ii. Rapid strep tests (10–30 minutes)—office procedure

      (a) Enzyme-linked immunosorbent assay (ELISA)

      (b) Latex-agglutination tests

      (c) Both 85–90% accurate.

    iii. Throat culture—incubator required

      (a) 95% accurate

      (b) 24–48 hr delay for results.

  d. Treatment

    i. Antibiotic

      (a) Penicillin 1st choice

      (b) Penicillin allergic

        (i) Erythromycin

        (ii) Cephalosporin

    ii. Supportive

      (a) Antipyretics, analgesics    (d) Rest

      (b) Warm saline gargles, lozenges    (e) Discuss contagious nature.

      (c) Fluids

  e. Factors for return to athletics

    i. Afebrile

    ii. Antibiotics started.

  f. Complications

    i. Peritonsillar abscess

    ii. Scarlet fever

   iii. Rheumatic fever

   iv. Acute glomerulonephritis.

 3. **Infectious mononucleosis**—an acute, generally self-limited, viral lymphoprolif-erative disease with autoimmune features.

  a. **Etiology: Epstein-Barr Virus (EBV)**

   i. Communicable transmission; excreted in saliva

    (a) Many cases with no known prior contact.

   ii. **30–50 day incubation period.**

  b. **Epidemiology:** Attack rate highest from ages 15–25, with 25–50% of these infected developing classic syndrome. 90% of Americans infected with EBV by age 30.

   i. Lower socioeconomic classes: infection generally at early age with subclinical disease.

  c. **Classic infectious mononucleosis syndrome**

   i. **Prodrome: 3–5 days**

    (a) Headache

    (b) Fatigue

    (c) Loss of appetite

    (d) Malaise

    (e) Myalgias.

   ii. **Classic signs and symptoms: days 5–15**

    (a) Moderate to severe sore throat with tonsillar enlargement

     (i) One-third of patients have tonsillar exudates.

    (b) Moderate fever ± sweats

    (c) Enlarged tender anterior and posterior cervical lymph nodes

     (i) Lymphadenopathy often generalized

    (d) Petechiae of palate

    (e) Swollen eye lids

    (f) Palpable enlarged spleen by second week in 50–70%

    (g) Jaundice 10–15%

    (h) Mild morbilliform rash 5–15%.

   iii. **Laboratory findings:**

    (a) **Serological diagnosis** with rapid slide test based on the classic heterophil antibody absorption test

     (i) Sensitive and accurate.

    (b) **Complete blood count (CBC)**

     (i) White blood cells count (WBC) moderately elevated: 10,000–20,000 WBC/mm$^3$

     (ii) Marked lymphocytosis: $\geq$ 50% of WBC

     (iii) Atypical lymphocytes: 10–20% of WBC.

    (c) Liver function tests reflect mild hepatitis in a great majority of cases.

  d. **Septic pattern of infectious mononucleosis** occurs in 10%.

   i. High fever and chills

   ii. Severe pharyngitis

   iii. Protracted acute phase.

  e. **Common complications**

   i. **Airway obstruction due to massive enlargement of tonsils and adenoids**

    (a) **May require emergency nasotracheal intubation**

    (b) **Definitive treatment is high-dose intravenous corticosteroids**

     (i) Tonsils and adenoids shrink within 2–4 hours.

   ii. **Concurrent Group A beta-hemolytic streptococcal pharyngitis: 5–30%**

    (a) Treat with penicillin or erythromycin.

(b) **Avoid ampicillin, which causes a florid erythematous maculopapular rash due to an antibody present in infectious mononucleosis.**
iii. **Ruptured spleen: 0.1–0.2%**
(a) **Occurs only in enlarged spleens, but most are not palpable**
(b) Occurs on days 4–21 of symptomatic illness
(c) May be **spontaneous or trauma related.**
(i) Collision sports are well-documented sources of trauma and strain leading to rupture.
(ii) May rupture during gentle activities or while straining at stool.
(d) Left upper quadrant pain with radiation to tip of left shoulder
(i) Exacerbated by deep inspiration
(ii) Generalized to entire abdomen
(iii) Clinical hypovolemia develops.
(e) **Usually marked white blood count elevation:** 15,000–30,000/mm$^3$
(f) **Medical emergency requiring immediate surgery** to salvage or remove the spleen.
iv. **Neurological complications:** Variety of *rare* CNS and peripheral disease, including encephalitis and Gullain-Barre syndrome
v. **Probably increased susceptibility to head trauma**
(a) **Brain tissue may be less compliant in some patients with infectious mononucleosis.**
(i) **Relatively minor blows to the head may cause significant head injury.**
f. **Treatment**
i. **Supportive therapy**
(a) Acetaminophen for headache, fever, myalgias
(b) Stool softeners to prevent straining at stool
ii. **Corticosteroid therapy**
(a) **Reserve for patients with specific indications:**
(i) Imminent airway obstruction
(ii) Severe mono-hepatitis
(iii) Neurologic complications
(iv) Hematologic complications
(v) Septic pattern with high fever and severe pharyngitis.
(b) Dose: 40–80 mg prednisone or prednisone equivalents on first day, tapering over 6–12 days.
g. **Return to athletics**
i. **Resume easy training 3 weeks after onset of illness if:**
(a) Spleen not markedly enlarged or painful
(b) Afebrile
(c) Liver functions normal
(i) Measure only if hepatomegaly, hepatic tenderness, or jaundice has been present.
(d) Pharyngitis and any complications resolved.
ii. **Resume strenuous exercise and contact sports 1 month after onset of illness if above conditions are met and there is no measurable splenomegaly.**
(a) **Consider ultrasound measurement:** Normal < 14 cm in length.
(b) May consider use of **"flack jacket" for football.**
4. **Pneumonia**
a. Symptoms
i. Fever
ii. Chills
iii. Productive cough
iv. Shortness of breath
v. Chest pain
vi. Fatigue.

    b. **Common etiologic agents: adolescents and young adults**
        i. Viral
        ii. Mycoplasma pneumoniae
        iii. Streptococcus pneumoniae.
    c. Evaluation
        i. Clinical exam
        ii. WBC
        iii. Sputum smear and culture
        iv. Chest x-ray.
    d. Treatment
        i. Empirical
           (a) Erythromycin
           (b) Parenteral procaine penicillin G
           (c) Follow-up in 24–48 hours.
        ii. Supportive
           (a) Antipyretic
           (b) Fluids
           (c) Rest
           (d) Antitussive optional.
    e. Factors for return to athletics
        i. Afebrile
        ii. Resolved shortness of breath.

5. **Otitis media**
    a. Symptoms
        i. Ear pain and/or congestion
        ii. Fever
        iii. Hearing difficulties.
    b. Etiologic agents
        i. Viral—30%
        ii. Streptococcus pneumoniae—50%
        iii. Hemophilus influenzae—20%.
    c. Treatment
        i. Antibiotics
           (a) Ampicillin or amoxicillin
           (b) Cefaclor (cost is 2–4 × ampicillin or amoxicillin) and other beta-lactamase resistant agents
           (c) Penicillin allergic:
              (i) Trimethoprim; sulfamethoxazole double strength or erythromycin-sulfisoxazole.
        ii. Antipyretics
           (a) ASA or acetaminophen.
        iii. Analgesics—NSAIDs.
    d. Factors for the athlete to return to athletics
        i. Afebrile
        ii. Nondraining, intact tympanic membrane for swimmers/divers.
6. **Otitis externa** ("swimmer's ear")
    a. Symptoms and signs
        i. Otalgia (ear pain)
        ii. Drainage from ear canal
        iii. Swollen ear canal
        iv. Hearing difficulties
        v. Dizziness.

    b. Etiologic agents

        i. Bacterial *(Pseudomonas aeruginosa)* major cause

        ii. Fungus.

    c. Treatment

        i. Cleanse ear canal with $H_2O$ or $H_2O_2$.

        ii. Evaluate for tympanic membrane rupture.

        iii. Antibiotic/antiinflammatory ear drops

            (a) Polymyxin b/hydrocortisone, i.e., Cortisporin

            (b) ¼% acetic acid/hydrocortisone: VoSoL HC.

        iv. May need ear canal wick to resolve inflammation/infection

        v. Avoidance of excessive exposure to water; (showering, swimming may clinically prolong course); may need ear plugs once resolved.

    d. Factors for return to athletics

        i. Dependent on sport

        ii. Absence of balance problems.

  7. **Acute labrynthitis**

    a. Signs and symptoms

        i. Sudden onset         iv. Tinnitus (ringing in ears)

        ii. Marked vertigo         v. Unilateral nystagmus is typical

        iii. Accompanying nausea/vomiting   vi. Hearing loss.

    b. Viral etiology

        i. Resolves spontaneously in 1–2 weeks (more severe 4–6 weeks); re-examine during this time to rule out central etiology, i.e., acoustic neuroma.

        ii. Return to participation based on subjective (how one feels) and objective (clinical exam for sport specific activities).

        iii. Treatment

            (a) Supportive—emotions

            (b) Bed rest

            (c) Meclizine (Antivert).

  8. **Sinusitis—bacterial infection of paranasal sinuses**

    a. Signs and symptoms

        i. Facial pain         iv. Fever

        ii. Purulent nasal drainage     v. Fatigue.

        iii. Facial edema

    b. Diagnosis

        i. Clinical exam

            (a) Transillumination of sinuses

            (b) Percussion of sinuses.

        ii. X-ray exam (4 views)

        iii. Culture—? accuracy since nasal flora often contaminate specimen.

    c. Etiologic agents

        i. **Streptococcus pneumoniae and Hemophilus influenzae = 60%**

        ii. Anaerobes, *Streptococcus pyogenes, Branhamella catarrhalis,* and others = 40%

    d. Treatment

        i. Antibiotics—oral

            (a) Amoxicillin

            (b) Cephalosporins

            (c) Trimethoprim/sulfamethoxazole, double strength

            (d) Erythromycin if allergic to penicillin.

        ii. Decongestant—topical × 2–4 days (Neosynephrine, 0.25%) then systemic

        iii. Hot packs
        iv. Antipyretic/antiinflammatory; ASA or NSAIDs.
   e. Effect on athletic performance is related to decreased air exchange, effects of fever, body fatigue.
   f. Return to participation when
       i. Afebrile
       ii. Therapy initiated.

**B. Chronic**
  **1. Cystic fibrosis**
    a. Longer survival secondary to improved antibiotic therapy for pulmonary disease— ↑ likelihood of athletic participation.
    b. Effects of exercise conditioning seen in cystic fibrosis:
       i. Increased exercise tolerance
       ii. Increased peak $O_2$ consumption
       iii. Lower heart rate.
    c. Improved feeling of well-being
    d. Symptom-appropriate activities and physical training should be chosen.
    e. Exerciser needs free access to salt or salty foods due to excess sweat electrolyte losses.
    f. Limit free water unless accompanied by increased salt intake.

  **2. Rhinitis—noninfectious**
    a. Common causes—not limited to athletes
       i. Allergy
       ii. Noninfectious/nonallergic
         (a) Rhinitis medicamentosa
           (i) Antihypertensive medication
           (ii) Aspirin sensitivity
           (iii) Topical decongestant abuse (rebound rhinitis)
           (iv) Cocaine abuse.
         (b) Endocrine
           (i) Hypothyroidism
           (ii) Pregnancy
           (iii) Oral contraceptives.
         (c) Anatomic
           (i) Nasal polyp: → most common cause is ASA allergy
           (ii) Deviated nasal septum
           (iii) Nasal tumor.
         (d) Vasomotor rhinitis.
    **b. Symptoms of noninfectious rhinitis**
       i. Obstruction of nasal airflow
       ii. Clear nasal discharge
       iii. Nasal itching
       iv. Sneezing
       v. Associated itching and puffiness of eyes.
    c. Treatment
       i. Allergic rhinitis
         (a) Avoidance/environmental control
         (b) Pharmacologic
           (i) Antihistamine for discharge, sneezing
           (ii) Decongestant for obstruction
           (iii) Antihistamine/decongestant combination
           (iv) Topical cromolyn sodium

(v) Topical corticosteroid
- Beclomethasone
- Flunisolide

(vi) Systemic corticosteroid: Medrol Dosepak

(vii) **Caution** when any of above used with athletes, since any agent may be on banned drug list for competition, particularly at high levels of competition

(viii) Hyposensitization with immunotherapy.

    i. Noninfectious/nonallergic

    (a) Treat underlying cause

    (b) Review medication.

3. **Asthma** (See Chapter 24, Exercise-induced Bronchospasm).

III. **Hematologic Problems**

A. **"Pseudoanemia," iron deficiency, and anemia in athletes**

1. **Athletic pseudoanemia: A dilutional phenomenon**

    a. Intense endurance exercise training causes:

        i. Increased total body red blood cell mass

        ii. Increased total body hemoglobin

        iii. Proportionately greater increase in plasma volume.

    b. Therefore, **standard hematologic measures decrease due to dilution, whereas the total amount of red blood cells and hemoglobin actually rises:**

        i. Decreased red blood cell count

        ii. Decreased hematocrit

        iii. Decreased serum hemoglobin.

    c. **Benign condition: no treatment indicated.**

    d. Differential diagnosis: true anemia in the athlete.

2. **Iron deficiency in the athlete**

    a. Common problem in endurance athletes and others in whom "making weight" or maintaining a low percent body fat is important.

    b. **Results from a combination of**

        i. **Insufficient iron intake**

        (a) Too little iron in diet

          (i) Especially if athlete is consuming $< 2000$ kcal/day.

        ii. **Inadequate iron absorption**

        (a) Evidence exists for an iron absorption defect in iron-depleted runners

        iii. **Accelerated iron loss** in the endurance athlete

        (a) Iron loss in distance runners is twice as great as in nonexercising populations.

        (b) Sources of loss:

          (i) Hematuria: microscopic and gross

          (ii) Hemoglobinuria (footstrike hemolysis may contribute)

          (iii) Myoglobinuria

          (iv) Profuse sweating

          (v) Gastrointestinal bleeding: microscopic and gross.

3. **Stages of iron deficiency and iron deficiency anemia** (Table 1)

    a. **Stage I: "Prelatent" iron deficiency**

        i. **Absent or markedly diminished iron stores**

        (a) Serum ferritin $< 20$ ng/ml highly suggestive

          (i) Athlete with prelatent iron deficiency may have a spuriously elevated serum ferritin due to heavy training.

**TABLE 1.** Stages of Iron Deficiency*

| Stage | Characteristic | Serum Ferritin | Serum Iron | Total Iron Binding Capacity | Transferrin Saturation | Hemoglobin | Bone Marrow Iron Stores |
|---|---|---|---|---|---|---|---|
| I. Prelatent | Marrow iron depletion | ↓ | N | N | N | N | ·0-trace |
| II. Latent | Serum iron depletion with iron-deficient erythropoiesis | ↓ | ↓ | ↑ | ↓ | N-low N | 0 |
| III. Manifest | Iron deficiency anemia | ↓ | ↓ | ↑ | ↓ | ↓ | 0 |

* Adapted from: Clement DB, Sawchuk LL: Iron status and sports performance. Sports Med 1:65–74, 1984; Cook J: Clinical evaluation of iron deficiency. Semin Hematol 19:6–18, 1982; Parr RB, Bachman LA, Moss RA: Iron deficiency in female athletes. Phys Sportsmed 12:81–86, 1984.

      ii. Erythropoiesis occurs but RBCs may be iron-deficient.
    b. **Stage II: "Latent" iron deficiency**
      i. **Absent iron stores. Serum hemoglobin and other red blood cell parameters reduced but within normal range.**
      ii. **Serum iron reduced and total iron binding capacity elevated**
        **(a) Transferrin saturation is below 16%.**
      iii. **Erythropoiesis continues or is slowed. RBCs are iron deficient.**
    c. **Stage III: "Manifest" iron deficiency**
      i. **Characterized by true anemia**
      ii. Serum hemoglobin below 12 g/100 ml in women and 14 g/100 ml in men
        (a) In **black athletes** the diagnosis of anemia must be made in light of the fact that normal hemoglobin in black children is 1 g/100 μl lower than in white children, regardless of dietary or socioeconomic differences.
      iii. RBC count, hematocrit, and RBC indices also reduced.
  4. **Effects on performance**
    a. **Iron deficiency anemia**
      i. Decreases performance by decreasing oxygen transport:
        (a) Decreases maximum aerobic capacity ($VO_2$max)
        (b) Decreases anaerobic threshold
        (c) May decrease efficiency of submaximal exercise
        (d) May decrease exercise time to exhaustion.
      ii. **Body's compensatory mechanisms for mild anemia**
        (a) Increased ventilation
        (b) Increased heart rate and cardiac output
        (c) Increased red blood cell 2,3-diphosphoglycerate.
    b. **Iron deficiency without anemia**
      i. **Reduced myoglobin**
        (a) Necessary for storage and transport of oxygen in muscle.
      ii. **Reduced cytochrome C**
        (a) Results in reduced oxidative metabolism and lactate accumulation from anaerobic metabolism.
  5. **Treatment of iron deficiency and iron deficiency anemia**
    a. **Dietary iron sources generally provide inadequate quantities of iron to treat established deficiency or anemia.**
    b. **Oral iron supplementation**
      i. Ferrous salt yielding 65 mg elemental iron one to three times daily, depending on the magnitude of the deficiency

(a) Ferrous sulfate is cheapest.

(b) Ferrous fumarate and ferrous gluconate produce less gastrointestinal irritation.

(c) Start dose low and increase gradually to avoid gastrointestinal side effects.

ii. **Absorption enhancers**

(a) **Heme-iron contained in red meat, poultry, and fish is more readily absorbed from the gut than nonheme-iron and enhances the absorption of nonheme iron as well.**

(b) **Ascorbic acid enhances the absorption of nonheme-iron when given concurrently.**

(i) Dose: 250 mg ascorbic acid with each dose of ferrous salt

(ii) Commercial preparations available that combine ascorbic acid into a single dose with a ferrous salt.

6. **Overtreatment with iron**

a. **Self-treatment with large doses of iron over long periods of time by an athlete is not warranted and may be dangerous.**

i. **Hemochromatosis** may result.

b. **Athletes of Mediterranean heritage should be screened for thalassemia before iron therapy is started.**

c. **Black athletes should be evaluated for sickle cell disease before iron therapy is started.**

IV. **Genitourinary Problems**

A. **"Athletic pseudonephritis" and hematuria in athletes**

1. **Effects of exercise on renal function**

a. **Decreased renal blood flow**

i. Begins within first 10 minutes of exercise as blood flow to muscles increases.

ii. Exercise at 50% of $VO_2max$ reduces renal blood flow 30%.

iii. **Exercise at high intensity may cause up to 75% reduction in renal blood flow.**

b. **Decreased glomerular filtration rate**

i. Intense exercise may cause 50% reduction.

ii. **Dehydration** may have further effect.

2. **"Athletic pseudonephritis"**

a. **Increased excretion of protein, red and white blood cells, and cellular and noncellular renal tubular casts as the result of strenuous exercise.**

i. Proteinuria may be lesser presentation.

b. **Transient finding which disappears spontaneously after one to several days rest.**

c. **Mechanisms:** Kidneys respond to reduced renal blood flow and glomerular filtration rate caused by exercise with increased glomerular permeability to protein and blood cells and decreased renal tubular protein reabsorption.

d. **Dehydration** alone may cause similar urinary sediment and protein changes.

e. Urinary sediment changes in athletic pseudonephritis **correlate with intensity of exercise and state of hydration.**

3. **Routine urinary screening is no longer recommended**

a. Not cost effective

b. Rarely reveals unsuspected disease

       c. Frequently triggers expensive unnecessary evaluation
       d. If urine obtained in an athlete for other reasons reveals abnormal sediment, rest the athlete two days and repeat the test.

**B. Exercise and male sex hormones**
    **1. Physiologic effects of intense exercise**
       a. Testosterone ↑ or ↓
          i. Decreased:
            (a) Marathon runners
            (b) Inversely related to mileage trained
            (c) Symptoms of decreased shaving and decreased libido observed.
          ii. Increased:
            (a) Moderate exercise
            (b) Secondary to catecholamine effect on testes.
       b. Prolactin level ↓ in runners (> 64 km/wk) though remains in normal physiologic range.
       c. Luteinizing hormone ↔
       d. Follicle-stimulating hormone ↔
       e. Endogenous opioid peptides (EOPs) are increased with exercise; EOPs = endorphins, enkephalins.
          i. Chronic administration of EOPs in human studies can:
            (a) Suppress gonadotropin
            (b) Elevate prolactin
            (c) Suppress/sexuality; satisfy urges/needs at supratentorial level of brain.
          ii. Acute affect of EOPs are unknown.
    **2. Sex hormones and cardiovascular risk in intensely trained men**
       a. Estradiol/testosterone ratio is lower in physically trained men.
          i. Is cardiac risk decreased with relative increase in estrogen effect?
    **3. Fertility**
       a. Decreased theoretically
          i. High testicular temperature—impairs spermatogenesis.
          ii. Penile frostbite (rare)—may interfere with sexual function.
       b. Men whose sexual function was adequate developed no long-term fertility problems during physical conditioning.

**D. Testicular trauma**
    1. Mechanism is **blunt** trauma usually in contact sport.
    2. Symptoms
       a. Pain
       b. Swelling of scrotum.
    3. Type of injury:
       a. Contusion—most common
          i. Soft tissue swelling of scrotum
          ii. Treatment is ice, elevation, rest, oral analgesics, and support of scrotum.
       b. Rupture—most serious
          i. Disruption of tunica albuginea covering vascular components of testis
          ii. Bleeding in scrotum with massive acute swelling
          iii. Exam to include transillumination of scrotum and Doppler probe for spermatic blood flow
          iv. Ultrasound of scrotum may be indicated
          v. Avoid aspiration of scrotum unless suspect severe vascular compromise secondary to tense swelling
          vi. Treatment is emergency surgery—injury is seen in high impact accidents, i.e., cycling.

    c. Rupture of pampiniform plexus the venous network of spermatic cord
        i. Engorgement of these veins = varicocele
        ii. Treatment is ice, elevation, rest, oral analgesics and scrotal support

## V. Gastrointestinal Problems

### A. Anxiety and stress reaction

1. Performance anxiety
2. Inhibitory effect on gastrointestinal function activity
   a. Decreased acid secretion in stomach
   b. Motor activity slowed
   c. Blood flow is reduced.
3. Continued anxiety may result in acid hypersecretion.
4. Symptoms—not unique to athletes
   a. Diarrhea—secondary to hyperactivity of GI tract
   b. Dyspepsia, "knot in stomach."
5. Associated conditions
   a. Irritable bowel syndrome
   b. Peptic ulcer disease.
6. Treatment
   a. Reassurance/education
   b. Behavior modification
   c. Relaxation exercises.

### B. Acute gastroenteritis

1. Incidence: second only to upper respiratory tract infections in adolescents/young adults.
2. Etiologic agents
   a. Viral—most common
      i. Rotavirus
      ii. Norwalk agent.
   b. Bacterial
   c. Protozoan: *Giardia lamblia.*
3. Peak incidence: winter in cities; summer in rural or outdoor sports.
4. Symptoms:
   a. Diarrhea        d. Abdominal cramps
   b. Vomiting       e. Myalgia.
   c. Fever
5. Treatment
   a. Usually self-limited, 2–3 days
   b. Clear fluids, electrolyte-containing fluids, (i.e., Gatorade) are cornerstone; replace fluid loss, liter for liter
   c. Assess degree of dehydration (body weight, urine output, blood pressure) prior to strenuous practice or game
   d. Antimotility drugs may be effective for abdominal cramps but also may prolong carrier state of some organisms.
      i. Imodium (loperamide)
      ii. Diasorb (nonfibrous attapulgite)
      iii. Lomotil (diphenoxylate HCl with atropine).
   e. **"Traveler's diarrhea"** may respond to:
      i. Trimethoprim/sulfamethoxazole, double strength, BID
      ii. Peptobismol, 1 oz, q1h, until symptoms abate or 8 oz are consumed.
6. Return to competition limited only by hydration status, infective nature of problem, symptom complex (i.e., frequent diarrhea), and re-conditioning.

C. **The spleen and splenectomized athletes**
 1. Lack of spleen
   a. Not a contraindication to participation by itself.
   b. Pneumovax-23 recommended secondary to increased risk of *pneumococcal pneumonia* infection.
      i. 0.5 cc subq or IM
      ii. Bacterial polysaccharides of 23 pneumococcal types.
D. **Diarrhea and gastrointestinal bleeding in runners**
 1. **Runner's diarrhea ("Runner's Trots")**
   a. Diarrhea stimulated by intense endurance running (with or without accompanying gastrointestinal bleeding)
      i. **Descriptive data** from a study of 425 runners in a 10K race[22]
         (a) **Incidence: 30% of runners in race**
         (b) Characteristics of syndrome:
            (i) 85% passed semiformed or watery stools
            (ii) 60% low abdominal pain or rectal urgency; generally relieved by defecation
            (iii) 51% multiple stools
            (iv) 13% large volume stools
            (v) **12% frank blood in stool.**
   b. **Proposed mechanism: increased intestinal motility stimulated by intense running.**
      i. Running produces increases of motilin and other gastrointestinal peptides.
      ii. Bowel ischemia may also be etiologic (see section V.D.2.c., below).
 2. **Gastrointestinal bleeding**
   a. **Grossly bloody diarrhea stimulated by intense performance**
      i. May be large amounts of red, maroon, or clotted blood
      ii. Often accompanied by severe abdominal pain.
   b. Incidence of microscopic increases in fecal hemoglobin after intense running even more common.
      i. Also noted in endurance bicyclists.
   c. **Proposed mechanism: relative bowel ischemia**
      i. Up to 80% of normal intestinal blood flow may be shunted away during intense exercise.
         (a) May produce local areas of bowel necrosis.
         (b) Heat stress may also contribute.
   d. **May mimic acute appendicitis or Crohn's disease.**
 3. **Prevention and therapy**
   a. **Antidiarrheal medications** may be helpful in cases of diarrhea that appear to be a form of functional bowel syndrome.
   b. **Dietary manipulations**—of empirical value
      i. Athletes on a low-fiber diet may improve by adding fiber to absorb intraluminal fluid.
      ii. Athletes on a high-fiber diet may improve by reducing fiber in an attempt to decrease stimulation of intestinal motility.
         (a) Many athletes prefer a high-fiber diet because it stimulates intestinal motility, thus reducing intraluminal contents. This preference is valid only up to a point.
      iii. Eliminate foods that trigger functional bowel symptoms in the individual athlete.
   c. **Improve hydration before and during performance.**
      i. Increased plasma volume may decrease ischemia.

d. **Decrease training and competition level 20% to 40% in both mileage and intensity; then build back up slowly.**

VI. **Immunological Issues**

A. **Immunizations**

1. **Tetanus**

a. Booster every 10 years after primary series: t.d.s. intramuscular

b. Booster every 5 years for dirty wound

c. Tetanus immunoglobulin (250 units) and booster if immunization is not maintained.

2. **Measles (rubeola)**

a. Recent campus outbreaks

b. Risk population—vaccination recommended

i. Born after 1957 with no history of immunization

ii. Immunized prior to 12 months of age

iii. Immunized between 12–15 months of age, with a direct exposure to clinically diagnosed measles.

c. Screening

i. Document natural infection by history

ii. Proven immunity with rubeola titer—hemagglutination inhibition (HI) testing.

d. Revaccination

i. To all or to nonimmune?

(a) No ill effects of vaccine in previously immunized testing positive (HI)

(b) MMR may be given without increased risk.

ii. Revaccination recommended for all prior to entering middle school.

iii. Reimmunization cost ($30/dose) may become a public health issue.

3. **Influenza**

a. Athletes are **not** in recommended group to receive yearly vaccine

b. **May** consider vaccination for fall and winter team sports

i. Close contact increases risk.

ii. Rapid spread may significantly disrupt season.

iii. Advisable if supply of vaccine is sufficient to meet needs of the elderly and chronically ill first.

4. **Rubella**

a. Indications

i. All children over age 12 months

ii. Susceptible prepubertal, adolescent, and adult females of child-bearing age

iii. Susceptibility status—determined by serologic testing. Adequate hemagglutination inhibition. Titer for rubella = protection.

## REFERENCES AND RECOMMENDED READING

1. Brown RL, Frederick EC, Falsetti HL, et al: Overtraining of athletes: A round table. Phys Sportsmed 11(6):93–110, 1983.
2. Busse WW, Anderson CL, Hanson PG, et al: The effect of exercise on the granulocyte response to isoproterenol in the trained athlete and unconditioned individual. J Allergy Clin Immunol 65:358–364, 1980.
3. Clement DB, Sanchuk LL: Iron status and sports performance. Sports Med 1:65–74, 1984.
4. Costill DL, Flynn MG, Kirwan JP, et al: Effects of repeated days of intensified training on muscle glycogen and swimming performance. Med Sci Sports Exerc 20:249–254, 1988.
5. Daniels WL, Sharp DS, Wright JE, et al: Effects of virus infection on physical performance in man. Military Medicine 150:8–14, 1985.

6. Dressendorfer RH, Wade CE, Scaff JH: Increased morning heart rate in runners: A valid sign of overtraining? Phys Sportsmed 13(8):77–86, 1985.
7. Eichner ER: The anemias of athletes. Phys Sportsmed 14(9):122–130, 1986.
8. Eichner ER: Gastrointestinal bleeding in athletes. Phys Sportsmed 17(5):128–140, 1989.
9. Eichner ER: Infectious mononucleosis: Recognition and management in athletes. Physician Sportsmed 15(12):61–72, 1987.
10. Fogoros RN: "Runner's trots:" Gastrointestinal disturbances in runners. JAMA 243:1743–1744, 1980.
11. Glasser W: Positive Addiction. New York, Harper & Row, 1976.
12. Green RL, Kaplan SS, Rabin BS, et al: Immune function in marathon runners. Annals Allergy 47:73–75, 1981.
13. Hanson P: Illness among athletes: An overview. In Strauss RH (ed): Sports Medicine. Philadelphia, W.B. Saunders, 1984, pp 79–90.
14. Larson DC, Fisher R: Management of exercise-induced gastrointestinal problems. Phys Sportsmed 15(9):112–126, 1987.
15. Maki DG, Reich RM: Infectious mononucleosis in the athlete: Diagnosis, complications and management. Am J Sports Med 10:162–173, 1982.
16. Mandell AJ: The second wind. In Sachs MH, Sachs ML (eds): Psychology or Running. Champaign, IL, Human Kinetics, 1981, pp 211–223.
17. Mellion MB: Medical syndromes unique to athletes. In Mellion MB (ed): Office Management of Sports Injuries & Athletic Problems. Philadelphia, Hanley & Belfus, 1988, pp 129–145.
18. Morgan WP: Negative addiction in runners. Phys Sportsmed 7(2):56–70, 1979.
19. Morgan WP, Costill DL, Flynn MG, et al: Mood disturbance following increased training in swimmers. Med Sci Sports Exerc 20:408–414, 1988.
20. Nash H: Can exercise make us immune to disease? Phys Sportsmed 14(3):250–253, 1986.
21. Priebe JR: Exercise and renal function. Sports Med 1:125–153, 1984.
22. Priebe WM, Priebe JA: Runner's diarrhea—prevalence and clinical symptomology. Am J Gastroenterol 79:827–828, 1984.
23. Reese RE, Douglas RG, Edelson PJ: Immunization. In Reese RE, Douglas RG (eds): A Practical Approach to Infectious Disease. Boston, Little, Brown, 1986, pp 723–737.
24. Sappi E, Vorjo P, Eskola J, et al: Effect of strenuous physical stress on circulating lymphocyte number and function before and after training. J Clin Lab Immunol 8:43–46, 1982.
25. Shields CE: How I manage infectious mononucleosis. Phys Sportsmed 11(1):57–59, 107–110, 1988.
26. Simon HB: Exercise and infection. Phys Sportsmed 15(10):135–141, 1987.
27. Torg JS, Beer C, Brund LA, et al: Head trauma in football players with infectious mononucleosis. Phys Sportsmed 8(1):107–110, 1980.

# Chapter 21: Women in Sports

## ROSEMARY AGOSTINI, MD

Women have made incredible strides in sports in this past decade. Two American women recently reached the summit of Mt. Everest. The effects of Title IX, a law passed by Congress in 1972 that mandated equal opportunity for females in all areas of education, including athletics, were joyfully demonstrated in the strength, power, agility, and beauty of women athletes in the 1988 Summer Olympic Games in Seoul.

There are specific issues that are important to consider in active women and women athletes. These issues are addressed in the following chapter.

I. **Gynecological Concerns**

   A. **Definitions**

      1. **Menstruation:** the cyclic physiological discharge through the vagina of blood or tissue from the nonpregnant uterus. **Normal cycle**—first day of flow up to, but not including, the onset of menstrual flow in the next cycle (range 21–36 days).

         a. **Preovulatory (follicular) phase**—first day of flow to ovulation

         b. **Postovulatory (luteal) phase**—begins at ovulation.

      2. **Menarche:** onset of first menstrual bleeding

         a. **Evaluate girls**

            i. Age 16 if they have not started menstruating.

            ii. Age 14 if they have not started menstruating and are not developing secondary sexual characteristics.

            iii. Note: Be aware that there is some concern about an increased incidence of scoliosis and decreased bone density in young women with delayed puberty.

      3. **Anovulation:** absence of egg release. Women may have irregular, cyclic periods, or no period.

      4. **Oligomenorrhea:** menstrual cycle interval greater than 36 days.

      5. **Amenorrhea:** absence of menstrual cycle. No menstrual cycle in consecutive 6-month period. Generally implies state of hypoestrogenemia.

   B. **Significance of menstrual irregularities**

      1. **Anovulatory bleeding:** hormonal environment of unopposed estrogen. This has been associated with endometrial hyperplasia and increased risk of cancer of the endometrium and breast.

      2. **Amenorrhea:** low estrogen, absent progesterone. Significance—decreased bone density, atrophic vaginitis, and urethritis.

   C. **Amenorrhea**

      1. **Prevalence**

         a. Up to 5% of the general population

         b. Up to 20% of exercising women

         c. Up to 50% of elite athletes.

      2. **Etiology**

         a. **Pregnancy**

         b. **Stress**—psychologic, physiologic

         c. **Prolactin secreting tumors**

         d. **Hyperandrogenism**

  e. **Premature ovarian failure**
  f. **Hypothalamic/exercise related**
   i. Weight loss/thinness
   ii. Percentage of body fat
   iii. Age
   iv. Previous menstrual abnormalities
   v. Dietary factors.
3. **Patient evaluation**
 a. **History**
   i. Menstrual cycle
   ii. Physical activity
    (a) Daily frequency
    (b) Intensity
    (c) Duration of training
    (d) Any changes in the above.
   iii. Sexual activity
   iv. Nutritional history
   v. Weight gain/loss—6 months and 12 months prior to onset of symptoms
   vi. History suggestive of eating disorders
   vii. Pregnancy
   viii. Conflicts and support systems
    (a) Home
    (b) Work
    (c) Social
   ix. Coping skills.
 b. **Physical exam**
   i. General examination
   ii. Tanner stage: breast development and axillary and pubic hair
   iii. Galactorrhea
   iv. Vaginal dryness, urethritis (suggests decreased estrogen)
   v. Acne and hirsutism (suggest androgen excess)
   vi. Pregnancy (enlarged uterus)
   vii. Presence of normal sexual organs.
 c. **Diagnostic examinations**
   i. Pregnancy test—if indicated.
   ii. TSH—rule out hypothyroidism.
   iii. Prolactin level—rule out microadenoma of the pituitary.
   iv. Progesterone challenge—10 mg of medroxyprogesterone acetate (Provera) × 5 days. If patient has a withdrawal bleed within 2–7 days of stopping the Provera, this indicates adequate levels of estrogen. If there is no withdrawal bleed, continue work-up.
   v. Estrogen and progesterone replacement. No bleeding = end-organ problems. If there is withdrawal bleeding, next step.
   vi. FSH/LH levels—if elevated, diagnosis is primary ovarian failure. If the woman is under age 30, she should have a karyotype determination. The presence of mosaicism requires laparotomy and excision of gonadal tissues, because there is a 25% chance of malignant tumor formation.
   vii. Referral to a gynecologist to further evaluate secondary causes of amenorrhea, i.e., macroadenoma of the pituitary or hypothalamus.
 d. **Treatment**
   i. Pregnancy: prenatal care/voluntary termination
   ii. Elevated prolactin level: CT scan or MRI

   iii. Treat hypothyroidism: Synthroid

   iv. Anovulation: Provera 10 mg p.o. × 10 days per month

   v. Amenorrhea

    (a) If very thin—weight gain

    (b) If intensely exercising (i.e., running) decrease running, increase weight lifting, swimming, etc.

    (c) Cyclic estrogen and progestin: usually estrogen 0.625 mg p.o., q.d., days 1–25

     Hydroxyprogesterone acetate (Provera) 10 mg p.o., q.d., days 16–25

    (d) If patient also requests contraception, a birth control pill containing 30–35 $\mu$g of ethinyl estradiol and 0.4 to 1.0 $\mu$g of progestin should be used.

 **4. Estrogen and osteoporosis**

  **a. Menstrual cycle changes related to exercise are often associated with lower basal estrogen levels. Low estrogens:**

   **i. Increase calcium resorption from bone**

   **ii. Decrease calcium absorption from intestines**

   **iii. Decrease calcium reabsorption from kidneys.**

  b. Basic skeleton (calcium deposition in bones) is laid down by age 30–35.

  **c. Theoretically, in order to delay the development of osteoporosis and reduce its severity, one should evaluate and treat menstrual cycle abnormalities in youth.**

**D. Dysmenorrhea**

 **1. Definition:** abdominal cramps caused by inadequacy of uterine blood flow during myometrial contractions stimulated by prostaglandin F2 alpha produced in the endometrium.

 **2. Treatment**

  a. Nonsteroidal anti-inflammatory of your choice

  b. Oral contraceptives.

**E. Endometriosis**

 **1. Definition:** functioning endometrial tissue that exists outside the endometrial cavity.

 **2. Symptoms**

  a. Pain

  b. Infertility

  c. May be asymptomatic.

 **3. Treatment**

  a. Medical

   i. Danazol

   ii. Oral contraceptives

   iii. Gonadotropin releasing hormone (GnRH) analogues—leuprolide

   iv. Progestins.

  **b. Surgical**

   i. Fulguration of endometriotic implants

   ii. Resection of endometriotic tissue or cyst

   iii. Hysterectomy with bilateral salpingoophorectomy

   iv. Laser treatment.

**F. Premenstrual syndrome**

 **1. Definition:** collection of distressing physical, psychological, and behavioral symptoms that occur cyclically in the week before menses and only in ovulatory cycles.

 **2. Symptoms**

  a. Mood changes

  b. Depression

    c. Breast tenderness
    d. Fluid retention
    e. Abdominal bloating
    f. Appetite changes.
  3. **Diagnostic studies**
    a. Premenstrual health history
    b. Psychiatric history
    c. Three-month diary.
  4. **Treatment approach**
    a. Initiate or increase a conditioning or exercise program.
    b. Decrease stress.
    c. Avoid caffeine.
    d. Avoid high salt foods.
    e. Eat low calorie foods, e.g., carrots.
    f. Eat complex carbohydrates, e.g., muffins.
    g. Spironolactone 25–100 mg q.d. premenstrually.
G. **Contraception** for the active woman is generally the same as that for other women. Ideal methods of birth control do not exist. Methods include:
  1. **Barrier methods**
    a. Diaphragm with spermicide
    b. Sponge
    c. Cervical cap
    d. Condoms.
  2. **Oral contraceptives**
    a. To control the time of the menstrual cycle, use a 1/35 mcg type pill (rather than the triphasic) and add extra pills to prevent a menstrual cycle from occurring during an important athletic event.
  3. Tubal ligation
  4. Vasectomy.
H. **Infertility**
  1. **Definition:** inability of a couple to conceive after no contraception = 1 year.
  2. **Prevalence:** ?20% or similar to general population.
  3. **Etiology**
    a. Shortened luteal phase
    b. Oligomenorrhea/amenorrhea
    c. Anovulation
    d. Low weight/% body fat
    e. Other factors
      i. Scarred fallopian tubes
      ii. Endometriosis.
    f. Comment: 40% of infertility problems can be attributed to decreased or absent spermatogenesis and problems with sperm numbers or function.
  4. **Treatment**
    a. Decrease training mileage or change training.
    b. Decrease running; increase weight training or swimming.
    c. Increase body fat if a woman is thin.
    d. Evaluate and treat anovulation, oligomenorrhea, and amenorrhea as previously described.
    e. Record basal body temperature to evaluate ovulation.
    f. Sperm count of partner: high-intensity, long-distance male runners may have a lower sperm count and they should also be counseled to decrease mileage and increase body fat.

I. **Heavy bleeding**
1. **Definition:** normal menstrual flow equivalent to 40 ml/cycle. One full tampon or pad is equivalent to 3.5 ml blood. If one menstrual cycle has greater than 10–12 full pads, the woman is at risk for iron deficiency anemia.
2. **Menorrhagia:** excessive uterine bleeding occurring at regular intervals.
   a. In athletes this is usually due to anovulation. Treatment is medroxyprogesterone acetate (Provera) 10 mg × 10 days per cycle.
   b. Oral contraceptives if birth control is desired.
3. **Metrorrhagia:** uterine bleeding occurring at completely irregular intervals.
   a. **Warrants endometrial sampling** to rule out endometrial hyperplasia or adenocarcinoma before initiating progestational therapy (Provera 10 mg p.o. × 10 days per cycle).
J. **Breast exam**
1. **All** women should perform a monthly breast exam after the menstrual period.
2. A good support bra is recommended.
3. If a woman has **fibrocystic or tender breasts,** decrease caffeine and salt intake.
   a. Other therapy
      i. Vitamin E
      ii. Bromocriptine
      iii. Danazol.

II. **Exercise and Pregnancy**

A. **Most pressing concern is how exercise will affect the fetus.**
B. **Prevalence**—one study reported 50% of reproductive age women in Vermont exercise regularly,[2] and many of these women will want to continue to exercise during pregnancy.
C. **History**
1. **Exercise**
   a. Type
   b. Frequency
   c. Duration
   d. Intensity.
2. Pregnant women
   a. Starting an exercise program?
   b. Recreational athlete?
   c. Elite/high performance athlete?
D. **Major Concerns**
1. **Hyperthermia:** what is the effect of elevated body temperature on the fetus?
   a. Conditioned maternal thermoregulatory mechanisms appear capable of dissipating the heat production by both the metabolically active fetus and mother **during moderate aerobic exercise.**
   b. The increased maternal plasma volume during pregnancy helps maintain optimal fetomaternal heat transfer and dissipation.
2. **Hypoxia:** Will exercise shunt blood from the uterus to the exercising muscle?
   a. Because of increased hemoglobin concentration during pregnancy, and thus increased blood oxygen-carrying capacity, and a flow redistribution within the uterus favoring fetal blood flow at the expense of the myometrial flow, the fetus does not appear to be compromised.
3. **Decreased fetal weight:** Will the athletic mother's potentially lower body weight and smaller weight gain compromise the fetus?

    a. One study shows a decrease of newborn weight by 500 g of women who were able to continue exercise at near preconception levels through the third trimester.[2] A number of other studies report no change in neonatal weight.

4. **Contraindications to exercising during pregnancy.** (The pregnant woman with the following diagnoses should be evaluated and treated individually.)
    a. Heart disease
    b. Diabetes, severe or poorly controlled
    c. Hypertension, uncontrolled
    d. Previous miscarriage
    e. Incompetent cervix
    f. Anemia, moderate to severe
    g. Renal disease
    h. Vaginal bleeding.

5. **Special concern: cardiac patients, especially those with hemodynamically significant mitral or aortic valve disease are at high risk.**
    a. Cardiac output decreases during pregnancy making exercise dangerous.

6. **Benefits of exercise in pregnancy**
    a. Weight control
    b. Improved muscle tone
    c. Improved fitness
    d. Enhanced self-esteem
    e. Decreased varicose veins
    f. Decreased backache
    g. Better sleep
    h. Sense of control
    i. Possibly easier pregnancy, labor and delivery.

E. American College of Obstetrics and Gynecology (ACOG) Guidelines (Table 1)
1. **Meet the needs of the previously sedentary woman**
2. **Provide a framework to start an exercise program in pregnancy**
3. **Do not take into consideration the high performance athlete who becomes pregnant**
4. **Issues in ACOG Guidelines to be considered further**
    a. No exercise in a supine position is recommended after 4 months of gestation. Concern is impingement on the aorta and/or inferior vena cava with possible orthostatic hypotension and decreased blood flow to the placenta. This is not a common problem.
    (Please note some women deliver in the supine position and monitoring during that time shows no effect in blood pressure, fetal heart rate, etc. Brief periods of exercise in the supine position are probably not harmful.)
    b. No bouncing movement (no reason or data exist to indicate ill effects).
    c. Duration, intensity, and frequency of exercise
      i. Duration: 15–60 minutes
      ii. Intensity: 60–90% of maximum heart rate (maximum heart rate = 220 – age)
        (a) If starting exercise, approximately 140 beats per minute
        (b) If previously exercising, approximately 160 beats per minute.

F. **Signals to stop exercising**
1. Common sense
    a. Shortness of breath
    b. Dizziness
    c. Headache
    d. Muscle weakness
    e. Chest pain or tightness
    f. Back pain
    g. Hip or pubic pain
    h. Difficulty walking
    i. Generalized edema
    j. Decreased fetal activity
    k. Uterine contraction
    l. Vaginal bleeding
    m. Amniotic fluid leakage.

G. Summary
Lotgering, et al.: "Although the increased demands of pregnancy might compete with those of exercise, under most circumstances the maternal organism can meet the combined demands of gestation and exercise through a remarkable reserve of physiological adjustments."

**TABLE 1.** American College of Obstetricians and Gynecologists Guidelines for Exercise During Pregnancy and Postpartum

EXERCISE GUIDELINES. The following guidelines are based on the unique physical and physiological conditions that exist during pregnancy and the postpartum period. They outline general criteria for safety to provide direction to patients in the development of home exercise programs.

*Pregnancy and Postpartum*

1. Regular exercise (at least three times per week) is preferable to intermittent activity. Competitive activities should be discouraged.
2. Vigorous exercise should not be performed in hot, humid weather or during a period of febrile illness.
3. Ballistic movements (jerky, bouncy motions) should be avoided. Exercise should be done on a wooden floor or a tightly carpeted surface to reduce shock and provide a sure footing.
4. Deep flexion or extension of joints should be avoided because of connective tissue laxity. Activities that require jumping, jarring motions or rapid changes in direction should be avoided because of joint instabililty.
5. Vigorous exercise should be preceded by a 5-minute period of muscle warm-up. This can be accomplished by slow walking or stationary cycling with low resistance.
6. Vigorous exercise should be followd by a period of gradually declining activity that includes gentle stationary stretching. Because connective tissue laxity increases the risk of joint injury, stretches should not be taken to the point of maximum resistance.
7. Heart rate should be measured at times of peak activity. Target heart rates and limits established in consultation with the physician should not be exceeded.
8. Care should be taken to gradually rise from the floor to avoid orthostatic hypotension. Some form of activity involving the legs should be continued for a brief period.
9. Liquids should be taken liberally before and after exercise to prevent dehydration. If necessary, activity should be interrupted to replenish fluids.
10. Women who have led sedentary lifestyles should begin with physical activity of very low intensity and advance activity levels very gradually.
11. Activity should be stopped and the physician consulted if any unusual symptoms appear.

*Pregnancy Only*

1. Maternal heart rate should not exceed 140 beats per minute.
2. Strenuous activities should not exceed 15 minutes in duration.
3. No exercise should be performed in the supine position after the fourth month of gestation is completed.
4. Exercises that employ the Valsalva maneuver should be avoided.
5. Caloric intake should be adequate to meet not only the entire energy needs of pregnancy, but also of the exercise performed.
6. Maternal core temperature should not exceed 38°C.

American College of Obstetricians and Gynecologists: Exercise During Pregnancy and the Postnatal Period (ACOG Home Exercise Programs). Washington, DC, ACOG, 1985, p 4, with permission.

III. **Eating Disorders** (see Chapter 14)

    A. **Anorexia nervosa** (Table 2)

        1. **Definition:** syndrome of self-imposed starvation and distorted body image

        2. **Prevalence:** 1% of the general population; up to 6.5% of the ballet, gymnastic athletic population

        3. **Etiology:** complex interaction of biologic, psychologic and sociocultural factors.

**TABLE 2.** Diagnosis of Anorexia Nervosa

| SHARED FEATURES (ATHLETE AND ANORECTIC) |
| --- |
| Dietary faddism |
| Controlled calorie consumption |
| Specific carbohydrate avoidance |
| Low body weight |
| Resting bradycardia and hypotension |
| Increased physical activity |
| Amenorrhea or oligomenorrhea |
| Anemia (may or may not be present) |

| DISTINGUISHED FEATURES | |
| --- | --- |
| *Athlete* | *Anorectic* |
| Purposeful training | Aimless physical activity |
| Increased exercise tolerance | Poor or decreasing exercise performance |
| Good muscular development | Poor muscular development |
| Accurate body image | Flawed body image (believes herself to be overweight) |
| Body-fat level within defined normal range | Body fat level below normal range |
| Increased plasma volume | Electrolyte abnormalities if abusing laxatives and/or |
| Increased $O_2$ extraction from blood | diuretics |
| Efficient energy metabolism | Cold intolerance |
| Increased $HDL_2$ | Dry skin |
| | Cardiac arrhythmias |
| | Lanugo hair |
| | Leukocyte dysfunction |

McSherry JA: The diagnostic challenge of anorexia nervosa. American Family Physician 29:144, 1984, with permission.

B. **Bulimia**
   1. **Definition:** syndrome of secretive binge-eating episodes followed by self-induced vomiting, fasting, and purging with laxatives and/or diuretics
   2. **Prevalence:** up to 10% of college age students.
C. **Weight loss in athletes**
   1. Excessive weight loss in athletes may be different from that seen in anorectics and bulimics. It may be situationally related to athletic performance or making weight.
   2. Etiology: no deep seated chronic problems.
   3. Treatment: instruct athlete to spend mealtime with teammates, counseling visits.

IV. **Musculoskeletal Problems**

Injuries are sports specific rather than gender specific; i.e., injury types and rates are similar for men and women in the same sport but different for women participating in different sports.
   A. **Patellofemoral knee pain** (see Chapter 40)
      1. **Definition:** retropatellar or peripatellar knee pain
      2. **Symptoms**
         a. Creptitus
         b. Aching
         c. Pain going up and down stairs
         d. Stiffness after sitting long periods of time
         e. Subjective feeling of instability
      3. **Etiology: Additional predisposition in female athlete due to:**
         a. Weakness of the vastus medialis may be seen more often in females because of the influence of broader gynecoid pelvis on mechanics of the knee.

B. **Ligamentous laxity**

The only time women may be at increased risk for ligamentous and musculoskeletal injuries is during the third trimester of pregnancy, when **relaxin,** a hormone that makes the pelvic area flexible for delivery, is released, and all the ligaments become more lax.

C. **Stress fractures** (see Chapter 41)

1. **Definition:** pathological fractures, partial or complete, in bone that has been weakened by long-term recurrent microtrauma

2. **Factors that may predispose women athletes to stress fractures include:**

a. Amenorrhea/hypoestrogenemia    c. Low estrogen levels

b. Anorexia nervosa    d. Reduced calcium intake

V. **Osteoporosis**

A. **Definition:** decreased bone mass and increased susceptibility to fracture in the absence of other recognizable causes of bone loss

B. **Prevalence**

1. Affects more than 20 million people in the United States

2. Causes 1.3 million fractures per year

3. Costs $3.8 billion.

C. **Etiology**—Not entirely understood but appears to include:

1. Deficiency of estrogen

2. Deficiency of calcium

3. Problem with absorption of calcium.

D. **Clinical features**

1. Vertebral compression fractures

2. Hip fractures

3. Wrist fractures.

E. **Risk factors**

1. Female

2. Advanced age

3. Menopause (natural or surgical)

4. White or Oriental

5. Diet low in calcium

6. Smoking

7. Alcoholism

8. Immobilization

9. Amenorrhea/hypoestrogenemia

10. Anorexia nervosa

11. Prolonged corticosteroid use.

F. **Factors that decrease absorption of calcium:**

1. Caffeine

2. Alcohol

3. Cigarette smoking

4. Lactose intolerance

5. Fiber intake.

G. **Two factors increase absorption of calcium**

1. Vitamin D

2. Estrogens.

H. **Exercise increases calcium content of bone**

I. **Treatment and recommendations:**

1. Calcium—1,000 mg/day for menstruating women; 1,500 mg/day for nonmenstruating women and postmenopausal women.

a. Best source of calcium is food (8 oz of milk, 4 oz of cheese, or 2 oz of hard cheese yields 200 mg of calcium).

b. Supplements: Tums, 1 tablet = 200 mg calcium; some have 500 mg of calcium.

2. **Practical guidelines:** Generally, athletes who ingest less than 2,000 calories of food per day should have diet supplemented with calcium and iron.

a. Appropriate dietary evaluation and counseling warranted.

3. **Amenorrheic/postmenopausal women**
   a. Increase calcium intake to 1,500 mg/day.
   b. Vitamin D or sunlight exposure.
   c. Estrogen replacement: 0.625 mg estrogen days 1 through 25, add medroxy-progesterone acetate (Provera), 10 mg per day, days 16–25.
   d. Weightbearing exercise

VI. **Psychological Concerns:** Too complicated to elaborate but too important to ignore. "Guidelines for Building Self Confidence" are presented as adopted from Dr. Charles Corbin.

A. **Ensuring successful performance:** "Nothing breeds confidence like success."
   1. Help establish realistic goals.
   2. Establish progressively more difficult tasks.
   3. Physically assist performance of progressively difficult tasks.
   4. Avoid situational vulnerability (at early stages of learning, avoid competition).
   5. Teach proper use of feedback.

B. **Use positive re-enforcement and positive role models.**
   1. Reward mastering an athletic skill.
   2. Be a positive role model (especially female models).
   3. Expose girls and women to respected highly skilled role models.
   4. Model approval (we should be careful our actions, not just our words, communicate approval).

C. **Use enhanced communication techniques.**
   1. Help females dream of success.
   2. Communicate clearly.
   3. Use praise as reward.
   4. Use persuasive techniques.
   5. Encourage positive self-talk.

D. Reduce anxiety.

   In summary, numerous factors affect women in sports and in all professions. We have come a long way, and we have an even longer way to go.

**Acknowledgments:** Many thanks go to Drs. Lorna Marshall, Karen Rosene, and Morris B. Mellion for their review and suggestions. I am also grateful for the editorial assistance of Dick Diedricks and typing assistance of Theresa Romane.

## REFERENCES AND RECOMMENDED READING

1. Agostini R: The athletic woman. In Mellion MB (ed): Office Management of Sports Injuries & Athletic Problems. Philadelphia, Hanley & Belfus, 1988.
2. Clapp JF III, Dickstein S: Endurance exercise and pregnancy outcome. Med Sci Sports Exerc 16:556–562, 1984.
3. Paisley JE, Mellion MB: Exercise during pregnancy. Am Fam Phys 38:142–150.
4. Shangold M, Mirkin G: Women and exercise. In Physiology and Sports Medicine. Contemporary Exercise and Sports Medicine Series. Philadelphia, F.A. Davis, 1988.
5. Walsh WM (ed): Symposium on the athletic woman. Clin Sports Med 3(4): 1988.

# Chapter 22: The Diabetic Athlete

KRIS BERG, EdD

I. **Introduction**
   A. Exercise was not typically emphasized in management of diabetes until recently, although it has been a component of overall treatment since the 1920s.
   B. **Acute effects of exercise in both types of diabetes are well understood, but chronic effects are not, particularly in type I patients.**
      1. Anecdotal (e.g., diabetic athletes) and biochemical evidence clearly suggests numerous long-term benefits.
         a. Weight loss
         b. Reduced risk of cardiovascular disease
         c. Increased insulin sensitivity
         d. Improved regulation of BG (blood glucose).
      2. Recent data show type I diabetics who were high school athletes have significantly **lower incidence** of **cardiovascular disease** as adults than type I diabetics who were not.
   C. **Diabetics are as trainable as nondiabetics if under reasonable metabolic control.**
      1. BG
      2. Ketone levels.

II. **Key Traits of Type I and II Diabetes Pertinent to Exercise**
   A. **Both types prone to hypoglycemia.**
   B. **Type I patients prone to ketoacidosis, whereas type II rarely experience this problem.**
   C. **Hypoglycemia and ketoacidosis can be minimized with appropriate monitoring of BG and ketones.**

III. **Benefits of Exercise**
   A. **Motivation to improve as an athlete may enhance diabetic management.**
      1. More frequent BG assessment.
      2. Closer attention to diet.
   B. **Consistent, good control of BG appears to minimize typical diabetic sequelae.**
      1. Retinopathy
      2. Microangiopathy
      3. Neuropathy
      4. Some degree of reversal of these conditions occurs with prolonged tight BG control.
   C. **Physical trainability and performance are probably optimized when BG is consistently good.**
      1. More normal substrate utilization
      2. Reduced protein degradation
         a. Greater muscle hypertrophy
         b. Possibly greater mitochondrial enzymes.
      3. Greater muscle and liver glycogen
      4. Increased body water
         a. Increased heat tolerance.

D. **Psychological effects of exercise**
   1. Improved self-esteem
   2. Improved self-confidence.
E. **Reduction in cardiovascular disease risk factors.**
   1. Reduced total cholesterol and LDL-C    4. Reduced blood pressure
   2. Increased HDL-C                         5. Increased fibrinolysis
   3. Reduced triglyceride level             6. Reduced stress.
F. **Increased insulin sensitivity**
   1. Reduced insulin or oral hypoglycemic medication doses often result.
      a. Occasionally, medication may be stopped in Type II diabetics.

IV. **Contraindications for Exercise**

A. **An exercise EKG is warranted if:**
   1. Over age 40
   2. If duration of diabetes exceeds 25 years or
   3. If a primary risk factor for cardiovascular disease exists.
B. **If peripheral neuropathy or microangiopathy exists, avoid exercise that traumatizes the feet.**
   1. Swimming and cycling are good alternatives to walking and jogging.
   2. **Examine the feet daily and keep them well lubricated.**
      a. Trim nails carefully.
      b. Avoid blisters, corns, and calluses.
         i. Wear properly fitting shoes and socks.
   3. **Treat foot injuries immediately to prevent complications.**
   4. Prevent thick callus formation by periodic filing with a pumice stone.
C. **Proliferative retinopathy precludes:**
   1. **Strenuous or jarring activity**         3. Scuba diving because of
      a. Weight lifting and training               increased water pressure.
      b. Contact sports                         4. Exercise while inverted
      c. Gymnastics                                a. Some yoga positions
      d. Running.                                  b. Standing on head
   2. Activity that raises the heart rate          c. Hanging upside down.
      dramatically and systolic blood
      pressure beyond 180 mm Hg.

V. **Exercise Guidelines**

A. **Good BG control should be established before starting an exercise program.**
B. **BG should be measured before and after exercise.**
   1. This allows patient and physician to study the BG response to various exercise conditions:
      a. Consecutive hard days of training
      b. Tournaments
      c. Reduced training days before competition.
   2. **The drop in BG during exercise is greater the higher it is at the onset of activity.**
   3. **If BG exceeds 250–300 mg/dl at the start of exercise, BG tends to rise, rather than fall, during exercise.**
      a. **If ketosis exists before exercise, ketone production rises.**
      b. These effects are due to the influence of counter-regulatory hormones:
         i. Low insulin
         ii. Catecholamines
         iii. Cortisol.

4. **Pregame anxiety mimics hypoglycemia, leading many diabetic athletes to overeat before competition.**
   a. They may treat what is perceived to be an insulin reaction.
   b. They may exaggerate reducing the dosage of insulin or oral hypoglycemic medication, peaking during the contest to avoid hypoglycemia, and possibly be hyperglycemic.
   c. These inappropriate steps may lead to:
      i. Accentuated ketoacidosis
      ii. Poor performance due to
         (a) Limited use of muscle glycogen/glucose
         (b) Reduced blood pH.

5. **Endurance training:**
   a. Increases fat utilization due to an increase in mitochondrial density and associated enzymes.
   b. Increases muscle and liver glycogen stores:
      i. Allowing the athlete to be active for a much longer time before needing supplemental carbohydrate.
   c. Reduces uptake of BG, which reduces the likelihood of hypoglycemia.

6. **Hypoglycemia is more likely to occur during exercise in the evening and least likely to occur in the morning because of a diurnal variation in growth hormone level.**
   a. If exercising in the evening, the amount of insulin taken that peaks after eating and during the rest of the evening should be reduced, or more food should be consumed before and possibly after exercise.
   b. Prior to actual competition in the evening, alteration in insulin or food intake should be experimented with several times to mimic the conditions (e.g., same time and similar energy expenditure) existing during evening competition.
   c. Because insulin sensitivity is affected for at least 4 hours and as long as 24 hours after exercise, hypoglycemia may occur during sleep. BG may have to be assessed in the middle of the night to prevent insulin reaction.

7. **Exercise performed within 1 hour of injection of regular insulin speeds its absorption and time to peak effect. The same effect occurs for about 2.5 hours after injection of intermediate insulin.**
   a. Type I diabetics typically inject insulin into the thigh, gluteal area, abdomen, triceps, or shoulder. The injection site can be altered, depending on the activity to prevent this effect.
   b. If exercise commonly is done soon after the injection of regular insulin, no alteration may be needed, because the athlete has probably learned to deal with the effect.
   c. **Elevation of body temperature also increases the rate of insulin absorption.**
      i. The duration of warm-up and the amount of clothing worn during warm-up should be reasonably consistent if exercise occurs within the first hour of injecting regular insulin.

8. **Consistent daily energy expenditure facilitates BG control.**
   a. Extra medication or lower food intake may be needed on days of reduced activity, whereas less medication or greater food intake may be needed for days of increased training duration or intensity.
   b. **When exercise lasts for several hours** (e.g., triathlons, mountaineering, cycling, tournament play) **the basal dose of insulin should be reduced in type I diabetics by as much as 50%. Supplemental food (about one carbohydrate exchange or 60 kcal) can be consumed every 30–45 minutes.**
      i. BG monitoring during the event has proven helpful to diabetics in such sports.

C. **Medication requirements are reduced in the early months of training (30–40% is typical) and remains lower as long as training occurs.**
   1. Mature exercising diabetic athletes usually take about 0.5–0.6 units of insulin/kg bodyweight, or even less, whereas the typical dosage is 0.5–1.0 units/kg.
   2. **Some type II patients may eventually need no oral hypoglycemic medication** due to the combined effect of fat loss and exercise on insulin sensitivity.
D. Achievement of good BG control facilitates development of muscle mass.
   1. Adequate insulin enhances normal uptake and utilization of amino acids.
   2. Inadequate insulin promotes protein degradation and water loss.
E. **Good BG control facilitates glycogen storage in skeletal muscle.**
   1. This reduces the likelihood of glycogen depletion occurring after consecutive days of vigorous training as well as during a prolonged endurance event.
   2. Recent evidence suggests that the amount of water stored with skeletal muscle glycogen has a strong effect on exercise capacity in the heat.
   3. Many marginally controlled diabetics have particular difficulty exercising in warm environments, partly because of reduced muscle glycogen and water.

VI. **Guidelines for Avoiding Hypoglycemia Associated with Exercise**

A. Hypoglycemia is a common fear among many diabetics regarding exercise. **Measure BG before exercise and:**
   1. If < 130 mg/dl, consume two CHO exchanges per 30–45 minutes of light-to-moderate exercise (< 60% VO$_2$max) and three exchanges if heavy exercise (> 70% VO$_2$max).
   2. If 130–180 mg/dl, consume one CHO exchange per 30–45 minutes of light-to-moderate exercise and two exchanges per 30–45 minutes of heavy exercise.
   3. **If 180–240 mg/dl, take no food before exercise.** If the exercise is heavy and the duration exceeds 30 minutes, take a second BG reading and use the criteria stated in 1 and 2 above.
   4. **If 250 mg/dl or higher, do not exercise as the action of counter-regulatory hormones may cause BG to rise during exercise as well as increase the ketone level.**
B. **Food should be readily available for supplemental feeding:**
   1. With the athletic trainer or coach
   2. In locker
   3. On bus
   4. On person (e.g., carried in pocket of running shorts, in a pack on bicycle).
C. **Decrease dosage of insulin that peaks during exercise.**
   1. Short-acting insulin normally taken before a meal might not be needed.
D. **Hypoglycemia occurs during and after exercise more frequently and severely in tightly controlled patients and those who have been type I diabetics for more than 10 years. It occurs in the latter group even when no clinical signs of autonomic neuropathy exist.**
E. **Avoid exercise in the evening or develop a plan to meet the reduced insulin needed if exercise cannot be avoided at this time of day.**
F. **After expending an unusually large amount of energy or if exercise is done in the evening, expect possible hypoglycemia at night and the next day.**
   1. **Extra BG monitoring is advisable.**
G. **Avoid exercising the muscles in the region where short-acting insulin was injected for 1 hour.**

## RECOMMENDED READING

1. A Round Table: Diabetes and exercise. Phys Sportsmed 7:49–64, 1979.
2. Berg K: Blood glucose regulation in an insulin-dependent diabetic backpacker. Phys Sportsmed 11:101–104, 1983.
3. Berger M, Berchtold P, Cuppers JJ, et al: Metabolic and hormonal effects of muscular exercise in juvenile type diabetics. Diabetologica 13:355–365, 1977.
4. Costill DL, Cleary P, Fink WJ, et al: Training adaptations in skeletal muscle of juvenile diabetics. Diabetes 28:812–822, 1979.
5. Felig P, Wahren J: Amino acid metabolism in exercising man. J Clin Invest 50:2703–2714, 1971.
6. Larsson Y, Persson B, Sterky G, Thoren C: Functional adaptation to vigorous training and exercise in diabetic and nondiabetic adolescents. J Appl Physiol 19:629–635, 1964.
7. Skyler J, Skyler D, O'Sullivan M: Algorithms for adjustment of insulin dosage by patients who monitor blood glucose. Diabetes Care 4:311–318, 1981.

# Chapter 23: The Hypertensive Athlete

MORRIS B. MELLION, MD
MARK E. McKINNEY, PhD

I. **Hemodynamics and Cardiovascular Anatomy**

  A. **Hemodynamics of hypertension**

    1. Blood pressure is the result of two factors: Blood pressure (BP) = **Cardiac output (CO)** × **Total peripheral resistance (TPR).**

    2. **The development of hypertension progresses through various stages, each marked by hemodynamic abnormalities (Fig. 1).**

      a. **Borderline hypertension**

        i. The earliest stage of hypertension

        ii. Also known as **latent** or **labile hypertension**

        iii. Associated with **increased CO and "normal" TPR**

          (a) TPR is normal compared to resting levels in nonhypertensive individuals, but is inappropriately high in the face of elevated CO.

            (i) In the nonhypertensive, TPR would fall to compensate for rise in CO, thereby maintaining normal blood pressure.

            (ii) Lack of TPR decrease due to impaired baroreceptor function

        iv. Accompanied by **increased serum catecholamine levels, renin levels, and renin blood flow**

        v. **Borderline hypertensives are hypersensitive to catecholamine secretion and mental stress, and have a hyperkinetic circulatory state.**

      b. **Mild established hypertension**

        i. **If borderline hypertension does not "resolve," it becomes mild, or established, hypertension.**

        ii. ↓CO, ↑TPR

        iii. **Decreased arterial lumen and disturbed autoregulation of blood flow in the periphery**

        iv. Often the first stage that is detected medically.

      c. **Established hypertension**

        i. ↓↓CO, ↑↑TPR

        ii. Increased afterload leads to **left ventricular hypertrophy (LVH).**

      d. **Severe hypertension and congestive heart failure**

        i. **CO can no longer increase in response to exercise or other physiological demands.**

        ii. **Marked LVH exists.**

        iii. **Loss of contractility leads to inability to clear fluid.**

          (a) Peripheral edema and cardiac edema are threats to cardiovascular function and electrolyte balance.

  B. **Hemodynamics and cardiovascular anatomy of exercise**

    1. **Dynamic exercise**

      a. **↑VO$_2$ = ↑CO · ↑A–VO$_2$**

        i. ↑CO (cardiac output) = ↑SV (stroke volume) × ↑HR (heart rate)

        ii. ↑A–VO$_2$ difference = Increased oxygen utilization.

      b. **BP = ↑↑CO · ↓TPR** (normotensive)

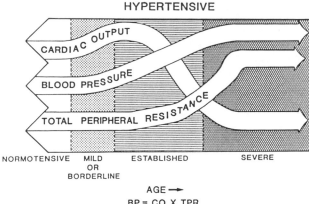

**HYPERTENSIVE**

NORMOTENSIVE    MILD        ESTABLISHED            SEVERE
                OR
              BORDERLINE

AGE ➝

BP = CO X TPR

**FIGURE 1.** The development of hypertension progresses through various stages, each marked by hemodynamic abnormalities. This illustration depicts the changes in cardiac output, total peripheral resistance and blood pressure over time in the untreated patient.

      i. ↑SBP (systolic BP) and ↑MAP (mean arterial pressure)

      ii. ↓TPR and DBP (diastolic BP)

  c. **Left ventricular size increases**

      i. Marked increase in LV diameter and lumen produces increased LV mass

      ii. Slight thickening of ventricular walls.

  d. Training effects, including increased SV and LVH, disappear after as little as 2 months of inactivity.

2. **Isometric exercise**

  a. **↑↑↑BP dramatically and rapidly**

      i. **SBP increases of 100–180 mm Hg** have been observed during weight-lifting.

  b. **↑↑HR**

  c. **Repetitive isometric exercise can lead to thickened LV walls (septal and posterior) and decreased lumen.**

      i. LVH can eventually result.

        (a) Concentric LVH.

      ii. **Even in normal athletes, prolonged high-intensity isometric exercise leads to decreased CO.**

        (a) Adolesecent and young adult athletes have a higher resting level of CO, but continued isometric exercise may lead to CO decrease.

        (b) May cause development of hypertension, due to increased afterload.

        (c) Anatomical changes may be more prevalent in black athletes.

3. **Hypertensive athletes and exercisers**

  a. **BP should be controlled before allowing the athlete/exerciser to participate in vigorous sports, since both dynamic and isometric exercise cause marked BP increases.**

  b. **Hypertensive athletes/exercisers do not shunt blood to the skin as effectively as normotensives.**

      i. Core temperatures can rise precipitously.

      ii. This makes exercise in the heat particularly dangerous for a hypertensive.

        (a) The fluid loss that accompanies exercise in the heat may also cause potassium loss, which can be especially dangerous for the hypertensive athlete/exerciser.

II. **Diagnosis and Hypertension**

    A. **Resting blood pressure**

        1. Hypertension is defined as **BP above 140/90 on a consistent basis.**

        2. **Early, or labile, hypertension, is usually marked by an increase in SBP.**

           a. Primarily due to ↑CO.

        3. **As hypertension progresses, DBP begins to increase.**

           a. **Primarily due to ↑TPR.**

           b. **DBP above 120 should be treated immediately and aggressively.**

           c. **Elevated DBP places the patient at risk for coronary heart disease, cerebral hemorrhage, and renal damage.**

        4. **Established hypertension is accompanied by end-organ damage.**

           a. Early renal damage may not be indicated by changes in serum creatinine or BUN.

           b. Mild proteinuria may be an indicator of early renal damage.

               i. May be hard to diagnose in athletes participating in contact sports.

    B. **Blood pressure during exercise**

        1. **Exercise stress testing can be used to differentiate types of hypertension.**

           a. Borderline hypertensives start at higher resting levels than normals but do not show abnormally high BP levels during maximal exercise.

           b. Some research suggests that labile hypertensives show less increase in pulse pressure than normotensives.

               i. May be due to less compliant vascular beds

           c. Rapid elevation in SBP indicates established hypertension.

           d. Established hypertensives show little or no decrease in DBP during maximal exercise.

    C. **"White coat" hypertension and other stress phenomena**

        1. Initial resting blood pressure may not accurately estimate true BP.

           a. Anxiety provoked by a medical examination can lead to artificially elevated BP, known as "white coat" hypertension.

           b. Other sources of mental stress can lead to elevated BP.

        2. **An average of several readings is a better estimate of true BP.**

           a. If initial BP is high, have athlete rest for 5 minutes and repeat BP check.

           b. If BP remains elevated, check BP at least once per week for at least 4 weeks before making the diagnosis of hypertension.

        3. **Averaged daily BP is a better predictor of later end organ damage than random office BP.**

           a. Ambulatory BP monitoring remains difficult and expensive.

           b. Athletes/exercisers can take their own BP as an alternative.

               i. The athlete/exerciser must be well-trained in the measurement of BP.

               ii. Emphasize the importance of *accurate* readings.

III. **Approaches to the Management of Hypertension**

    A. Although there are many diverse approaches to the management of hypertension, management of the hypertensive athlete (or the exercising adult with hypertension) generally involves a combination of several nonpharmacologic therapies, often with one or more antihypertensive medications.

    B. **Nonpharmacologic strategies** may provide a safe, effective foundation for any good antihypertensive regimen. Their strength lies in the fact that **risk of side-effects is low** to nonexistent, but their weakness is that for success **they depend on long-term compliance with major changes in deeply ingrained lifestyle behaviors.**

        1. **Nonpharmacologic approaches used without concurrent antihypertensive medications are most appropriate for the control of borderline or mild hypertension, but they may be useful as adjunctive therapies for all levels of hypertension.**

2. **Dietary modification**
   a. **Altering electrolyte intakes**
      i. **Decreasing sodium intake**
         (a) Goal: 2 g dietary sodium/day
         (b) Especially important in **"salt-sensitive"** hypertensives
             (i) 2/3 of black hypertensives are "salt-sensitive."
      ii. **Increasing potassium intake**
         (a) Lowers blood pressure in the hypokalemic patient.
         (b) May have antihypertensive effect in normokalemic patient, but more research is needed.
      iii. **Increasing calcium intake**
         (a) Many hypertensives, especially women, may be calcium deficient.
         (b) 1–2 g/day calcium supplementation may reduce blood pressure
      iv. **Increasing magnesium intake—controversial**
         (a) Possible benefit, but conflicting research results
         (b) Supplementation is important in patients who are magnesium-depleted from diuretics.
             (i) Potassium-sparing diuretics also spare magnesium.
   b. **Weight reduction**
      i. **Obesity increases both preload and afterload on heart, resulting in hypertensive effect.**
         (a) **Preload:**
             Obesity
             → ↑ intravascular volume
             → ↑ total peripheral resistance
             → ↑ left ventricular preload
             (i) Pattern common in borderline to mild hypertension.
         (b) **Afterload:**
             Obesity
             → ↑ central norepinephrine production
             → ↑ total peripheral resistance
             → ↑ left ventricular afterload.
         (c) Hypertensive with combined elevation of both preload and afterload is at high risk for accelerated left ventricular hypertrophy and congestive heart failure.
      ii. Weight reduction may alter both preload and afterload.
   c. **High fiber diet**
      i. Early research evidence suggestive that high fiber diet may lower blood pressure.
   d. **Low saturated fat diet**
      i. Early research evidence suggestive that low saturated fat diet may lower blood pressure.
   e. **Elimination or moderation of alcohol consumption**
      i. > 2 ounces of alcohol/day may be etiologic for hypertension.
3. **Relaxation techniques: Main value as adjunct therapy, but some individuals may have exceptionally good response.**
   a. Biofeedback
      i. Can be directly for blood pressure change or for general relaxation effects through change in other systems, such as muscle tension.
   b. Stress management
   c. Muscle relaxation techniques:
      i. Progressive relaxation, which employs tensing and releasing muscle groups, needs to be used with care in severe hypertensives.

ii. Audio-guided instructions provide a good home-use technique and are commercially available.

d. Meditation

4. **Exercise as therapy for hypertension**

a. Evidence

i. Epidemiological evidence demonstrates that vigorous exercise correlates with lower risk of developing hypertension.

ii. **Clinical trials** demonstrate:

(a) Endurance exercise conditioning may lower resting systolic blood pressure 5–25 mm and diastolic blood pressure 3–15 mm.

(i) Benefit more marked in borderline and mild hypertensives.

(ii) Multiple research studies, but most are uncontrolled and/or poorly designed.

(b) Difficult to differentiate the direct effect of exercise on blood pressure from the effect of weight loss that often accompanies exercise conditioning.

b. **Prescribing exercise: "F I T"**

i. **Frequency:** 3–5 sessions/week

ii. **Intensity:** 60–85% of predicted maximum heart rate

(a) In older or less fit patients start at 60–70%; in more fit patients start at 70–80%.

(b) Predicted maximum heart rate:

Men: 225 – Age

Women: 220 – Age.

iii. **Time** (duration): Initially 15–30 minutes; eventually 30–60 minutes/session.

iv. **Type of exercise: "Dynamic Isotonic Exercise"** = "Moving your body through space."

(a) Examples: walking, jogging, swimming, cycling, cross-country skiing, aerobic dance.

c. **Avoid intense isometric exercise**

i. **Massive blood pressure elevation in weight lifters working with heavy loads**

(a) Static load →

↑↑↑HR + ↓SV →↑↑CO

(i) Even in light isometric exercise the heart rate increase is disproportionately high for the load.

(ii) Static load → no Δ TPR.

ii. **Chronic effect: concentric left ventricular hypertrophy**

(a) → ↓ LV lumen due to increased wall thickness

(b) → ? effect on conduction.

iii. There are no good research data about the safety of isometric exercise in well-controlled hypertensives.

iv. Hypertensives should avoid inversion therapy (i.e., hanging in an inverted position).

IV. **Pharmacotherapy for the Exercising Hypertensive**

A. **General principles**

1. All current antihypertensives permit an essentially normal exercise response except beta-blockers.

a. Some do so better than others.

b. There is still a role for beta-blockers.

2. The choice of agent may depend on other considerations.

B. **Best choices for endurance athletes:**

1. **Angiotensin converting enzyme inhibitors** (captopril, enalapril, lisinopril)
   a. Block conversion of angiotensin I to angiotensin II.
      i. Block vasoconstriction caused by angiotensin II, therefore ↓ TPR.
      ii. Block sodium retention stimulated by angiotensin II.
   b. Hemodynamic effects during exercise:
      ↑stroke volume
      ↓heart rate
      ↓total peripheral resistance.
   c. Decrease "exaggerated" blood pressure effect during exercise.
   d. Anecdotal reports of postural hypotension in athletes stopping abruptly following intense endurance exercise.
      i. Emphasizes need for "cooling down" following exercise to prevent venous pooling.
2. **Alpha₁ receptor blockers** (prazosin, terazosin)
   a. Competitively block the postsynaptic $\alpha_1$ arteriolar smooth muscle receptors → ↓ TPR.
   b. Normalize central hemodynamics at rest and during exercise.
   c. Occasionally cause an exaggerated hypotensive response to the first dose.
      i. Response to first dose should be monitored.
3. **Central alpha agonists** (clonidine, quanabenz, quanfacine)
   a. Act on alpha₂ receptors in brainstem to block central sympathetic stimulation → ↓ HR and ↓ TPR at rest.
      i. Also block sympathetically mediated sodium retention.
   b. Normal hemodynamic response to exercise.
C. **Beta blockers** (listed in Table 1)
   1. **Useful in certain groups**
      a. **Intermittent exertion sports**
      b. **Untrained or partially trained athlete**
      c. **Arteriosclerotic heart disease patient.**
   2. **General effects of beta blockers**
      a. Acutely: beta blockers:
         → ↓ myocardial contractility + ↓ heart rate
         → ↑ diastole
         → ↑ coronary perfusion
         → ↑ exercise tolerance in CAD.
      b. **Hemodynamic effects during exercise:**
         i. ↓↓↓ HR with compensatory increase in oxygen extraction (A–VO₂ diff) and possible compensatory SV (more common with cardioselective agents)

$$\dot{V}O_2 = (HR \times SV)(A\text{-}VO_2 \text{ diff})$$
$$\downarrow \quad \downarrow\downarrow\downarrow \quad \uparrow \quad \uparrow$$

**TABLE 1.** Beta Blocking Agents Arranged by Cardioselectivity and Intrinsic Sympathomimetic Activity (ISA)

|  | No ISA | ISA |
|---|---|---|
| Cardioselective | Atenolol (Tenormin)<br>Metoprolol (Lopressor)<br>Carteolol (Cartrol)<br>Penbutolol (Levatol) | Acebutolol (Sectral) |
| Noncardioselective | Nadolol (Corgard)<br>Propranolol (Inderal)<br>Sotalol (Sotacor)<br>Timolol (Blocadren) | Alprenolol (Aptin)<br>Oxprenolol (Trasicor)<br>Pindolol (Visken) |

(a) Performance effect: **Well-trained subjects experience a greater drop in VO$_2$max than untrained subjects on beta blockers.**

    (i) More potential in the untrained for compensatory ↑ A–VO$_2$ diff and ↑ SV.

  ii. **↑ TPR**

    (a) Peripheral sympathetic effects:
    Alpha → vasoconstriction
    Beta$_2$ → vasodilatation.

    (b) Beta blockers (especially noncardioselective) may block peripheral vasodilatation and result in unopposed vasoconstriction.

      (i) Chronically, this effect may be blunted.

        • "Readjustment phenomenon" = TPR returns to normal functional levels over several years.

  iii. **Metabolic effects of beta blockers**

    (a) Block mobilization and utilization of free fatty acids.

    (b) Noncardioselective agents block glycogenolysis.

    (c) **Hypoglycemia may result,** especially during or after intense exercise.

    (d) Can increase serum cholesterol and LDL levels.

  iv. **Beta blockers increase perceived exertion in working muscles,** thus causing reduced endurance.

    (a) Probably due to metabolic effects

    (b) **No increase in cardiovascular perceived exertion.**

  v. Beta blockers decrease performance more in individuals with a high percentage of slow twitch muscle fibers.

    (a) This effect is more pronounced on propranolol (noncardioselective) than on atenolol (cardioselective).

  vi. Effect of **intrinsic sympathomimetic activity** in beta blockers on heart rate and cardiac output during intense exercise is unclear.

    (a) ISA may prove helpful, but presently there are only a few studies with conflicting results.

D. **Combined alpha and beta blocker** (labetolol)

  1. Three effects

    a. **Beta blockade →**

      i. ↓ HR → ↓ CO

      ii. ↓ renin.

    b. **Alpha$_1$ blockade** → ↓ vasoconstriction → ↓ TPR.

    c. **Beta$_2$ agonist** → ↓ TPR.

    d. **Beta effects are greater than alpha effects.**

  2. ↓ cardiac output 10–14% at rest and during exercise at 1 year.

    a. Cardiac output gradually returns to baseline over next 5 years due to ↑ in stroke volume.

    b. TPR remains ↓ 15–20%.

E. Diuretics

  1. **Acute effect:** Diuretics → ↓ plasma volume
                         → ↓ stroke volume
                         → ↓ cardiac output
                         → ↓ blood pressure

  2. **Long-term effects, normal dose range**

    a. **Small decrease in cardiac output,** but generally not during exercise.

      i. Larger doses may produce a larger decrease in cardiac output, which may persist during exercise.

  3. Small doses of diuretics (12.5 mg hydrochlorothiazide) may be useful as second-step therapy in exercising patients.

      a. Particularly important consideration in black athletes, who are more likely to be salt-sensitive hypertensives.

      b. → ↓ total peripheral resistance

          → ↓ blood pressure.

   4. Diuretics may produce cramping in athletes in spite of normal serum potassium.

   5. Exercise in the heat may produce potassium depletion and rhabdomyolysis.

F. **Calcium antagonists** (diltiazem, nicardipine, nifepidine, verapamil)

   1. Lower blood pressure by reducing calcium concentration in vascular smooth muscle cells → ↓ TPR.

   2. Many physicians have found this class of drugs useful as first-step therapy in athletes; however, there is a paucity of good research data in this population.

      a. Concerns that need clarification in the exercising hypertensive:

         i. Heart rate suppression: verapamil and diltiazem

         ii. Hemoconcentration during exercise: verapamil

        iii. Reflex tachycardia: nifedipine, nicardipine

        iv. Decreased left ventricular contractility: verapamil and diltiazem

         v. Intransigent pedal edema: nifedipine, nicardipine.

## REFERENCES AND RECOMMENDED READING

1. Blair SN, Goodyear NN, Gibbons LW, Cooper KH: Physical fitness and incidence of hypertension in healthy normotensive men and women. JAMA 252:487, 1984.
2. Creager MA, Massie BM, Faxon DP, et al: Acute and long-term effects of enalapril on the cardiovascular response to exercise and exercise tolerance in patients with congestive heart failure. J Am Coll Cardiol 6:163, 1985.
3. Dlin RA, Hanne N, Silverberg DS, BarOr O: Follow-up of normotensive men with exaggerated blood pressure response to exercise. Am Heart J 106:316, 1983.
4. Fagard R, Lijnen P, Vanhees L, Amery A: Hemodynamic response to converting enzyme inhibition at rest and exercise in humans. J Appl Physiol 53:576, 1982.
5. Kaiser P, Hylander B, Eliasson K, Kaiser L: Effect of beta-1-selective and nonselective beta blockade on blood pressure relative to physical performance in men with systemic hypertension. Am J Cardiol 55:79D, 1985.
6. Kaiser P, Tesch PA, Thorsson A, et al: Skeletal muscle glycogenolysis during submaximal exercise following acute beta-adrenergic blockage in man. Acta Physiol Scand 123:285, 1985.
7. Kaplan NM: Non-drug treatment of hypertension. Ann Intern Med 102:359, 1985.
8. Kenney WL, Zambraski EJ: Physical activity in human hypertension: A mechanisms approach. Sports Med 1:459, 1984.
9. Lund-Johansen P: Hemodynamic changes in long-term diuretic therapy of essential hypertension. Acta Med Scand 187:509, 1970.
10. Lund-Johansen P: Spontaneous changes in central hemodynamics in essential hypertension—a 10-year follow-up study. In Onesti G, Klimt TR (eds): Hypertension: Determinants, Complications and Intervention. New York, Grune and Stratton, 1979, p 201.
11. Lund-Johansen P: Hemodynamic changes at rest and during exercise in long-term prazosin therapy of essential hypertension. In Cotton DWK (ed): Prazosin—A New Antihypertensive Agent. Excerpta Medica. 1974, p 43.
12. Lund-Johansen P: Short- and long-term (six-year) hemodynamic effects of labetolol in essential hypertension. Am J Med 75:24, 1983.
13. McKinney ME, Mellion MB: Exercise and hypertension. In Mellion MB (ed): Office Management of Sports Injuries & Athletic Problems. Philadelphia, Hanley & Belfus, 1988, p 98.
14. Messerli FH: Cardiovascular effects of obesity and hypertension. Lancet i:1165, 1982.
15. Messerli FH, Ventura HO: Cardiovascular pathophysiology of essential hypertension: A clue to therapy. Drugs 30(suppl 1):25, 1985.
16. Paffenbarger RS Jr, Wing AL, Hyde RT, Jung DL: Physical activity and incidence of hypertension in college alumni. Am J Epidemiol 117:245, 1983.
17. Pearson SB, Banks DC, Patrick JM: The effect of beta-adrenoceptor blockade on factors affecting exercise tolerance in normal man. Br J Clin Pharmacol 8:143, 1979.
18. Tesch PA: Exercise and beta-blockade. Sports Med 2:389, 1985.
19. Tipton CH: Exercise, training, and hypertension. Exerc Sports Sci Rev 12:245, 1984.
20. Wilmore JH, Ewy GA, Freund BJ, et al: Cardiorespiratory alterations consequent to endurance exercise training during chronic beta-adrenergic blockade with atenolol and propranolol. Am J Cardiol 55:142D, 1985.

# Chapter 24: Exercise-induced Bronchospasm

NAPOLEON LEE, MD
ROGER H. KOBAYASHI, MD

I. **Introduction**

Exercise induced bronchospasm **(EIB)** is a very common and troublesome affliction of the pulmonary system, frequently impairing optimal athletic performance. **EIB** was first described in the second century A.D. by Aretaeus the Cappadocian. However, it was not until recently that efforts toward prevention and treatment have been made.

A. **Epidemiology** (Table 1)
1. 12% of total population experience EIB.
2. EIB can be detected in 41% of those with a history of allergic rhinitis.
3. 70–90% of all asthmatics have EIB.
4. It can occur at any age and is equally distributed among the two sexes.

B. **Definition**
1. **Clinical features**
EIB typically occurs after strenuous exercise. Following a near maximum (80%) exercise load of $\geq$ 5 minutes, the athlete experiences difficulty breathing, manifested by shortness of breath, coughing, chest tightness, and/or wheezing.
2. **Pulmonary function criteria**
a. $\geq$ 20% fall of $FEV_1$ from baseline (normal subjects may have $\leq$ 10% fall of $FEV_1$) after exercise.
b. $\geq$ 35% fall of forced expiratory flow, $FEF_{25-75}$.
c. $\geq$ 10% fall of peak expiratory flow rate (PEFR).
d. Increased functional reserve capacity (increase in residual volume [RV] and total lung capacity [TLC]), reflecting air trapping (Fig. 1).
3. **Severity**
a. Mild—15–20% decrease in $FEV_1$
b. Moderate—20–40% decrease in $FEV_1$
c. Severe—greater than 40% decrease in $FEV_1$.

C. **Factors influencing EIB**
1. **Type of exercise**
a. **Sports activities more likely to cause EIB**

|  |  |
|---|---|
| i. Running | iii. Playing offense in team sport |
| ii. Cycling | iv. Cross-country skiing. |

b. **Sports activities less likely to cause EIB**

|  |  |
|---|---|
| i. Kayaking | v. Gymnastics |
| ii. Swimming | vi. Downhill skiing |
| iii. Aerobics exercise | vii. Playing goalie in soccer |
| iv. Dancing | viii. Playing defense in team sport. |

2. **Duration of exercise**
a. Maximal fall of pulmonary function tests (PFT) occurs after 5–8 minutes of vigorous exercise.
b. However, if activity is extended, generally no further increase of bronchospasm is noted.

**TABLE 1.** Athletes at Risk for Exercise-induced Bronchospasm

Those known to have asthma
Those with allergic rhinitis (hay fever)
Those with a family history of asthma
Those with frequent chest symptoms, i.e., coughing, congestion
Those with viral bronchitis
One out of every 10 members on your team

3. **Degree of stress from exercise**
   Very strenuous exercise is more likely to induce EIB.
4. **Conditions affecting EIB**
   a. **Increase EIB** (Table 2)
      i. Cold air       iv. Allergens
      ii. Dry air       v. Viral infections.
      iii. Air pollution
   b. **Decrease EIB**
      i. Warm air
      ii. Humid air.

II. **Possible Mechanisms**

A. **Historical theories**
   1. **Hyperventilation** resulted in airway heat and water loss, thereby triggering EIB.
   2. **$CO_2$ loss** through hyperventilation may cause EIB. This is prevented by rebreathing expired air, replacing of $CO_2$ with 7% $CO_2$ inhalation, or by breathing slowly and deeply.
   3. **Release of mast cell mediators:** histamine, eosinophilic chemotactic factor of anaphylaxis (ECFA), and neutrophil chemotactic factor (NCF), which act on smooth muscles thus causing bronchospasm.

B. **Current theory**
   1. Increased ventilation results in **water loss.** This increases the osmolarity of the epithelial fluid, resulting in bronchospasm by cholinergic or inflammatory mediator release mechanisms.

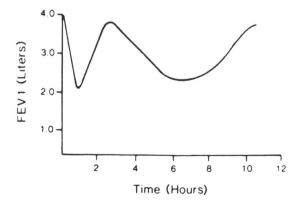

**FIGURE 1.** Patterns of bronchospasm in early phase (10 min to 2 hrs) and late phase (4–8 hours) exercise-induced bronchospasm. (From Kobayashi RH, Mellion MB: Exercise-induced asthma and related problems. In Mellion MB (ed): Office Management of Sports Injuries & Athletic Problems. Philadelphia, Hanley & Belfus, 1988, with permission.)

**TABLE 2.**  Factors That Might Aggravate Exercise-induced Bronchospasm

|  |
| --- |
| Cold air |
| Dry air |
| Air pollution, e.g., sulfur dioxide, smoke |
| Allergens |
| Viral infections |

2. **Mediators** (histamine, NCF, platelet activating factor, leukotrienes) are released after exposure to antigens and exercise.
3. **Mouth breathing** causes cooling of airways, thus triggering EIB.

III. **Diagnosis and Testing**
   A. **Clinical signs and symptoms** (Table 3)
      1. Similar to an acute asthma attack but of shorter duration.
      2. Very common among known asthmatics (70–90% have EIB).
      3. Cough, chest tightness or "burning," wheezing, and shortness of breath are frequently seen shortly after or during exercise.
      4. Prior chest disease such as bronchitis, emphysema, and bronchopulmonary dysplasia can exacerbate EIB.
      5. Athletes suffering from allergies or sinus disease may have an increased incidence of EIB.
   B. **Testing**
      1. **Equipment**
         a. For **general purposes:** simple equipment such as a peak flow meter is adequate and inexpensive in assessing lung status before and after exercise.
            i. Important to sustain vigorous exercise, i.e., sprinting for at least 5 minutes continuously.
            ii. Heart rate should exceed 140 beats/minute.
         b. **Standardized testings**—Pulmonary function tests ($FEV_1$, $FEF_{25-75}$, and PEFR) are measured before and after exercise at 1, 3, 5, 10, and 15 minute intervals.
            i. **Equipment:** simple spirometer (e.g., Breon spirometer).
            ii. **Free running**
               (a) **Advantages:** most asthmogenic; require minimal cardiovascular monitoring devices.
               (b) **Disadvantages:** difficult to maintain constant humidity, ambient temperature, and workload.
            iii. **Treadmill**
               (a) **Advantages:** cardiovascular monitoring and pulmonary function can be measured during exercise. Workload can be standardized.
               (b) **Disadvantages:** less asthmogenic; requires a laboratory with expensive equipment.

**TABLE 3.**  Signs and Symptoms of Exercise-induced Bronchospasm

|  |
| --- |
| Shortness of breath |
| Coughing |
| Chest "tightness" |
| Chest pain |
| Feeling "out of shape" |
| Wheezing |
| Lack of energy (especially in children) |

iv. **Cycloergometer**
  (a) **Advantages:** workload can be easily maintained, and cardiopulmonary monitoring can be easily accomplished. Other physiologic parameters can be simultaneously monitored.
  (b) **Disadvantages:** least asthmogenic; requires a laboratory with expensive equipment.

2. **Medications to avoid before studies**
   a. **Aerosols** containing beta agonists or anticholinergic agents are to be avoided at least **6 hours** prior to testing.
   b. **Oral medications** (theophylline, substained release beta agonists) are to be avoided at least **24 hours** prior to testing.
   c. **Cromolyn sodium** should be withheld for **24 hours.**
   d. **Steroid** preparations may be used unless the patient is also being evaluated for late phase asthma.
   e. **Antihistamines** and/or **decongestants** with antibronchospastic properties are probably best avoided.

3. **Precautions**
   a. Wait at least **3 hours** between testing episodes.
   b. Test no more than twice in one day since refractoriness may affect results.
   c. Some athletes may experience significant bronchospasm that may be difficult to reverse.
   d. Test with caution in those patients with heart disease, seizures, or in those taking beta blockers.
   e. Use albuterol or terbutaline inhaler after testing to reverse bronchospasms (2 to 4 puffs).

IV. **Therapy**

A. **Drugs** (Table 4)
   1. **β-Agonists**
      a. Albuterol (Proventil, Ventolin) is highly effective, of long duration, and easy to use.
      b. Terbutaline (Brethaire) is highly effective, easy to use, and of long duration.
      c. Bitolterol (Tornalate) is highly effective, of long duration, but somewhat inconvenient to use.
      d. Pirbuterol acetate (Maxair) is highly effective and long lasting.
      e. Metaproterenol (Metaprel, Alupent) is effective with moderate duration of action.
      f. Isoetharine (Bronkosol) is effective with short duration of action and is rarely used now.
   2. **Cromolyn sodium** (Intal) is effective but of short duration; blocks *late phase* asthma; has no bronchodilatory effect.
   3. **Theophylline**
      Effective. Effects of sustained-release forms may be enhanced if used regularly.
   4. **Steroids**
      Inhaled steroids (Vanceril, Beclovent, Azmacort, AeroBid) may be used but have only marginal effect on EIB.
   5. **Ipratropium bromide** (Atrovent) may have limited usefulness in preventing EIB.

B. **Banned drugs**
   Many drugs routinely or frequently used for asthma and allergy may be banned by the International Olympic Committee or the NCAA. These drugs are listed in Tables 5 and 6. Nevertheless, the team physician is advised to check with the U.S. Olympic Committee or the NCAA, since this list changes periodically.

**TABLE 4.** Medications Used to Treat Exercise-induced Bronchospasm

| Drugs | Dose | Comments |
|---|---|---|
| **β-agonists** | | |
| Albuterol (Proventil, Ventolin) | 2–4 puffs | Highly effective, long duration, easy to use. |
| Terbutaline (Brethaire) | 2–3 puffs | Highly effective, long duration , easy to use. |
| Bitolterol (Tornalate) | 1–2 puffs | Highly effective, long duration, inconvenient to use. |
| Pirbuterol acetate (Maxair)* | 2 puffs | Highly effective, long lasting, easy to use. |
| Metaproterenol (Metaprel, Alupent) | 2–3 puffs | Effective, moderate duration, easy to use. |
| Isoetharine (Bronkosol)* | 2–3 puffs | Effective, short duration, inconvenient to use. |
| **Cromolyn sodium** (Intal) | | Effective, short duration, easy to use, blocks *late phase* asthma. |
| **Theophylline** (sustained release) | 5–8 mg/kg, every 12 hrs | Effective; regular use may be more effective than occasional use before exercise. |
| **Steroids** (inhaled) | 2–4 puffs | Marginal effect on EIB. |
| **Ipratropium bromide** (Atrovent) | 2 puffs | Limited use in EIB. |

* Not approved for use by the International Olympic Committee and the National Collegiate Athletic Association.

1. **Sympathomimetic agents**
2. **Decongestants**
3. **Miscellaneous.**
C. **Nonpharmacological** (Table 7)
   1. **Conditioning** may reduce the severity of EIB, but it does not prevent it.
   2. **Short bursts of vigorous exercise** within a period of time may extinguish EIB and induce short-term refractoriness, e.g., seven 30-second periods of running ("wind sprints") separated by short intervals.
   3. **Warming up** prior to activity induces bronchodilation and refractoriness to EIB.
   4. **Warming down** after strenuous exercise decreases EIB.
   5. **Miscellaneous maneuvers**
      a. **"Running through"** EIB
      b. **Avoid hyperventilation**
      c. **Nasal breathing** humidifies, warms, and cleans the air.
      d. **Cold weather:** wearing mask or scarf around the nose and mouth creates warm, moist air and may diminish EIB.
      e. Avoid strenuous exercise during periods when air pollution is high, or with significant viral infection.

**TABLE 5.** Drugs Banned for Use During Competition

All sympathomimetic amines (except beta₂ specific).

Includes virtually all oral decongestants and many topical decongestants for the eyes. The NCAA permits some decongestant use with a letter from the team physician.

Opiate analgesics and antitussives (nonopiates acceptable, e.g., dextromethorphan, diphenhydramine).

**TABLE 6.** Banned Sympathomimetic Vasoconstrictors

Ephedrine
Phenylephrine
Phenylpropanolamine
Pseudoephedrine
Tetrahydrozoline

**TABLE 7.** Nonpharmacologic Maneuvers That May Minimize Exercise-induced Bronchospasm

Conditioning.

Induction of "refractoriness" to EIB by short bursts of exercise.

Appropriate "warming up" before exercise and "warming down" following vigorous exercise.

Avoiding hyperventilation.

"Running through" the EIB.

V. **Exercise-induced Anaphylaxis** (Table 8)

A. **Introduction**

1. **Epidemiology**

There have been approximately 500 reported cases of exercise-induced anaphylaxis. Attacks range in frequency from once a year to as often as monthly. Numerous attacks may occur before medical care is sought or the diagnosis is made. Most of the cases occur in accomplished athletes who exercise regularly.

2. **Definition**

Exercise induced anaphylaxis is characterized by a sensation of warmth, pruritis, cutaneous erythema, urticaria ($>$ 10 mm in diameter), upper respiratory obstructive symptoms, and occasionally vascular collapse. Exercise-induced anaphylaxis is distinct from exercise-induced asthma, cholinergic urticaria, angioedema, and cardiac arrhythmia, which are all recognized as exertion-related phenomena.

3. **Risk factors** include:

a. Previous **history of atopy** (50% of all cases).

b. Family history of atopy (67% of all cases).

c. **Food ingestion:** certain foods such as shellfish, nuts, or celery have been associated with EIA.

d. **Weather conditions** (heat, high humidity).

**TABLE 8.** Exercise-induced Anaphylaxis

1. **Signs and Symptoms**

Generalized pruritus.

Generalized urticaria.

Angioedema (face, palms of the hands, and soles of the feet).

Upper respiratory symptoms.

Choking and difficulty swallowing.

Gastrointestinal symptoms, cramping, nausea, and diarrhea.

Headaches.

2. **Risk Factors**

Positive personal or family history of allergies.

Food ingestion: shellfish, celery, aspirin.

Weather conditions: seems more common with hot, humid weather.

Intensity of exercise: appears to be worse with highly vigorous exercise.

3. **Prevention/precautions**

Reduction in intensity of exertion.

Avoidance of exercise on hot, humid days.

Avoid eating before exercise.

Immediate availability of an individual capable of treating anaphylaxis.

Medications:

Pretreatment with antihistamines partially effective.

Pretreatment with beta-adrenergic agents and theophylline compounds of unproven benefit.

4. **Signs and symptoms** (four stages)
   a. **Prodromal** stage—associated with fatigue, generalized warmth, itchiness, and erythema.
   b. **Early** stage—marked by confluent urticaria, rash, and angioedema.
   c. **Established** stage—associated with choking, stridor, colic, nausea, vomiting, and/or hypotension.
   d. **Late** stage—marked by headache.
5. **Complications**
   Can be life-threatening.

B. **Mechanisms**
   During an exercise induced anaphylaxis attack, serum histamine levels have been shown to increase from baseline values, thus suggesting mast-cell involvement.

C. **Prevention** through modification of exercise program
   1. Decrease intensity of exertion.
   2. Avoid exercising during warm and humid days.
   3. Interrupt exercise at the earliest sign of itching.
   4. Avoid meals at least 4 hours before exercise. Avoid certain foods which may be associated with exercise-induced anaphylaxis.

D. **Treatment**
   1. Epinephrine, fluid replacement, and antihistamines are commonly used.
   2. Pretreatment with antihistamine will not prevent exercise induced anaphylaxis.
   3. Patient should have EpiPen or Ana-Kit immediately available. Companion should also be familiar with its use.
   4. Where life-threatening reactions have occurred, the athlete may have to switch to a less strenuous sport or, in some instances, abandon athletics altogether.

VI. **Cholinergic Urticaria**

A. **Introduction**
   1. **Definition**
      Generalized **small** urticarial papules occurring after a warm bath, shower, exercise, or fever. Also known as generalized heat urticaria.
   2. **Signs and symptoms**
      a. Urticaria is usually small papules that appear first in the upper thorax and neck, spreading caudally to involve entire body.
      b. Systemic reactions such as abdominal pain, syncope, or wheezing are **rare.**
      c. Cholinergic reactions (lacrimation, salivation, diarrhea) may be observed.
   3. **Risk factors**
      a. Heat
      b. Humidity.

B. **Mechanisms**
   1. Neurogenic reflex
   2. Mediator release (histamine, NCF).

C. **Prevention**
   1. Avoid heat and humidity.
   2. Antihistamine may prevent or decrease incidence.

D. **Therapy**
   Antihistamines are generally used; hydroxyzine (at a dose of 25–200 mg per day) is the drug of choice. Cyproheptadine may also be used (at a dose of 4–20 mg per day).

## VII. Summary

A. **Exercise-induced bronchospasm**
1. Common
2. Diagnosis often overlooked
3. Preventable and treatable.

B. **Exercise-induced anaphylaxis**
1. Rare
2. Potentially fatal
3. Extreme caution.

C. **Cholinergic urticaria**
1. Not uncommon
2. Bothersome to patient.

**Acknowledgments:** The authors would like to thank Win Cole for her secretarial assistance and Dr. Roger M. Katz for providing helpful criticism.

## *RECOMMENDED READING*

**General Review Articles**
1. Bierman C: Exercise-induced asthma. NER Allergy Proc 9:193–197, 1988.
2. Eggleston PA: Exercise-induced asthma. Clin Rev Allergy 1:19–37, 1983.
3. Katz R: Exercise induced asthma. American Journal of Asthma & Allergy for Pediatricians 1:71–74, 1988.
4. Kobayashi R, Mellion M: Office Management of Sports Injuries & Athletic Problems. Philadelphia, Hanley & Belfus, 1988, pp 117–127.

**Mechanisms**
5. Anderson SD, Schoeffel RE, Follet R: Sensitivity to heat and water loss at rest during exercise in asthma patients. Eur J Respir Dis 63:459–471, 1982.
6. Bar-Yishay E, Godfrey S: Mechanisms of exercise induced asthma. Lung 162:195–204, 1984.

**Testing**
7. Haynes RL, Ingram RH Jr, McFadden ER Jr: An assessment of pulmonary response to exercise in asthma and analysis of factors influencing it. Am Rev Respir Dis 114:739–752, 1976.
8. Jones RS, Buston MH, Wharton MJ: The effect of exercise on ventilatory function in the child with asthma. Br J Dis Chest 56:78–86, 1962.
9. Silverman M, Anderson S: Standardization of exercise tests in asthmatic children. Arch Dis Child 47:882–889, 1972.

**Pharmacology**
10. Anderson S, Seale JP, Ferris L, et al: An evaluation of pharmacotherapy for exercise induced asthma. J Allergy Clin Immunol 64:612–624, 1979.
11. Rohr AS, Siegel SC, Katz RM, et al: A comparison of inhaled albuterol and cromolyn in the prophylaxis of exercise induced bronchospasm. Ann Allergy 59:107–109, 1987.
12. Sly RM: β-adrenergic drugs in the management of asthma in athletes. J Allergy Clin Immunol 73:680–685, 1984.

**Exercise-induced Anaphylaxis**
13. Kidd JM, Cohen SH, Sosman AJ, Fink JN: Food dependent exercise-induced anaphylaxis. J Allergy Clin Immunol 71:407–411, 1983.
14. Sheffer AL, Austen KF: Exercise-induced anaphylaxis. J Allergy Clin Immunol 73:699–703, 1984.

**Cholinergic Urticaria**
15. Daman L, Lieberman P, Ganier M, Hashimoto K: Localized heat urticaria. J Allergy Clin Immunol 61:273–278, 1978.
16. Grant JA, Findlay SR, Theuson DO, et al: Local heat urticaria/angioedema: Evidence for histamine release without complement activation. J Allergy Clin Immunol 67:75–77, 1981.

# Chapter 25: The Athlete with Epilepsy

DONALD R. BENNETT, MD

I. **Overview of Epilepsy**
   A. **Definitions**
      1. **"Convulsive disorders (epilepsy)** are states characterized by sudden, brief, repetitive and stereotyped alterations of behavior which are presumed to be due to a paroxysmal discharge of cortical or subcortical neurons."[1]
      2. **Primary generalized epilepsies** are characterized primarily by absence and/or tonic-clonic seizures. Onset is usually in childhood. There is no evidence of structural brain abnormalities, and these patients are neurologically normal and with normal IQs. This type of epilepsy may be inherited or no cause can be determined.
      3. **Secondary generalized epilepsies** are characterized by several seizure types, usually generalized tonic-clonic, akinetic, or multi-focal. Onset is usually in childhood. Diffuse brain damage is present and patients are neurologically impaired and retarded.
      4. **Partial epilepsies** are characterized by simple or complex partial seizures with or without secondary generalization. This type of epilepsy can occur at any age. With the exception of infrequent types, such as benign rolandic epilepsy of childhood, they are caused by structural brain lesion such as a tumor.
      5. **Provoked seizures** are seizures, either generalized or partial, that occur at the time of an acute neurological insult such as a head injury, meningitis or encephalitis, hyperthermia, or with hypoglycemia or electrolyte abnormalities. Provoked seizures may also occur with sleep deprivation or after alcohol or drug withdrawal. Patients whose seizures are secondary to an acute brain injury such as head trauma are at risk for the development of unprovoked convulsions.
      6. **Unprovoked seizures** are seizures, either generalized or focal, that occur without a known precipitating cause. In children the risk of a second unprovoked seizure is 52%[2] and in adults ranges between 27 and 58%.[3,4]
   B. **Classification of epileptic seizures**[5]
      1. See Table 1
   C. **Epidemiology of epilepsy**
      1. There are approximately 375,000 epileptics between the ages of 5 and 24 years in the U.S.[6]
      2. Of these, approximately 277,000 attend normal schools, and many of them could participate in competitive sports.[6]
   D. **Drug treatment, seizure type, anticonvulsant serum half-lives, and therapeutic blood levels**[10]
      1. See Table 2
   E. **Anticonvulsant side effects**[10]
      1. See Table 3
   F. **Seizure control**
      1. Primary generalized epilepsy: Good control in 75–85% of patients.[7]
      2. Secondary generalized epilepsy: Much more difficult to control. No definite percentages are available.

**TABLE 1.** Classification of Seizures

I. Partial (focal, local) seizures
  A. Simple partial seizures (consciousness not impaired)
    1. With motor symptoms
    2. With somatosensory or special sensory symptoms
    3. With autonomic symptoms
    4. With psychic systems
  B. Complex partial seizures (with impairment of consciousness)
    1. Beginning as simple partial seizures and progressing to impairment of consciousness
      a. With no other features
      b. With features as in par. I.A.1–I.A.4
      c. With automatisms
    2. With impairment of consciousness at onset
      a. With no other features
      b. With features as in par. I.A.1–I.A.4
      c. With automatisms
  C. Partial seizures evolving to secondarily generalized seizures.
    1. Simple partial seizures evolving to generalized seizures
    2. Complex partial seizures evolving to generalized seizures
    3. Simple partial seizures evolving to complex partial seizures to generalized
II. Generalized seizures (convulsive or nonconvulsive)
  A. Absence seizures
    1. Absence seizures
    2. Atypical absence seizures
  B. Myoclonic seizures
  C. Clonic seizures
  D. Tonic seizures
  E. Tonic-clonic seizures
  F. Atonic seizures (astatic seizures)
III. Unclassified epileptic seizures
Includes all seizures that cannot be classified because of inadequate or incomplete data.

    3. Partial epilepsy: Total seizure control in 31–80% of patients, with complex partial seizures the most resistant.[8]
  G. **Relapse after anticonvulsant withdrawal**
    1. **Rate of relapse** is approximately 30%[9] for children and adolescents. Is somewhat higher for adults. Most recurrences occur within the 1st year of withdrawal.
    2. **Predictors for favorable outcome in children:**[10]
      a. Seizures begin after 2 years of age.
      b. Normal neurological examination and normal IQ.

**TABLE 2.** Anticonvulsants, Seizure Type, Half-life and Therapeutic Levels

| Drug | Seizure Type | Half-life | Therapeutic Levels |
|------|--------------|-----------|--------------------|
| Ethosuximide | Absence<br>Myoclonic | 20–60 hr for adults and children | 40–100 $\mu$g/cc |
| Carbamazepine | Partial seizures<br>Generalized tonic-clonic | 14–24 hr for adults and children | 4–12 $\mu$g/cc |
| Phenobarbital | Generalized tonic-clonic<br>Partial seizures | 46–136 hr for adults<br>37–73 hr for children | 15–40 $\mu$g/cc |
| Phenytoin | Generalized tonic-clonic<br>Partial seizures | 10–34 hr for adults<br>5–14 hr for children | 10–20 $\mu$g/cc |
| Primidone | Generalized tonic-clonic<br>Partial seizures | 6–18 hr for adults<br>5–11 hr for children | 5–12 $\mu$g/cc |
| Valproic acid | Absence<br>Myoclonic<br>Generalized tonic-clonic | 6–15 hr for adults<br>8–15 hr for children | 40–150 $\mu$g/cc |

**TABLE 3.** Anticonvulsant Side-effects

| Drug | Dose Related | Non-Dose Related | Idiosyncratic |
|---|---|---|---|
| Phenobarbital | Sedation<br>Behavioral changes<br>Ataxia<br>Hyperactivity | Decrease in attention span<br>Hyperactivity<br>Changes in sleep pattern | Allergic dermatitis<br>Stevens-Johnson syndrome<br>Hepatic failure |
| Primidone | Sedation<br>Behavioral changes<br>Ataxia<br>Hyperactivity | Nausea and vomiting | Allergic dermatitis |
| Phenytoin | Nystagmus<br>Ataxia<br>Incoordination<br>Cognitive<br>  impairment | Hirsutism<br>Gingival hyperplasia<br>Lymphadenopathy<br>Neuropathy<br>Folic acid deficiency/<br>  anemia | Allergic dermatitis<br>Hepatic failure<br>Lupus erythematosus-like reaction<br>Anemia and granulocyte<br>  suppression |
| Valproic acid | Nausea<br>Diarrhea<br>Tremor<br>Behavioral changes | Weight gain<br>Nausea<br>Nausea<br>Hair loss | Reye-like syndrome<br>Hepatic failure<br>Pancreatitis |
| Carbamazepine | Diplopia<br>Blurred vision<br>Behavioral changes<br>  and lethargy<br>Ataxia<br>Cardiac conduction<br>  disturbance<br>Dyskinesias | Diarrhea<br>Fluid retention | Granulocyte suppression<br>Aplastic anemia<br>Hepatic and renal failure<br>Allergic dermatitis<br>Stevens-Johnson syndrome<br>Thrombocytopenia |
| Ethosuximide | Fatigue<br>Headache<br>Dysequilibrium | Gastric discomfort<br>Nausea, vomiting and<br>  anorexia | Leukopenia<br>Thrombocytopenia<br>Stevens-Johnson syndrome |

    c. Primary generalized epilepsy.

    d. Seizure control for 4–5 years.

  3. **Predictors for favorable outcome in adults:**[10]

    a. Only one primary generalized seizure type.

    b. Younger than 30 years when first seizure occurred.

    c. Seizure control achieved early after onset.

    d. Normal serial EEGs while patient is taking anticonvulsants.

    e. Seizure free for 2–5 years.

**H. Mortality and morbidity**

  1. Seven percent of epileptics die as a result of accidents;[11] however, only 5% of these deaths can be attributed to injuries sustained during a seizure.[12] Bath tub drownings are responsible for most of the seizure-related deaths.

  2. The risk for drowning while bathing in the sea or swimming in a pool is four times greater for epileptic children than their peers.[13] This can be markedly reduced by careful supervision.

  3. The accident rate is about the same for epileptic and nonepileptic children.[14]

  4. A history of epilepsy does not indicate an increased predisposition to suffer a seizure immediately or soon after a head injury.[15,16]

  5. **The most frequent injuries sustained during a seizure,** primarily generalized tonic-clonic attacks, are:[17,18]

    a. Fractures of the humeral neck, femoral trochanter, clavicle, and ankle

    b. Vertebral compression fractures

    c. Shoulder and hip dislocations

    d. Head and cervical spine injuries.

## II. Exercise and Epilepsy

A. Seizures tend to occur when the patient is "off guard, sleeping, resting, idling."[19]

B. **A regular exercise program may have a beneficial effect on seizure control.**[20]

C. **Seizures or EEG epileptiform discharges occurring in epileptics during exercise or in the immediate postexertion period have rarely been reported.**[6,21–24]

    1. Both generalized and partial seizures, particularly complex, partial, have been documented.

    2. **There are no reports of status epilepticus triggered by exercise.**

D. If a patient's first seizure occurs during physical activity, particularly complex partial attacks, a structural brain lesion such as a tumor should be ruled out.[9]

E. There is no evidence that the pharmacokinetics of anticonvulsant drugs are altered by a regular exercise program, although research in this field is limited.

F. Sports-related injuries are not increased in the epileptic.[14,15]

G. The "sudden death syndrome" in epileptics is not associated with physical activity.[25]

H. Epileptics, including those who because of physical or mental handicaps are unable to participate in regular competitive sports, should be encouraged to participate in exercise programs and games, including the Special Olympics Programs.

## III. The Athlete with Epilepsy

A. Granting permission for epileptics to participate in competitive sports, particularly collision or contact sports, is a difficult decision for physicians, parents, and school officials. Reservations are based on the following **concerns:**

    1. A seizure during contests or practice would predispose the player to a serious injury, particularly of the brain or spinal cord.

        a. Although a theoretical possibility, confirmatory data to support this are lacking, with the exception of swimming. (see par. I.H.2; II.F.)

    2. Single or cumulative head blows may adversely affect seizure control or cause an immediate or early post-traumatic seizure (see par. I.H.4).

        a. Reports suggest that this should not be a concern.

        b. However, because of the inherent dangers, **boxing** should be excluded.

B. **All-inclusive lists of sports that epileptics may participate in have not been promulgated. This is because each case has to be judged on its own merits, comparing the potential risks versus the benefits. What is good for one athlete may not be good for another. These judgmental decisions have been addressed by several committees.**

    1. **The Committees on Children with Handicaps and Sports Medicine of the American Medical Association**[26] recommends that children be allowed to participate in physical education and interscholastic athletics including contact and collision sports provided there is:

        a. Proper medical management, good seizure control, and proper supervision.

        b. Avoid situations or sports in which a dangerous fall could occur, such as rope climbing, activity on parallel bars, and high diving.

        c. Swimming should be supervised; however, underwater swimming is not acceptable.

    2. **The Professional Advisory Board of the Epilepsy Foundation of America**[27] in response to a question whether an epileptic should be allowed to take scuba diving at the Instructor level stated:

        a. "Persons with epilepsy whose seizures are controlled can and should lead full lives without any personal restrictions."

   b. "The risk for a person who has had epilepsy that is now controlled whether receiving medication or not are somewhat greater than for a person without a history of seizures. The magnitude of these risks is small."
   c. "It is also the right of the individual to evaluate these risks and undertake any activity for which he feels the risks are reasonable."
   d. "In the case of such a person becoming a scuba diver, we do not believe that such an individual . . . should involve other persons who do not have such risk factors without their specific knowledge and consent."
   3. Other sports such as auto racing, mountaineering, and sky diving could be substituted for scuba diving in the above statement.

IV. **Guidelines for Determining Participation and Follow-up of Epileptics on Anticonvulsant Medication in Competitive Sports**
   A. **Contact or collision sports (boxing excluded)**
      1. **Participation**
         a. Determine if athletic interest is genuine. If not, encourage the athlete to participate in other sports.
         b. The athlete, parents, or legal guardian, as well as school authorities, should understand the inherent risks.
         c. **Neurological criteria:**
            i. No evidence of progressive neurological disease.
            ii. **Seizure-free on anticonvulsant drug(s) for at least 1 year.**
            iii. The absence of significant abnormalities on the neurological examination, particularly in motor and coordination skills, that could hamper performance.
            iv. Athlete is compliant in taking anticonvulsant medication as documented by several recent therapeutic blood levels.
            v. Absence of dose-related, nondose-related, and idiosyncratic side-effects of the anticonvulsants (see Table 3).
            vi. If there are concerns or unanswered questions, request a neurological examination.
      2. **Follow-up**
         a. Periodic anticonvulsant blood levels.
            i. Obtain in a.m. before 1st daily dose.
            ii. If subtherapeutic, athlete cannot participate until level is therapeutic.
            iii. If at toxic level, wait until it is in therapeutic range.
         b. Periodic complete blood counts. Other blood studies such as liver function tests will depend on the potential toxic effects of the anticonvulsants prescribed.
         c. Anticonvulsants should not be taken just prior to practice or before a game, nor should they be taken on an empty stomach. Frequency of daily dose is dependent on the half-life of the drug (see Table 2). Workout an appropriate dose-time schedule.
         d. The athlete should inform the team physician when medications are used to treat other ailments, because certain drugs may alter the metabolism of the anticonvulsants.
         e. Stress the importance of the need for proper amount of sleep as well as good nutrition.
         f. Emphasize strict avoidance of alcohol, stimulant medications, anabolic steroids, and recreational drugs.
         g. **An epileptic even though he/she has been seizure-free for 2 years or longer should be maintained on anticonvulsants during his/her competitive career.**

   h. In sports that require periodic drug screens of athletes, the authorities should be notified in advance of the anticonvulsant(s) being taken by the athlete.
  3. **Seizure recurrence**
   a. **If a seizure occurs during competition or practice, the athlete should be taken to an emergency room.**
    i. Perform a neurological examination.
    ii. Obtain a head CT scan, if:
     (a) There is a suspicion of a head injury, or
     (b) The neurological examination is abnormal, particularly if focal deficits such as a hemiparesis are found, or if
     (c) The athlete is slow to respond, i.e., the postictal period is prolonged.
    iii. Obtain anticonvulsant blood levels.
   b. If seizure is not related to competition:
    i. Perform a neurological examination.
     (a) If abnormal, and this represents a change from the baseline examination, obtain a CT scan of the head.
    ii. Obtain serum anticonvulsant levels.
   c. Disposition
    i. Subtherapeutic anticonvulsant levels:
     (a) Adjust dose until therapeutic blood levels are obtained on several determinations over a 4-week period.
     (b) Emphasize the need for compliance.
     (c) May return to competition once therapeutic levels have been established.
     (d) If subsequent seizures occur with subtherapeutic levels, the athlete should not be allowed to continue in contact or collision sports.
    ii. Therapeutic blood levels:
     (a) Should not be allowed to participate in contact or collision sports unless cleared by a neurologist.
     (b) If further seizures occur, should not be allowed to continue in contact or collision sports.
 B. **Other sports**
  1. **Participation**
   a. Criteria should not be as strict as with contact or collision sports.
   b. The occurrence of an occasional seizure should not preclude participation unless it occurred during a sport in which there is an increased risk for injury such as gymnastics or swimming.
   c. Neurological criteria (see par. IV.A.1.c.i,ii–vi).
  2. **Follow-up.**
   a. See par. IV.A.2.a–h.
  3. **Seizure recurrence**
   Further participation will depend on the sport and the athlete's compliance in taking his medication.

V. **Guidelines for Participation and Follow-up of Athletes in Competitive Sports with a Past History of One or More Seizures Who Are Not Taking Anticonvulsant Drugs**

 A. **May participate if:**
  1. No evidence of progressive neurological disease.
  2. There are no neurological abnormalities, particularly in motor and coordination skills, that could hinder performance.
  3. The athlete has been seizure-free off anticonvulsant medications for **2 years** or longer.

**TABLE 4.** Causes of Seizures By Age

| Causes | Approximate Peak Periods |
|---|---|
| Birth trauma; congenital malformations; metabolic abnormalities, infections | Neonatal |
| Birth trauma; congenital malformations; infections | Birth to 5 years |
| Idiopathic (genetic) | 5 to 15 years |
| Brain trauma | 15 to 40 years |
| Cerebrovascular disease | Older than 40 years |

    B. **Follow-up.**
        1. If seizures recur, then follow guidelines in par. VI.B. and C.

VI. **An Athlete's First Seizure**
    A. **Evaluation**
        1. Establish the type of seizures (Table 1) from the history and observations of witnesses. Determine if it was provoked or unprovoked (par. I.A.5. and 6.).
        2. Attempt to establish a cause (Table 4)[9] from:
           a. General physical and neurological examination
           b. CBC, urinalysis, blood chemistries to include glucose, BUN, Ca, Mg, and serum electrolytes
           c. Electroencephalogram (awake and sleep recording)
           d. Head CT scan or MRI when indicated
           e. A neurological consultation is required when a definite cause cannot be found.
    B. **Treatment**
        1. Unprovoked
           a. Start on appropriate anticonvulsant based on seizure type. Anticonvulsants with sedative properties should be avoided.
        2. Provoked
           a. Primary brain injury
           If seizure is caused by a head injury, meningitis, etc. from which the athlete completely recovers, it is best to treat prophylactically with anticonvulsants so long as the athlete continues to compete, particularly in contact or collision sports.
           b. Secondary event
           If seizure is caused by an event that is not likely to occur again, such as heat stroke, sleep deprivation, hypoglycemia, drug or alcohol withdrawal, etc., prophylactic anticonvulsant treatment may not be required.
    C. **Disposition**
    Before the athlete can return to competition, he/she must:
        1. Show no evidence of a progressive neurological disease.
        2. Be seizure-free for both unprovoked and provoked seizures for at **least 12 months;** however, there may be circumstances that could reduce this observation period. However, a neurological consultation is required before this can be done.
        3. For those started on anticonvulsant medication, they must have therapeutic blood levels on several occasions.
        4. Absence of anticonvulsant side-effects.
    D. Follow-up (see par. IV.2.).

## REFERENCES

1. Kurland LT, Kurtzke JF, Goldberg ID (eds): Epidemiology of Neurologic and Sense Organ Disorders. Cambridge, MA, Harvard University Press, 1973.
2. Canfield PR, Canfield CS, Dooley JM, et al: Epilepsy after a first unprovoked seizure in childhood. Neurology 35:1657–1660, 1985.
3. Hauser WA, Anderson VE, Loewensen RB, et al: Seizure recurrence after a first unprovoked seizure. N Engl J Med 307:522–528, 1982.
4. Johnson LC, DeBolt WL, Long MT, et al: Diagnostic factors in adult males following initial seizures: A 3-year follow-up. Arch Neurol 27:193–197, 1972.
5. Gastaut H: Clinical and electroencephalographic classification of epileptic seizure. Epilepsia 11:102, 1970.
6. Bennett DR: Sport and epilepsy: To play or not to play. Sem Neurol 1:345–357, 1981.
7. Delgado-Escueta AV, Treiman DM, Walsh GO: The treatable epilepsies. N Engl J Med 308:1508–1514, 1983.
8. Mattson RH, Cramer JW, Collins JF, et al: Comparison of carbamazepine, phenobarbital, and primidone in partial and secondary tonic-clonic seizures. N Engl J Med 313:141–151, 1985.
9. Bennett DR: Epilepsy in the athlete. In Jordan B, Tsaris P, Warren R (eds): Rockville, MD, Aspen Publishers, Ch 10, pp 346–373 (in press).
10. Penry JK: Epilepsy: Diagnosis, Management, Quality of Life. New York, Raven Press, 1986.
11. Hauser WA, Annegers JF, Elveback LR: Mortality in patients with epilepsy. Epilepsia 21:399–412, 1980.
12. Zielinski JJ: Epilepsy and mortality rate and cause of death. Epilepsia 15:191–201, 1974.
13. Pearn J, Nixon J, Wilkey I: Freshwater drowning and near-drowning accidents involving children. Med J Aust 2:942–946, 1976.
14. Aisenson MR: Accidental injuries in epileptic children. Pediatrics 2:85–88, 1948.
15. Livingston S, Berman W: Participation of epileptic patients in sports. JAMA 224:236–238, 1973.
16. Jennett BW: Early traumatic epilepsy: Incidence and significance after non-missile injuries. Arch Neurol 30:394–398, 1974.
17. Lidgren L, Walloe A: Incidence of fracture in epileptics. Acta Orthop Scand 48:356–361, 1977.
18. Pedersen KK, Christiansen C, et al: Incidence of fracture of the vertebral spine in epileptic patients. Acta Neurol Scand 54:200–203, 1976.
19. Lennox WG, Lennox MA: Epilepsy and related disorders. 2:823–824, 1960.
20. Department of Health, Education and Welfare: Plan for Nationwide Action on Epilepsy Washington, DC, Government Printing Office, pp 29–43.
21. Kocczyn AD: Participation of epileptic patients in sports. J Sports Med 19:195–198, 1979.
22. Gotze W, Kubicki ST, Munter M, et al: Effect of physical exercise on seizure threshold (investigated by electroencephalographic telemetry). Dis Nerv Syst 28:664–667, 1967.
23. Kuijer A: Epilepsy and exercise, electroencephalographical and biochemical studies. In Wada JA, Penry JK (eds): Advances in Epileptology: The Tenth Epilepsy International Symposium. New York, Raven Press, 1980, p 543.
24. Ogunyemi A, Gomex MR, Klass DW: Seizures induced by exercise. Neurology 38:633–634, 1988.
25. Jay GW, Leestma JE: Sudden death in epilepsy. Acta Neurol Scand 82(suppl):1–66, 1981.
26. American Academy of Pediatrics Committee on Children with Handicaps and The Committee on Sports Medicine: Sports and the child with epilepsy. Pediatrics 72:884, 1983.
27. Dreifuss FE: Epileptics and scuba diving (Letter to the Editor). JAMA 253:1877–1878, 1985.

# Chapter 26: The Athlete with Headache

DONALD R. BENNETT, MD

I. **Headaches, an infrequent complaint of athletes, may be symptomatic of serious or even life-threatening systemic or neurological disease. It is therefore imperative that the team physician establish the cause as soon as possible.** In order to accomplish this, he/she should be familiar with the diagnostic criteria for the various headache types.[1] In addition, the following information obtained from the history and physical and neurological examinations, as well as laboratory tests, will help to establish a differential diagnosis.

A. **History: From the patient's history or from observers, determine:**
  1. If the headache onset occurred during physical activity and if so what type.
  2. If the headache onset was related to head or neck trauma or sudden movement of these structures.
  3. If the intensity of the pain was maximum at the onset or was slow to evolve.
  4. If the pain was localized or generalized.
  5. If there is a past and/or family history of headaches, and if so what type.
  6. If there were any adverse environmental factors at the time of the headache onset, such as heat, high humidity, high altitude, etc.
  7. The type of equipment worn at onset of headache such as helmets, headbands, goggles, mouth pieces, etc.
  8. A drug and dietary history.
  9. **Whether other neurological symptoms preceded, occurred at the time, or followed the onset of the headache. Important signs and symptoms are:**
    a. Alteration of consciousness or a behavioral change including amnesia.
    b. Visual changes such as amaurosis, scintillating scotoma, or diplopia.
    c. Nausea and vomiting.
    d. Vertigo.
    e. Gait abnormalities or problems with coordination.
    f. Focal motor or sensory abnormalities such as a hemiparesis or hemisensory loss.
    g. Problems with communication such as aphasia.
    h. Convulsive activity.
B. **Physical and neurological examinations.** The following are the essential components of an initial screening evaluation when the athlete is seen soon after the onset of headache. This format can also be used to evaluate athletes with recurrent headaches who are asymptomatic at the time of the examination.
    a. Vital signs, to include blood pressure, pulse, respirations, and temperature.
    b. Inspect the head for signs of external trauma.
    c. Determine by percussing the head if there is localized tenderness.
    d. Check for nuchal rigidity.
    e. Evaluate state of hydration.
    f. Perform a thorough cardiopulmonary examination.
    g. Document the athlete's state of orientation to time, place, person, and the quickness and appropriateness of his/her responses to questions.
    h. Determine if there are any memory deficits or problems with communication.

     i. Note size and symmetry of pupils and reaction to direct and consensual light.

     j. Check for visual field defects or abnormalities of ocular motility, including paresis of cranial nerves 3, 4, and 6.

     k. Look for the presence of nystagmus.

     l. Look for papilledema.

     m. Determine if strength, reflexes, and sensations are normal and symmetrical.

     n. Perform the Babinski reflex.

     o. Evaluate the athlete's gait.

C. **Laboratory studies.** The selection of appropriate laboratory studies is dependent on the initial clinical impression. These studies are covered in the subsequent section on headaches occurring during exercise or competition.

II. **The Differential Diagnosis of Headaches Occurring During Exercise or Competition**

A. **"Benign" exertional headaches**

1. **Diagnostic criteria**

     a. Precipitated by sports that require a sudden brief, maximum expenditure of energy such as weight lifting.[2-4]

     b. Is of sudden onset with the pain maximum at the beginning.

     c. Is located bilaterally, occipital greater than frontal, and is often throbbing.

     d. Is of short duration, usually 5 min, but may be followed by a dull posterior or suboccipital pain that lasts for 24 hr.

     e. Is not usually associated with other neurological symptoms or signs.

     f. May be recurrent. If so, nonsteroidal anti-inflammatory drugs may be helpful in preventing future attacks.

2. Comment: Approximately 10% of patients with this type of headache harbor intracranial lesions such as brain tumors, vascular anomalies, or Arnold Chiari-Type I malformations.[5] Therefore an athlete with this type of headache should be evaluated neurologically. **This workup should include an MRI study of the head and cervical spine. If these studies are normal, he/she may return to competition.**

B. **"Effort migraine"**[6]

1. **Diagnostic criteria**

     a. The duration of the exercise is longer than with "benign" exertional headaches. For example, a 200- or 440-yard dash.

     b. Is retro-orbital and usually unilateral.

     c. Onset is usually at the end of the activity.

     d. May be associated with a visual aura, hyperventilation, nausea, or vomiting.

     e. Lasts for approximately 1 hr.

     f. There may be a history of migraine.

     g. May recur.

2. Comment: **This type of headache is usually self-limited and no treatment is necessary. If it occurs frequently, then a neurological consultation should be obtained. It may be prevented by a graded warm-up period.**

C. **Vascular headache with prolonged exercise**

1. **Diagnostic criteria**

     a. Diffuse throbbing headache with prolonged exercise such as long-distance running or swimming.

     b. Most frequent in poorly conditioned athletes.

     c. May occur in well-conditioned athletes when exercising in unaccustomed high altitudes.

     d. Heat stress, dehydration, and hypoglycemia are precipitating conditions.

     e. Transient or persistent neurological deficits may occur.[7,8]

      f. Headache may persist for up to 24 hr after the exercise is completed.

      g. Athlete may have a history of migraine.

  2. **Comment: Achieving increased conditioning levels and long gradual warm-up can be preventative.[9] If athlete has associated neurological signs or symptoms with this type of headache, he/she should be seen by a neurologist.**

D. **Headache related to an acute increase in systemic blood pressure**

  1. **Diagnostic criteria**

      a. Usually bilateral and throbbing.

      b. Commonly associated with nausea and vomiting.

      c. Visual symptoms may be present.

      d. Duration variable—may be only 15 min or less or prolonged.

      e. Recurrent.

      f. Demonstration of significantly elevated blood pressure during attack, i.e., 260–300/120+ mmHg.

      g. Patients frequently have baseline hypertension.

  2. **Comment: Athletes with recurrent headaches associated with exercise and documented significant hypertension during the episode require further investigation to rule out a pheochromocytoma.[10]**

      a. Remember, there is an increased incidence of this tumor in von Recklinghausen's disease. The decision on further participation will depend on determining the cause.

E. **Headache secondary to spontaneous intracranial hemorrhage[11]**

  1. **Subarachnoid hemorrhage**

    a. **Diagnostic criteria**

      i. Sudden onset of explosive headache.

      ii. Headache usually generalized.

      iii. Maximum headache intensity reached in a period of several minutes and is persistent.

      iv. May be associated with change in consciousness and/or focal neurological signs, as well as nausea and vomiting.

      v. Nuchal rigidity may not be detected until 4–6 hr post-bleed.

      vi. Most likely causes are ruptured intracranial aneurysm or arteriovenous malformations.

    b. Comments (see below).

  2. **Intracerebral hemorrhage**

    a. **Diagnostic criteria**

      i. Sudden onset of explosive headache.

      ii. Usually lateralized or may be located posteriorly.

      iii. Maximum intensity reached within minutes and persists.

      iv. Usually associated with a disturbance of consciousness, focal neurological signs, nausea, and vomiting.

      v. Nuchal rigidity may or may not be present.

      vi. Most frequent causes are pre-existing hypertension or a ruptured arteriovenous malformation.

    b. Comments (see below).

  3. **Intraventricular hemorrhage**

    a. **Diagnostic criteria**

      i. See par. II.E.2.a.i.–v.

      ii. Disturbances of consciousness more frequent and pronounced than with intracerebral hemorrhage.

      iii. Most likely cause is pre-existing hypertension. However, condition has occurred in nonhypertensive weight lifters.[12] The headache in these athletes simulated "benign" exertional headaches (see par. II.A.); however, they persisted and were associated with disturbances of consciousness.

   b. Comments (see below).

  4. **Comments:** Headaches secondary to intracranial hemorrhage have been reported in joggers,[11] a squash player,[11] and weight lifters.[12] Two patients developed a hemorrhage in brain tumors while jogging.[13] They had been asymptomatic prior to hemorrhage. Although the reported cases of intracranial hemorrhage occurred in recreational exercises, the possibility exists that spontaneous intracranial hemorrhage can occur in competitive athletes. **For the team physician the hallmarks for suspecting an intracranial hemorrhage are:**

    a. **Abrupt onset of a severe headache**

    b. **Persistence of severe headache**

    c. **Alteration of consciousness**

    d. **Focal neurological signs**

    e. **If suspected, the athlete should be taken immediately to the nearest hospital with neurosurgical coverage.**

F. **Headache secondary to cerebral ischemia**

  1. **Focal ischemia**

    a. **Diagnostic criteria**

      i. Most cases of transient focal ischemia or infarction have been reported in runners.[6-8,14-16]

     ii. Headache is usually abrupt in onset, reaching its intensity within 15–30 min.

    iii. Generally localized to the side of vascular compromise, i.e., left side with left middle cerebral artery ischemia.

    iv. Focal neurological deficits may precede the onset of headache as in migraine. With this condition, the deficits progress over a period of 10–20 min and then are followed by headache.

     v. Focal neurological deficits time-locked with headache onset and maximum at the beginning and which clear within 5–10 min suggest an embolic cause.

    vi. Progression of neurological deficits with increasing headache intensity, in the absence of intracranial hemorrhage, suggests arterial thrombosis or dissection. Venous thrombosis secondary to dehydration, sickle cell disease, or polycythemia can present with similar signs and symptoms.

   vii. The onset of headache with neurological abnormalities following sudden neck movements suggests an arterial dissection.[17-20]

  viii. **Any athlete with headache and associated neurological signs should be immediately taken to the nearest hospital with neurosurgical coverage.**

    ix. **An MRI or CT scan should be done immediately.** Other studies to consider depending on the suspected cause are:

      (a) CBC and sed rate      (d) Chest x-ray and EKG

      (b) Chemistry profile      (e) Echocardiogram.

      (c) Serum electrolytes

     x. The decision on further participation in athletics will depend on the cause. It is recommended that neurological or neurosurgical consultation be obtained before this decision is made.

  2. **Global ischemia**

    a. **Diagnostic criteria**

      i. Generalized headache, frequently pulsating with and without loss of consciousness (syncope).

        ii. Usually of less than 1 hr in duration, caused by hypertension.

        iii. Absence of focal neurological deficits.

        iv. Caused by decreased cerebral blood flow secondary to hypotension.

    b. Precipitating events may be dehydration, increase in core temperature, Valsalva maneuver (weight lifters), and orthostatic hypotension secondary to decreased systemic resistance following exhaustive exercise.[21]

    c. The team physician should evaluate the athlete for possible predisposing cardiopulmonary diseases.

### G. Headaches secondary to head or neck trauma

  **1. Intracerebral hematomas**

    a. **Diagnostic criteria**

        i. Documented head trauma with or without loss of consciousness.

        ii. Headache may be present immediately or be delayed.

        iii. Intensity of headache increases with time.

        iv. As intensity increases, alteration of consciousness, focal neurological signs, nausea and vomiting, signs of increased intracranial pressure, or seizures usually appear.

    b. **For team physicians, an increasing intensity of a headache following a blow to the head is the major diagnostic clue to the possible presence of an intracranial hematoma. The athlete should be transported immediately to the nearest hospital with neurosurgical coverage. Time is of the essence particularly in the diagnosis and treatment of acute epidural and subdural hematomas.**

  **2. Trauma-induced migraine[22]**

    a. **Diagnostic criteria**

        i. **Head injury is minor** and usually not associated with loss of consciousness or signs and symptoms of a concussion.

        ii. Following a symptom-free interval, usually of several minutes, visual, motor, sensory, or brainstem symptoms begin and last for 15–30 min.

        iii. As these symptoms resolve, a diffuse or focal headache begins and lasts for 12–24 hr, with decreasing intensity over time.

        iv. Nausea and vomiting often accompany the headache.

        v. The athlete may have a personal or family history of migraine.

        vi. Attacks may recur with subsequent head trauma or occur spontaneously.

    b. Comment: This type of symptom complex occurring during an athletic event, particularly in collision or contact sports, can simulate a serious neurological emergency. **Therefore, with the first episode the athlete should be taken to the hospital for diagnostic tests, including a head CT scan and observation. Once the diagnosis is established, the athlete can return to competition.** Because this syndrome is so unpredictable, i.e., not following every blow to the head, prophylactic antimigraine drugs are not recommended.[22]

    c. The decision on future participation in contact or collision sports is based on the results of a complete neurological evaluation.

  **3. Post-traumatic headaches**

    a. **Diagnostic criteria**

        i. Recurrent headache with onset within minutes or several days post-trauma.

        ii. Loss of consciousness may or may not have been present at the time of trauma.

        iii. More frequent after trivial than after major head injuries.

        iv. Pain described as either:

(a) A steady pressure with cap-like distribution.

(b) Tenderness around impact site.

(c) Episodic aching or throbbing pain, usually unilateral.

   v. Pain is intensified by exertion, stress, coughing, or change in position.

  vi. May be associated with nonspecific complaints of dizziness, fatigue, blurring of vision, and difficulty with concentration (postconcussion syndrome).

 vii. The neurological examination is normal.

viii. Unusual to persist longer than 2 months.

  b. Comment: This type of headache **is uncommon in athletes**. If persistent, then a neurological evaluation is indicated. If no evidence of neurological disease, a graded exercise program or a more prolonged warm-up period may be of help in preventing the return of the headache with exercise.

H. **External compression headache**

  1. **Diagnostic criteria**

    a. Results from application of external pressure to the forehead or scalp from tight headbands, helmets, or goggles.[23,24]

    b. Is felt in the area subject to pressure.

    c. Is a constant pain.

    d. Is prevented by avoiding the precipitating cause.

    e. Is not associated with cranial or intracranial disease.

  2. **Comment: May trigger a migrainous headache if compression is prolonged.**

I. **Headache secondary to temporomandibular dysfunction**

  1. **Diagnostic critera**

    a. Recurrent headaches with pain located in the temporomandibular joints or in the temporalis muscles.

    b. Associated signs are:

      i. Temporomandibular joint noise on jaw movement

     ii. Limited or jerky jaw movements

    iii. Pain on jaw functioning

    iv. Locking of jaw on opening

     v. Clenching of teeth

    vi. Gnashing of teeth (bruxism)

   vii. Tongue, lip or cheekbiting.

    c. Most common cause in athletes is stress, malocclusions, overbites, and improperly fitted mouth guards.[25]

    d. Pain usually occurs after exercise.

    e. Normal neurological examination.

    f. Comment: Athletes with frequent headaches due to temporomandibular dysfunction should be evaluated by an oral surgeon. A stress management program may also be helpful.

J. **Environment-induced headaches**

  1. **Altitude headache**

    a. **Diagnostic criteria**

      i. Occurs within 24 hr after rapid ascent to altitudes above 3,000 M. Rarely occurs at elevations of less than 2,500 M.

     ii. Headache is usually generalized and throbbing in quality.

    iii. Intensity of headache is increased by exertion, coughing, or change in positions.

    b. Effort migraine (see par. II.B.) is more frequent at high altitude even in the best-conditioned athletes.

    c. Headache may be the initial symptom of acute mountain sickness.

      d. Comment: At lower altitudes the headache usually lasts only 24 to 48 hrs. If severe, acetazolamide (Diamox) may provide relief. **If other symptoms of acute mountain sickness such as shortness of breath and disorientation develop, then immediate descent to lower altitudes is mandatory. The best prevention is gradual aclimatization.**

   2. **Other environment-induced headaches**

      a. **Diagnostic criteria**

         i. Generalized headache, often throbbing.

        ii. Gradual in onset.

       iii. May resemble migraine.

       iv. Usually no focal neurological deficits.

        v. **Can be precipitated by dehydration, exhaustion, hypoglycemia, heat intolerance, hypoxia. May be the presenting manifestation of heat stroke.**

      b. Comment: Should not present any problems in diagnosis. Treatment is based on identifying the cause. **Also, remember that headache simulating classic or complicated migraine has been reported with decompression sickness.**[26]

 K. **Headaches associated with substance use or withdrawal**

   1. **Diagnostic criteria**

      a. Headache is usually generalized in type and dull, but may be pulsating especially with caffeine withdrawal.

      b. Not associated with other neurological signs or symptoms unless drug is taken in toxic doses.

      c. **Birth control pills** can precipitate recurrent migraine attacks.

      d. Other substances that can cause headaches are.

         i. Stimulants, particularly amphetamines

        ii. Alcohol

       iii. Anabolic steroids

       iv. Chronic analgesic abuse

        v. Nitrates or nitrites

       vi. Monosodium glutamate.

      e. The most common substances that cause **withdrawal headaches** are **caffeine** (remember caffeine is a constituent in many over-the-counter as well as prescribed analgesics), **alcohol,** chronic use of **ergotamine preparations** for treatment of migraine, **hallucinogenic drugs,** and chronic use of **analgesics.**

      e. **Comment: Should be suspected when there is no obvious cause for recurrent nonexercise-induced headaches.** A careful drug history, particularly about the use of over-the-counter analgesics, is important. In some cases, a blood and urine drug screen may be indicated.

III. **Recurrent Non-exercise-induced Headaches in Athletes**

 A. The most common are:

   1. Muscle contraction headaches

   2. Migraine

 B. Refer to any standard neurological textbook or the classification of headaches by the Headache Committee of the International Headache Society for diagnostic criteria and therapy.[1]

 C. The team physician should perform a general physical and neurological examination.

 D. If there are other associated neurological symptoms or abnormalities found on the neurological examination, the athlete should have a neurological consultation. In some cases, a head CT scan or MRI should be obtained prior to the referral, particularly if a structural CNS lesion is suspected.

E. Treatment is dependent on establishing the cause.
  1. **The team physician should not prescribe medications that may interfere with physical or mental performance, particularly if the athlete's headaches are frequent and prophylactic treatment is indicated.** Examples of this are the use of beta-blockers or Elavil for the prevention of migraine headaches.

## REFERENCES

1. Classification and Diagnostic Criteria for Headache Disorders, Cranial Neuralgias and Facial Pain. Cephalagia 8:1–96, 1988.
2. Powell B: Weightlifter's cephalgia. Ann Emerg Med 11:449–451, 1982.
3. Fremaux R: Weightlifter's Cephalgia Treatment Questioned (Letter to the Editor). Ann Emerg Med 12:112, 1983.
4. Paulson GW: Weightlifter's headache. Headache 23:193–194, 1983.
5. Rooke ED: Benign exertional headaches. Med Clin North Am 52:801–808, 1968.
6. Massey EW: Effort headache in runners. Headache 22:99–100, 1982.
7. Miller RG: Transient focal cerebral ischemia after extreme exercise. Headache 17:196–197, 1977.
8. Seelinger DF, Coin GC, Carlow TJ: Effort headache with cerebral infarction. Headache 15:142–145, 1975.
9. Lambert RW, Burnet DL: Prevention of exercise-induced migraine by quantitative warm-up. Headache 25:317–319, 1985.
10. Paulson GW, Zipf RE, Beekman JF: Pheochromocytoma causing exercise-related headache and pulmonary edema. Ann Neurol 5:96–99, 1974.
11. Chester JF, Conlon CP: Case reports: Some cerebrovascular complications of exercise. Br J Sports Med 17:143–144, 1983.
12. Leibrock LG, Streib EW: Personal communication, 1986.
13. Downey R, Antunes JL, Michelsen WJ: Hemorrhage within brain tumors during jogging. Ann Neurol 7:496, 1980.
14. Kelly WF, Roussak J: Stroke while jogging. Br J Sports Med 14:229–230, 1980.
15. Phillips J, Horner B, Doorly T, Toland J: Cerebrovascular accident in a 14-year-old marathon runner. Br Med J 286:351–352, 1983.
16. Abdon NJ, Landin K, Johansson BW: Athlete's bradycardia as an embolizing disorder? Symptomatic arrhythmias in patients aged less than 50 years. Br Heart J 52:660 666, 1984.
17. Fields WS: Nonpenetrating trauma of the cervical arteries. In Bennett DR (ed): Sports Medicine. Sem Neurol 1:284–290, 1981.
18. Katirji MB, Reinmuth OM, Latchow RE: Stroke due to vertebral artery injury. Arch Neurol 42:242–248, 1985.
19. Sherman DG, Hart RG, Easton JD: Abrupt change in head position and cerebral infarction. Stroke 12:2–6, 1981.
20. Tramo MJ, Hainline B, Petito F, et al: Vertebral artery injury and cerebellar stroke while swimming. Case report. Stroke 16:1039–1042, 1985.
21. Bjurstedt G, Rosenhamer G, Balldin G, Katkov V: Orthostatic reactions during recovery from exhaustive exercise of short duration. Acta Physiol Scand 119:25–31, 1983.
22. Bennett DR, Fuenning SI, Sullivan G, Weber J: Migraine precipitated by head trauma in athletes. Am J Sports Med 8:202–205, 1980.
23. Pestronk A: Pestronk S: Goggle migraine (Letter to the Editor). N Engl J Med 226:227, 1983.
24. Jacobson RI: More "goggle headache": Supraorbital neuralgia (Letter to the Editor). N Engl J Med 308:1363, 1983.
25. Kaufman A, Kaufman RS: Use of the MORA to reduce headaches on members of the U.S. Olympic Luge Team. Basal Facts 5:129–133, 1983.
26. Anderson B Jr, Heyman A, Wahlen RE, Saltzman HA: Migraine-like phenomena after decompression from hyperbaric environment. Neurology 15:1035–1040, 1965.

# Chapter 27: The Athlete's Heart

JERRY W. HIZON, MD
WM MacMILLAN RODNEY, MD

## I. Introduction

Athletes can have cardiac changes secondary to chronic exercise.[1] When evaluating an athlete, these changes must be considered, as well as certain diseases that may predispose the athlete for sudden death (Tables 1 and 2). A careful assessment of an athlete at risk for sudden death may prevent this tragedy.

## II. Review of Cardiac Conditioning and Efficiency

**The heart's response to exercise depends on the type of stress that is applied. The stress can be either a volume load, a pressure load, or a combination.**

A. **Increase volume load**
   1. **In exercise that increases the volume load, the heart compensates with an increase in the ventricular cavity (left ventricular end diastolic volume [LVEDV]), whereas the wall thickness remains at normal diameter.**
   2. **Typical exercises that produce an increased volume load to the heart are isotonic, aerobic exercises** such as running, swimming, bicycling, and cross-country skiing.

B. **Increase pressure load**
   1. **When an increased pressure load is applied to the heart, there is an increase in the ventricular wall thickness without any significant changes to LVEDV.**
   2. **These "static athletes"** (weight lifters and shot putters, for example) **must maintain elevated cardiac outputs for a briefer period of time under greatly elevated vascular resistance.**
   3. **Law of Laplace:** This adaptation of increased wall thickness to compensate for increase pressure load satisfies the Law of Laplace:
$$\text{Wall stress} = \frac{\text{Intraventricular pressure}}{\text{Wall thickness} \times 2}$$

C. **Combination load**
   1. **Practically speaking, most static althletes also engage in dynamic training and, conversely, many dynamic athletes do some static training.** Hence the clinician often sees a spectrum of changes rather than a strict dichotomy.
   2. Furthermore, many intermittent exercisers (so-called "weekend warriors") may be engaging in regular exercise to comply with prescribed aerobic conditioning, a minimum of 3–4 hours per week. They may also demonstrate cardiac compensations consistent with the athletic heart syndrome.
   3. The prevalence of athletic heart syndrome among an average family practice of 1400–1500 patients is low.

## III. History

A. **Exercise history**
   1. Initially it is helpful to note the type, length, and intensity of the athlete's workout or training regimen. Specifically ask if there have been any reasons that the athlete has had to interrupt or stop an exercise program.

**TABLE 1.** Cardiac Conditions Contraindicating Participation in Competitive Athletics*

1. Obstructive hypertrophic cardiomyopathy.
2. Congenital coronary artery abnormalities.
3. Cystic medical necrosis of the aorta (Marfan's syndrome).
4. Pulmonic stenosis with RV pressure greater than 75 mm of mercury.
5. Aortic stenosis with a gradient greater than 40 mm of mercury across the valve.

* Reprinted with permission from Hara JH, Puffer JC: The preparticipation physical examination. In Mellion MB (ed): Office Management of Sports Injuries & Athletic Problems. Philadelphia, Hanley & Belfus, 1988.

B. **Problems with exertion**
   1. Discuss with the athlete any problems with exercising or exertion. Especially ask if he or she has ever had syncope, arrhythmias, or dyspnea on exertion. Has the athlete ever been told not to exercise previously been refused medical clearance to participate in athletics? Does the athlete have any reservation about exercising to maximal level for fear of some adverse health consequence?
C. **Family history**
   1. Any known family history of sudden death while exercising, or early coronary heart disease (CAD). Early CAD is defined as an MI, angina, CAD requiring coronary artery bypass grafting (CAB) or percutaneous transluminal coronary angioplasty (PTCA) prior to age 50 years old.
D. **General medical history**
   1. Also noteworthy is any history in the athlete of general medical conditions that may increase the risk of sudden death such as hyperlipidemia, diabetes mellitus, smoking or recreational drug use, especially cocaine, amphetamines, or anabolic steroids.
   2. Note that **sickle-cell trait** has recently been described as a risk factor for sudden death in physical training.[2] A study of a large series from the U.S. Armed Forces examined sudden deaths among enlisted recruits. At this stage, this is an interesting observation that requires further study. Nevertheless, athletes with sickle-cell trait should not be excluded from physical training at this time. The absolute risks were 3 cases per 10,000 for recruits with hemoglobin AS as compared to approximately 1 death per 10,000 among recruits without hemoglobin AS. The review of systems should concentrate on cardiovascular, pulmonary, and neurologic systems.

IV. **The Cardiovascular Examination**

The cardiac examination is frequently normal in athletes. In the dynamic athlete, a large pulse amplitude and a diffuse left ventricular precordial impulse may be noted.
   A. The **heart rate commonly will be bradycardic** (less than 60 beats per minute [bpm]), and rates as low as 25 bpm have been noted in certain highly trained athletes.

**TABLE 2.** Cardiac Conditions That Would Not Specifically Contraindicate Participation*

1. Mitral valve prolapse in absence of significant ventricular arrhythmias or severe mitral regurgitation.
2. Small shunts associated with atrial septal defect (ASD), ventricular septal defect (VSD), or patent ductus arteriosus (PDA).
3. Wolff-Parkinson-White syndrome (WPW) in absence of documented atrial fibrillation with rapid ventricular response.
4. Primary ventricular arrhythmias in the absence of underlying coronary, myocardial, or valvular disease.

* Reprinted with permission from Huston TP, Rodney WM: Clinical Features of the Athletic Heart Syndrome. In Mellion MB (ed): Office Management of Sports Injuries & Athletic Problems. Philadelphia, Hanley & Belfus, 1988.

B. **Blood pressures** in athletes may be low compared with nonathletes. **It is not uncommon for diastolic blood pressures to be zero in well-conditioned athletes.** Utilization of Phase 4 Korotkoff sounds as the diastolic end-point eliminates many of these pseudo-low diastolic readings. Borderline hypertension that is exacerbated with exercise probably demonstrates labile hypertension.

C. **Auscultation**

1. **Ventricular gallops and soft systolic murmurs are commonly heard.** There is high interobserver variability in studies on auscultation of well-trained athletes, and this corresponds to the subjective nature of this aspect of the cardiac exam. Midsystolic murmurs have been noted in 30–50% of dynamic athletes. Generally, these murmurs are graded I or II/VI.

2. **Cardiac murmurs that are III/VI or greater in intensity should be referred for echocardiograms.**

3. Also, murmurs that become louder with Valsalva maneuvers should also be investigated.

4. Similarly, third and fourth heart sounds are common.[3] Third heart sounds are more common than fourth, but even fourth heart sounds have been detected in a range of 20–60%.

5. A midsystolic click consistent with **mitral valve prolapse** is common, especially in female athletes.

D. On **palpation** of the precordium, cardiomegaly may be noted but usually does not simulate cardiac illness.

E. The **chest x-ray** occasionally shows modest cardiomegaly (cardiothoracic ratio of 0.5 or greater) with or without a globular appearance. Pulmonary venous engorgement may even accompany some of these cases.

F. Unusual **body habitus** may predispose an athlete to sudden death.

1. Tall, thin-appearing athletes might have Marfan's syndrome (cystic medial necrosis of the aorta) (Table 3).

2. Obesity has been documented to be an independent risk factor for sudden death and other cardiovascular mortality.[4] Those who are more than 20% over ideal body weight may indeed benefit from additional investigations such as electrocardiograms.

V. **Electrocardiogram**

A. **Alterations in repolarization are a prominent manifestation of the training effect.** ST-segment and T-wave changes are seen most frequently, but not exclusively, in dynamic athletes. There are four primary patterns of altered repolarization.

**TABLE 3.**   Suggested Screening Format for Marfan's Syndrome*

Screen all men over 6 feet and all women over 5 feet 10 inches in height with electrocardiogram and slit lamp examination when any two of the following are found:

1. Family history of Marfan's syndrome[†]
2. Cardiac murmur or midsystolic click.
3. Kyphoscoliosis.
4. Anterior thoracic deformity.
5. Arm span greater than height.
6. Upper-to-lower body ratio more than one standard deviation below the mean.
7. Myopia.
8. Ectopic lens.

* Reprinted with permission from Hara JH, Puffer JC: The preparticipation physical examination. In Mellion MB (ed): Office Management of Sports Injuries & Athletic Problems. Philadelphia, Hanley & Belfus, 1988.
† This finding alone should prompt further investigation.

1. ST-segment elevation with peaked T-waves.
2. ST-segment depression with depressed J points.
3. "Juvenile" T-wave pattern (right precordial J-point elevation with inverted T-waves).
4. T-wave inversion in the lateral precordium.

B. ST-segment elevation
   1. *The frequency of ST-segment elevation varies, but in general the more highly trained the athlete is, the more likely one will find it.* Elevation of the ST-segment has been shown to develop and increase in direct relation to training intensity. As with the rhythm changes, **it normalizes with exertion** and is thought to be due to a change of autonomic input to the heart.[5]

C. T-wave
   1. The T-wave changes one sees consist of tall and peaked waves (usually associated with J-point elevation) or of T-wave inversions. Both of these occur in limb and/or precordial leads. These T-wave inversions have been associated with normal arteriograms. An increase in left ventricular mass has been noted when athletes with T-wave inversions are compared to athletes without the inversions. Similar to peaked T-waves, inverted T-waves appear as a direct effect of training, and they readily normalize with sympathetic maneuvers. These observations support a probable vagotonic etiology and, therefore, a benign prognosis. A third and less common T-wave change is a biphasic T-wave with terminal negativity in leads V3 to V6.[6]

D. Voltage
   1. **Conditioned athletes can have large voltages, which are a manifestation of the physiologic enlargement that occurs with conditioning.** Increased P-wave amplitude, as well as evidence of right ventricular hypertrophy (RVH) and left ventricular hypertrophy (LVH), are found. The prevalence of LVH has reached up to 85% in various surveys. RVH is slightly less frequent. Ventricular hypertrophy of either chamber occurs less frequently in static athletes when compared to dynamically conditioned athletes. The amplitude of the voltages has been observed to increase as training progresses. A 25% increase in voltage amplitude was observed during the 11 weeks of training in one prospective study.[7] Table 4 summarizes the ECG changes found in athletes.

VI. **Rhythm Disturbances Seem to be Limited to Dynamic Athletes** (Table 5)

   A. The most common abnormality is **sinus bradycardia,** with the prevalence frequently exceeding 50% in several large studies.[8–11] **The degree of bradycardia correlates with**

**TABLE 4.** ECG Changes in the Athletic Heart Syndrome

Voltages seen in AHS:
    Increased P-wave amplitude
    LVH (85% in various surveys)
    RVH (less frequent than LVH).

Repolarization:
    ST-segment elevation with peaked T-waves
    ST-segment depression with depressed J-points
    "Juvenile" T-wave pattern (right precordial J-point elevation with inverted T-waves)
    T-wave inversion in the lateral precordium.

T-waves:
    Tall, peaked T-waves with elevated J-points
    T-wave inversion
    Biphasic T-wave with terminal negativity in leads V3 to V6.

**TABLE 5.**  Frequencies of Rhythm Disturbances on Resting Electrocardiograms
of the General Population and Athletes*

| Arrhythmia | General Population (%) | Athletes (%) |
| --- | --- | --- |
| Sinus bradycardia | 23.7 | 50–85 |
| Sinus arrhythmia | 2.4–20 | 13.5–69 |
| Wandering atrial pacemaker | — | 7.4–19 |
| First degree block | 0.65 | 6–33 |
| Mobitz I | 0.003 | 0.125–10 |
| Mobitz II | 0.003 | Not reported |
| Third degree block | 0.0002 | 0.017 |
| Nodal rhythm | 0.06 | 0.031–7.0 |
| Ventricular pre-excitation | 0.1–0.15 | 0.15–2.5 |
| Atrial fibrillation | 0.004 | 0–0.63 |

* Reproduced with permission from Huston TP, Puffer JC, Rodney WM: The athletic heart syndrome. N Engl J Med 313:24–32, 1985.

the intensity of the training. There is ongoing discussion over the reason for the bradycardia. Some studies indicate the excess vagal predominance ("vagotonia") is responsible, whereas others claim that there may be an intrinsic cardiac adaptation. ("Vagotonia" could represent either an increase in vagal tone or a decrease in sympathetic tone.)

B. **Sinus dysrhythmias** are commonly seen in athletes, ranging from 13.5 to 69% in dynamic athletes.[9,11] Atrial and ventricular tachycardias have been known to occur in otherwise healthy athletes, but not in controlled trials. Hence, it is questionable if these tachycardias are a result of training (i.e., part of the athletic heart syndrome).

C. **Atrioventricular blocks** are the third most common rhythm abnormalities seen. Given the vagal influence on AV node conduction, this is not surprising. A prolonged conduction time has been observed in controlled studies and also has been shown to develop *de novo* as athletes embark on training programs. Cessation of training results in disappearance of the AV block.

1. Most common is the **first degree block,** detected in 10–37% resting and ambulatory ECGs.

2. **Second degree block (Mobitz I)** is clearly related to training.[12] Long-term follow-up of these cases reveals no association with evolving cardiac disease.

3. **Mobitz Type II and third degree heart block** are seen less frequently. Again, these AV blocks seem to disappear with cessation of training.

4. **Junctional rhythms** might also be anticipated from the theory of excess vagal tone. Several studies have revealed a prevalence of 7–20% seen in athletes versus nonathletes.[12]

5 **Many other disturbances** of rhythm and conduction may occur. Examples include anecdotal reports of bundle branch block, pre-excitation, atrial fibrillation, paroxysmal supraventricular tachycardia, ventricular tachycardia, and ventricular fibrillation.[13] **We emphasize the need for immediate discontinuation of athletic activity if any of these conditions is observed.** Without controlled or prospective studies, they cannot be considered a result of training. Furthermore, the common thread that links documented athletic heart disturbances is a relative increase in vagal tone. This mechanism could not account for these additional abnormalities.

6. Isolated **premature ventricular contraction** and/or contractions are seen in athletes.

a. **Certainly higher grade forms of ventricular rhythm abnormalities (such as multiformed premature ventricular contractions (PVCs), ventricular** tachycardia, etc.) **require workup.** Furthermore, there are data to suggest that otherwise healthy, asymptomatic young adults probably do have a normal range of unifocal PVCs. Some use 100 PVCs in a 24-hour period as the upper limit of normal for athletes.[13]

b. Athletes who present to the physician or trainer with an ECG demonstrating an isolated PVC should be carefully screened for cardiac abnormalities. **If all of the risk factors are negative, exercise testing may be the most helpful single test to demonstrate the effect of exercise on ventricular ectopy.** If other risk factors exist, echocardiography, Holter monitoring, and/or cardiac consultation may be considered.

VI. **Morphologic Adaptations**

Conditioned dynamic athletes frequently have morphologic changes in their hearts that are needed for maximum efficiency. There is debate whether static isometric exercise will also cause these changes, but clearly these adaptations in both types of athletes are usually not pathologic. As summarized in Table 6, there are several changes found typically in conditioned athletes; some closely simulate pathologic states such as dilated or hypertrophic cardiomyopathy. However, in these cases the probability of cardiac disease is extremely low, and further invasive testing usually is not indicated. Echocardiograms are not routinely ordered for the asymptomatic athlete.

A. **Left ventricular end diastolic diameter (LVEDD)** is usually increased and can be observed to change as training progresses, an average of 9.8% with training (Table 7).[14]

   1. This compensation is the response to the volume overload as stated previously in the Law of LaPlace.
   2. Since the systolic diameter does not change, **the stroke volume will increase.** And, since cardiac output is the product of the heart rate and stroke volume, the athlete's heart substantially increases achievable cardiac output. This is how the athlete's heart contributes to the entire sequence of physiologic adaptation, culminating in an increase in maximal myocardial oxygen uptake ($VO_2max$) and, ultimately, athletic performance.

**TABLE 6.**  Echocardiographic Changes in Isotonic and Isometric Athletes*

| Measurement | Isotonic | Isometric |
|---|---|---|
| Left ventricular end-diastolic diameter | ↑ | ↑, no Δ |
| Left ventricular end-diastolic diameter per square meter or per kilogram | ↑ | no Δ |
| Left ventricular end-systolic diameter | ↑, ↓, no Δ | ↑, ↓, no Δ |
| Left ventricular end-diastolic volume | ↑ | no Δ |
| Left ventricular posterior-wall thickness | ↑ | ↑ |
| Left ventricular mass | ↑ | ↑ |
| Left ventricular mass per square meter or per kilogram | ↑ | no Δ |
| Interventricular septal thickness | ↑ | ↑ |
| Interventricular-septum/posterior-wall ratio | ↑, no Δ | ↑, no Δ |
| Right ventricular diameter | ↑ | — |
| Left atrial diameter | ↑ | — |
| Ejection fraction | no Δ | no Δ |
| Cardiac output (resting) | no Δ | no Δ |
| Stroke volume | ↑ | ↑, no Δ |
| Velocity of circumferential fiber shortening | ↑, ↓, no Δ | no Δ |

* Reproduced with permission from Huston TP, Puffer JC, Rodney WM: The athletic heart syndrome. N Engl J Med 313:24–32, 1985.
↑ denotes increase, ↓ denotes decrease, and no Δ = no change.

**TABLE 7.**   Ventricular Dimensions in Athletes and Nonathletes as Assessed by Echocardiography in Published Studies*

| Echocardiographic Variable | Nonathlete Controls | | Athletes | | Percent Difference (%) |
|---|---|---|---|---|---|
| | Mean Value | Number of Subjects | Mean Value | Number of Subjects | |
| Ventricular septal thickness (mm) | 9.1 | 313 | 10.4 | 461 | +14.3 |
| Posterior free wall thickness (mm) | 9.0 | 439 | 10.7 | 740 | +18.9 |
| LV end-diastolic diameter | 49.1 | 394 | 53.9 | 701 | + 9.8 |
| Estimated LV mass (g) | 175 | 252 | 256 | 381 | +46.3 |
| RV internal transverse diameter (mm) | 17.7 | 146 | 22.0 | 147 | +24.3 |

* Reprinted with permission from the American College of Cardiology. Maron BJ: Structural features of the athletic heart as defined by echocardiography. J Am Coll Cardiol 7:190–203, 1986.

   B. **Right ventricular end diastolic diameter (RVEDD)** is generally increased in dynamic athletes.[15-17] The reason for this is generally thought to be the same as with the increased LVEDD.
   C. **Left atrial enlargement** of a mild degree occurred in over half of all studies surveyed. In conditioned athletes, the right atrial transverse axis has been increased by up to 22% when compared to nonathletes.
   D. **The left ventricular free wall and the septum undergo hypertrophy in response to both static and dynamic exercise.** An average wall thickness increase of 14% in static athletes, 19% in dynamic athletes.[18] Usually this is within normal limits but a thickness of up to 15 mm occasionally has been reported.[9] This is also noted in childhood athletes.[19] The ventricular septum hypertrophies with a documented thickness of up to 16 mm. This again is to compensate for the increased chamber diameter by reducing the wall strain. These changes, however, revert with deconditioning in as little as 4 days.

VII. **Exercise Testing in Athletes**

   Treadmill or bicycle ergometry exercise testing is helpful to determine how an athlete responds to the stress of dynamic exercise. If there are no contraindications, athletes may undergo a symptom-limited maximal exercise test. The desirability of universal exercise ECG screening will vary from one community to another.[20] The problems regarding exercise testing research have recently been reviewed.
   A. When indicated and if there are no contraindications, athletes should undergo symptom-limited maximal exercise tests. Since there is a wide scatter around age-predicted maximal heart rates, subjects should be allowed to exercise to a maximal perceived exertion as outlined by the Borg scale (i.e., exercising to a 20 on a scale of 6 to 20).
   B. Many of the rhythm and wave changes seen in dynamic athletes at rest resolve during exercise.
   C. Conditioned athletes have a work capacity much higher than nonathletes. Maximal $VO_2$'s near 70 ml $O_2$/kg/min can commonly be attained.
   D. **If athletes can exercise to maximal effort without difficulty, then the clinician can conclude that abnormal ECG changes are likely to represent the athletic heart syndrome. This is helpful to clear certain athletes for maximal training.**
   E. Routine screening for coronary artery disease in asymptomatic athletes is not recommended, since there is a high rate of false positives, especially in women. These false positive results would incorrectly label athletes as having CAD when they do not.

VIII. **Mitral Valve Prolapse**

    A. **General:** There has been much discussion regarding the etiology and significance of mitral valve prolapse syndrome (MVPS). It occurs in approximately 6–10% of healthy females. It has many names (mitral click syndrome, Barlow's syndrome, click murmur syndrome, etc.). It is thought to be secondary to a redundancy in either the mitral valve, the valvular ring, or the chordae tendineae, causing the valve to "balloon or parachute" back into the left ventricle. This causes a click and/or murmur. Some experts feel that the heart findings are only part of a larger constellation of signs and symptoms which also involves the autonomic nervous system.

    B. **Physical exam:** A midsystolic click is heard best with the bell applied lightly to the left side of the chest wall, approximately midclavicular near the level of the fourth intercostal space. The true syndrome has, besides the midsystolic click, a late systolic murmur. In advanced stages, a true mitral regurgitation murmur is auscultated. The click will move closer to S1 when standing, and farther away with squatting.

    C. **ECG:** MVPS often produces nonspecific ST-segment and T-wave abnormality in various leads. The T-wave can often be inverted in leads II, III, and VF, and the finding may resemble diaphragmatic myocardial infarction. There are various cardiac rhythms associated with MVPS, especially frequent PVCs and atrial tachyarrhythmias. In severe cases, complete AV block and ventricular fibrillation is possible. The risk of sudden death has been estimated to occur in about 1.2% of these severely affected patients, but we feel this is extremely rare in primary care settings. Therefore, asymptomatic MVP is not a contraindication for athletic participation.

    D. **Echocardiography:** MVP can be readily demonstrated with two-dimensional echocardiography, with the mitral leaflets moving retrograde in systole. A cardiac echo is very sensitive, but false positives can occur in normal individuals.

    E. **MVP in athletes:** A midsystolic click or murmur is frequently heard during preparticipation examinations. It occurs more in women and especially in athletes with Marfan's syndrome.

        1. If an athlete has no other cardiac risk factors or symptoms other than the click and/or murmur, most authorities agree that no more needs to be done, except to note it on the exam form for future reference. Athletes do not usually benefit from beta blockers (Inderal, etc.) and can have problems with exercise if placed on beta blockade inappropriately. They usually do not require prophylactic antibiotics prior to dental procedures as once thought.

        2. If an athlete has other cardiac risk factors or symptoms (palpatations, atypical chest pain, or exercise limitations, for example), then a cardiac echo should be performed to evaluate the mitral valve. A maximal treadmill exercise test is helpful to evaluate the athlete and determine if the athlete can participate safely. Another alternative is Holter monitoring to rule out arrhythmias. If the patient has Marfan's syndrome, he should not participate in athletics. To decrease the risk of sudden death during athletics, the patient should be referred for complete cardiac workup.

IX. **Sudden Death in Athletes**

**The ability to engage in athletics does not necessarily protect against sudden death.** Sudden death in athletes is occasionally attributable to cardiomyopathy and/or coronary artery disease. In studies by Maron, **97% of young athletes who died unexpectedly while exercising had structural cardiovascular abnormalities.**[21]

    A. **Hypertrophic cardiomyopathy** was the most common reason, with **anomalous origin of the coronary arteries** also being a predisposing factor.

B. **Atherosclerotic coronary heart** disease was relatively uncommon. In one study of 83 nontraumatic prehospital sudden deaths, 50% were cardiac in origin, with coronary artery disease, rheumatic-valvular disease, and cardiomyopathies the most common.[22]

C. **Marfan's syndrome**, as seen in Olympic athlete Flo Hymen, is a syndrome that should be considered if the athlete has a suggestive habitus.

D. The rhythm disturbance that causes sudden death in athletes is usually thought to be **ventricular fibrillation.**[23]

E. The **drug-related sudden deaths** in athletes are thought to be secondary to ventricular fibrillation induced by sympathomimetics, i.e., cocaine and methamphetamines.

F. **Mitral valve prolapse** in absence of significant ventricular arrhythmias or severe regurgitation is not considered a specific predisposition.

G. Recently an intussusception of a coronary artery served to remind us of our current inability to screen for every potentially lethal condition.[24]

## X. Management Summary

In treating athletes, you will encounter the normal cardiac variance produced by conditioning and training. You must interpret signs and symptoms within the context of dynamic and static athletics. The athlete may have physical, electrocardiographic, and echocardiographic findings that would be considered abnormal in an untrained individual. Simultaneously, the experienced clinician is aware of the fact that disease can occur even in healthy and exceedingly fit individuals. For the asymptomatic athlete with routine physical findings and an ECG typical of the athletic heart, vigorous reassurance is strongly recommended. In some cases, an exercise treadmill test may be helpful in emphasizing and underlining normalcy. The clinician should, however, be wary of the poor predictive value of a positive result (i.e., false-positive effect).

If the athlete is symptomatic, further investigation may be useful. The first level of this investigation should be an attempt to witness the symptoms. Most frequently, this can be done on an exercise treadmill test. Nevertheless, there are many symptoms that merely require a more thorough history and physical examination. The finding of chest-wall pain or costochondritis does not merit an expensive treadmill investigation.

In summary, the American medical profession is in an extremely cautious posture regarding the underdiagnosis of disease. Nevertheless, when confronted with the physical and electrocardiographic findings previously described, we should re-emphasize the high probability of health. It is recommended to state categorically that the athlete is absolutely "super normal" unless one has convincing evidence of possible organic heart disease.[25] The athletic heart syndrome should be kept in mind when evaluating highly trained athletes. This will appropriately stratify those that need further investigation, while preventing cardiac neurosis and/or financial morbidity when this strategy is not followed. Abnormalities detected in the absence of well-developed conditioning effect are less likely to be benign.

## REFERENCES

1. Blake JB, Laarraba RC: Observations upon long distance runners. Boston Med Surg J 148:95, 1903.
2. Kark JA, Posey DM, Schumacher HR, Ruehle CJ: Sickle-cell trait as a risk factor for sudden death in physical training. N Engl J Med 317:781–787, 1987.
3. Lembo NJ, Dell'Italia LJ, Crawford MH, O'Rourke RA: Bedside diagnosis of systolic murmurs. N Engl J Med 1572–1578, 1988.
4. Messerli FH: Overweight and sudden death: Increased ventricular ectopy in cardiopathy of obesity. Arch Int Med 147:1725–1728, 1987.

5. Zeppilli P, Pirrami MM, Sassara M, Fenici R: Ventricular repolarization disturbances in athletes: Standardization of terminology, ethiopathogentic spectrum and pathophysiological mechanism. J Sports Med Phys Fitness 21:322–335, 1981.

6. Fenici R, Caselli G, Zeppilli P, Piovano G: High degree A-V block in 17 well-trained endurance athletes. In Lubich T, Venerando A (eds): Sports Cardiology. Bologna Aulo Gaggi, 1980, pp 523–537.

7. DeMaria AN, Neumann A, Lee G, Fowler W, Mason DT: Alternations in ventricular mass and performance induced by exercise training in man evaluated by echocardiography. Circulation 57:2370–2374, 1978.

8. Parker BM, Londeree BR, Cupp GV, Dubiel JP: The noninvasive cardiac evaluation of long-distance runners. Chest 73:376–381, 1978.

9. Cohen JL, Gupta PK, Lichstein E, Chadda KD: The heart of a dancer: Noninvasive cardiac evaluation of professional ballet dancers. Am J Cardiol 45:959–965.

10. Paulsen W, Boughner D, Ko P, et al: Left ventricular function in marathon runner: Echocardiographic assessment. J Appl Physiol 51:881–886, 1981.

11. Minamitani K, Miyagawa M, Konco M, Kiamura K: The electrocardiogram of professional cyclists. In Lubich T, Venerando A (eds): Sports Cardiology. Bologna, Aulo Gaggi, 1980, pp 315–325.

12. Zeppilli P, Fenici R, Sassara M, et al: Wenckebach second-degree A-V block in top-ranking athletes: An old problem revisited. Am Heart J 100:281–294, 1980.

13. Grauer K, Gums J: Ventricular arrhythmias, Part I. Prevalence, significance, and indications for treatment. JABFP 1:135–142, 1988.

14. Maron BJ: Structural features of the athlete heart as defined by echocardiography. J Am Coll Cardiol 7:190–203, 1986.

15. Zeppitti S, Sandric S, Cecchetti F, et al: Echocardiographic assessments of cardiac arrangements in different sports activities. In Lubich T, Venerando A (eds): Sports Cardiology. Bologna, Aulo Gaggi, 1980, pp 723–724.

16. Roeske WR, O'Rourke RA, Klein A, et al: Noninvasive evaluation of ventricular hypertrophy in professional athletes. Circulation 53:286–292, 1976.

17. Hauser AM, Dressendorfer RH, Von M, et al: Symmetric cardiac enlargement in highly trained endurance athletes: A two dimensional echocardiographic study. Am Heart J 109:1038–1044, 1985.

18. Snoechke LHEH, Abelling HFM, Lambregts JAC, Schmitz JJF, Reneman RS: Echocardiographic dimensions in athletes in relation to their training programs. Med Sci Sports Exerc 14:428–434, 1982.

19. Cahill NS, O'Brien M, Rodahl A, et al. A pilot study on left ventricular dimensions and wall stress before and after submaximal exercise. Br J Sports Med 13:122–129, 1979.

20. Detrano R, Lyons KP, Marcondes G, Abbass N, Froelicher VF, Jones A: Methodologic problems in exercise testing research: Are we solving them? Arch Int Med 148:1289–1295, 1988.

21. Maron BJ, Roberts WC, McAllister HA, Rosing DR, Epstein SE: Sudden death in young athletes. Circulation 62:218–229, 1980.

22. Raymond JR, Von den Berg EK, Knapp MJ: Nontraumatic prehospital sudden death in young adults. Arch Int Med 148:303–308, 1988.

23. Nirod P, Polikar R, Peterson KL: Hypertrophic cardiomyopathy and sudden death. N Engl J Med 318:1255–1257, 1988.

24. Rogers CC: Strong statements on kids and sports. Phys Sports Med 13(8):32, 1985.

25. Huston TP, Puffer JC, Rodney WM: The athletic heart syndrome. N Engl J Med 313:24–32, 1985.

# Chapter 28: Managing Skin Problems in Athletes

## LOREN H. AMUNDSON, MD

### I. Introduction

Physicians who manage skin problems in athletes must be aware of their effect upon participation and performance. Skin problems are common in athletes, and it is important that the sports-oriented physician possess skill in their diagnosis and treatment.

The physician should also be aware of the many environmental factors that affect the skin and, in addition, the damage that can be caused by inappropriate care. The importance of daily skin care should be stressed and should include fresh clean underclothing and socks, and clean clothing and equipment for practice and competition. Equipment may cause many sports-related skin problems due to trauma during athletic training and competition.[1] Suggested preventive techniques are often not adhered to by athletes.

To manage skin problems effectively for the athlete, it is necessary to understand principles of skin care, to be familiar with the pharmacology of topical and systemic agents, and to understand various physical modes of therapy, such as cryotherapy. Glucocorticoids represent the most commonly used topical agents, and it is incumbent upon the sports physician to understand fully the indications and complications of corticosteroid therapy, when used topically, intralesionally or parenterally.

### II. Injuries and Physical Factors

#### A. Heat

##### 1. Sunburn

###### a. History
   i. Usually obtaining the history not a problem.
   ii. Suntan lotions are often used to speed up tanning of the skin. Although these agents may produce an artificial tan for a few days, they offer no protection against sunburn, especially in swimmers.

###### b. Diagnosis
   i. Usually not a problem.
   ii. Onset of redness and blistering may be delayed several hours after sun exposure.

###### c. Treatment
   i. First and second degree sunburn respond well to analgesics and cool compresses.
   ii. Taken before[2] or started immediately after a significant sun exposure, and taken in high doses for 24 hours, aspirin may reduce the severity of the burn and provide adequate analgesia.[3]
   iii. Systemic steroids can be used to combat acute distress of more extensive burns.

###### d. Complications
   i. Sun exposure may lead to a herpes labialis flareup, necessitating 10–14 days for complete resolution.

**TABLE 1.** Topical Photosensitive/Photoallergic Substances*

| | |
|---|---|
| Acne medications<br>  vitamin A acid (Retin-A) | Plants (furocoumarins) |
| | Soap deodorants (photoallergic) |
| Coal tar derivatives | halogenated salicylanilides |
|   acridine | (tri- and tetrachlor-; brominated) |
|   anthracene | bithionol |
|   phenanthrene | hexachlorophene |
|   pyridine | dichlorophene |
| | carbanilides |
| Cosmetics | |
|   indelible lipsticks | Sunscreens |
|   perfumes and aftershave lotions | para-aminobenzoic acid (PABA) |
|     having essential oils | digalloyl trioleate (Sunstick) |

| Pigments and dyes | |
|---|---|
| yellow cadmium sulfide | eosin |
| proflavine, acriflavine | anthraquinone |

* Modified from Mellion MB (ed): Office Management of Sports Injuries & Athletic Problems. Philadelphia, Hanley & Belfus, 1988.

    ii. Photosensitive and photoallergic reactions (Tables 1 and 2).

    iii. "Sun poisoning" may occur if the exposure is severe, presenting with a toxic clinical picture and necessitating supportive care and IV fluids.

    iv. Long-term skin damage, leading to increased incidence of solar elastoses, actinic keratoses, and skin cancer.

  e. **Prevention**

    i. Reduce skin exposure, especially 10 am–2 pm.

    ii. Protective clothing, wide-brimmed hats, and the like.

    iii. Sun-blocking agents, such as zinc oxide.

    iv. Sunscreens with a sun protection factor (SPF) above 15 are very effective. These must be applied before exposure and reapplied every few

**TABLE 2.** Systemic Photosensitive/Photoallergic Substances*

| | |
|---|---|
| Anthistamines<br>  diphenhydramine (Benadryl) | Psoralens<br>  methoxypsoralens |
| Dyes | Sulfa drugs and analogues |
|   eosin | sulfonamides |
|   fluorescein | hypoglycemics |
|   trypaflavine | sulfonylurea (Dymelor) |
|   rose bengal | tolbutamide (Orinase) |
|   methylene blue | chlorpropamide (Diabinese) |
| | diuretics |
| | thiazides (HydroDIURIL) |
| Food additives | phenothiazines |
|   saccharin | chlorpromazine (Thorazine) |
|   cyclamates | promethazine (Phenergan) |
| | prochlorperazine (Compazine) |
| Miscellaneous | |
|   birth control agents | |
|   chlordiazepoxide HCl (Librium) | Other antibiotics |
|   furosemide (Lasix) | tetracycline |
| | doxycycline (Vibramycin) |
| | nalidixic acid (NegGram) |
| | griseofulvin |

* Modified from Mellion MB (ed): Office Management of Sports Injuries & Athletic Problems. Philadelphia, Hanley & Belfus, 1988.

hours after sweating and swimming. Oily sunscreens may produce folliculitis.

    v. Tanning booths (UV-A) are currently popular. The long range effects of UV-A are suspect for causing skin damage, and the use of tanning booths cannot be recommended.

### 2. Erythema ab igne
#### a. History
    i. Seen after prolonged use of local heat for treatment of persistently painful joints or muscles.
#### b. Diagnosis
    i. Characteristic localized hyperpigmentation and reticulated erythema.
#### c. Treatment
    i. Discontinue use of heat as a modality. The erythema and pigmentation usually disappear after several months.
    ii. Introduce other interventions.
#### d. Prevention
    i. The key.

## B. Cold
### 1. Hypothermia (see Chapter 12)
### 2. Erythema pernio
#### a. History
    i. Seen following exposure to cold, wet environment.
#### b. Diagnosis
    i. Lesions may occur 12–24 hours after injury, most common on lower extremities.
    ii. Edematous red to blue plaques are seen, which usually disappear in 1 to 2 weeks.
#### c. Treatment
    i. Usually not necessary.
#### d. Prevention
    i. Modify environmental exposure if frequent or recurrent.

### 3. Dry skin
#### a. History
    i. Occurs after prolonged cold exposure in winter sports, secondary to loss of hydration in the keratin layer.
#### b. Diagnosis
    i. Skin appears dry and roughened, may crack, chap, and lead to dermatitis.
    ii. Common names for dry skin include dry skin eczema, winter itch, asteatotic eczema, eczema craquelé.
#### c. Treatment
    i. Moisture (bathing) followed by lubricants and emollients (Table 3).
#### d. Prevention
    i. Improved general skin care.
    ii. Humidification of home environment.

## C. Friction and pressure
### 1. Abrasion
#### a. History
    i. Friction is the usual etiologic agent.
#### b. Diagnosis
    i. Usually not a problem.
    ii. Localized, denuded, oozing skin that is tender.

**TABLE 3.**  Lubricants and Emollients for Dry Skin*

| Ointments/Creams | Lotions |
|---|---|
| Lanolin-based | Cetaphil |
|   Aquaphor | Wondra |
|   Nivea | Aloe Vera |
|   Eucerin | Esoterica Dry Skin |
|   Keri | Eucerin |
| Petroleum based | Vaseline Intensive Care |
|   Lanolor | Wibi |
|   Keri Creme | Alpha Keri |
|   Lubriderm | Lachydrin |
|   Cold Cream USP | UltraMide |
|   Hydrophilic ointment USP | |
|   Vaseline Dermatology Formula | |

* Modified from Mellion MB (ed): Office Management of Sports Injuries & Athletic Problems. Philadelphia, Hanley & Belfus, 1988.

    iii. A variety of terms apply: turf burn, mat burn, cinder burn, road rash, raspberry, strawberry.

  c. **Treatment**

    i. May include cleansing with water or hydrogen peroxide followed by application of an antibiotic ointment and dry gauze dressing.

    ii. Films, foams, hydrocolloids, and hydrogels are available.

    iii. One effective treatment utilizes DuoDERM, a hydrophilic dressing applied after washing the wound with soap and water.[4] Once applied, there is little or no pain. It may need to be replaced during the healing process, which is usually complete within a week. Follow recommended directions for best results.

    iv. Other occlusive dressings include Tegaderm, Synthoderm, Vigilon, OP-Site and Bio-clusive. These are less effective in larger abrasions as they lose their adhesive quality when damp.

  d. **Prevention**

    i. Protection from trauma to susceptible areas when possible.

    ii. Early therapy reduces secondary infection.

2. **Blisters**

  a. **History**

    i. Usually occur in athletes wearing shoes.

    ii. May occur in other areas of friction.

    iii. More common if skin is moist.

    iv. Less common if skin is dry, greasy, or very wet.

  b. **Diagnosis**

    i. Usually not a problem.

  c. **Treatment**

    i. Aspiration and adhesive taping, using the epidermal layers of the blister as an occlusive dressing.

    ii. Removal of the blister with application of an adherent such as Tuf-Skin (causes initial discomfort) followed by a piece of moleskin large enough to cover the blister (plus overhang) and left in place until healing is complete.

    iii. Removal of the blister and application of DuoDERM as described earlier.

  d. **Prevention**

    i. Hardening the skin with 10% tannic acid soaks.

    ii. Proper footwear and padding with socks.

    iii. Application of Vaseline to skin or sites of friction in shoes.

        iv. Use of talc to reduce moisture.

        v. Use of adhesive tape or moleskin over potential or previous blister sites.

3. **Chafing**
  a. **History**
    i. Results from mechanical irritation, regardless of location.
    ii. Aggravated by sweating and protective equipment.
    iii. Frequent in runners and bikers.
  b. **Diagnosis**
    i. Superficial denudation of skin, even to the point of bleeding.
    ii. Axillae and groins bear the brunt of insult.
    iii. May affect nipples in runners and bikers.
  d. **Treatment**
    i. Air, cool compresses, heat lamps, mild steroid creams.
  d. **Prevention**
    i. Clean, loose clothing.
    ii. Talc or ZeaSORB to keep areas dry.
    iii. Lubricating creams such as Cramer's Skin Lube or Eucerin to reduce friction.
    iv. Sports bra may be necessary for runners and bikers.

4. **Calluses and corns**
  a. **History**
    i. Result from pressure (or less commonly friction) that the skin was not designed to sustain.
    ii. Most common on the feet.
    iii. May occur on hands of golfers and gymnasts, over ischial rami of bikers.
  b. **Diagnosis**
    i. Usually not a problem.
    ii. Corns may be misdiagnosed as warts (pearly eye of corn vs. multiple black dots, vessels of wart). Both may occur at pressure points.
  c. **Treatment**
    i. Intermittent paring and trimming.
    ii. Sanding with pumice stone.
    iii. Use of salicylic acid plasters.
    iv. The less surgical the eradication, the better.
  d. **Prevention**
    i. Modification of causative factors, such as footwear (including use of metatarsal bars), hand grips, and cycle seats.

D. **Hemorrhage**
  1. **Soft tissue**
    a. **History**
      i. Usually obtaining this history is not a problem.
    b. **Diagnosis**
      i. Subcutaneous ecchymoses occur frequently in tips of great and second toes, often seen in tennis and basketball players due to fast starts and stops. Also seen in long-distance runners.
      ii. Black heel ("talon noir") may be seen on the plantar surface of the heel, even in seasonal athletes.
    c. **Treatment**
      i. Usually not necessary.
    d. **Prevention**
      i. Thicker socks, moleskin, and emollient creams prior to practice and competition.

2. **Hematoma**
   a. **History**
      i. Usually not a problem to obtain a history.
   b. **Diagnosis**
      i. Blood blister, or contusion in more superficial tissues.
      ii. Thickening and tenderness when hematoma is located in muscles; usually seen in collision/contact sports.
   c. **Treatment**
      i. Evacuate blister and treat as a blister (described earlier).
      ii. Rest, ice, compression, and elevation (RICE therapy) indicated for more extensive hematomas.
      iii. More aggressive therapy (including physical therapy) may be indicated for muscle hematomas to prevent long-term disability and complications such as myositis ossificans.
   d. **Prevention**
      i. Adequate training, equipment, and on-site care.

3. **Nails**
   a. **History**
      i. Usually obtaining the history is not a problem.
   b. **Diagnosis**
      i. Onycholysis of nail.
      ii. Subungual hemorrhage.
   c. **Treatment**
      i. Supportive care for avulsed nail, using the nail as a dressing.
      ii. Evacuate hemorrhage with a hot wire or by twirling a needle or pointed scalpel to effect drainage.
   d. **Prevention**
      i. Usually not practical.

4. **Lacerations**
   a. **History**
      i. A variety of lacerations occur in the competitive athlete.
   b. **Diagnosis**
      i. Usually not difficult.
      ii. Assess for deeper tissue damage.
   c. **Treatment**
      i. Assurance of tetanus status.
      ii. Appropriate surgical wound care provides the best protection against infection while promoting early healing.

5. **Moisture**
   a. **History**
      i. Hyperhidrosis common in athletes
      ii. May affect manual dexterity and aggravate several pedal skin problems.
   b. **Diagnosis**
      i. Usually straightforward.
   c. **Treatment**
      i. Usually not necessary
      ii. Treat primary skin problem if present.
   d. **Prevention**
      i. Drysol (20% aluminum chloride in anhydrous ethyl alcohol) can be applied to completely dried palms and soles at bedtimes. Follow product directions closely.

**TABLE 4.**   Physical Urticarias*

| Inciting Factor | Suggested Therapy |
| --- | --- |
| Solar | Sunscreens |
| Cold | Cyproheptadine |
| Heat | $H_1$ antihistamines |
| | Cyproheptadine |
| Cholinergic | Cyproheptadine |
| | Hydroxyzine |
| Exertion, pressure | $H_1$ antihistamines |
| | $H_2$ antihistamines |
| | Hydroxyzine |

Combinations of medications (such as $H_1 + H_1$ or $H_1 + H_2$ antihistamines) sometimes indicated.

* Modified from Mellion MB (ed): Office Management of sports Injuries & Athletic Problems. Philadelphia, Hanley and Belfus, 1988.

6. **Urticarias**
   a. **History**
      i. Physical exertion, pressure, cold, heat, solar, aquagenic, and cholinergic factors may lead to exercise-related forms of urticaria.
      ii. Hives are most often caused by drugs or foods, but also occur as a result of diverse types of infection and by a variety of physical agents.
   b. **Diagnosis**
      i. Hives are the classical wheal or wheal-and-flare reactions that may occur anywhere on the body, are usually itchy, and frequently are surrounded by an erythematous halo while showing central clearing.
   c. **Treatment**
      i. Therapy includes a variety of medications as outlined in Table 4.
   d. **Prevention**
      i. Prevention is difficult, short of total avoidance of inciting factors.
7. **Bites and stings**
   a. **History**
      i. Unattended insect bites frequently lead to infection and must be monitored by athlete and those responsible for the athlete, especially in athletic environments combining sweat, dirt, and occlusion.
   b. **Diagnosis**
      i. Usually straightforward.
   c. **Treatment**
      i. For those athletes demonstrating systemic sensitivity to stinging insects (bees, wasps, and others), the physician must instruct the athlete as to risks and make injectable adrenalin available to those responsible for on-field evaluation and care.
      ii. Several self-contained "bee sting kits" are available commercially, and one belongs in the field athletic bag.
   d. **Prevention**
      i. For those athletes sensitive to a variety of insect bites, common mosquito repellents containing diethyltoluamide deter most would-be invaders.
E. **Other**
   1. **Ingrown nail**
      a. **History**
         i. Tight-fitting footwear.
         ii. Trimming toenails too deeply at corners.
         iii. Most commonly seen in tennis, basketball, and long-distance running.

b. **Diagnosis**
   i. Configuration of nail approaches a semicircle in cross-section.
   ii. Periungual inflammation, often with development of excessive granulation tissue (pyogenic granuloma).
   iii. Painful involvement of nail, affecting athletic performance.
c. **Treatment**
   i. Warm soaks and antibiotics to resolve inflammatory periungual tissue.
   ii. Removal of leading edge of ingrown nail (wedge to entire nail).
   iii. Pyogenic granuloma can be handled by application of silver nitrate, freezing with liquid nitrogen, shaving of the lesion with curettement of the base, snipping across the base with a scissors, or by tying off pedunculated lesion with suture material. Generous ooze of blood usually necessitates hemostasis.
d. **Prevention**
   i. Cut the great nail straight across without snipping off the protruding corners.
   ii. Proper footwear (size, width, and socks) and foot care (bathing, cleaning under nails).

2. **Dermatofibroma**
   a. **History**
      i. Results from microtrauma to the skin, along with the residuals of localized infections such as folliculitis.
      ii. Most seen where repeat shaving of hair and taping occur, commonly on the legs.
   b. **Diagnosis**
      i. Small, slightly elevated, firm papule, often brownish to purple in color.
      ii. Lesion "dimples" when pinched.
   c. **Treatment**
      i. Usually not necessary.
   d. **Prevention**
      i. Usually not possible.
      ii. Appropriate minor wound care may be preventive.

3. **Green hair**
   a. **History**
      i. Discoloration of hair, most often greenish in tint, due to copper deposition in hair matrix.
      ii. Seen most commonly in blonde swimmers.
   b. **Diagnosis**
      i. Awareness is key.
   c. **Treatment**
      i. Therapy with 3% peroxide bleach (2–3 hour session) is helpful.[2]
      ii. Local application of a commercial chelating agent (Metolex) is helpful.
   d. **Prevention**
      i. Shampooing after swimming usually prevents this problem.

III. **Contact Dermatitis**

A. **Allergic**
   1. **History**
      a. Exposure to offending agents, which include poison ivy, clothing dyes (blue and black), nickel-containing metals, all "caine" containing medicaments, and benzoin preparations (tincture of benzoin, Tuf-Skin).
      b. Other potent skin sensitizers include ethylenediamine and neomycin.

2. **Diagnosis**
   a. Common symptoms and findings include itching leading to scratching, reddening of the skin with the development of papules, even blisters when process is acute.
   ii. More chronic cases show thickening and lichenification.
3. **Treatment**
   a. Remove offending agent.
   b. Cool, wet compresses (water, Domeboro solutions).
   c. Antipruritic (non-"caine"-containing) lotions and creams, including topical steroids.
   d. Rarely, a short course of systemic steroids may be indicated.
4. **Prevention**
   a. Avoid offending agent when possible.
   b. Clear nail polish applied to metal may prevent nickel dermatitis.
   c. Daily skin care and clean equipment may reduce likelihood.

B. **Irritant**
1. **History**
   a. Usually due to physical and mechanical agents.
   b. Common irritants include adhesive tape, lime, dry ice, artificial turf, cold-pack chemicals (from a leak in "liquid ice"), a variety of clothing fibers, poorly fitting gear, rubber-containing straps and pads, leather gloves, shoes and chin straps, and a number of skin products.
2. **Diagnosis**
   a. See "Allergic dermatitis" (above).
   b. History and location of lesions usually diagnostic.
3. **Treatment**
   a. See "Allergic dermatitis" (above).
4. **Prevention**
   a. See "Allergic dermatitis" (above).

IV. **Infections**

A. **Bacterial**
1. **Pyodermas**
   a. **History**
      i. Sweat, dirt, and occlusion by equipment.
      ii. Break in skin.
      iii. Irritation from skin lubricants, elbow and forearm pads, whirlpool baths, and athletic tape.
      iv. Contact with infected athletes.
   b. **Diagnosis**
      i. Thin-walled vesicles, leading to yellowish crusts, typical of impetigo.
      ii. Infected hair follicles seen in furunculosis.
      iii. Papulovesiculopustular lesions in areas covered by swimwear, occasionally heralded by mild systemic symptoms typical of hot-tub folliculitis, caused by *Pseudomonas* organism.
      iv. Other *Pseudomonas* infections include "green" lesions of nails, periungual tissue, and interdigital webs.
   c. **Treatment**
      i. Temporary cessation of athletic activities by those infected often indicated for pyodermas.
      ii. Impetigo responds to warm wet compresses, 5–10% benzoyl peroxide solution, or topical antibacterial ointments such as Bacitracin. Oral

penicillin or erythromycin may be indicated Pustular impetigo caused by staphylococcus may warrant penicillinase-resistant penicillins or first-generation cephalosporins.

    iii. Furuncles may develop into boils and require stab-wound drainage. Widespread, recurrent, and resistant lesions indicate need for culture and antibiotics.

    iv. Hot-tub folliculitis course is benign and self-limited. Antibiotics not indicated.

    v. *Pseudomonas* infection of finger webs and nails respond to topical gentamicin (Garamycin).

2. **Keratolysis**
   a. **History**
      i. Usually seen on soles of tennis and basketball players, also runners.
      ii. Precipitated by hyperhidrosis, aggravated by occlusive footwear, caused by *Corynebacterium* species.
   b. **Diagnosis**
      i. 1 to 3 mm discrete craters on soles.
   c. **Treatment**
      i. 5% formalin soaks.
      ii. Oral erythromycin.
   d. **Prevention**
      i. Proper footwear and footcare.

3. **External otitis (swimmer's ear)**
   a. **History**
      i. Aquatic participants.
   b. **Diagnosis**
      i. Weepy, tender, external ear canals.
      ii. Most often bilateral involvement.
   c. **Treatment**
      i. Otic wick saturated with acetic acid (VoSol), antibacterial (Coly-Mycin S Otic), or corticosteroid (VoSol Otic) ear drops.
      ii. Promote measures that assure a more aerobic environment for the external ear, including removal of excess cerumen.
   d. **Prevention**
      i. Use of VoSol or Burow's solution (Domeboro) after swimming and showers, especially if recurrent.
      ii. Use of hair dryer after swimming and showers to dry external ear canals.

B. **Fungal**
   1. **History**
      a. Macerating effects of chronic perspiration reduce the natural barriers of the stratum corneum.
      b. Common locations for dermatophytoses include the feet ("athletes foot") and groin crease ("jock itch").
      c. *Candida* infections likely to occur in warm moist areas of skin, including the above.
      d. Tinea versicolor seen more commonly in swimmers and divers.
   2. **Diagnosis**
      a. All fungi can be diagnosed by proper KOH preparations of skin scrapings. Cultures occasionally indicated.
      b. All topical fungal infections share characteristics typical of papulosquamous skin disorders.

    c. Locations often diagnostic.

    d. Classic 1–2 mm satellite lesions, just beyond main area of dermatitis, typical of candidiasis.

    e. Tinea versicolor, usually limited to chest wall, usually fluoresces gold to orange under Wood's light.

    f. Clinical findings often altered by self-treatment, including OTC preparations.

3. **Treatment**

    a. Miconazole (Monistat-Derm) and clotrimazole (Lotrimin) effective for dermatophytoses and candidiasis.

    b. Oral griseofulvin occasionally indicated for dermatophytoses.

    c. 3% selenium sulfide shampoo (Selsun), applied and left on for 3–5 minutes after a shower, and repeated daily for 5 days, constitutes a satisfactory course of therapy for tinea vesicolor.

4. **Prevention**

    a. Shower daily and after practice and competition.

    b. Daily changes of socks and shorts.

    c. Absorbing foot powder, absorbent (leather) footwear.

    d. Daily cleansing of athletic, shower and dressing facilities.

C. **Viral**

1. **Warts**

    a. **History**

        i. Most common on hands and feet.

        ii. Low rate of infectivity.

        iii. Often recalcitrant to therapy, but are self-limited.

    b. **Diagnosis**

        i. Surfaces include crypts or invaginations, resembling a cauliflower sprig, which are irregular and rough.

        ii. Plantar warts look different due to the weight-bearing surface, but black dots representing thrombosed capillary tips diagnostic after paring off roof of lesion.

        iii. A greater confluence of plantar warts present as a mosaic.

    c. **Treatment**

        i. A variety of methods are available, including liquid nitrogen, carbon dioxide stick, intermittent application of strong acids, home therapy with weak acids (Duofilm), gentle electrodesiccation, and currettage under local anesthesia.[5]

        ii. Less common methods include 0.025% Retin A gel and 2–5% 5FU.[4]

        iii. Mosaic warts best treated with commercial 40% salicylic acid plaster, applying new plasters every few days following bathing and gentle rubbing, to remove remaining debris.

        iv. Do not use elliptical excision of warts.

        v. Strong acids, liquid nitrogen, and cautery should not be used during the athletic season.

        vi. For therapy of troublesome, painful plantar warts during the athletic season, weekly injection (1–3 weeks) of 1% Xylocaine into the base may shell out the wart.

2. **Molluscum contagiosum**

    a. **History**

        i. Skin trauma known to be a causative factor.

        ii. Hands and face are common locations, including upper body of boxers and wrestlers.

b. **Diagnosis**
  i. Small, translucent, umbilicated papules (2–4 mm) that may be single, grouped, or inoculated along a scratch (Koebner's lines) are characteristic.
c. **Treatment**
  i. A variety of therapies that extrude the molluscum body are successful, including a tiny stab of the papule with a pointed scalpel blade, spark from an electric needle, application of liquid nitrogen, or continued diligent application of dilute acid preparations (Duofilm).
d. **Prevention**
  i. Often difficult.
  ii. Transmission through contact sports can be prevented if athlete withhheld from practice and competition until cleared.

3. **Herpes simplex**
a. **History**
  i. May be recurrent, especially following sun exposure (face) or trauma (hands).
  ii. Most frequent locations are face and hands.
  iii. May affect mucosal surfaces.
  iv. May spread by contact.
b. **Diagnosis**
  i. Typical, grouped 1–2 mm vesiculobullous lesions on mildly inflammatory base are diagnostic.
  ii. An initial attack may be accompanied by pain, adenopathy, and fever.
  iii. Recurrent lesions may be heralded by pain, pruritus, or dysesthesia.
c. **Treatment**
  i. Therapies abound, including wet compresses, rubbing alcohol, ethyl ether, tincture of benzoin, or 4% zinc solution.
  ii. 5–10% benzoyl peroxide and other drying agents are also used in the acute blistering phase, followed by a variety of bland creams or ointments when the lesions begin crusting.
  iii. Acyclovir (Zovirax) is now available for topical, oral, and systemic use. Oral form may be indicated for athletes with recurrent herpes, especially those conditions producing an unusual degree of distress or requiring repeated time away from competition.
d. **Prevention**
  i. Withhold athlete from contact and competition while lesions are active.
  ii. Another effective preventive measure includes scrubbing of the wrestling mat after each practice and competition.

V. **Infestations**

A. **Pediculosis**
  1. **History**
    a. Head and pubic lice occur in athletes, most commonly the latter and under circumstances of inadequate hygiene and close physical contact (usually off the field of competition).
    b. Localized itching a helpful clue.
  2. **Diagnosis**
    a. Lice and nits easily visualized on scalp and pubic areas with magnification.
    b. Pubic lice may infest eyelashes and axillary hair (similar hairshaft diameter).

    3. **Treatment**
        a. Single application of a Kwell product or Nix (permethrin cream rinse) usually curative.
        b. Reinfestation not uncommon.
        c. Nightly application of generous amounts of petrolatum to eyelashes will clear those lesions, as Kwell should not be used near the eyes.
        d. Wash clothing and bedclothes during treatment.
    4. **Prevention**
        a. Cleanliness.
  B. **Scabies**
    1. **History**
        a. Still at epidemic levels in this country.
        b. Inadequate hygiene and close physical contact (as with pediculosis).
        c. May be spread by fomites such as towels, uniforms, and equipment.
        d. Generalized itching, worse at night.
    2. **Diagnosis**
        a. Maintain a high index of suspicion.
        b. Skin changes may include burrows, small vesicles, papules, and a variety of excoriated lesions, usually interdigitally and in skin creases and lines of clothing pressure.
        c. Itchy papules of the breast areolae or penis are essentially pathognomonic.
    3. **Treatment**
        a. A single application of Kwell lotion, applied after a bath in the evening from neck to toes and left on overnight, is usually curative.
        b. Treat all family and sexual contacts.
        c. Physician may need to personally supervise the application of the scabicide.
        d. Systemic antipruritics (Periactin, Atarax) indicated until inflammatory skin changes have been replaced with normal epithelium (often several weeks).
        e. Judicious use of mild topical steroids may be helpful, but extent of need often makes use impractical and expensive.
    4. **Prevention**
        a. Cleanliness.

VI. **Effects of Exercise on Preexisting Dermatoses**
  A. **Acne**
    1. **History**
        a. Aggravation by sweat, dirt, and occlusive sports equipment.
    2. **Diagnosis**
        a. Rarely a problem.
    3. **Treatment**
        a. Objectives are twofold; short-term cosmetic results and long-term prevention of scarring.
        b. In spite of athletic lifestyles and environment, improvement can be achieved, even during the athletic season, by judicious use of benzoyl peroxide, retinoic acid derivatives, and topical or systemic antibiotics.
        c. Sunshine is helpful.
        d. The athlete with significant cystic acne may need special attention, including injection of early cysts with $\frac{1}{4}\%$ triamcinolone acetonide (to abort maturation), hot compresses, and a small incision to drain contents when fluctuant, or referral to a dermatologist if Accutane, a derivative of vitamin A, is considered for systemic "curative" use.

4. **Prevention**
   a. Loose-fitting, dry, clean, absorbent cotton clothing.
   b. Avoidance of abrasive skin cleansers and consistent picking at acne lesions.
B. **Eczema (Atopy)**
   1. **History**
      a. Aggravation during athletic endeavors more likely if elements of atopy have been present since infancy or childhood.
   2. **Diagnosis**
      a. Usually not a problem.
      b. Areas of chronic thickening and excoriation in flexural creases at the elbows and knees often flare during competition.
      c. Fall and winter sports participants at greater risk of flareup.
   3. **Treatment**
      a. Adequate rest, generous oral hydration, home humidification, use of systemic antipruritic medications, and relief from emotional tension are all helpful, both for treatment and prevention.
      b. Avoidance of excessive soap during bathing.
      c. Frequent use of bland emollients such as Vaseline or Eucerin.
      d. Judicious use of topical corticosteroids.
      e. Stress need for continuing, gentle topical care.
   4. **Prevention**
      a. See "Treatment."
      b. These athletes are also at risk to develop exercise-related urticaria, exercise-induced bronchospasm (EIB, asthma), allergic rhinitis, and aspirin sensitivity.
C. **Dyshidrosis**
   1. **History**
      a. These athletes usually exhibit ongoing hyperhidrosis.
      b. Affects athletes of all ages.
   2. **Diagnosis**
      a. Deep-seated vesicles affecting the hands and feet, or both, commonly located along the sides of the digits and on the palms and soles.[6]
      b. Bullae are occasionally produced, and, when they occur, secondary infection is more likely in the active athlete.
      c. Athletes uncomfortable during flareups.
   3. **Treatment**
      a. Wet soaks or compresses (Domeboro) in the acute stage, followed by topical steroids and lubricating emollients (Eucerin) for more chronic cases.
      b. Continuing therapy necessary as acute flareups disconcerting to competitive athlete—the hands of a golfer or gymnast, the feet of a runner, basketball or football player.
   4. **Prevention**
      a. Continuing therapy as described under "Treatment."
D. **Seborrhea**
   1. **History**
      a. Itchy dandruff signifies seborrheic dermatitis.
   2. **Diagnosis**
      a. Inflammatory changes involving the scalp, salmon-orange in color, may also affect the central forehead and face, ear canals, mid-chest, axillae, umbilicus, groin, and intergluteal cleft.
      b. Flareups common during tense athletic seasons.

   3. **Treatment**
      a. Key to therapy is frequent scalp shampooing. This alone will often make the dermatitis elsewhere easier to control.
      b. Topical steroid lotions are used as an adjuvant to scalp care.
      c. If other areas of the skin require therapy, mild corticosteroid creams or Cetacort lotion is helpful.
   4. **Prevention**
      a. Daily scalp and body care.

VII. **Conclusion**

The physician who cares for athletes can effectively diagnose and treat most skin disorders seen in these patients. Many are preventable and most respond to therapy without significant side-effects. Encouraging compliance to the treatment regimen augments the chance of successful outcome and is less likely to be a problem if the physician is dedicated to sports and the physician and athlete have a sound doctor-patient relationship. The certified athletic trainer can also have a positive influence on prevention, early diagnosis, and supervision of therapy.

*REFERENCES*

1. Amundson LH, Caplan RM: Dermatology II. Monograph, Edition 109, Home Study Self-Assessment Program. Kansas City, American Academy of Family Physicians, June 1988.
2. Basler RSW: Skin lesions related to sports activity. Primary Care 10(3):479–494, 1983.
3. Liteplo MG: Sports-related skin problems. In Vinger PF, Hoerner EF (eds): Sports Injuries: The Unthwarted Epidemic. Boston, John Wright, 1982, pp 188–202.
4. Amundson LH, Mellion MB: Common skin problems. In Mellion MB (ed): Office Management of Sports Injuries & Athletic Problems. Philadelphia, Hanley & Belfus, 1988, pp 146–159.
5. Amundson LH, Caplan RM: The skin and subcutaneous tissues. In Taylor RB (ed): Family Medicine, 3rd ed. New York, Springer-Verlag, 1988, pp 366–394.
6. Amundson LH, Caplan RM: Dermatology I. Monograph, Edition 108, Home Study Self-Assessment Program. Kansas City, American Academy of Family Physicians, May 1988.

# PART III

# INJURY PREVENTION, DIAGNOSIS, AND TREATMENT

## Chapter 29: Musculoskeletal Injuries in Sports

W. MICHAEL WALSH, MD
RONNIE D. HALD, RPT, ATC
LAURA E. PETER, MS

I. **General Classification of Musculoskeletal Sports Injuries**—Can be broken down into **traumatic** and **overuse** injuries.

  A. **Traumatic injuries**—resulting from specific episode(s) of trauma, whether recent (acute) or in the more distant past (subacute or chronic).
    1. **Bone:** Traumatic injury to bone most commonly results in **fracture,** though rarely there can be another process, such as **subperiosteal hematoma.** Various descriptive terms used with fractures include:
      a. **Closed fracture:** Fracture that does not produce open wound in skin.
      b. **Open fracture:** Open wound in skin communicates with fracture site.
      c. Descriptive terms for direction of fracture line:
        i. Fracture at right angles to long axis of bone is called **transverse.**
        ii. Fracture line at other angle to long axis of bone is called **oblique.**
        iii. Bone twisted apart creates **spiral** configuration of fracture.
      d. **Comminuted fracture:** Bone is broken into three or more pieces.
      e. **Avulsion fracture:** A "pull-off" fracture; a piece of bone is pulled off by ligament or tendon attachment.
      f. **Greenstick fracture:** Incomplete fracture in children. One side of a bone is broken, whereas the other side appears bent.
      g. **Torus fracture:** Localized buckling in the cortex of the bone, common in children.
      h. **Epiphyseal fracture:** Fracture that involves the growth center at the end of a long bone in children.
    2. **Joint:** Traumatic injury to joint and supporting structures (capsule, ligaments) often results in an instability episode referred to as **dislocation** or **subluxation.** Rarely, some other process occurs from a direct blow, such as joint contusion or hemarthrosis.
      a. **Dislocation:** Complete displacement of joint surface so that they no longer make normal contact at all. Important to distinguish **first time** or **recurrent** dislocation.
      b. **Subluxation:** Partial displacement of joint surfaces, usually transient in nature. Important to distinguish **first time** or **recurrent** subluxation.
      c. Dislocation or subluxation implies damage to ligaments or other supporting structures of joint. Important to ascertain injury to those tissues; discussed below.

3. **Ligament:** Traumatic injury to ligament referred to as **sprain.** Sprains classified as:
   a. **1st degree:** Tear of only a few ligament fibers. Mild swelling, pain, disability. No instability of joint created.
   b. **2nd degree:** Tear of a moderate number of ligament fibers, but ligament function is still intact. Moderate amount of swelling, pain, disability. Little to no instability of joint.
   c. **3rd degree:** Complete rupture of ligament. Severe swelling and disability. Definite joint instability. Instability may be classified as:
      i. **1+:** Joint surfaces normally stabilized by ligament can be displaced 3–5 mm from their normal position.
      ii. **2+:** Joint surfaces can be separated by 6–10 mm.
      iii. **3+:** Joint surfaces can be separated by greater than 10 mm.
4. **Muscle-tendon unit:**
   a. Traumatic injury to muscle or tendon due to **indirect force** (i.e., contraction of muscle itself) is referred to as **strain.** Strains are classified as:
      i. **1st degree:** Tear of only a few muscle or tendon fibers. Mild swelling, pain, disability. Can also be characterized by patient's ability to produce strong, but painful, muscle contraction.
      ii. **2nd degree:** Disruption of a moderate number of muscle or tendon fibers, but muscle-tendon unit still intact. Moderate amount of pain, swelling, disability. Characterized by patient's weak and painful attempts at muscle contraction.
      iii. **3rd degree:** Complete rupture of muscle-tendon unit. May be at origin, muscular portion, musculotendinous junction, within tendon itself, or at tendon insertion. Characterized by patient's extremely weak but painless attempts at muscle contraction.
   b. Traumatic injury to muscle due to **direct force** may produce **deep muscle contusion.**
      i. Typically, quadriceps or brachialis muscles involved in contact or collision sports.
      ii. May lead to **myositis ossificans** and therefore permanent loss of function.
5. Other soft tissues
   a. Traumatic injury to bursa with bursal swelling referred to as **traumatic bursitis,** usually due to bleeding into bursa.
   b. Traumatic injuries to other soft tissues include various **contusions** and **hematomas.**
   c. Lacerations may involve musculoskeletal tissues.
   d. Shearing injuries: avulsions, abrasions, blisters.
B. **Overuse injuries**—Noted to account for more than 50% of injuries seen in primary care practices.
   1. **General overuse concepts:** If viewed as a function of Newton's third law of motion, athletic injury can be described as resulting from equal and opposite reactions, which in turn result in macro- or microtrauma.
      a. Macrotrauma: Equal and opposite forces exceed the strength of a specific anatomic structure, and therefore the structure fails (See "Traumatic injuries," par. I.A., above).
      b. Microtrauma: Microscopic subliminal injury from repeated activity. Repetitive microtrauma can be cumulative over time and can result in local tissue breakdown. Local tissue breakdown can in turn result in inflammation, characterized by pain and dysfunction.

2. **Predisposition:** Equally important are factors that predispose the athlete to overuse injury. These can be intrinsic or extrinsic:
   a. **Intrinsic:** malalignment of limbs, muscular imbalances, other anatomical factors
   b. **Extrinsic:** training errors, faulty technique, incorrect surfaces and equipment, poor environmental conditions
3. **Degenerative processes** may influence traumatic injuries as well, but more commonly have effect on overuse injuries. Normal degenerative processes occur in many musculoskeletal tissues with aging. May add to likelihood of certain injuries. Common examples are rotator cuff and Achilles tendon problems.
4. **General classification:** Overuse injuries can be classified as four stages, according to pain:
   a. **Stage 1:** pain after activity only
   b. **Stage 2:** pain during activity; does not restrict performance
   c. **Stage 3:** pain during activity, restricts performance
   d. **Stage 4:** chronic, unremitting pain, even at rest.
5. **Bones:** Overuse injury of bone may be **stress fracture** or **apophysitis.**
   a. **Stress fracture:** Most often found in lower extremity, but can also be found in the spine (see "Spondylolysis and Spondylolisthesis," Chapter 38) and in the upper extremity when it is subjected to weightbearing (e.g., gymnastics, weight training).
   b. **Apophysitis:** In skeletally immature athletes, traction injuries can occur to the apophysis. Appear to result from repeated stress at tendinous insertion into bony growth center, followed by reactive bone formation. Most common apophysitis is Osgood-Schlatter's disease (see Chapter 40).
6. **Joints:** Overuse joint injuries are almost invariably the result of mechanical factors. While they may create a condition that could be called "arthritis," it may be more valid when treating athletes to think of it as a **synovitis.**
   a. Synovitis may be generalized, with swelling, warmth, pain, and occasionally redness.
   b. Certain synovitis may be more localized, e.g., synovial plica of knee, peripatellar synovitis in extensor mechanism malalignment of knee (see Chapter 40).
7. **Ligament:** There are few examples of pure overuse injuries to ligaments. Theoretically, they may occur whenever a ligament is subjected to repeated stress. Examples may include:
   a. **Medial elbow injuries:** Part of this spectrum may include overuse injury to the medial collateral ligament of the elbow, resulting from repetitive throwing with valgus loading.
   b. **Breaststroker's knee:** Probably the most common example of pure ligament injury through overuse. Typically involves medial collateral ligament of knee at femoral attachment, secondary to breaststroke kick.
   c. **Plantar fasciitis:** Technically, a ligament connecting bone to bone, the plantar fascia is commonly involved in overuse syndromes of the foot (see Chapter 42).
8. **Muscle-tendon unit:** Overuse injury of muscle-tendon unit may be **myositis, tendinitis,** or **tenosynovitis.**
   a. Myositis overuse injuries of muscle tissue are rather nondescript. Can involve practically any muscle in the body. More distinct syndromes are known when overuse symptoms occur at muscular origin and attachment to bone/periosteum. Those syndromes include:
      i. Lateral epicondylitis of the elbow
      ii. Medial epicondylitis of the elbow

        iii. Chronic groin strain

        iv. Shin splints.

   b. Tendonitis: inflammatory reaction within the tendon tissue itself. Closely related to the concept of normal aging and degenerative changes within tendons (tendonosis), which may predispose to microtrauma. Common examples are:

        i. Bicipital tendonitis

        ii. Rotator cuff tendonitis

        iii. Achilles tendonitis.

   c. Tenosynovitis (peritendinitis, tenovaginitis): inflammatory change involves tissue surrounding the tendon itself. Classic physical finding is crepitation or "dry leather creaking" sensation over involved tendon as tendon is moved through its sheath. Common locations include:

        i. Extensor tendons of forearm

        ii. Tibialis anterior in the lower leg.

9. Other soft tissues: The most common overuse musculoskeletal injury involving other soft tissue is **bursitis.**

   a. Bursae lie between tissue planes and help to reduce frictional stress between those structures.

   b. Common sites for mechanical bursitis in athletes include:

        i. Subacromial bursa

        ii. Greater trochanteric bursa of the hip

        iii. Retrocalcaneal bursa just anterior to the Achilles tendon insertion.

## II. General Treatment of Musculoskeletal Injuries

  A. Basic athletic first aid (see Chapter 30 for complete discussion)—represented by the mnemonic "PRICES"

    1. Protection          4. Compression

    2. Rest              5. Elevation

    3. Ice               6. Support.

  B. Other treatment methods

    1. **Oral anti-inflammatory medication:** Non-steroidal anti-inflammatory drugs (NSAIDs) are commonly used in treating musculoskeletal sports injuries. Many different types and brands exist. Their use is usually based on clinician's empiric results rather than on objective scientific studies. Choice should always be tempered by known sideeffects (e.g., renal damage). Best thought of as adjunctive treatment to other modes.

    2. **Physical modalities:** Cold, heat, ultrasound, iontophoresis, and electrical muscle stimulation are commonly employed. See Chapter 30 for discussion.

    3. **Therapeutic exercises:** Most important, but most commonly underutilized means of treating musculoskeletal sports injuries. Important to correct not only deficits that may result from injury, but also those that predispose to injury.

    4. **Injection therapy:** Most commonly injected material is corticosteroid, with or without local anesthetic. **Studies have demonstrated direct harmful effect of steroid on articular cartilage and weakening effect on tendon.**

      a. **Should never inject corticosteroid into:**

        i. **Young athletes' joints.**

        ii. **Major joint (e.g., knee, shoulder)** in athlete of any age when there is not already objective degenerative change.

        iii. **Major load-bearing tendons,** e.g., patellar tendon, Achilles tendon. **To do so may hasten rupture.**

    b. Acceptable to inject corticosteroid into:
       i. Muscular trigger points.
      ii. Bursae.
     iii. Small non-weight-bearing joints, e.g., acromioclavicular joint.
     iv. **Muscular** attachments to bone, e.g., lateral epicondyle. **Total number** of injections should be limited.
      v. Ligament attachments to bone where subsequent rupture of ligament would not be disastrous, e.g., plantar fascia attachment to calcaneus.
     vi. Tendon **sheath,** but not the tendon itself, e.g., for de Quervain's disease at wrist.
    vii. Already degenerated joint in older athlete.
  5. **Braces, supports, and other devices:** A variety of products have been developed to aid in the treatment of athletic injuries. These range from simple compressive sleeves for various joints to expensive custom-made braces. These are discussed in the chapters on anatomical parts and individual sports and in Chapter 43.

III. **Selected Musculoskeletal Evaluation Techniques:** Certain musculoskeletal parameters are so commonly evaluated in athletic injuries that they are presented here for easy reference from other chapters:

  A. **Flexibility testing:** Flexibility is limited by the length of a muscle across a joint. Lack of flexibility in two-joint muscles (muscles that cross two joints) is often indicated as a cause of musculoskeletal problems. In testing for flexibility, one must consider whether the restriction seen is due to muscular tightness, or other sources of restriction, such as lack of joint range of motion or pain.
    1. **Heel cord flexibility** (Fig. 1): Athlete sits with knee extended and is asked to actively dorsiflex the ankle. Measurement is made goniometrically. Normal value is considered to be at least 10 degrees beyond plantigrade. This may also be done with the knee flexed to assess tightness within the soleus (normal value is at least 20 degrees beyond plantigrade).
    2. **Hamstrings flexibility** (Fig. 2): Athlete lies supine with hip maintained at 90 degrees flexion and is asked to extend the knee actively without repositioning the hip. Measurement is made goniometrically. Normal value is considered to be less than 10 degrees short of full extension.
    3. **Quadriceps flexibility** (Fig. 3). Athlete lies prone and knee is flexed passively by examiner. Normal value is considered to be full knee flexion without tilting of the pelvis.
    4. **Iliotibial band flexibility** (Fig. 4): Athlete lies on the opposite side, near the edge of the examining table, facing away from the examiner. On the side to be examined, the hip is slightly extended and passively adducted by gravity. Take care not to let iliotibial band slip anterior or posterior to the greater trochanter, or to allow lateral tilting of the pelvis. Normal is considered to be when the knee drops level or below the level of the table. This test is also referred to as the modified Ober's test.[2]
  B. **Strength testing:** Although there are many ways to assess strength, the authors prefer the manual muscle "break" test technique.[5] This requires the athlete to generate a maximal contraction of the muscle in the shortened range, and the examiner then applies an opposite force in an attempt to move the athlete from the testing position. A common muscle testing rule is not to apply forces across adjacent joints, but athletes are generally able to support adjacent joints adequately, thus allowing the examiner to apply more force to the area in question. Strength is usually graded on a 0–5 scale (0 = zero, 1 = trace, 2 = poor, 3 = fair, 4 = good, 5 = normal). Most athletic applications of the scale are in the upper range of this scale

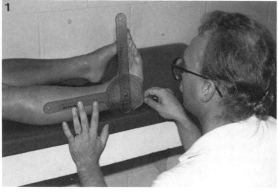

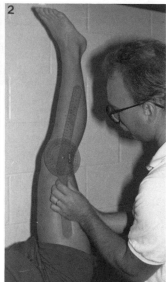

FIGURE 1.    Heel cord flexibility.
FIGURE 2.    Hamstrings flexibility.
FIGURE 3.    Quadriceps flexibility.
FIGURE 4.    Iliotibial band flexibility.

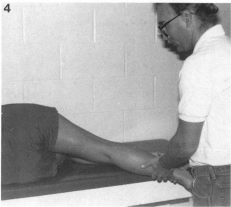

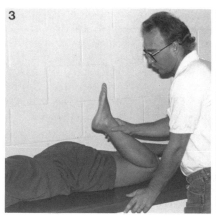

and are subjective in nature. Although more objective methods are available, the manual muscle test continues to be the most easily administered. The hip flexion, hip abduction,[5] and supraspinatus[4] strength tests are included, since weakness may indicate a new condition or an unrehabilitated condition more distal in the kinetic chain. The ankle dorsiflexion strength test is included because of its relationship to patellofemoral problems.[1]

1. **Hip flexion strength** (Fig. 5): Athlete sits at edge of table with arms crossed. Athlete flexes hip and examiner performs a manual muscle "break" test. If a break occurs, observe whether the weakness identified is located in the hip or the abdominals.

2. **Hip abduction strength** (Fig. 6): Athlete lies on opposite side, facing away from the examiner. Athlete abducts hip and examiner performs a manual muscle "break" test. If a break occurs, observe whether the weakness identified is located in the hip or the abdominal obliques.

3. **Ankle dorsiflexion strength** (Fig. 7): Athlete sits with knee extended and is asked to dorsiflex ankle. Examiner performs a manual muscle "break" test.

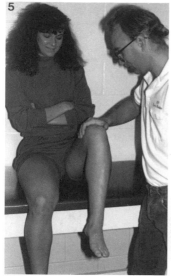

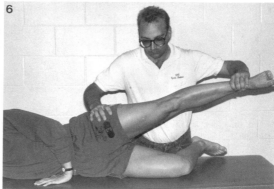

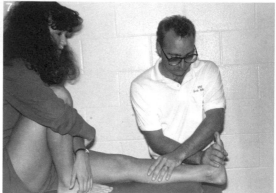

**FIGURE 5.** Hip flexion strength.
**FIGURE 6.** Hip abduction strength.
**FIGURE 7.** Ankle dorsiflexion strength.
**FIGURE 8.** Supraspinatus strength.

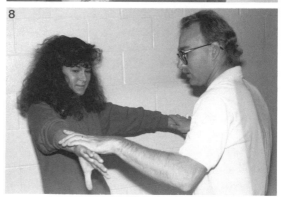

4. **Supraspinatus strength** (Fig. 8): Athlete sits or stands with shoulders abducted to 90 degrees, horizontally adducted to 30 degrees, and in a "thumbs down" position (fully internally rotated). Examiner performs a manual muscle "break" test, taking care to eliminate substitution from the trapezius.

## REFERENCES

1. Black JE, Alten SR: How I manage infrapatellar tendinitis. Phys Sportsmed 12:86, 1984.
2. Davies GJ, Malone T, Bassett FH: Knee examination. Phys Ther 60:1565, 1980.
3. Kendall H, Kendall F, Wadsworth G: Muscles: Testing and Function. Baltimore, Williams & Wilkins, 1971.

4. Jobe FW, Moynes DF: Delineation of diagnostic criteria and a rehabilitation program for rotator cuff injuries. Am J Sports Med 10:336, 1983.
5. Nicholas JA, Strizak AM, Veras G: A study of thigh weakness in different pathological states of the lower extremity. Am J Sports Med 4:241, 1976.

## *Other Suggested Readings*

1. Baker BE: Current concepts in the diagnosis and treatment of musculo-tendinous injuries. Med Sci Sports Exerc 16:323–327, 1984.
2. McKeag DB: The concept of overuse. Primary Care 11:43–59, 1984.
3. Peterson L, Renstrom P: Sports Injuries. Chicago, Year Book Medical Publishers, 1986.
4. Puffer JC, Zachazewski JE: Management of overuse injuries. AFP 38:225–232, 1988.

# Chapter 30: Comprehensive Rehabilitation of the Athlete

## GUY L. SHELTON, PT, ATC

I. **Goals of Rehabilitation**
   A. Return athlete to participation as soon as safely possible.
      1. **Decrease recovery time/promote healing.**
         a. Decrease swelling, congestion and msucle spasm (pain).
         b. Facilitate nutrient supply for rebuilding injured tissue.
      2. **Decrease morbidity.**
         a. Minimize deconditioning—range of motion (ROM), strength, endurance.
         b. Recondition—injured and uninjured areas.
      3. **Prevent further injury/reinjury.**
         a. Allow adequate healing time.
         b. Protection.

II. **Steps in Treatment**
   A. Common treatment MISCONCEPTIONS:
      1. Treat with medication only.
      2. Ice for 24–48 hours, then heat.
      3. Wrap for support, not compression.
      4. Don't use crutches unless pain is intolerable.
      5. Immobilization instead of rehabilitation.
      6. Time heals all.
      7. Return to play is based on calendar timetable.
   B. **Prevention**
      1. First step in treating injuries.
      2. An ounce of prevention is worth a pound of cure.
   C. **Triage**
      1. **Evaluate**
         a. Within your skill and knowledge level.
      2. **Assessment**
         a. On the field "diagnosis."
         b. Not necessarily specific but detailed enough to make the proper initial decision.
      3. **Decision**
         a. What next step to take?
            i. Return to play?
            ii. Hold out?
            iii. Refer for further evaluation?
               (a) Urgent?
               (b) Routine?
         b. **Be conservative!**
   D. **Emergency care—basic athletic first aid: "PRICES":**
      1. **'P'rotection** from further injury.
         a. Crutches for any lower extremity injury when the athlete is unable to walk normally (no pain, limping, or buckling).

      b. Splint or sling to immobilize extremity when more serious injury is suspected.

      c. Stretcher should be used to move injured athlete if any serious injury is suspected or there is any doubt about the injury.

  2. **'R'est**—avoid aggravating injury further.

      a. **Absolute rest**

         i. Complete rest from activity.

        ii. Best until serious injury ruled out.

      b. **Relative rest**

         i. Partial participation based on symptoms.

        ii. Used only in minor injuries until further evaluation is made.

  3. **'I'ce**—cold

      a. Decreases swelling, pain, inflammatory response, nerve conduction velocity, and muscle spasm.

      b. Cold applied for **up to 30 minutes,** depending on degree of symptoms.

      c. **Ice bag best;** gel packs and cold water immersion good.

  4. **'C'ompression**

      a. Circumferential wrap limits swelling in injured area.

      b. May also provide some support.

  5. **'E'levation**

      a. **Gravity** helps decrease swelling.

  6. **'S'upport**

      a. Implies a more **functional type of protection** (taping, bracing).

      b. Used when injury is minor and athlete can return to play.

E. **Definitive diagnosis and treatment**

  1. Thorough clinical **examination.**

  2. **Special tests** where applicable.

  3. **Referral** to appropriate medical specialty.

  4. **Diagnosis needs to be specific** so best treatment plan can be determined.

  5. **Treatment**

      a. **Immobilization**

         i. Used for certain fractures and sprains.

        ii. Should not be used with a less serious injury **just** to keep athlete from participating.

       iii. **Always should be followed by functional treatment.**

      b. **Surgical**

         i. Should be used for specific indications.

        ii. Sometimes indicated in acute injuries.

       iii. Often considered only after failed conservative care.

       iv. **Always should be followed by functional treatment.**

      c. **Functional (rehabilitative)**

         i. Activity-oriented goals require **active treatment.**

        ii. **Most important** form of treatment.

       iii. **Integral part of both immobilization and surgical treatment.**

F. **Rehabilitation—functional treatment**

  1. **Pyramid of recovery** (see Figs. 1 and 2)

      a. **Building blocks** of therapeutic exercise.

      b. **Primary treatment** in most cases.

      c. **Total athlete concept:** When an injury occurs, the **entire athlete is affected.** The longer the recovery period, the greater the potential for **systemic deconditioning.** The injured area deserves primary consideration but the other parts of the athlete cannot be neglected.

         i. **Local treatment**—injured area itself.

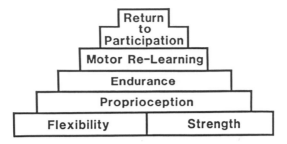

## PYRAMID OF RECOVERY
### (Therapeutic Exercise)

### FIGURE 1.

ii. **Limb treatment**—limb functions as a kinetic chain.
iii. **System treatment**—uninjured limbs, cardiovascular system, and overall agility and timing.

2. **Specifics of therapeutic exercise**
   a. **Flexibility** (see Figs. 3 through 11 for selected flexibility exercises).
      i. Joint range of motion
         (a) Respect healing structures.
         (b) Should be regained with **minimal aggravation of symptoms.**
      ii. Muscle elasticity
         (a) Inflexibility decreases muscle function at extreme positions, decreases adaptability of muscle-tendon unit, and increases joint compression forces.
         (b) Repetitions should be **prolonged and static** with moderate tension felt in muscle.

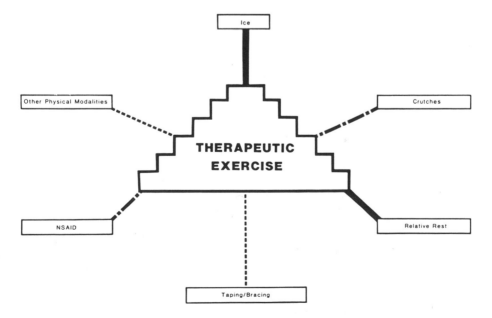

**FIGURE 2.**   Relationship of therapeutic exercise to adjunct treatments.

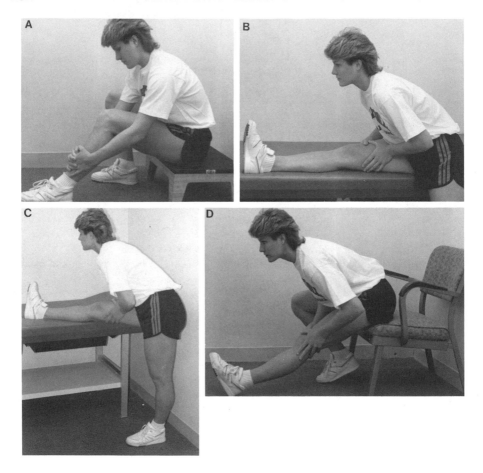

**FIGURE 3.** *A,* Assisted knee flexion from a low seat. Low seat keeps hip lower than knee and minimizes substitute movement of lifting hip instead of flexing knee. *B,* Hamstring stretching—long sitting at edge of table or couch. *C,* Hamstring stretching standing. *D,* Hamstring stretching from chair with foot on floor.

        (c) Degree of flexibility varies, so adequate time should be allowed each session **based on individual levels of flexibility.**
   b.  **Strength** (see Figs. 12 through 20 for selected strength exercises).
      i.  General considerations:
        (a) Muscle must be **overloaded** to facilitate strengthening.
        (b) Exercises need to be **specific** with regard to ultimate activity.
        (c) Rate of **progression** is determined by initial level of fitness, healing stage of injury, and individual differences.
     ii.  **Exercise prescription**
        (a) **Intensity**
           (i) Must be adequate to **create overload.**
          (ii) **Lower intensity during early rehabilitation to avoid symptoms.**
        (b) **Frequency**
           (i) Number of sessions per day/days per week.
          (ii) **Higher frequency while intensity is low.**

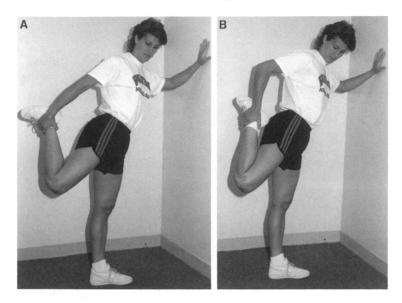

**FIGURE 4.** *A,* Quadriceps stretching. Keep heel away from buttocks initially. *B,* Quadriceps stretching. As flexibility and comfort progress, gradually pull heel to buttocks as long as symptoms do not increase.

    (c) **Duration/repetitions**
        (i) **Higher number of repetitions while intensity is low.**
        (ii) Watch fatigue and symptoms.
    (d) **Mode/specific techniques**
        (i) Must be adjusted to **patient's tolerance.**
        (ii) **Modification** of standard techniques and equipment must be made for certain injuries.

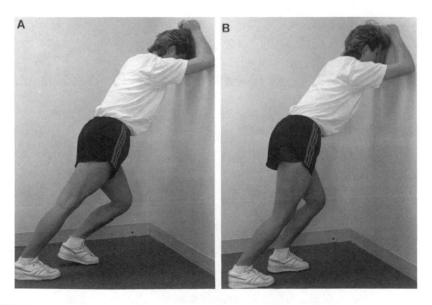

**FIGURE 5.** *A,* Heelcord stretching—knee straight. Used to stretch the gastrocnemius muscle. *B,* Heelcord stretching—knee bent. Used to stretch the soleus muscle and Achilles tendon.

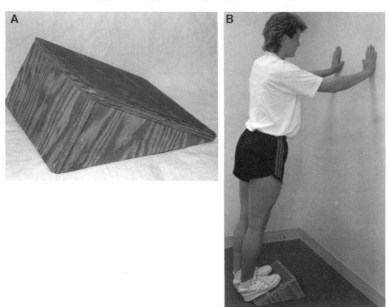

**FIGURE 6.** *A,* Slant board (12″ × 12″ × 6″ high) to increase stretch on calf. *B,* Heelcord stretching using slant board.

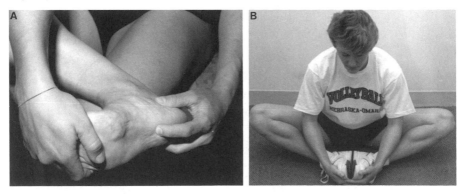

**FIGURE 7.** *A,* Plantar fascia stretch. Done manually to increase flexibility as a treatment for plantar fasciitis. *B,* Adductor stretch.

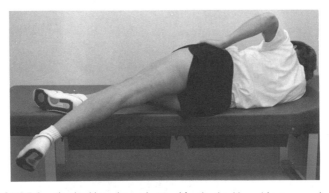

**FIGURE 8.** Iliotibial band stretch. Used for iliotibial band friction syndrome.

**FIGURE 9.** Wrist extensor stretch. Used for lateral epicondylitis.

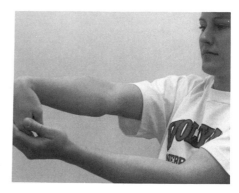

iii. **Types of strengthening exercise**
  (a) **Isometric**
    (i) Muscle contraction against **immovable resistance.**
    (ii) Muscle contraction **intensity can be varied** from very light to maximum.
    (iii) Usually **well tolerated** fairly soon after injury.

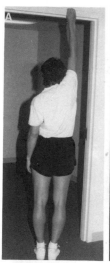
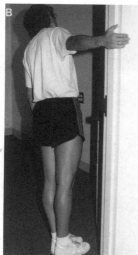
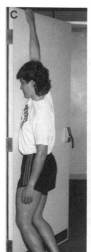
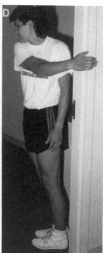

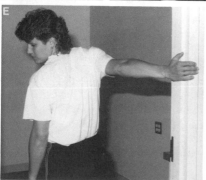

**FIGURE 10.** *A,* Shoulder flexion stretch using doorway to anchor hand. *B,* Distraction stretch for glenohumeral joint. Useful as early stretching exercise in impingement syndrome and rotator cuff problems. *C,* Overhead version of exercise in Figure 10B. This is a more advanced technique and should be achieved gradually. *D,* Horizontal adduction with distraction. Useful in impingement syndrome as acute symptoms decrease. *E,* Horizontal abduction stretch.

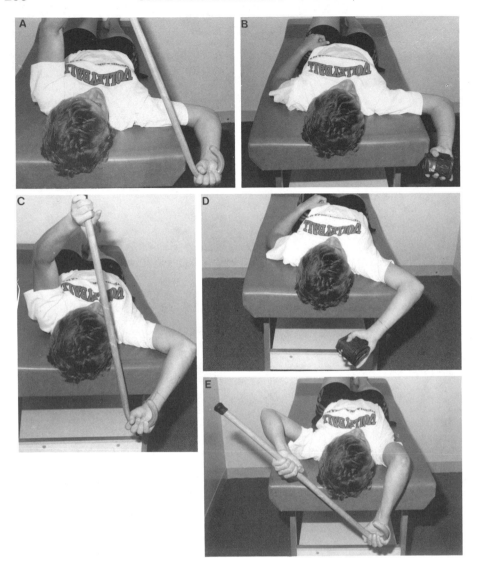

**FIGURE 11.** *A,* Supine external rotation stretch in 90° abduction using wand to provide stretch. *B,* Supine external rotation stretch in 90° abduction using weight to provide stretch. *C,* Supine external rotation stretch in 135° abduction using wand to provide stretch. Progression of stretch in Figure 11A. *D,* Supine external rotation stretch in 135° abduction using weight to provide stretch. Progression of stretch in Figure 11B. *E,* Supine external rotation stretch in 180° abduction. Progression of stretch in Figure 11D. Very helpful with shoulder problems in throwing athletes.

        (iv) Strengthening effects are **specific to joint position.**
        (v) Resistance provided manually or against a solid object.
    (b) **Isotonic** (most common)
        (i) Muscle contraction against **constant resistance** through a range of motion.
        (ii) **Speed of movement can vary.**
        (iii) With **concentric** contractions, muscle shortens during contraction.

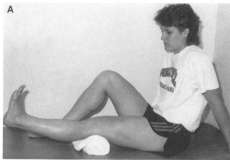

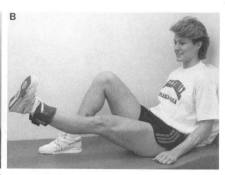

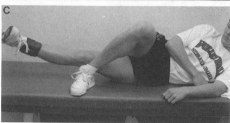

**FIGURE 12.** *A,* Terminal knee extension. Used in regaining full active knee extension and early quadriceps strengthening. May be done as initial phase of leg raise. *B,* Straight leg raise with external rotation. Used for quadriceps strengthening. External rotation component used in athletes with patellofemoral problems. Biases strength toward vastus medialis obliquus (VMO). *C,* Hip adduction sidelying. With quadriceps set at onset, this can provide additional stimulus to the VMO to improve patellofemoral stability.

(iv) With **eccentric** contractions, muscle lengthens during contraction.
(v) **Eccentric contractions are an important component of many sports activities.**
(vi) Resistance may be provided by limb weight, strap-on weights, barbells, machines, hydraulics, and elastic bands or tubing.
(c) **Isokinetic**
  (i) Muscle contraction against device that holds **speed of movement constant.**

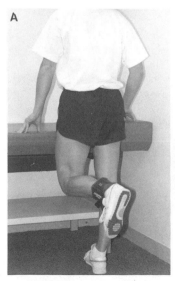

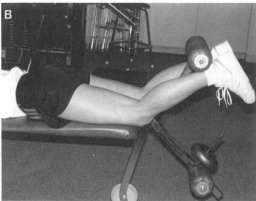

**FIGURE 13.** *A,* Knee curls standing. For hamstring strengthening. *B,* Knee curls prone using curl machine. More advanced hamstring strengthening exercise.

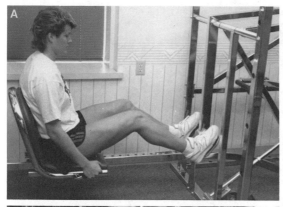

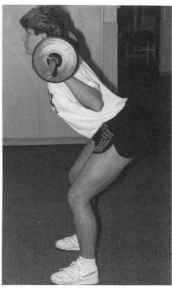

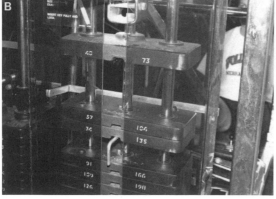

**FIGURE 14** *(left)*. *A,* Leg press. Closed kinetic chain strengthening for quadriceps and hip extensors. A more physiologic method than knee extensions for quadriceps strengthening. *B,* Modified weight stack for leg press. Allows less-flexed starting position and thus less patellofemoral stress.

**FIGURE 15** *(right)*. Mini-squat. Partial depth is preferred over the traditional parallel squat. Keeping shins vertical lessens shear forces at knee. Used in intermediate and advanced phases.

        (ii) Resistance **varies according to effort provided by patient (accommodating resistance).**
        (iii) Speed specific exercise program possible.
        (iv) Helpful in intermediate and advanced rehabilitation programs.
        (v) Intensity can be quite high so **symptoms must be monitored.**
        (vi) Equipment cost quite high.
    c. **Proprioception** (see Figs. 21 through 23 for selected proprioception exercises).
      i. Synergistic muscle action
      ii. **Reaction time**—quickness
      iii. Balance boards, weighted balls and implements, and basic coordination and agility exercises.
    d. **Endurance** (see Fig. 24 for selected endurance exercises).
      i. Muscle endurance—repetitions.
      ii. Cardiorespiratory fitness—aerobic.
    e. **Motor relearning**
      i. Advanced coordination and agility drills.
      ii. Progressive running drills (Table 1).
      iii. Progressive throwing/racquet drills (Table 2).
      iv. Sports specific fundamental drills.
      v. Progressive return to activity.

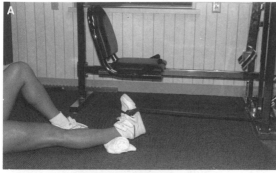

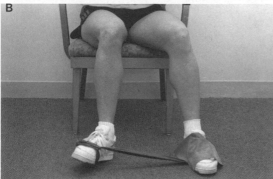

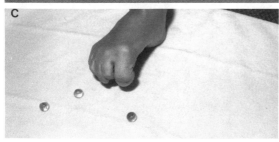

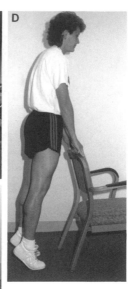

**FIGURE 16.** *A,* Ankle dorsiflexion. Used for ankle rehabilitation. Also helpful for patellar tendinitis when eccentric phase is emphasized. *B,* Ankle eversion. Used to strengthen dynamic stabilizers with inversion ankle injuries. *C,* Toe curls. Marbles or small, smooth stones are grasped by the toes. Used to strengthen foot intrinsic muscles. *D,* Toe raises. Used to strengthen calf. Start on both legs, progress to only one leg.

**TABLE 1.**   Progressive Running Program

| Step | Progression Criteria |
| --- | --- |
| Bicycle | 30–45 minutes. |
| Walk | 2 miles in 30 minutes or less. |
| Jog | Jog 50 yards, walk 50 yards up to ¼ mile, increase total distance to 1 mile, then increase jogging and decrease walking until jogging 1 mile straight through. |
| Run | Increase jogging to 2–4 miles, then increase pace to preinjury level. |
| Sprint | Take 10–15 yards to build up to ½ speed, sprint at ½ speed for 40 yards, take 15–20 yards to slow down and stop. Gradually work up from ½ to ²/₃ to ¾ to full speed. Do 10–20 sprints per session. |
| Figure 8 | Gently jog to a large (20–30 yards) figure 8. Gradually run the 8 faster. Then decrease the size of the 8 by 2–3 yards at a time so that the cutting is progressively sharper. Work down to a 4–5 yard 8. Do 10–20 figure eights at a session. |
| Basic drills | Work into jumping rope, power jumping activities, stairs, backward running, side step running, side crossover running, quick starts and stops, cutting, and other basic drill activities important to the athlete's specific sport. |
| Sports drills | Target these fine-tuning drills to the specific activity the athlete wants to resume. |

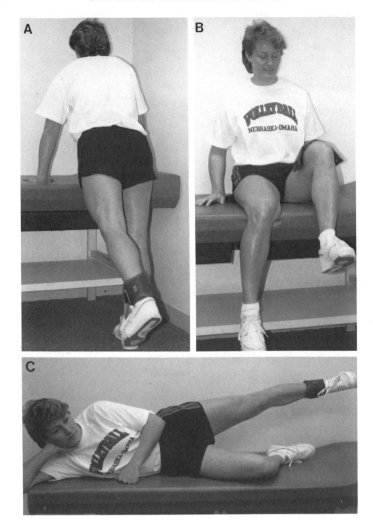

**FIGURE 17.** *A,* Standing hip extension. *B,* Sitting hip flexion. *C,* Sidelying hip abduction.

**TABLE 2.** Progressive Pitching Program

| Step | Progression Criteria |
| --- | --- |
| Short toss | Toss ball 10–15 feet for accuracy using good throwing mechanics. |
| Long toss | Stand in short center field. Throw ball so that it rolls to second base. Then throw so that ball reaches second base in four bounces, then three bounces, then two and finally one. Use good mechanics and throw for accuracy. |
| Mound toss | From the mound throw at ½ speed toward the plate. Emphasize accuracy and mechanics. |
| Straight throws | Throw straight pitches progressively faster up to ¾ speed. |
| Breaking throws | Throw curve and slider pitches progressively faster up to ¾ speed. |
| Speed | Increase speed on all pitches toward full speed while maintaining good mechanics and accuracy. |
| Special pitches | Add any specialty pitches to program. |
| Fielding | Work on fielding ground balls and throwing to various bases from gradually more awkward positions. |

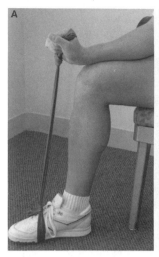
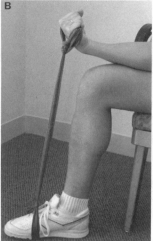
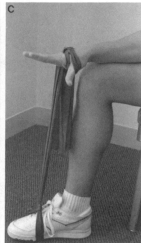

FIGURE 18. *A*, Wrist extension using elastic band. *B*, Wrist flexion using elastic band. *C*, Forearm pronation using elastic band.

    f. **Evaluation for return to participation**
        i. **Family or referring physician**
           (a) Provides clearance to begin to workout.
           (b) Statement of **adequate healing.**

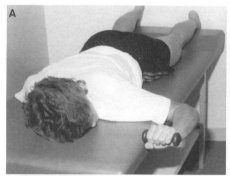
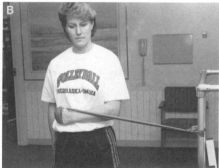
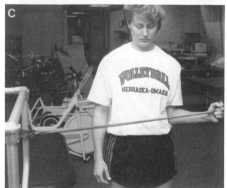

FIGURE 19. *A*, Shoulder external rotation prone for rotator cuff strengthening. *B*, Standing internal rotation using elastic band. *C*, Standing external rotation using elastic band.

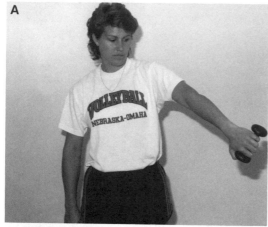

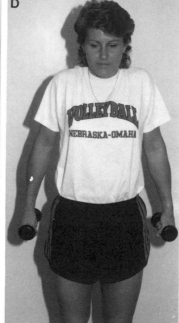

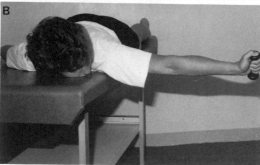

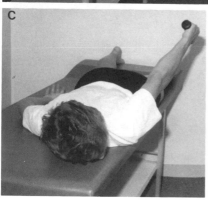

**FIGURE 20.** *A,* Isolated position for the supraspinatous muscle for rotator cuff strengthening. *B,* Horizontal abduction prone with arm externally rotated for rotator cuff strengthening. *C,* Shoulder extension prone. *D,* Shoulder shrug/scapular adduction for scapulothoracic stability.

    ii. **Team physician, athletic trainer, coach, or combined** must document athlete's **readiness to return and perform.**
       (a) **Fully rehabilitated**—strength, flexibility, endurance, coordination, agility.
       (b) Athlete must **demonstrate full speed performance** in all phases.
       (c) **No symptoms** at any point.
       (d) **Full confidence**—no favoring or hesitation.
  g. **Timetable for return to participation**
    i. Should be **based on individual's symptoms and tolerance** to progressive activity—"One day at a time."

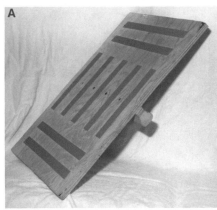

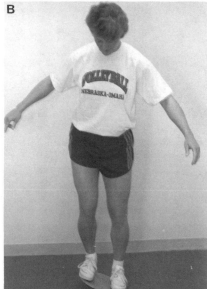

**FIGURE 21.** *A,* Uniaxial balance board. (16" × 24" with 2 " to 2.5" tall pivot on bottom). *B,* Uniaxial balance board in use. Foot position can be varied to balance side to side or front to back.

ii. A fixed length of time to recover from an injury does not exist and should not be used.

G. **Adjunctive treatment to therapeutic exercise** (see Fig. 2)
   1. **Functional taping and bracing**
      a. Taping and bracing are adjuncts to healing and rehabilitation.

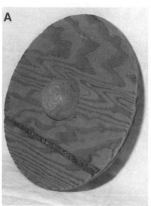

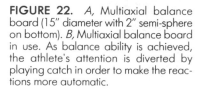

**FIGURE 22.** *A,* Multiaxial balance board (15" diameter with 2" semi-sphere on bottom). *B,* Multiaxial balance board in use. As balance ability is achieved, the athlete's attention is diverted by playing catch in order to make the reactions more automatic.

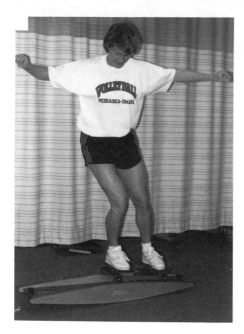

**FIGURE 23.** Fitter. Used for proprioception training and can be adjusted to various levels of resistance.

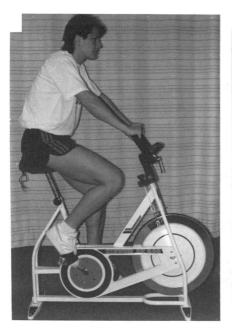
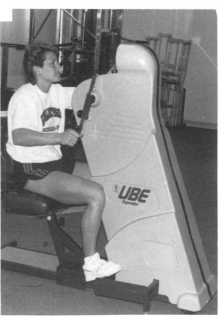

**FIGURE 24.** *(Left),* Stationary bicycle riding. Seat height, pedalling resistance, pedalling speed and pedalling phase effort can be adjusted for treatment of various injuries. *(Right),* Upper Body Exercise (UBE) Ergometer (Cybex, Ronkonkoma, NY). Used for upper extremity endurance training and maintenance of aerobic capacity during rehabilitation.

b. They **do not provide a short cut** to participation.
c. Tape or brace may **limit extremes of motion** and increase **proprioceptive feedback** to the injured area.
d. **An unhealed or unrehabilitated injury is more likely to be reinjured, no matter how well taped or braced.**

2. **Modalities**
   a. General considerations
      i. **Adjunctive,** not primary or long-term treatment.
      ii. Used to **control symptoms** and facilitate healing.
      iii. Helps allow patient to rehabilitate more effectively.
      iv. **Should not be used indiscriminately.**
   b. **Cold**
      i. Therapeutic effects
         (a) Vasoconstriction.
         (b) Decreased tissue metabolism.
         (c) Decreased inflammatory response.
         (d) Decreased pain.
         (e) Decreased muscle spasm.
      ii. **Advantages**
         (a) Effective to decrease inflammation.
         (b) **Relatively safe** for patient self application.
      iii. Disadvantages
         (a) Possible patient intolerance to cold.
         (b) Messy.
         (c) Cold injury risk.
      iv. Technique of application
         (a) Ice bags, gel packs, cold water immersion, ice massage, fluid-filled sleeve around injury are all effective; chemical cold packs, freon gas-filled sleeve around injury are much less effective.
         (b) **10–30 minutes treatment time.**
         (c) **Followed by at least an equal time off.**
         (d) Treatment customized based on method of cooling used, patient's tolerance, and cold intensity.
      v. Safety
         (a) Start with mild cold and progress colder as tolerated.
         (b) Inspect area before, during, and after treatment for signs of cold injury.
         (c) Thorough home instructions for patient self-application.
   c. **Heat**
      i. Therapeutic effects
         (a) Vasodilation.
         (b) Increased tissue metabolism.
         (c) Decreased pain.
         (d) Increased local circulation.
         (e) Increased tissue extensibility.
      ii. Advantages
         (a) Increased circulation may promote healing.
         (b) Relatively comfortable for patient.
         (c) Relatively safe for patient self-treatment.
      iii. Disadvantages
         (a) Risk of skin injury (burn).
         (b) If applied too soon following injury, may increase swelling and other symptoms.

        iv. Technique of application
            (a) Hot pack, heating pad, hot water bottle, warm soaks, whirlpool may all be effective.
            (b) 20 minutes average treatment time.
        v. Safety
            (a) Start with mild warmth and progress as tolerated.
            (b) Inspect area before, during and after treatment.
            (c) Electrical safety when electrical modalities used.

    d. **Contrast treatment**
        i. Therapeutic effects
            (a) Alternate vasoconstriction and vasodilation.
            (b) Creates vascular exercise to help reduce swelling.
        ii. Advantages
            (a) Benefits of heat with protection of cold.
        iii. Disadvantages
            (a) Heat component may be used too soon and increase swelling.
        iv. Technique of application
            (a) Alternate warm and cool.
            (b) Warm: cool ratio of 1:1 to 4:1.
        v. Safety
            (a) As with heat and cold as above.

    e. **Ultrasound**
        i. Therapeutic effects
            (a) Thermal
                (i) **Deep heating** effects up to 2.5 cm.
            (b) Mechanical
                (i) Increase **extensibility** of connective tissue.
                (ii) **Phoresis** of therapeutic medications (cortisone, salicylates).
            (c) Analgesic
                (i) **Decreases nerve conduction velocity.**
        ii. Technique of application is **best left to professionals** trained in the proper use of, safety with, and contraindications to these techniques.

    f. **Electrical stimulation**
        i. Transcutaneous electrical nerve stimulation (TENS)
            (a) Pain control post-injury and post-surgery.
        ii. Functional electrical stimulation
            (a) **Facilitate** muscle contraction for re-education.
            (b) **Supplement** voluntary muscle effort.
            (c) Helpful with **selective retraining** of muscles.
        iii. **Iontophoresis**
            (a) Introduce therapeutic medications (usually lidocaine or dexamethasone) into areas for anti-inflammatory and other effects depending on medication used.
            (b) Small local burns from direct current a risk.
            (c) Must check for **allergy** to medications used.
        iv. Technique of application is **best left to professionals** trained in the proper use of, safety with, and contraindications to these techniques.

    g. **EMG biofeedback**
        i. **Facilitates patient's re-education efforts.**
        ii. Allows patient to monitor and quantify exercise efforts.
        iii. Often used after function electrical stimulation.

        iv. Technique of application is **best left to professionals** trained in the proper use of, safety with, and contraindications to these techniques.

    h. Modality summary

        i. **Therapeutic exercise the most important modality.**

        ii. All others adjunctive.

        iii. If something is not helping, do something different.

H. **Protective equipment**

  1. **Standard equipment** must fit properly.

  2. **Modified standard equipment** may be adapted for specific injury.

  3. **Special equipment** created to provide protection for a specific injury.

I. **Patient education**

  1. Successful rehabilitation cannot be accomplished without the **cooperative efforts of the patient.**

  2. Patient must know how to best help himself/herself.

  3. **More than just handing the patient a list of instructions** (not a cookbook).

  4. Patient must be **"sold"** on the idea of the rehabilitation program.

  5. Method of "selling" (teaching method) should be based on patient's **learning style.**

    a. **Demonstrate deficits** that exist.

    b. **Explanation of injury** and treatment methods.

    c. **Testimonials.**

  6. **Initial instruction**

    a. **Instruction and demonstration** of rehabilitation techniques by **clinician.**

    b. **Patient** is asked to **demonstrate** newly learned techniques and **echo** other instructions.

    c. Patient's technique and understanding are **fine-tuned** by the clinician.

    d. Patient's **questions are answered; follow up questions are encouraged.**

    e. **Written handouts** are provided to **supplement, not replace,** instructions and demonstrations.

    f. **Follow up visit** is scheduled.

  7. **Subsequent follow-up visits**

    a. Open-ended question—"How are you doing?"

    b. Rehabilitation program **echoed and re-demonstrated** by patient.

    c. What helps? What hurts?

    d. Current **functional level assessed.**

    e. Exercise **technique corrected** where necessary.

    f. Rehabilitation **program modified** as re-evaluation dictates.

    g. New and modified techniques are echoed and reviewed and new handouts provided.

B. **This level of care and concern for the patient takes time and effort on the part of the clinician**

    a. Physician may not have the time or expertise in rehabilitation techniques to deal with these details.

    b. Physical therapist and/or certified athletic trainer

        i. **Possesses skills and expertise** in rehabilitation.

        ii. **Motivates** patient.

        iii. **Troubleshoots** problems the patient encounters during the rehabilitation process.

III. **Rehabilitation Principles for Specific Injury Types**

A. **Fractures**

  1. **Respect immobilization** or protection.

    2. Exercise involved area based on type of fracture and type of immobilization or protection.

    3. Exercise **uninvolved areas.**

    4. Fully rehabilitate all areas once specific injury is healed.

B. **Sprains**

    1. Flexibility, joint ROM as specific injury dictates.

    2. **Dynamic joint stability**—synergistic muscle contraction.

    3. **Don't disrupt healing** static stabilizers.

    4. Consider kinetic chain.

C. **Strains**

    1. **Flexibility**—improves muscle's ability to adapt to extremes.

    2. **Strength**—restores muscle's contractile capabilities.

    3. Adjacent areas—kinetic chain.

D. **Contusions**

    1. Treat as strains.

    2. **Beware of myositis ossificans.**

       a. **Inadequate recognition/suspicion** of initial injury

       b. **Repeated injury** before full healing has occurred

       c. **Overly aggressive physical therapy**—heat, passive stretching.

E. **Overuse**

    1. **Relative rest**

       a. Avoid irritating amounts and types of activity.

    2. **Control inflammation**

       a. NSAIDs

       b. Ice massage

       c. Phonophoresis

       d. Iontophoresis

       e. Injection??—last resort.

    3. **Correct contributing and acquired deficits**

       a. Conditioning

       b. Training errors

       c. Mechanical factors.

# Chapter 31: Head and Neck Injuries

RICHARD L. CARTER, MD
ARTHUR L. DAY, MD

## I. Physical Examination

In all head and neck injuries, the physical and neurological examination must begin with evaluation of the athlete's airway, breathing pattern, and circulation status. Once respiratory and cardiovascular systems are stable, attention can then be directed towards the rest of the examination.

### A. Head

1. **Scalp and face**
   a. **Scalp**
      i. Lacerations, abrasions—assess complete extent of laceration, assess and arrest scalp bleeding, and examine for foreign material and underlying skull fracture.
      ii. Bruises: assess for subcutaneous blood collections behind the ear (Battle's sign), periorbital area (raccoon sign), external ear canal, and behind the ear drum (hemotympanum).
   b. **Face**
      i. Mouth: note the adequacy of airway; inspect for fractured teeth or other foreign material.
      ii. Eyes: inspect for subconjunctival hemorrhage, orbital rim bruises, or lacerations and function of pupils.

2. **Brain**
   a. **Level of consciousness**
      i. Assess for transient (concussion) or sustained loss or alteration of consciousness, and loss of memory for event (amnesia)
      ii. Most injuries are minor, with no or transient disorientation. Some may be accompanied by loss of memory for events occurring after the accident (post-traumatic amnesia) or loss before the injury (retrograde amnesia). Persistent loss of consciousness or focal neurologic deficits (weakness, numbness, pupillary abnormalities) greatly increase the likelihood of significant brain injury or blood clot development.
   b. **Motor response**
      i. Evaluate for purposeful and symmetrical movements of arms, legs, and face.
      ii. Abnormal flexion or extension movements of the arms or legs are an ominous sign and reflect loss of brain control, with reversion to more primitive brain reflex activities and control.
   c. **Eye movements**
      i. Evaluate for eye opening and pupillary responses and their symmetry.
      ii. Particularly note progressively dilating pupil in accompaniment with deterioration of level of consciousness.
   d. **Respirations**
      i. Evaluate depth, pattern, and ease of breathing.
      ii. Irregular breathing patterns may indicate severe brain or brainstem injuries.

**TABLE 1.** The Glasgow Coma Scale

| Eye Opening (E) | Motor Response (M) | Verbal Response (V) |
|---|---|---|
| | Glasgow Coma Scale = E + M + V | |
| Spontaneous – 4 | Obeys commands – 6 | Oriented – 5 |
| To speech – 3 | Localizes painful stimuli – 5 | Confused conversation – 4 |
| To pain – 2 | Withdraws from painful stimuli – 4 | Inappropriate words – 3 |
| No response – 1 | Abnormal flexion response (decortication) – 3 | Incomprehensible sounds – 2 |
| | Abnormal extensor response (decerebration) – 2 | No response – 1 |
| | No reseponse – 1 | |

**TABLE 2.** Prognostic Value of the Glasgow Coma Scale

| Glasgow Coma Scale Score | Percentage of Patients Dead or Vegetative State |
|---|---|
| 3–4 | 80% |
| 5–7 | 54% |
| 8–10 | 27% |
| 11–15 | 6% |

   e. **Glasgow Coma Scale** (Tables 1 and 2)
      i. The Glasgow Coma Scale is used to quantitate the initial findings of the neurologic examination. Scores are given for the patient's eye opening, motor function, and response to verbal communication. These scores are then added, according to the values of the scale (Table 1), and may then be useful in predicting neurologic outcome (Table 2).
   f. **Signs and symptoms that demand emergency evaluation include:**
      i. Increasing headache
      ii. Persistent nausea or vomiting
      iii. Progressive or continued impairment of consciousness
      iv. Seizures
      v. Pupillary inequality
      vi. Inequality or deficiency of motor activity
      vii. Alteration of ventilation patterns.

B. **Neck**
   1. **History:** Normal mental function should allow detailed history about the presence or absence of limb tingling, weakness, or neck pain. Any of these complaints may be an indication of an underlying fracture or ligamentous injury in an otherwise neurologically normal patient. Any athlete who complains of or exhibits weakness or altered sensation in his/her arms and legs, or who has sustained a head injury and is not awake and alert, must be presumed to have an unstable neck injury until proven otherwise by x-ray examination and/or subsequent physical examination.
   2. **Physical examination:** Examination should include detailed testing of motor, sensory, and reflex systems of both arms and legs, as well as the skin and soft tissue structures.
      a. **Lacerations:** may be accompanied by cranial nerve, blood vessel (carotid artery, jugular vein), airway (trachea), or swallowing tube (esophagus) injuries.
      b. **Deviation of the trachea** to one side may indicate a chest injury with a collapsed lung (pneumothorax).
      c. **Spinal tenderness or pain:** An awake or alert athlete with a head or neck injury may describe pain voluntarily. Alternatively, pain may be elicited by palpation of the spinous processes of the cervical spine.

d. **Range of motion:** If the patient does not exhibit historical or physical findings reflecting neck or spinal cord injury, neck range of motion may be evaluated. The athlete himself should actively perform flexion, extension, and rotation movements without assistance from medical personnel. If pain or paresthesia should occur, a neck injury must be considered and further neurologic evaluation deferred to the appropriate facility and physician.

II. **Specific Injuries**

A. **Head**

1. **Scalp lacerations, abrasions**

   a. Definition: includes abrasions, contusions, hematomas, and lacerations of the face and scalp.

   b. Clinical findings: Significant scalp lacerations should be inspected carefully for persistent bleeding, foreign bodies, or signs of underlying skull fracture.

   c. Treatment: Abrasions and contusions can be treated with gentle cleansing, topical antibiotics, and cold compresses. Lacerations should be shaved and cleansed thoroughly, and closed in a single-layer using sterile suture and technique. Devascularized material should be excised prior to closure.

2. **Skull fracture**

   a. **Definition:** Skull fractures may be described as **linear** (in a line), **comminuted** (in multiple pieces), or **depressed** (fragment in-driven toward brain). Any skull fracture that communicates with a scalp laceration, a sinus, or the middle ear is called a **compound** fracture. **Basilar** skull fractures involve the skull base.

   b. **Clinical findings:** All scalp lacerations should be investigated for underlying evidence of fracture of the cranial vault, for depression of bone fragments, or for the leakage of spinal fluid. Certain types of fractures may predispose to the development of an intracranial hematoma or to infections of the nervous system (meningitis). Bruises or bleeding in certain areas such as behind the ear, in the ear canal, or around the eye suggests a basilar skull fracture. Blood or spinal fluid exiting from the ear (otorrhea) or nose (rhinorrhea) also occur with basilar fractures. Hearing loss, lack of smell, or facial paralysis may develop from these fractures due to damage to nerves as they penetrate the skull base.

   c. **Treatment: Closed skull fractures** usually require observation only, especially when the neurological status is normal. **Compound fractures** often require thorough debridement in the operating room. **Compound depressed skull fractures** are always treated surgically with wide debridement and elevation of the bone fragment. Prophylactic antibiotics and anticonvulsant medicines are often given to patients with depressed skull fractures.

   Athletes with **basilar skull fractures** are usually admitted for observation, as they often will have accompanying spinal fluid leakage. This leakage may require craniotomy to seal the defect. Plain x-rays and CT scans of the head are usually indicated in any patient in whom a skull fracture or significant brain injury is suspected.

3. **Brain injuries**

   a. **Concussion**

      i. **Definition:** a clinical syndrome characterized by immediate and transient impairment of neurologic function, such as alteration of consciousness, disturbance of vision, equilibrium, etc., due to mechanical forces upon the brain. Concussions are usually graded based on the length of mental impairment and the loss of memory before and after the injury.

ii. **Clinical findings: The characteristic feature of a concussion is total return of neurologic normality without subsequent deterioration.** Examination should include complete mental status assessment, especially focusing on memory and orientation. The gait should also be tested.

iii. **Treatment:** In mild concussions, no loss of consciousness may be observed, and observation only is indicated. Increasingly long periods of impairment of consciousness may necessitate hospitalization and CT scanning. CT scan should always be normal following uncomplicated concussion.

Individuals may develop **a postconcussive syndrome,** with complaints of persistent headache, concentration difficulty, irritability, and depression. Improvement will occur with time, and there is no specific therapy for the syndrome.

Any athlete with amnesia should generally not be allowed to return to the athletic activity on that particular day.

b. **Contusions**

i. **Definition:** While concussion implies that the brain has not been structurally injured, a contusion implies a more extensive injury, with **actual "bruising" of the brain.**

ii. **Clinical findings:** Individuals suffering prolonged "concussions" or neurological deficits often have contused their brain. **CT scan demonstrates small foci of blood within the brain,** usually directly beneath the injured scalp and skull area.

iii. **Treatment:** Usually do not require surgical decompression unless brain edema is large. A higher incidence of prolonged or persistent neurologic deficit or seizures follows this type of injury.

c. **Hematomas**

i. **Epidural hematoma**

(a) **Definition:** a collection of blood between the skull and the dural membranes covering the brain. **Eighty-five percent are due to an injury of the middle meningeal artery.** This vessel travels in a groove in the temporal and frontal areas of the skull. Some skull fractures traverse this groove, simultaneously tearing the artery.

(b) **Clinical findings:** The classic history originates with a mild head injury that produces a skull fracture and a brief period of unconsciousness. After awakening from the concussion phase of the injury, the athlete then progressively returns to coma. **Time span between the lucid interval and coma is usually short (hours),** due to the high-pressure bleeding from the arterial injury. The declining level of consciousness may soon be followed by dilation of the pupil, paralysis, and death.

(c) **Treatment:** These lesions have very high morbidity and mortality rates if untreated. They are easily diagnosed by CT scanning. **Prompt surgical evacuation usually prevents permanent neurologic injury.**

ii. **Subdural hematomas**

(a) **Definition:** blood collections beneath the skull and outside the brain that arise between the arachnoid membrane and the dura, in the subdural space.

(b) **Clinical findings:** Subdural hematomas may present in a variety of fashions. When alert, individuals will usually complain of headaches. There is often immediate or progressive decline of consciousness, with eventual coma or death if untreated. There are three types, depending on the time in which the participant presents relative to the inciting injury.

   (i) **Acute subdural hematoma:** Blood clot generally accompanies simultaneous brain injury. Blood accumulates rapidly at the time of injury, and, together with the associated brain injury, produces immediate neurologic dysfunction.

   (ii) **Subacute hematomas:** present 24 hours or more after the head injury. The brain has usually not been injured substantially by the accident; otherwise, the hematoma would have been identified earlier.

   (iii) **Chronic subdural hematomas:** presents 2 or more weeks after the original injury: most often seen in the elderly, partially due to atrophy of the brain with aging.

(c) **Treatment:** CT scanning readily provides a diagnosis in acute and chronic types. Once identified, such lesions invariably require **surgical drainage.** Acute subdural hematomas often have a much poorer prognosis because of the associated high-velocity brain injury. Chronic hematomas are usually quite responsive to treatment without associated or prolonged brain dysfunction.

iii. **Intracerebral hematomas**

(a) **Definition:** bleeding within the brain substance itself.

(b) **Clinical course:** similar to cerebral contusions but often more severe because of the larger hematoma size.

(c) **Treatment:** Often requires surgical evacuation to reduce intracranial pressure. Readily diagnosed by CT scan.

4. **Vascular injuries**

   a. **Dissecting aneurysms:**

   i. **Definition: Direct blows or severe neck stretching or turning may injure the carotid artery, which may lead to hemorrhage into the wall of that vessel.** The lumen of the artery may become narrowed and subsequently occlude or discharge blood clots upward toward the brain.

   ii. **Clinical findings:** May present with sudden neurologic deficits such as unilateral paralysis, loss of speech, etc., suggesting stroke. Prior to these signs, aneurysm may cause unilateral headache or mild drooping of one eyelid, due to partial injury of nerves surrounding the carotid artery.

   iii. **Treatment: CT scans are often normal initially but will show the stroke eventually. Cerebral arteriography is required to establish the diagnosis.** Anticoagulation is usually successful in preventing neurological complications until the artery has time to heal.

   b. **Carotid cavernous fistula**

   i. **Definition:** Injury to the carotid artery in the skull, often in association with basilar skull fracture, in which the injured vessel actually ruptures into the surrounding venous structure (the cavernous sinus).

   ii. **Clinical findings:** The venous system within the cavernous sinus becomes filled with high-pressure arterialized blood, which then drains into the orbit, producing orbital swelling, double vision (diplopia), visual failure, and facial pain. Dramatic enlargement and redness of the conjunctiva, paralysis of eye movement, and pulsations of the eye are often evident.

   iii. **Treatment:** Diagnosis requires **arteriography** to confirm the presence of the arterial injury. The artery-vein connection (fistula) must be eliminated to cure this lesion, which can often be accomplished without open surgical intervention.

B. **Specific neck injuries**
  1. **Myofascial sprain**
      a. **Definition:** Injury (tearing) of the muscle and ligamentous components of the neck.
      b. **Clinical findings:** Sprains are the most common from of neck injuries. Mechanisms of injury include flexion, extension, compression, rotation, or combinations of these motions. Symptoms include pain and decreased range of motion of the neck in all planes of movement. Paraspinous muscle spasms may be evident, and pain may radiate into the intrascapular area. There is absence of neurologic dysfunction such as numbness or weakness. Differential diagnosis includes cervical spine instability, mild nerve root compressive syndromes, cervical arthritis, fibromyositis, etc.
      c. **Treatment:** X-ray studies often reveal normal or straightened alignment without evidence of fracture or dislocation. Therapy is conservative and usually involves nonsteroidal anti-inflammatory drugs, muscle relaxants, and cervical immobilization with a cervical collar.
  2. **Herniated nucleus pulposus** (ruptured discs, herniated discs, "slipped" disc)
      a. **Definition:** extrusion of the center of the disc (nucleus pulposus) through a tear in the fibrous outer coverings of the disc (annulus fibrosus), with subsequent nerve root and/or spinal cord compression.
      b. **Clinical findings:**
          i. **Mechanisms** include cervical compression, axial loading, and hyperflexion injuries. Predisposing factors may include a history of repetitive minor neck injuries or axial loading forces, as is often seen in competitive divers, down-linemen, and wrestlers.
          ii. **History:** Presenting complaints include sharp neck pain with radiation into an upper extremity. The pain is often exacerbated by Valsalva maneuvers (breath-holding, straining, or coughing) and neck movement. There may be associated numbness, weakness, and parasthesiae in a dermatomal (nerve) distribution into the arm. In severe cases, there may be complete loss of motor function below the level of the injury, including arm and leg paralysis, loss of bladder, bowel, or sexual function. Spurling's maneuver (turning the head with the neck extended) often reproduces sharp radicular pain into the affected extremity in the distribution of the compressed nerve root. Babinski's signs (upgoing toes when the plantar surface of the foot is stroked) are often present if the spinal cord is compressed.
          iii. **Physical examination:** Reveals decreased range of motion of the neck, paraspinous muscle spasms, and neurological deficits, including weakness, numbness, and reflex changes compatible with the nerve root affected (Table 3).
          iv. **Differential diagnosis** includes nerve root tumors, nerve root compression from cervical arthritis or fracture, and brachial plexus injuries.

**TABLE 3.** Neurologic Deficits with Cervical or Nerve Root Injuries (From Fractures, Disc Ruptures, etc.)

| Disc Space | Nerve Root Affected | Distribution of Motor Deficit | Sensory Abnormalities (Usually Numbness) | Reflex Abnormalities |
|---|---|---|---|---|
| C4–5 | C5 | Deltoid | Lateral aspect of shoulder | None |
| C5–6 | C6 | Biceps | Thumb | Biceps |
| C6–7 | C7 | Triceps | Middle finger | Triceps |

c. **Treatment:** Cervical spine films may reveal disc space narrowing, but are usually normal. MRI, CT scan, or myelography is often required to demonstrate the neural compression by the bulging and displaced disc fragment. EMG studies may demonstrate nerve root irritability.

Therapy includes cervical collar and traction, in combination with nonsteroidal anti-inflammatory drugs, pain medicines, and muscle relaxants. Surgery may be indicated when symptoms persist or progress despite conservative measures, or in the presence of major neurologic deficits. An anterior cervical fusion is often the treatment of choice, with postoperative collar immobilization.

3. **Spinal stenosis**
   a. **Definition:** narrowing of the cervical spinal canal; may predispose athlete to spinal cord or nerve injury after relatively minor trauma.
   b. **Clinical findings:** often asymptomatic until direct blow to forehead (forced hyperextension) or occiput (hyperflexion) produces neurologic signs. The narrowed spinal canal diameter restricts the spinal cord's ability to decompress itself. Wrinkling of the ligaments within the canal (ligamentum flavum), bone spurs (osteophytes) due to athletic-related injuries, or congenital narrowing may contribute to compromised canal diameter.

      Athletes may develop immediate quadriparesis, with arm weakness greater than leg weakness, secondary to contusion (bruising) of the central portion of the spinal cord (central cord syndrome). Milder cases may produce "burning" of one or both hands, allowing diagnostic confusion with burners or stingers secondary to brachial plexus stretch (see section below).
   c. **Treatment:** X-rays will show the narrowing of the cervical spine canal and may also define any arthritic changes and bone spur formation. Treatment initially consists of observation, as most patients improve without surgery. Steroids may be of benefit to reduce spinal cord swelling. Some patients may require anterior cervical fusion and removal of the osteophyte, or laminectomy to decompress a congenitally narrow cervical spinal canal.

4. **Cervical instability**
   a. **Ligamentous instability**
      i. **Definition:** Injury and disruption of the ligaments (anterior and posterior longitudinal ligament, intraspinous ligament, etc.) supporting the vertebral bodies. May occur with or without associated cervical fractures. May result in dislocations without associated fractures, causing catastrophic neurologic injury.
      ii. **Clinical findings:** the most common complaint is neck pain, usually exacerbated by neck extension or flexion. The neurological examination may initially be normal. Whether associated with fractures, ligamentous injuries can lead to varying degrees of neurologic dysfunction, ranging from mild weakness to complete quadraplegia.
      iii. **Treatment:** X-rays should be obtained in all athletes with complaints of significant neck pain. If x-rays do not reveal bony abnormalities, flexion and extension films must be obtained. These are best done by having the athlete himself perform these maneuvers in an active fashion. Pain or paresthesiae will usually limit neck motion and forewarn of any potential neurologic damage.

         Patients with mental status changes may also have ligamentous injuries. In this situation, the neck must be immobilized with a cervical collar, with postponement of flexion/extension films until the mental examination has returned to normal. **Flexion/extension films should**

never be performed when routine spine films show evidence of severe
trauma with subluxation, locked facets, etc.

In cases of cervical dislocation or neurologic deficit, the spine must be
reduced and stabilized. Cervical tongs should be applied to distract the
vertebrae into their normal position and to maintain their alignment
thereafter. Surgical therapy may be required to maintain and insure proper
future neck position. Myelography, MRI, and CT scanning are useful in
defining the extent of the injury to the spinal cord and nerve roots.

5. **Fractures**
   a. **Definition:** Injury to the bony components of the spine, usually resulting in
      compression of the vertebral bodies. These injuries may be classified as **stable**
      (integrity of spine still preserved) or **unstable)** (excess movement between
      adjacent osseous elements).
   b. **Clinical findings**—same as for cervical instability.
   c. **Treatment**—same as for cervical instability. Should be managed as if
      potential for spinal cord injury is present (see next section).

6. **Acute spinal cord injury management: A conscious athlete who complains of
   neck pain, numbness, or weakness should be treated as if he/she harbors an
   underlying unstable spinal injury. Any unconscious participant should be
   considered to have a potential spinal cord injury until proven otherwise.**

   **In moving such athletes, it is imperative to stabilize the cervical spine.** If
   possible, a hard collar should be placed prior to initial movement. One person
   in charge should be assigned the task of immobilizing the head and neck, while
   at least four others take care of the trunk and other body parts (Fig. 1). All
   obstructive elements to the face such as face guards should be removed, but the
   helmet should be left on during transport. Large bolt cutters should be available
   to cut away all obstructive athletic gear.
   a. Acute spinal cord injury transport on the field.[1]
      i. At least four, but better five or six, people should be assembled for the
         transport team.
      ii. One person should be in charge and should be positioned at the head of
          the injured athlete to call the moves.
      iii. The person in charge should control the head and shoulders by cradling
           the head between his forearms, clasping the trapezius, clavicle, and
           scapula if possible, or the inside of the shoulder pads and the trapezius.

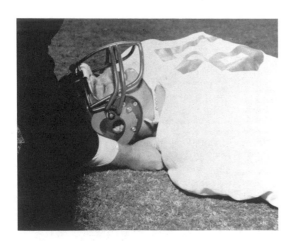

**FIGURE 1.** The method of immobilizing the head to the trunk. The
person in charge holds the
trapezius-clavicle-scapula area
with his hands and holds the head
between his forearms. (From Watkins RG, et al: Cervical spine injuries
in football players. Spine State Art
Rev 4(2):391–408, 1990, with permission.)

     iv. An additional person on the transport team can help to support and fix the head to the chief's forearms during the move.

     v. Other members of the team should be positioned one on each side of the shoulders and one on each side of the waist, and if available a member should support the legs and feet.

     vi. At the direction of the person in charge, the members of the team should reach under the athlete, clasp hands, and lift the injured athlete in unison onto the back board.

  b. Intubation

If the athlete is seriously injured and requires intubation, care must be taken not to hyperextend the cervical spine. Airway and circulatory systems must be stable before he can be safely transported.

  c. Prone position ("log roll")

If the athlete is initially injured in the prone position, he should be log-rolled and placed in the supine position (Fig. 2), followed by placement of the collar. Rolling onto a long spine board should be done whenever possible, so that immobilization of the entire spine may be accomplished.

  d. Immobilization

Most emergency transport teams have spinal boards equipped with cervical/head immobilizing units. If none is available, sand bags or other weights may be placed on either side of the head.

After cervical immobilization, the athlete should be transferred to an appropriate neurosurgical facility as soon as possible. Haste should never be sought at the expense of excellent immobilization.

7. **Brachial plexus injuries ("burners," "stingers")**

  a. **Definition:** Stretch-injury to the nerves of the upper extremity, caused by forceful downward distraction of the shoulder while the head is distracted to the opposite side.

  b. **Clinical findings:** Immediately after impact, the athlete complains of burning pain radiating into one arm and hand. The injury usually affects the upper trunk of the brachial plexus, with sensory loss or paresthesia into the thumb and index finger, and motor loss of the deltoid, spinati, and bicep muscles. The pain typically resolves in seconds or minutes. More severe or repetitive injuries may lead to persistent or permanent neurologic deficits.

  c. **Treatment:** no further contact until symptoms completely resolved. Atypical cases or mechanisms must be differentiated from cervical spine injury.

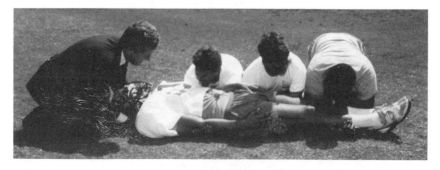

**FIGURE 2.** Multiman carry. The chief immobilizes the head and neck and calls the signals. Three men on each side of the body (the three on the near side are not pictured) join hands and lift. The spine board is introduced underneath. (From Watkins RG, et al: Cervical spine injuries in football players. Spine State Art Rev 4(2):391–408, 1990, with permission.)

## REFERENCES

1. Watkins RG, Dillin WH, Maxwell J: Cervical spine injuries in football players. Spine: State Art Rev 4:391–408, 1990.
2. Cloward RB: Acute cervical spine injuries. Clin Symp 32:1, 1980.
3. Committee on Head Injury Nomenclature of the Congress of Neurological Surgeons: Glossary of head injury including some definitions of injury of the cervical spine. Clin Neurosurg 12:388, 1966.
4. Friedman WA: Head injuries. Clin Symp 35:4, 1983.
5. Maroon JC: Burning hands in football spinal cord injuries. JAMA 238:2049–2051, 1977.
6. Schneider RC: Head and Neck Injuries in Football: Mechanisms, Treatment and Prevention. Baltimore, Williams & Wilkins, 1973.
7. Schneider RC, Kennedy JC, Plant ML: Sports Injuries: Mechanisms, Prevention, and Treatment. Baltimore, Williams & Wilkins, 1985.
8. Shields CL Jr, Fox JM, Stauffer ES: Cervical cord injuries in sports. Phys Sportsmed 6:71, 1978.
9. Torg JS: Athletic Injuries to the Head, Neck, and Face. Philadelphia, Lea & Febiger, 1982.
10. Vegso JJ, Bryant MH, Torg JS: Field evaluation of head and neck injuries. In Torg JS (ed): Athletic Injuries to the Head, Neck, and Face. Philadelphia, Lea & Febiger, 1982, pp 39–52.

# Chapter 32: Eye Injuries in Sports: Evaluation, Management, and Prevention

GERALD R. CHRISTENSEN, MD

I. **Introduction:** Eye injuries occur in all sports and in all age groups for which data are collected in North America.

A. **Incidence of sports eye injuries**

   About 1.5% of all selected sports injuries involve the eye or ocular adnexa and almost all are preventable. Baseball and basketball are the leading causes of eye injuries. However, as a percentage of total sports injuries, the highest incidences of eye injuries occur in racquet sports, soccer, swimming, and boxing. Of all sports eye injuries, 30% to 40% seen by ophthalmologist are associated with racquet sports.

   The mechanisms of sports eye injuries are varied, including lacerations from sharp flying objects and shattered protective eye wear; blunt trauma to the globe, orbit, or head; and exposure to radiant (ultraviolet) energy.

B. **Certification of the athlete for participation**

   This involves evaluating the athlete for eye injury risk factors in his/her particular sport.

   1. **General considerations:** Ideally, the athlete should have a visual acuity of 20/20 or better in each eye, either unaided or with modest correction.

      a. **Visual risk factors:** These include a best corrected visual acuity of less than 20/40 in either eye and/or a spectacle correction for myopia or hyperopia that is greater than six diopters. The disability from high corrective spectacle lenses can sometimes be mitigated by contact lenses; however, contact lenses themselves can be a risk factor. **Contact lenses should never be used as a substitute for an eye protective device.**

      b. **Anatomical risk factors** refer to diseases, degenerations, or structural weakness of the eye itself. This includes myopia greater than six diopters, thin sclera, history of retinal degenerative disease, and any history of previous eye surgery that weakens the coats of the eye, especially cataract or refractive surgery. **Athletes with such risk factors should be evaluated by an ophthalmologist prior to engaging in high- or extremely high-risk sports.**

   2. **Special considerations** need to be given to the one-eyed athlete, a person with visual acuity in the fellow eye of 20/200 or less. He/she should be evaluated by an ophthalmologist before deciding to participate in a particular sport. In most cases where there is loss of one paired organ, collision and contact sports are not recommended; however, many one-eyed athletes can safely participate in some of these activities. Conversely, most noncontact racquet sports are not recommended for anyone without adequate eye protection.

   3. **Routine visual testing:** Visual acuity should be measured periodically and reported to the team physician. Testing for distance visual acuity is done with a Snellen card or a commercial vision tester with the distance correction in place and each eye measured separately. Anyone testing less than 20/40 in either eye should be referred to an ophthalmologist.

## II. Examination of the Injured Eye

### A. History

1. **Types of injury:** The history is most important in order to determine the exact mechanism of injury. This is necessary in evaluating the injury itself and also for developing protective gear and gathering statistical data regarding particular sports and their hazards.

2. **Signs and symptoms:** Inquiry should be made regarding specific ocular complaints that might have particular diagnostic significance relative to eye injury. These include red eye, pain, decreased vision, diplopia, flashing lights, and a past history of eye disease or surgery.

### B. Gross inspection: Many eye injuries in sports are contusions or lacerations, conditions that distort the gross appearance of the normal anatomy.

1. **Eyelids and orbit:** Evaluate for symmetry between the two sides and especially look for ptosis of the upper eyelid or proptosis of the globe on the injured side. Ecchymosis of the eyelids and subconjunctival hemorrhage is frequently associated with orbital hemorrhages and proptosis.

2. **Cornea and sclera:** Examine carefully for signs of perforation and rupture indicated by darkly pigmented uveal tissue presenting through a laceration. These injuries can result in distortion of the pupil and other asymmetries of the iris. Always apply fluorescein stain to identify superficial corneal epithelial defects.

3. **Anterior chamber:** Look carefully for signs of microscopic bleeding or hyphema. When present, blood will generally be found layered out in the anterior chamber angle inferiorly, forming a crescent of blood at the 6 o'clock position.

### C. Functional testing

1. **Visual acuity** is the single most important test in evaluating eye injuries. If formal materials for visual acuity testing are not available, vision can be evaluated with any reproducible object such as printed material, fingers, or lights. Visual acuity testing is done with the distance correction in place and for each eye separately. Decreased visual acuity suggests a variety of disorders, including disruption of the refractive surfaces of the eye such as seen in corneal or lens injury, clouding of the ocular media, or injury to the retina or optic nerve.

2. **Extraocular muscle balance** is tested with a penlight to determine if the eyes are in parallel alignment. This is determined when the pupillary light reflex falls on corresponding areas of both corneas. Muscle function is tested in both eyes simultaneously, having the patient look to gaze right; gaze left; gaze up and right; gaze up and left; gaze down and right; and gaze down and left. Any suggestion of restriction of movement or report of diplopia suggests the possibility of an injury to the soft tissue of the orbit or interference of extraocular muscle function from paresis or entrapment. Failure of the eyelids to open or close normally suggests the possibility of a motor nerve deficit or soft tissue injury.

3. **Sensory nerve testing.** Especially in cases of blunt trauma involving the orbit, always test the sensory nerve functions throughout the distribution of the maxillary branch of the trigeminal nerve ($V^2$). Orbital floor fractures frequently disrupt this nerve, producing hypesthesia on the surface of the face.

4. **Pupillary testing:** Generally the pupil should be round, symmetrical, and react to direct and consensual light. Pupillary paresis following blunt injury to the globe is not uncommon and presents as a sluggish response to any stimulation. A pupillary reflex that is reduced to direct but not consensual light is suggestive of an injury involving the retina or optic nerve (Marcus-Gunn pupil).

5. **Intraocular pressure:** Intraocular pressure is best tested with the Schiotz tonometer; however, it its absence, pressure can be estimated by palpating the globe and using the palpated tension in the fellow eye for comparison. Care should be taken to avoid compression of a ruptured or perforated globe by this test. Intraocular pressure may be elevated with hemorrhage or swelling of the orbital contents and may be decreased in certain cases of blunt injury to the globe.

D. **Funduscopic examination:** This can be done with any device that is designed to pass a light beam through the length of the eye and focus on the surface of the retina and optic nerve disc.

1. **Assessment of the media:** Clear ocular media are necessary to produce the normal red reflex pattern seen when directing an ophthalmoscope light through the pupil. The reflex depends on a normal transparent cornea and lens, with smooth unblemished surfaces and clear aqueous and vitreous humor. Wrinkling of the cornea or defects on its surface and subluxation of the lens will interfere with this normal phenomenon. Even modest bleeding into the ocular media can alter or obscure the red reflex, and on occasion this may be the only sign of occult rupture of the globe.

2. **Fundus anatomy:** The normal image from the posterior pole of the eye, as seen with the ophthalmoscope, consists of the diffuse choroidal microcirculation viewed through the normally transparent retinal tissue. Retinal edema resulting from any interruption of circulatory dynamics will produce a loss of retinal transparency and an obscuration of background choroidal circulation. Such changes not only alter the intensity of the red reflex but obliterate the image detail of the choroid. Retinal edema occurs in contusion injuries to the globe and is also seen in retinal detachments from any of a variety of mechanisms.

III. **Sports Injuries**

A. **Abrasion:** Abrasion is the result of a loss of surface epithelium and is most significant when it occurs on the cornea. The cornea must maintain a smooth mirror-like anterior surface, utilizing its epithelial layers, in order to function as an optical-quality refracting surface. Disruption of this smooth surface near the central visual axis will interfere with the visual acuity.

1. **Signs and symptoms** are pain, photophobia, conjunctival injection, tearing (epiphora), and decreased visual acuity if the central corneal area is involved.

2. **Examination:** Fluorescein solution stains denuded and devitalized areas. In some cases a topical anesthetic may be necessary to facilitate examination, and additional ocular injury must be ruled out.

3. **Treatment:** Healing is best facilitated by the management of pain and discomfort and controlling lid movement. Postinjury infection is uncommon; however, topical antibiotics may be useful in some cases. Patching, if adequate to prevent movement of the eyelids, will generally be sufficient to manage the discomfort. In a large abrasion where there is significant pain and photophobia, a topical cycloplegic drug such as 2% homatropine is helpful and can be applied before patching. Generally, avoid topical corticosteroid preparations except in extreme cases.

4. **Prognosis:** Uncomplicated corneal epithelial injuries will heal completely within 24 to 48 hours without scarring. Even though frequently contaminated they rarely become infected. **Chronic use of topical anesthetics for pain management will interfere with corneal re-epithelialization and is absolutely contraindicated.** Topical steroids may enhance corneal fungal and viral infections and consequently

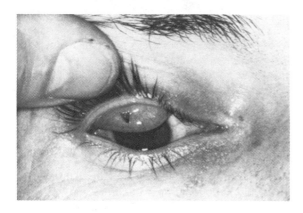

**FIGURE 1.** Foreign body in the upper tarsal conjunctiva. (From Tucker W: Ophthalmic emergencies. Office Procedures State Art Rev 1(1):106, 1986, with permission.)

should be used with extreme caution. Recurrent epithelial erosion is occasionally a complication from abrasion injuries, and the patient needs to be advised that this difficulty may occur.

B. **Foreign body**
   1. **Signs and symptoms:** Same as for abrasions.
   2. Examination: Injuries with tiny foreign bodies may require magnification to be properly visualized and removed. In the cornea, their localization can be enhanced by fluorescein stain, and the use of topical anesthetic may be necessary to facilitate the examination. In addition, both upper and lower conjunctival fornices should be examined carefully for the presence of foreign body. The upper eyelid should be everted and the conjunctival surface over the tarsal surface specifically inspected for the presence of foreign body (Fig. 1).
   3. **Treatment:** For corneal foreign bodies, apply a short-acting topical anesthetic and remove the foreign material with a cotton tip applicator or disposable hypodermic needle. Rust rings, if present, should be removed as well (Fig. 2). Successful removal of a foreign body converts the injury into an abrasion, which is then subsequently treated as described in III.A.
   4. **Prognosis:** Same as for corneal abrasion. In cases with minimal epithelial defects, patching may not be necessary.

C. **Lacerations:** Lacerations may occur in association with blunt trauma as well as from sharp objects, and can result from the propulsion and shattering of eye protective equipment.

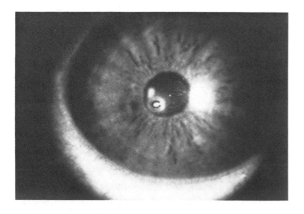

**FIGURE 2.** Corneal foreign body surrounded by a rust ring. (From Tucker W: Office Procedures State Art Review, 1986, with permission.)

1. **Eyelids**
   a. **Signs and symptoms:** Swelling, hemorrhage, and anatomical disruption of the lids. However, the damage may be subtle and the appearance normal.
   b. **Examination** includes evaluation of the normal anatomical relationship of the lid margins and front surface of the globe, as well as the symmetry with the uninjured side. Opening and closing function are assessed specifically, especially to verify that the lids can be spontaneously closed. Specific attention needs to be directed to rule out the possibility of upper-lid ptosis and lacerations in the lacrimal drainage system. In addition, the globe must be thoroughly inspected for signs of damage.
   c. **Treatment:** Lacerations require individual suturing of the lid tissue layers and additional specific repairs to injuries involving the integrity of the lacrimal drainage apparatus.
   d. **Prognosis:** Because of a rich vascular supply to the eyelids, healing is rapid and deformities are minimal in cases where there is minimal tissue loss and good anatomical approximation.
2. **Globe**
   a. **Signs and symptoms:** Decreased visual acuity, pain, discomfort, distortion or displacement of the pupil, and loss of the fundus red reflex of the fundus.
   b. **Examination:** Evaluate the anterior segment of the globe for signs of **subconjunctival hemorrhage.** The pupil should be round, central, and symmetrical with the fellow eye. **Lacerations of the cornea** frequently incarcerate iris tissue, causing distortion and displacement of the pupil (Fig. 3). **Scleral lacerations** also may displace the location of the pupil due to herniations of the uveal tract through the defect. **Prolapsed uveal tissue** presents as a dark brown or black mass, even in fair-complected, blue-eyed individuals. **Lacerations of the globe** that extend to involve the lens zonules may result in subluxation of the crystalline lens. **Intraocular bleeding** is also a frequent complications, causing obscuration of the ocular media and loss of the red fundus reflex. The intraocular pressure may be decreased; however, many lacerations are self-sealing and pressure levels can vary.
   c. **Treatment:** Once a lacerated glove is suspected, manipulation should be minimized. The patient needs to be transported to the care of an ophthalmologist, taking care to avoid further injury to the eye. The patient should be moved in either the supine or upright position (avoid a prone or head-down position) with the eye protected by a rigid ocular shield (Fig. 4). If necessary, a makeshift ocular shield can be fashioned from a disposable

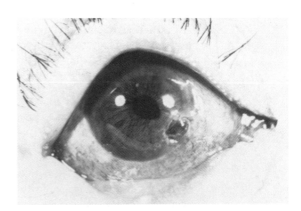

**FIGURE 3.** Corneal laceration with prolapsed iris and irregular pupil. (From Tucker W: Office Procedures State Art Rev, 1986, with permission.)

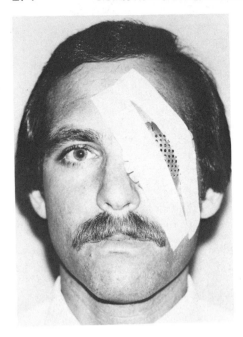

**FIGURE 4.** Protective metal shield. (From Tucker W: Office Procedures. State Art Rev, 1986, with permission.)

drinking cup. Repair is accomplished by reapproximation of the laceration and surgical clearing of any opacity of the ocular media.

   d. **Prognosis:** The prognosis is generally guarded but varies with the location and severity of the injury. Injuries of the cornea and limbus can produce an irregular astigmatism as a result of healing contractures. A loss of corneal transparency may also occur in the area of scarring. Injuries involving the lens will generally produce a cataract, which often can be managed in the usual surgical fashion. Lacerations involving areas posterior to the ciliary body have a much more guarded prognosis, often necessitating complex surgical procedures and frequently a poor visual result.

D. **Contusion injuries:** Blunt or contusion injuries to the globe are the most common sports injury to the eye and may be associated with abrasions and lacerations. Contusion injuries result from facial blows directly to the orbital contents or from sudden pressure increases transmitted to the eye from the surrounding orbital tissue.

  1. **Orbit**

    a. **Orbital hemorrhage:** Edema and hemorrhage within the orbit frequently coexist with facial fractures and injuries to the globe. Uncomplicated orbital hemorrhage from blunt trauma is a result of extensive force to create such an injury. The resulting swelling of the orbital contents increases the tissue pressure surrounding the globe and forces the globe outward into a position of proptosis.

      i. **Signs and symptoms:** If the globe has escaped injury, the vision may be unaffected. Restrictions to ocular motility, if present, are frequently associated with diplopia, which can be demonstrated especially in extremes of gaze. Intraocular pressure may be increased, sometimes to levels that compromise retinal circulation, resulting in pulsation of the retinal arterioles at the optic nerve head. (Pulsation of the venules is not a diagnostic sign and is frequently a normal finding.) Proptosis, if present, can be associated with upper-lid retraction and inability to completely close the lid.

   ii. **Examination:** Record the visual acuity and conduct an inspection to rule out injury to the eyeball. Examine the binocular eye movements (versions) by observing both eyes simultaneously moving through the six cardinal positions of gaze (see II.C.2.). This examination is best accomplished with a small penlight. Look for loss of parallel alignment of the eyes during this maneuver, especially at extremes of gaze, and inquire as to the presence of diplopia. Test for proptosis (exophthalmos) by measuring the distance from the lateral edge of the orbit to a plane aligned with the apex of the cornea and compare this measurement with the uninjured side. Conduct appropriate studies to rule out orbital fracture.

   iii. **Treatment** is generally symptomatic, except in unusual circumstances of massive hemorrhage that may require surgical drainage or decompression. Rest and analgesics are indicated, and cold compresses may control further edema and bleeding.

   iv. **Prognosis**—good.

 b. **Orbital fracture (blowout fracture)**

   i. **Signs and symptoms**—Fracture injuries to the orbit most commonly involve the floor (roof of the maxillary sinus) and the medial wall (wall of the ethmoid sinus). The floor fractures are the most likely to be symptomatic. The triad suggesting orbital floor fractures consists of diplopia, obscured maxillary sinus cavity on x-ray, and hypesthesia of the face. Large fenestrated fractures of the floor allow the orbital contents to be displaced from the orbit into the maxillary sinus thereby causing the globe to be displaced posteriorly and downward. These injuries are frequently associated with significant bleeding into the maxillary sinus. Fractures of the orbital floor can interrupt the second branch of the trigeminal nerve ($V^2$) leading to hypesthesia where it innervates the face. Linear nonfenestrated fractures can cause tissue entrapment of orbital contents resulting in restricted motility of the globe especially in elevation. Such a situation results in a tethering of the globe to the orbital floor. Version testing will elicit diplopia which becomes worse (farther apart) on upward gaze. In nonfenestrated fractures proptosis rather than enophthalmos may be present if there is sufficient contusion with hemorrhage and edema.

   ii. **Examination:**—The visual acuity is recorded, followed by an examination of extraocular muscle function as described in II.C.2. With the eyes in the primary gaze position inspect the globe for evidence of retropositioning backwards into the orbit with displacement of the posterior pole of the globe inferiorly. This gives the appearance of the globe in a position of enophthalmos with the visual axis directed slightly upwards. Attempts to elevate both eyes by directing gaze further upwards will accentuate the misalignment if there is entrapment of the orbital tissue in a floor fracture. In the presence of enophthalmos of the globe there is a relative ptosis of the upper lid present. Maxillary nerve function is tested by comparing the sensation of light touch over the distribution of this nerve on both the normal and affected side. Appropriate radiologic studies may reveal clouding of the maxillary sinus cavity as well as actual fracture defects in the orbital floor on the injured side.

   iii. **Treatment**—Surgical repair of these injuries is directed toward restoring the normal topography of the orbital floor. This can be accomplished by mobilizing any tissue trapped within the fracture and replacing any defect in the orbital floor either by placing an explant underneath the periosteum of the orbital bones or by stabilizing the periosteum by filling the adjacent sinus cavities with temporary packing material. Surgical treatment is usually necessary only when there is an actual interruption or herniation of orbital tissue. Diplopia may be transient following these injuries so surgical intervention should be deferred until a significant portion of the contusion injury has resolved. Conversely, in cases with little contusion injury and obvious interruption or herniation of orbital tissue there is no need to delay definitive repair.

    iv. **Prognosis**—Will vary depending on the degree of injury. Obviously it is best when there is minimal orbital tissue damage. Prolonged tissue entrapment and inflammation can result in fibrosis and contractures which can lead to permanent functional disabilities.

2.  **Globe**—Contusions of the globe cause a sudden increase of intraocular pressure which can result in swelling, bleeding, tearing and displacement of the structures within the eye. Intraocular hemorrhage is an important sign that the eye has sustained significant injury and there is a high probability that damage to the eye has occurred. Management of intraocular hemorrhage depends upon the location and extent of the hemorrhage.

    a.  **Hyphema**—refers to the presence of blood in the anterior chambers and is an important diagnostic and prognostic sign (Fig. 5). Frequently, it occurs in microscopic quantities and, consequently, can be easily overlooked in a cursory examination. **Such bleeding indicates that there has been an intraocular injury of sufficient intensity to result in a vascular disruption. It is important that this situation be identified as delayed rebleeding from such injuries can occur which may be both massive and destructive.** Such rebleeds have been referred to as so called "eight-ball hemorrhages."

       i. **Signs and symptoms**—Since many hyphema are of small volume, the visual acuity may be unaffected by its presence. There may be only mild injection of the globe with moderate transient discomfort and photophobia. Gradually the blood will settle into the inferior angle of the anterior chamber forming a crescent shaped precipitate that can easily be overlooked unless examined for specifically. In addition to the hyphema other damages associated with contusion injuries may also be found. These include pupillary paralysis, pupillary contour irregularities as well as tearing of the uveal tract.

      ii. **Examination**—Unless the hyphema is of such quantity to occlude the pupillary axis the visual acuity may be relatively unchanged. Slit lamp

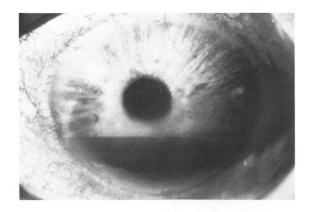

**FIGURE 5.** Layered hyphema due to trauma. (From Tucker W: Office Procedures Stat Art Rev, 1986, with permission.)

examination is necessary to identify turbid microscopic hyphema before it has had time to settle out inferiorly in the chamber angle.

  iii. **Treatment**—is directed toward the prevention of rebleeding. Hemostasis following the initial injury is due to formation of a fibrin clot within the lumen of the damaged vessel. **Physical activity should be severely restricted** and the use of anti-fibrinolytic drugs considered. Rebleeding, if it occurs, is most frequent during the first four days following injury.

  iv. **Prognosis**—Generally excellent, especially if the blood clears rapidly and there is no associated rebleeding or concurrent ocular damage.

     b. **Vitreous hemorrhage**—When it is due to trauma, requires significant force and is generally associated with additional injury to the eye.

       i. **Signs and symptoms**—Vitreous hemorrhage frequently arises from tearing of the retinal arterioles or the choroidal vasculature. The blood obscures the light path through the vitreous cavity of the eye and reduces the visual acuity. On ophthalmoscopic examination the fundus detail is blurred or disappears entirely and may be seen only as a "black reflex." Isolated vitreous bleeding is not associated with other symptoms such as pain or discomfort.

       ii. **Examination**—consists of measurement of the visual acuity and a careful funduscopic examination with emphasis on the red fundus reflex and clarity of fundus detail.

       iii. **Treatment**—is generally conservative. Severe cases may require surgical removal of the blood and vitreous. Such procedures are often being done at the time of repair of associated ocular injuries.

       iv. **Prognosis**—Guarded.

     c. **Retinal hemorrhages and edema** can occur as a result of direct trauma to the eye by transmission of the force to the retinal surface from a contusion injury to the globe. Occasionally, these same changes can be due to the retinal capillary instability seen in situations of violent exercise performed in conditions of decreased oxygen saturation. Elevated venous pressure from Valsalva maneuvers can also produce retinal edema and hemorrhages. Such findings have been documented in such activities such as mountain climbing and weight lifting.

       i. **Signs and symptoms:** It is not uncommon to have multiple areas of retinal hemorrhage and edema that are asymptomatic, especially if the affected areas are confined to the peripheral retina. Involvement with the macula will result in decreased visual acuity and/or a distortion of the visual perception of form (metamorphopsia).

       ii. **Examination:** Includes visual acuity measurement and testing for metamorphopsia with the Amsler grid. Ophthalmoscopic examination will reveal both the flame-shaped hemorrhages typically seen in the superficial retina, as well as the round-blot hemorrhages characteristic of those occurring within the deeper layers. Retinal edema results in a loss of retinal transparency, giving the appearance of an opacity within the retina that blocks the normal red fundus reflex.

       iii. **Treatment** is symptomatic.

       iv. **Prognosis** is variable, depending on the location, extent, and severity of the involvement.

     d. **Dislocated lens** is the result of tearing of the lens zonules, with loss of support for the lens in its normal position. Zonular injury confined to an isolated sector may result in a subluxation or a movement of the lens away from the site of the injury, causing the lens to de-center but otherwise to remain in a relatively normal position. More extensive damage may displace the lens entirely, causing it to fall into either the anterior or posterior chamber.

       i. **Signs and symptoms:** Visual acuity will be affected by even the slightest shift in the position of the crystalline lens. Lens decentration causes irregular astigmatism, and complete dislocation results in the condition of aphakia. In both cases, a different refractive correction is required to reestablish the visual acuity. Shifts of lens position, even though slight, can also cause a loss of iris stability and a resulting tremulousness to slight ocular movements or vibrations (iridodonesis). With significant subluxation the lens may be displaced to the extent that its edge (equator) may come to lie within the pupillary axis.

   ii. **Examination:** The visual acuity may be initially reduced but can frequently be corrected by a change in refraction, which may vary significantly from the previous correction. Slit-lamp examination may reveal iridodonesis, especially at the pupillary margins following rapid eye movement. Pupillary dilatation can aid in the assessment of the lens position.

   iii. **Treatment** is variable and may necessitate surgical removal of the lens.

   iv. **Prognosis** varies with the extent of the injury.

  e. **Chamber angle recession** refers to the appearance of a gross anatomical deepening of the chamber angle as a result of a laceration of the face of the ciliary body, followed by posterior displacement of the muscles of accommodation. This is generally a result of blunt trauma to the globe causing a sudden increase in pressure within the anterior chamber, which is transmitted to the lens—iris diaphragm, propelling it backwards. The dynamics of this injury are similar to that of lens dislocation; however, in angle recession the lens position is usually normal. Following a blow to the eye, the lens and iris together react in the same fashion as the diaphragm of a drum. The bowing posteriorly results in the angle damage. In a few cases, the force of the injury is sufficient to produce an associated injury to the trabecular meshwork that eventually leads to glaucoma.

   i. **Signs and symptoms:** In cases when there is development of glaucoma, the onset is almost invariably delayed from the time of the injury and progresses slowly. As with other forms of chronic glaucoma, visual loss is insidious, beginning with the peripheral areas of the visual field involved initially. Angle recession glaucoma should always be suspected in cases of **unilateral** chronic glaucoma.

   ii. **Examination** consists of the usual methods for evaluating chronic glaucoma. These include measurement of intraocular pressure and visual field examination, with special attention to the peripheral field defects commonly seen in chronic glaucoma.

   iii. **Treatment:** Angle recession glaucoma is frequently not responsive to the usual antiglaucomatous drugs and may require surgical treatment.

   iv. **Prognosis** varies with the extent of the pressure elevation, the length of time it has been present, and the responsiveness to treatment.

  f. **Retinal detachment** is the result of the development of holes or tears within the retinal tissue associated with areas of vitreous body degeneration, liquefaction, and traction. This allows a segment of the retina to separate from the underlying retinal pigment epithelium, producing an immediate loss of visual function within the detached segment. In the absence of treatment, the entire retina will eventually become involved, and a total retinal detachment will develop. Any form of blunt or perforating trauma can produce retinal detachment as well. Indirect trauma such as severe head injury, myopia, and vitreous traction are risk factors that can affect patients with certain predispositions for detachment.

   i. **Signs and symptoms:** Retinal detachment almost invariably begins at the retinal periphery and results in a positive scotoma (a blind spot perceived by the patient) at the edge of the visual field. As the detachment progresses, there may be physical stimulation to the retina, resulting in the visualization of "lightning flashes" or "flying sparks." The enlarging scotoma may be seen as a waving, black curtain encroaching on the central vision. If the macular area of the retina becomes involved, the central visual acuity will be markedly reduced.

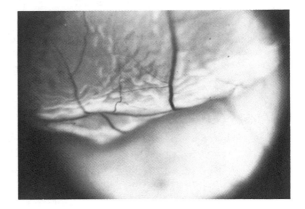

**FIGURE 6.** Retinal detachment. (From Tucker W: Office Procedures State Art Rev, 1986, with permission.)

ii. **Examination:** As areas of detached retina become elevated from the underlying retinal pigment epithelium, the retinal tissue undergoes a loss of transparency (Fig. 6). This results in the inability to visualize the normal underlying vascular pattern during the ophthalmoscope examination. As the retina becomes more elevated, it will be necessary to add additional convex or plus lenses to the ophthalmoscope viewing port in order to maintain a sharp focus on the internal surface in the detached areas. Since detachments begin in the far periphery, it is necessary to dilate the pupil widely in order to visualize the disorder during its early stages. Visual field defects will also be present in areas corresponding to the retinal detachment.

iii. **Treatment:** In cases when retinal holes or tears exist in the absence of detachment, cryosurgery and laser surgery may be adequate to seal the holes and prevent further progress of the disease. Surgical intervention is almost invariably necessary after actual separation of the retina has occurred.

iv. **Prognosis** depends on the extent of the involvement. The chance for recovery of good central vision is generally poor if the retina becomes detached in the area of the macula.

E. **Burns** associated with sports injuries are generally confined to **radiation exposure from sunlight.** Because of the additive effects of reflection from water surfaces and snow, they are most commonly seen in sports related to this environment. Ultraviolet radiation burns the conjunctiva and cornea surfaces in the same manner that it does the skin. The result is necrosis with loss of individual surface epithelial cells and burning injury to the underlying substantia propria (dermis).

1. **Signs and symptoms:** The most prominent signs of ocular burn by ultraviolet light are intense pain and photophobia that develop after a significant delay following exposure. The visual acuity may be somewhat reduced due to the roughening of the corneal epithelial surface. Fluorescein stain of the cornea reveals scattered areas of punctate epithelial defects on the surface. **Pain is intense and disproportionately severe in relation to the corneal epithelial involvement.** The relative amount of pain and the delay in the onset of symptoms from the time of exposure are classic signs for ultraviolet burn. Patients will also complain of intense photophobia.

2. **Examination:** The typical fluorescein staining pattern, intense pain, photophobia, and history of exposure with delay of onset of symptoms confirm this diagnosis. Because of the severe pain, it may be necessary to use a topical anesthetic to allow the patient to cooperate with the examination.

3. **Treatment** is directed toward pain relief and should include the use of systemic analgesics, topical corticosteroid preparations, and cycloplegic drugs. As with other painful corneal disorders secondary to surface damage, the chronic use of topical anesthetic agents is absolutely contraindicated as part of the management plan.
4. **Prognosis** is excellent.

IV. **Injury Prevention**

A. **Selected excerpts from the International Federation of Sports Medicine (IFSM) Position Statement on Eye Injuries and Eye Protection:**
   1. Sports eye injuries are relatively frequent and almost completely preventable.
   2. Loss of sight of any degree has serious financial consequences for both individuals and society.
   3. **All** athletes should be prescribed eye protection when appropriate to the sport.
   4. Athletes who are "one-eyed" **must** have a diagnostic evaluation and appropriate eye protection prescribed.
   5. Glass lenses, ordinary plastic lenses, and open eye guards (class III sports eye protectors) do **not** provide adequate protection for those involved in active sports and in some cases may increase the risk for injury both in frequency and severity.

B. **Classification of eye injury risk in sports when protective eye wear in not used:**
   1. **Low risk**—sports that do not involve a thrown or hit ball, a bat, a stick, or close aggressive play with body contact. Examples are track, field, swimming, gymnastics, and rowing.
   2. **High risk**—sports that involve a high-speed ball or puck, use of a bat or stick, or close aggressive play with intentional or unintentional body contact or collision. These include hockey (ice, field, and street), the racquet sports, lacrosse, baseball, football, basketball, handball, soccer, and volleyball. Adequate eye protective devices are available for these sports.
   3. **Extremely high risk**—sports that are combative and for which adequate eye protective devices are not available. Examples include boxing and full-combat karate. Functional one-eyed athletes should be discouraged from participation in these sports.

C. **Other risk factors for sports eye injuries:**
   1. **Physical development and skill level**
      a. **Beginners** may have an increased risk because of lack of necessary refinement of the skill of the sport.
      b. **Advanced players,** especially in some high-risk sports, may play more aggressively and be at greater risk for an eye injury.
   2. **Existing visual impairment** will increase the risk of injury, especially in activities included in the high-risk and extremely high-risk groups.
   3. **Pre-existing eye disease** may present an increased risk factor to athletes in all risk groups. Conditions that may lead to serious eye disorders or get worse following even minor trauma to the eye include retinal detachment, retinal degeneration, severe myopia, thin sclera, and prior eye surgery, plus other systemic eye diseases and serious injuries.
   4. **Functional one-eyed athlete:** This risk must factor in the serious disability that can result from an injury to the remaining good eye. Most people with one normally functioning eye do not demonstrate significant disability in their athletic performance as a result of their vision. With the exception of extremely high-risk sports, one-eyed athletes should be able to safely participate in all other sports while utilizing adequate protective eye wear.

D. **Types of eye protectors**
 1. **Total head protector:** A combination of helmet and face shield designed to protect the eyes, teeth, jaw, and larynx—for use in high-risk sports that require total head protection. These include football, hockey and lacrosse.
 2. **Full face protector:** Designed for use in conjunction with eye protectors for high-risk sports that do not require protection for the brain. This category includes fencing and some positions in baseball and softball.
 3. **Helmet with separate eye protectors:** For use in sports with low risk for injuries to the lower face and neck, including bicycle riding, snowmobiling, skiing, and auto and bobsled racing.
 4. **Helmet only:** These protectors are designed to protect the brain only. They afford very little protection to the face or eyes and are used in boxing and cycling.
 5. **Sports eye protectors:** Used only to protect the eyes and are recommended in all high-risk sports for which additional head and face protection is impractical. They are recommended for all racquet sports as well as baseball, soccer, basketball, and softball.
E. **Necessary components for impact-safe sports eye wear**
 1. Frames that firmly hold and totally encircle the lenses.
 2. Impact-resistant lenses, preferably made of polycarbonate plastic.
 3. Strong nose bridge and nose pads firmly attached to the frame.
F. **Classification of eye protectors**
 1. **Class I**—Eye protector in which the face, frame, and lenses are molded as a single unit, with the temples and straps attached separately.
 2. **Class II**—The lenses are molded and installed in a frame that is a separate unit. This presents the risk of the lenses popping out of the frame under certain conditions.
 3. **Class III**—Single-unit face frame containing no lenses. This device is not recommended for use in high-risk sports.
G. **Classification of spectacles**
 1. **Street wear spectacles**—Those designed to correct refractive error only and are not recommended for use as sports eye protection.
 2. **Safety glasses**—When made of polycarbonate plastic and equipped with clear side shields, they generally provide adequate eye protection for high-risk sports.
 3. **Sports eye protectors**—Best when designed for a specific sport and made of polycarbonate plastic.

# Chapter 33: Maxillofacial Injuries

HAROLD K. TU, DMD, MD
LEON F. DAVIS, DDS, MD
THOMAS A. NIQUE, DDS, MD

I. **Introduction**

Injuries of the maxillofacial region are common in sports, especially when protective head and mouth gear are not worn. The injuries may be classified into three major categories: (1) soft tissue injuries, (2) dentoalveolar trauma, and (3) facial skeletal trauma. Overall treatment objectives are the restoration of function and facial appearance. Treatment priorities should be consistent with maintaining airway, control of hemorrhage, treatment of shock, management of associated injuries (e.g., cervical spine), and definitive care of facial injuries. Rehabilitation after definitive treatment will vary with the type of injury, as well as the type of sport to be resumed. Rehabilitation protocol and athletic restrictions should be established in consultation with the athlete's physician.

II. **History**

   A. Document the history of the injury and all related clinical findings, including the cause of the trauma (e.g., baseball, hockey stick).
   B. Take a complete medical history, with special attention to medications and allergies.

III. **Initial Care**

The primary consideration is maintenance of airway, prevention of shock (although rare from facial injuries) through prompt hemorrhage control, and the assessment and management of loss of consciousness. Early physical examination and continuous neurologic evaluation are essential.

   A. **Airway maintenance**

   In the conscious patient without evidence of neck injury, airway maintenance can be accomplished by sitting the patient upright and slightly forward. Blood clots, vomitus, and foreign objects (dentures) may be cleared by sweeping a finger deep into the back of the throat. Maintaining airway in the unconscious patient or suspected cervical spine injury requires the use of appropriate airway technique: jaw thrust, oral airway, nasoendotracheal tube, and coniotomy or tracheostomy. These techniques should be performed by those with proper training.

   B. **Hemorrhage**

   Hemorrhage is sometimes difficult to control due to the abundant blood supply in the maxillofacial region. Direct pressure and prevention of airway obstruction is the initial treatment.

   C. **Cervical spine injuries**

   These must be suspected in all athletes with significant maxillofacial injuries and/or who are unconscious. Constant cervical traction or use of sandbags or cervical collar to immobilize the neck during any manipulation or transportation is required. Use of cervical collars should be performed by those with proper training.

IV. **Physical Assessment of Injuries**

   A. **Cervical spine injuries**

   Check for neck pain, neurologic deficits (motor or sensory), and limitation of motion.

B. **Laryngeal injuries**

Check for change in voice (usually hoarseness), cervical emphysema (subcutaneous air), or loss of thyroid cartilage prominence (Adam's apple).

C. **Facial injuries**

The signs and symptoms range from laceration, discomfort, edema (swelling), and ecchymosis (bruising) to gross deformity. Visually inspect for facial asymmetry, areas of swelling, discoloration, and obvious deformity, which are clues to the area of involvement. Assess the occlusion or bite of the teeth. Bimanual manipulation of the facial bones can show areas of bone discontinuity and mobility. Suspected upper-jaw fracture can be diagnosed by grasping the upper teeth and determining evidence of gross movement of the upper jaw and midface. Assess jaw opening and determine if it is associated with pain, limitation, or deviation.

D. **Radiographs**

1. Lateral cervical spine view in indicated patients should be obtained prior to other x-rays (unless there is a life-threatening injury) to determine cervical spine fractures.

2. **Facial series**

   a. Oblique view: helps to evaluate the mandible and lower third of the face.
   b. Panoramic view: helps to evaluate the mandible, teeth, maxillary sinus, and condyle.
   c. Lateral view: helps to evaluate the nasal bones.
   d. Submental view: helps to evaluate the zygomatic arch.
   e. Waters view: helps to evaluate the maxilla, zygoma, sinuses, and orbits.

C. **Special imaging techniques**

Tomograms, CT scan, and MRI may provide additional information, at the direction of the consultant.

V. **Soft Tissue Injuries**

A. **Incidence**

Soft tissues of the scalp, forehead, cheeks, nose, lips, and the internal structures of the mouth constitute some of the most common sports injuries. Not surprisingly, ice hockey, squash, and racquetball lead in the frequency of facial soft tissue injuries, but no sport is immune, including swimming.

B. **Mechanisms**

Injury occurs when the athlete is struck by a wayward projectile, as a hockey puck or baseball, or is struck by other athletic equipment, including hockey sticks, squash racquets, face guards or helmets, and shoe cleats, or the athlete strikes a stationary object such as a diving board, basketball backboard, or hockey cage, or collides with parts of another body, such as faces, elbows, knees, and fingers.

C. **Prevention**

Many of these injuries could be prevented with **proper protection,** such as face masks in hockey or racquetball. The use of mouthguards, primarily designed to prevent injuries to the teeth and jaws, is also effective in minimizing soft tissue injuries around the mouth and tongue.

D. **Classifications**

Soft tissue injuries can be classified into three categories of (1) **contusion,** (2) **abrasion,** and (3) **laceration.** Lacerations include **punctures.**

E. **Examination and treatment**

The area of injury is readily apparent, particularly if bleeding is occurring. **It is important to remember that any trauma severe enough to injure the soft tissues may also have injured the underlying bony structure.** Hemorrhage is controlled with the application of pressure, using sterile gauze 4 × 4s. Once the hemorrhage has been controlled and hemostasis is present, the wound should be inspected. The wound should be thoroughly cleaned, making sure to remove any debris by irrigation with saline. Contusions are easily treated by thoroughly cleansing the area, applying an antibiotic ointment, and then a gauze dressing. As a temporizing measure, minor lacerations may be closed with Steri-strips, then protected with an occlusive dressing of gauze and tape.

Since **lacerations and abrasions of the facial area are cosmetically serious,** appropriate medical attention is needed to minimize disfiguring scars that may occur. Lacerations of the face must be sutured. Sutures no larger than 5-0 are mandatory. Care should be taken that deep wounds are closed in appropriate layers. Lacerations of the lip that cross the vermilion border and are not repaired appropriately can result in significant disfiguring scars. During the laceration closure, it is extremely important that the vermilion border be properly aligned. Almost all lacerations can be closed with local anesthesia.

**Intraoral lacerations** deserve the same attention as facial lacerations.

E. **Athletic restrictions**

If the laceration is minor and can be stabilized well with Steri-strips or temporary sutures, then the athlete may return to competition with definitive treatment delayed until completion of the contest, providing the wound is completely protected with an occlusive dressing. Subsequent participation requires similar protection until healing is complete. External lacerations in swimmers require a waterproof dressing if further participation that day is desired.

VI. **Dentoalveolar Injuries**

A. **Description**

Dentoalveolar injuries involve the teeth and supporting structures

B. **Mechanism of injury**

**Anterior teeth usually bear the brunt of most sports related dentoalveolar injuries** (e.g., bat, ball, hockey puck). Individual teeth may be luxated (loosened), partially or totally avulsed (knocked out), or impacted. Lacerations of the face, lips, and mucosa are often present and, despite their sometimes extensive appearance, careful debridement and meticulous closure will achieve anatomical reapproximation and minimal scarring.

C. **Examination**

1. Regional examination to rule out other facial injuries should be carried out.
2. Intraoral examination to determine the presence of missing and fractured teeth, lacerations, and foreign objects (e.g., gravel) should be carefully done.
3. Panoramic x-ray study may be, most useful, but additional dental films may provide more detail. Chest films should be obtained if an avulsed tooth cannot be found, as aspiration into the lungs is possible.

D. **Treatment**

1. Most dentoalveolar injuries can be prevented with the use of proper face and mouthguards. Custom mouthguards can be fabricated by a dentist, or commercial mouthguards can be obtained in most sports stores.
2. Repair the dentoalveolar damage prior to management of facial or lip lacerations.
3. The reimplantation of a recently avulsed tooth should always be attempted. How an athlete or trainer handles the avulsed tooth can have a significant effect on the overall prognosis.
   a. Handle the tooth by the crown. Do not rub it to remove dirt.
   b. Gently rinse the tooth in tap water to remove blood and dirt.
   c. Replace the tooth in the socket and have the patient bite down on a gauze or moist tea bag to keep the tooth in place. Refer to a dentist. If a tooth cannot

be replaced in the socket quickly, then place in a cup of warm, mild salt water, the patient's saliva, or milk. With an adult, the tooth can be placed under the tongue, or in the cheek pouch.

    d. Most alveolar (tooth-bearing bone) fractures can usually be reduced with digital pressure and stabilized by using a splint.

    e. Antibiotics are indicated when avulsed teeth are contaminated. Penicillin is the antibiotic of choice (Pen VK 500 mg PO qid for 10 days).

    f. Anti-tetanus prophylaxis should be considered when the tooth has contacted soil and the athlete's immunization has been 5 years previously or longer. Tetanus toxoid 0. 5 cc should be given.

  E. **Athletic restrictions**

    1. Contact drills or competition should be restricted during the period when the patient is in stabilization splint. Appropriate face and mouthguards should be worn to prevent further injury.

VII. **Nasal Fractures**

  A. **Description**

Isolated nasal fractures are the most common sports-related facial fracture and the nose is probably the most commonly injured structure of the face (Fig. 1).

  B. **Mechanism of injury**

The prominence of the nose and its low impact-tolerance make it especially susceptible to sports injury. Nasal injuries are seen particularly in contact sports such as rugby, football, and boxing. The fracture most commonly seen in sports injuries is lateral displacement of the nasal bones. The severity may range from a slightly depressed greenstick fracture (commonly seen in adolescents and younger) to displacement and/or disruption of the bony and cartilaginous components of the nose.

  C. **Examination**

    1. **Signs and symptoms**

      a. Epistaxis (nosebleed)

      b. Nasal airway obstruction

      c. Nasal asymmetry

      d. Crepitus (crackling) over nasal bridge

      e. Possible periorbital and subconjunctival ecchymosis

      f. Possible cerebral spinal fluid leak

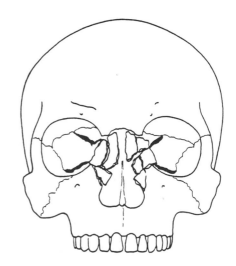

**FIGURE 1.** Frontal view of the skull showing common isolated nasal fractures.

g. Septal deformity

h. Septal hematoma (possible).

2. **X-ray studies**

a. Waters view

b. PA and lateral skull films

c. Nasal bone films.

D. **Treatment**

1. Control of nasal hemorrhage with pressure or intranasal packing.

2. Examine for the presence of septal hematoma. If present, this must be drained.

3. Protect from further injury and refer.

4. Non- or minimally displaced nasal fractures can be treated with closed reduction and intranasal packing with external splinting. Complex nasal fractures may require open reduction and internal fixation.

E. **Athletic restrictions**

1. Workouts and strenuous exercises are to be restricted while the patient has intranasal packing, usually 3 to 4 days.

2. The athlete should be restricted to noncontact drills and competition for the first 3 to 4 weeks. Protective headgear should be worn for 2 to 3 months.

VIII. **Maxillary Fractures**

A. **Description**

These fractures, also known as midface fractures, essentially involve the upper jaw and associated bony structures. They are classified as Le Fort I, II and III fractures, depending whether the nasal or cheek bones are involved (Fig. 2).

B. **Mechanism of injury**

Usually involves a direct blow to the middle portion of the face. This can occur from a hockey stick, bat, punch, a projectile such as a ball, or collision. Any sport with these potentials is a risk, although these fractures are uncommon.

C. **Examination**

1. **Common signs and symptoms**

a. Lengthening of face

b. Mobility of maxilla and midface

c. Open bite deformity—malocclusion (teeth apart in front)

d. Ecchymosis (bruising) in buccal vestibule

e. Epistaxis (nosebleed)

f. Nasal deformity

g. Flattening and splaying of the naso-orbital region.

2. **X-ray studies**

a. Waters view

b. PA and lateral skull films

c. CT scan.

D. **Treatment**

1. **Temporary treatment:** The patency of airway is of primary concern in these injuries, followed by rapid transfer for definitive diagnosis and treatment. The airway in a conscious patient may be best managed in a forward-sitting position, allowing dependent drainage of saliva and blood to occur externally. A cervical spine injury should be suspected and precautions taken (see par. III.C.). Nasal packing for bleeding is discouraged unless cerebrospinal leakage can be ruled out.

2. **Definitive treatment** will involve reduction, fixation, and immobilization of the fractures (refer to par. IX.D.). Complex midface fractures may require extensive surgery and possibly secondary reconstruction.

3. **Rehabilitation** is similar to mandibular fractures (see par. IX.D.).

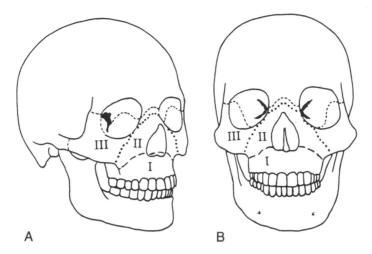

**FIGURE 2.** *A,* Left and *B,* frontal views of the skull showing Le Fort I, II, and III fractures of the upper jaw.

IX. **Mandibular fractures (fractures of the lower third of face)**

A. **Description**

Mandibular fractures are the third most common facial bone fractures related to sports injury. These fractures involve the lower third of the facial skeleton and are classified as to their anatomic location (Fig. 3) and whether they are simple, comminuted, or compounded.

B. **Mechanism of injury**

The face is susceptible to injury in sports in which it is exposed or involved, especially if protective devices are not worn, e.g., hockey, boxing, football. Mandibular fractures are usually not isolated. More than half of the patients have multiple fractures.

The anatomic region of the mandible where fracture is most likely to occur obviously depends on the direction and amount of the force, but most commonly the mandibular angle and condyle are involved.

C. **Examination**

1. **Common signs and symptoms**
   a. Change in the bite
   b. Mobility of mandibular in segments
   c. Pain on function

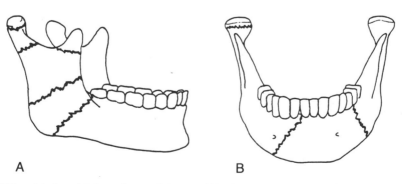

**FIGURE 3.** *A,* Left and *B,* frontal view of the mandible showing common mandibular fracture or an injury to the temporomandibular joint.

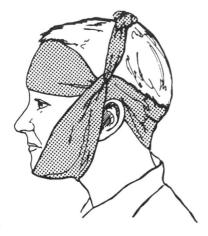

**FIGURE 4.** Barton (barrel) bandage for temporary immobilization in the treatment of a mandibular fracture or an injury to the temporomandibular joint.

    d. Inability to chew or open mouth widely
    e. Numbness or change in sensation of the lower lip
    f. Bruising of gums and floor of mouth
    g. Deviation of lower jaw on opening.
  2. **X-ray studies**
    a. Panorex
    b. Lateral obliques of mandibular angles
    c. PA mandible film
    d. Towne's view.
D. **Treatment**
  1. **Reduction, fixation, and stabilization** are the essential elements of fracture management.
    a. Temporary immobilization can be obtained by a Barton or barrel bandage (Fig. 4) or an Ace wrap from under the chin around the occiput. In most cases, this is adequate stabilization until definitive care can be provided.
    b. Definitive treatment in most cases involves reduction and appropriate fixation of the fracture. The use of intermaxillary fixation (wiring jaws together) continues to be a common technique. However, indicated use of rigid internal fixation (bone plates) obviates the need for intermaxillary fixation. This is especially advantageous for those athletes wanting to return to their sport at the earliest opportunity.
    c. Rehabilitation may be delayed for 4 to 6 weeks when the jaws are immobilized.
       The patient will require a high-protein, carbohydrate liquid diet during the period of intermaxillary fixation. Close monitoring of the patient's weight loss is required and a 5 to 10% weight loss is commonly seen. Weight loss exceeding 10% will require further nutritional supplementation.
       During the period of intermaxillary fixation, activities such as weight lifting, running, and contact workouts should be avoided, as it may be difficult to breathe and the fracture may be displaced. Repetitive mild activities, such as stationary bike, swimming, light weights to maintain muscle tone, and conditioning, are recommended.
       Once the jaws are unwired, the athlete can resume training with minimal restrictions. Resumption of direct contact sports (e.g., boxing, football) should be delayed an additional 1 to 2 months, with special headgear and mouthguard customized to provide further protection. Physical therapy to improve jaw opening is recommended. When bone plates are used, rehabilitation may

begin as early as 10 to 14 days after surgery, with return to full activity one month earlier as a result of the plates.

E. **Mandibular condyle fractures (in most cases associated with mandibular fractures)**
  1. **Common signs and symptoms**
     a. Tenderness and pain in the preauricular area (front of the ear), especially on opening
     b. Deviation of the jaw
     c. Limitation of jaw motion
     d. Change in the bite.
  2. **X-ray studies**
     a. Panorex
     b. Towne's view
     c. Lateral oblique mandible films
     d. Tomograms of the condyle.
  3. **Treatment** (refer to par. IX.D.).
     The period of intermaxillary fixation (wired jaw) is usually 2 to 3 weeks.
  4. **Rehabilitation**
     These patients require a much shorter period of immobilization, approximately 2 to 3 weeks, and early physical therapy is required to prevent joint ankylosis. Close follow-up is especially important in children and adolescents, as condylar injury may affect their jaw growth (refer to par. XII.E. and G.).

X. **Zygomatic Complex (ZMC) Fractures**
  A. **Description**
     Zygomatic complex fractures occur as the result of a force striking the prominence of the zygomatic bone or cheekbone (Fig. 5).
  B. **Mechanism of injury**
     A direct blow, such as from a hockey stick, bat, baseball (e.g., to the cheekbone). ZMC fracture is the second most common facial bone fracture seen in sports-related injuries. Classification of this type of fracture is based on displacement and severity of the fracture. Since the ZMC is intimately associated with the orbit, one should evaluate for ocular injuries.
  C. **Examination**
     1. **Common clinical signs and symptoms**
        a. Flatness of the cheek
        b. Limited mandibular opening

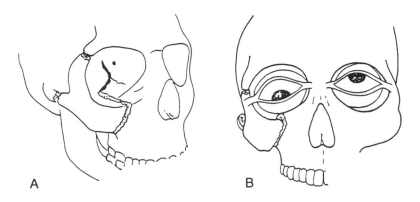

A          B

**FIGURE 5.** *A*, Left and *B*, frontal views showing zygomatic complex fracture.

    c. Paresthesia or anesthesia (numbness) of the affected cheek

    d. Periorbital edema (swelling) and ecchymosis (bruising) or emphysema (air in tissue)

    e. Subconjunctival hemorrhage

    f. Enophthalmos (eye sunken in)

    g. Diplopia (double vision)

    h. Step defects (bone discontinuity) at inferior and lateral orbital rims and zygomatic buttress

    i. Intraoral buccal (inside cheeks) ecchymosis

    j. Limitation of ocular movement

    k. Pupillary height discrepancy.

  2. **X-ray studies**

    a. Waters view

    b. Submental (below the chin) vertex

    c. PA and lateral skull films

    d. CT of head or orbital apex tomograms are indicated when there is suspected ocular injury.

D. **Treatment**

  1. Protect from further injury and transfer for definitive care.

  2. Fractures of the zygomatic bone are usually reduced readily. The fractured complex is elevated into position through various approaches (intraoral or temporal), and the zygomatic bone reduces into place and remains stable.

  3. Healing is usually complete in 6 to 8 weeks. Special headgear designed to protect the cheekbone should be worn for 3 to 4 months. Visual problems such as diplopia (double vision) may be a complication of zygomatic fractures. Athletes involved in sports requiring eye-hand coordination, such as baseball, tennis, and racquetball, may suffer delay in return of their previous skill level. Any visual problems should be evaluated by an ophthalmologist.

XI. **Orbital Floor Fracture ("blowout" fracture,** see also p. 294)

A. **Description**

This is an isolated fracture of the orbital floor (eye socket). It is a rare fracture involving a segment of orbital floor (bone) and a portion of the periorbitis (eye fat) into the maxillary sinus, with or without muscle entrapment. The orbital rim is intact in a pure "blow-out" fracture (Fig. 6).

B. **Mechanism**

It is caused by a rapid increase in intraorbital pressure. The force is usually a blunt object (tennis ball, racquetball), only slightly larger than the inlet, directed at the

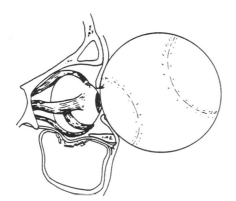

**FIGURE 6.** Orbital floor fracture ("blowout" fracture) caused by the force of the baseball striking the eye. The orbital rim is left intact.

globe and lids. The sudden increase in pressure fractures the bony orbit at areas of weakness, usually along the orbital floor.

C. **Examination**
1. **Common signs and symptoms**
    a. Decreased mobility of the globe (decreased ability to look around)
    b. Diplopia (double vision)
    c. Periorbital edema, ecchymosis, or emphysema
    d. Subconjunctival ecchymosis (bruising)
    e. Enophthalmos (eye sunken in)
    f. Unilateral epistaxis (nose bleeding)
    g. Unequal pupillary height as compared to opposite side.
2. **X-ray studies**
    a. Waters view
    b. Tomograms of the orbit and maxillary sinus.

D. **Treatment**
1. **Immediate:** Protect from further injury and refer for definitive care.
2. Definitive care may require open exploration from a lower lid incision, with reconstruction of orbital floor.
3. **Rehabilitation** is similar to zygomatic complex fractures (see par. X.D.3.).

XII. **Temporomandibular Joint Injuries**

A. The **temporomandibular joint (TMJ)** is a sliding hinge joint and articulates the mandibular condyle and temporal bone of the skull. It is functionally associated with the dentition and the contralateral joint. The joint is separated into upper and lower compartments by a fibrocartilage meniscus. The joint is stabilized by ligaments.

B. **Mechanism of injury**
Injury to the TMJ can result from any blow to the mandible due with forces being transmitted to the condyle. The injury usually includes:
1. Hemarthrosis (intracapsular bleeding)
2. Capsulitis (inflammation of the capsular ligaments)
3. Internal derangement (meniscal displacement)
4. Subluxation/dislocation (condylar displacement with or without voluntary reduction)
5. Fracture (see par. IX.E.).

C. **Examination**
1. Limitation of opening (normal > 40 mm)
2. Deviation to the side of injury on opening
3. Pain on opening and biting
4. Malocclusion (change in the bite)
5. Joint noise (clicking, popping, crepitus)
6. Unable to close (dislocation and meniscus displacement).

D. **Radiographs**
1. Panoramic and Towne's view
2. TMJ arthrogram to evaluate meniscal displacement.

E. **Treatment**
1. Temporary immobilization can be accomplished with an Ace bandage wrapped around the chin over the top of the head (see Fig. 4).
2. Limitation of opening for 7 to 10 days.
3. Soft diet.
4. Moist heat to the area.
5. Aspirin or actaminophen 650 mg PO q4h for 7 to 10 days, or ibuprofen 600 mg PO qid for 7 to 10 days.

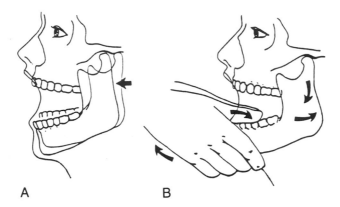

A           B

**FIGURE 7.** Manual reduction of *A*, temporomandibular joint dislocation. *B*, Using both hands, hook thumbs inside the mouth, away from the teeth, and exert firm downward and posterior force. Anesthetic may be necessary.

     6. Dislocation can be reduced manually by grasping each side of the jaw with the thumb hooked inside the mouth (away from the teeth) and exerting firm downward and posterior force (Fig. 7). In some cases, a local anesthetic injection of the joint, oral sedation with Versed 3–5 mg or IV, or a general anesthetic may be required.

F. **Rehabilitation**
     1. Physiotherapy consists of repetitive, passive opening exercises using tongue blades as an aid. The gradual addition of tongue blades increases the opening and documents the progress.
     2. Thermotherapy, coolant therapy, electrical stimulation, massage, and relaxation therapy can all be useful adjunctive therapy.

G. **Athletic restrictions**
     1. Following acute injury, physical contact activities should be restricted until acute signs and symptoms have diminished, usually in 7 to 10 days.
     2. Heavy weight lifting should be restricted during the acute period.
     3. Athletes on muscle relaxants should be restricted from workouts and competition.
     4. Athletes undergoing arthroscopy should follow the same restrictions as those suffering from acute injury.
     5. Athletes undergoing arthroplasty can usually expect a 4- to 6-week recovery before returning to conditioning and light drills. Resumption of direct contact sports (e.g., boxing, football) should be delayed an additional 2–3 months with special headgear and mouthguard to provide further protection.

## REFERENCES

1. Rowe NL, Killey HC: Fractures of the Facial Skeleton, 2nd ed. Edinburgh, Churchill-Livingstone, 1968.
2. Rowe NL, Williams JL: Maxillofacial Injuries, Vol 1. New York, Churchill-Livingstone, 1985.
3. Converse. Reconstructive Plastic Surgery, Vol 2, 2nd ed. Philadelphia, W.B. Saunders, 1964.
4. Hawkins RW, Lyne ED: Skateboarding fractures. Am J Sports Med 9:99, 1981.
5. Kendrick RW: Some "sporting" injuries. Int J Oral Surg 1(Suppl 10):245, 1981.
6. Koplich B, Koplik M: Mouthguards prevent most oral injuries in contact sports. NY J Dent 44:84, 1974.
7. Morton JG, Burton JF: An evaluation of the effectiveness of mouthguards in high-school rugby players. NZ Dent J 75:151, 1979.

# Chapter 34: Shoulder Injuries

MICHELE J. JULIN, PA-C, MS
MONTY MATHEWS, MD

I. **History.** Historical information is invaluable in the investigation of a shoulder problem. The following areas should be queried:

  A. Sport

  B. Specific activity

  C. Chronic (overuse) vs. acute (traumatic)

  D. Do symptoms increase with activity and/or improve with rest?

  E. Instability. Has the shoulder ever slipped out or felt like it could slip out of place?

  F. Weakness

  G. Pain—character and location

  H. Crepitation

  I. Radicular symptoms.

II. **Physical Examination**

  A. **Observation**

    1. **Deformity**

      a. Position of humeral head

        i. Anterior

        ii. Inferior

        iii. Posterior.

      b. Alignment of clavicle

        i. Prominence of distal tip at clavicle.

        ii. General alignment of shaft

        iii. Position of medial tip of clavicle at sternoclavicular joint.

      c. Position of scapula—winging

      d. Effusion.

    2. **Muscular atrophy**

      a. Asymmetry

        i. May indicate nerve damage.

        ii. May indicate disuse atrophy.

        iii. Secondary to pain, instability, or decreased range of motion.

    3. **Skin appearance**

      a. Swelling

      b. Ecchymosis

      c. Color

      d. Venous distention.

  B. **Palpation**

    1. **Tenderness**

      a. Acromioclavicular joint

      b. Sternoclavicular joint

      c. Clavicle shaft

      d. Humeral head

> > i. Bicipital groove
> > ii. Greater and lesser tuberosity.
> e. Anterior, lateral and posterior glenohumeral joint
> f. Ligaments—especially acromioclavicular and coracoclavicular
> g. Tendons—especially biceps and rotator cuff
> h. Scapula
> i. Brachial plexus.

> 2. **Crepitation**
> > a. Acromioclavicular joint
> > b. Glenohumeral joint
> > c. Long head of biceps.
> 3. **Effusion**
> 4. **Radial pulse**
> 5. **Skin temperature.**

C. **Movement**
> 1. **Active/passive range of motion of shoulder**
> > a. Forward flexion
> > b. Extension
> > c. Adduction
> > d. Abduction
> > e. Internal rotation
> > f. External rotation
> > g. Horizontal adduction.
> 2. **Active/passive range of motion of cervical spine**
> > a. Flexion
> > b. Extension
> > c. Lateral motion
> > d. Rotation.
> 3. Assess whether motion is painful.
> 4. Assess if apprehension or subluxation is associated with any shoulder movement, especially forward flexion with external rotation.
> 5. Manual muscle testing
> > a. **Supraspinatus** (abduction) (Fig. 1A)
> > > i. Patient abducts arm to 90 degrees, internally rotates arm until thumbs point down, and angulates shoulders forward 30 degrees. Examiner pushes the arms downward against resistance. Pain and weakness are considered a positive test for supraspinatus injury.
> > b. **Subscapularis** (internal rotation) (Fig. 1B)
> > > i. Internal rotation against resistance, with arm adducted and elbow flexed to 90 degrees. Patient attempts to internally rotate while examiner forces external rotation.
> > c. **Infraspinatus and teres minor** (external rotation) (Fig. 1C)
> > > i. External rotation against resistance with arm adducted and elbow flexed to 90 degrees. Patient attempts to external rotate while examiner forces internal rotation.
> > d. **Biceps**
> > > i. Shoulder forward-flexed to 90 degrees with elbow at 0–15 degrees of flexion, palms supinated. Patient tries to maintain position as examiner attempts to force arms downward.

D. **Specific tests**
> 1. **Joint stability**
> > a. **Glenohumeral**

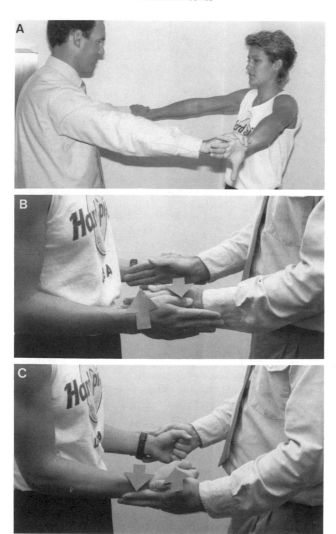

**FIGURE 1.**   *A,* Supraspinatus test; *B,* subcapularis test; *C,* infraspinatus and teres minor test.

    i. **Anterior apprehension/instability test**
       (a) May be performed with patient in supine, sitting, or standing position.
       (b) Slowly abduct and externally rotate the shoulder (Fig. 2).
       (c) Position patient's arm with shoulder in 90 degrees of abduction and 90 degrees of elbow flexion. Place your hand on the glenohumeral joint with your fingers palpating the humeral head posteriorly and the thumb anteriorly. With anterior-directed stress to the humeral head, lever it anteriorly. Repeat maneuver at varying degrees of abduction, feeling for anterior laxity or subluxation.
       (d) Patient apprehension suggests prior subluxation or dislocation.
       (e) Pain may suggest rotator cuff tear or glenoid labrum tear.
       (f) Compare with opposite side.

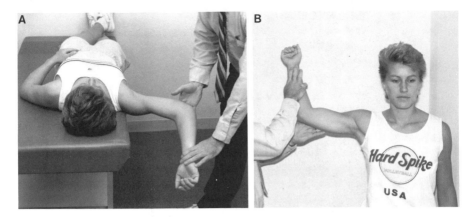

**FIGURE 2.** *A,* Anterior apprehension test in the supine position; *B,* anterior apprehension test in the standing position.

ii. **Posterior apprehension/instability test**
   (a) May be performed with patient supine or sitting.
      (i) Supine position—place patient's shoulder in 90 degrees of abduction and 90 degrees of elbow flexion. Apply pressure to mid-humerus in an attempt to displace humeral head posteriorly (Fig. 3A).
      (ii) Supine—position shoulder at 90 degrees of forward flexion and internal rotation, and elbow at 90 degrees flexion. Direct posterior pressure at elbow in attempt to sublux humeral head posteriorly.
      (iii) Supine or sitting—position patient's arm with shoulder in 90 degrees of abduction and 90 degrees of elbow flexion. Place your hand on the glenohumeral joint with your fingers palpating the humeral head posteriorly and thumb anteriorly. With posterior-directed stress to the humeral head, lever it posteriorly. Repeat maneuver at varying degrees of abduction, feeling for posterior subluxation.
   (b) Apprehension of pain felt by patient suggests prior subluxation or dislocation.

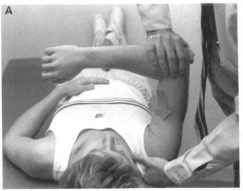
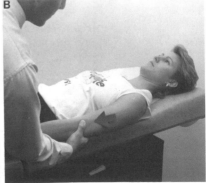

**FIGURE 3.** *A,* Posterior apprehension test in the supine position; *B,* inferior apprehension test.

(c) Compare to opposite side.

(d) A mild degree of posterior displacement is considered normal.

iii. **Inferior apprehension or instability test** (Fig. 3B)

(a) Performed with patient in supine position.

(b) Have patients stabilize themselves by grasping table edge with opposite arm. Pull caudally on arm in 0 degrees of shoulder adduction and elbow flexion. Feel for inferior subluxation. Observe presence of sulcus between humeral and acromion.

(c) Apprehension or pain may indicate prior subluxation or dislocation.

iv. **Acromioclavicular joint**

(a) Downward pressure over distal one-third of clavicle may cause pain and motion of AC joint (Fig. 4A).

(b) Anteroposterior compression over anterior clavicle and scapular spine may cause pain and motion of the AC joint (Fig. 4B).

v. **Sternoclavicular joint** (Fig. 4C)

(a) Pressure or traction on medial clavicle may produce pain and motion of the sternoclavicular joint.

vi. **Scapulothoracic joint** (Fig. 4D)

(a) Observe joint motion with rotation of the humerus at varying degrees of abduction. For every 2 degrees of glenohumeral joint motion, there should be 1 degree of scapulothoracic motion.

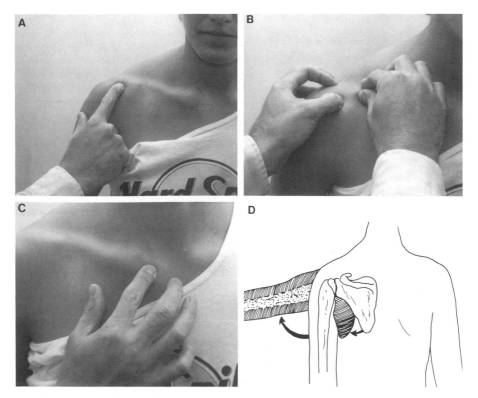

**FIGURE 4.** *A*, Tenderness over the distal third of clavicle may suggest injury to the clavicle or acromioclavicular joint; *B*, motion of distal clavicle on the acromion suggests significant laxity of the acromioclavicular joint; *C*, sternoclavicular joint; *D*, scapulothoracic joint. For every 2 degrees of glenohumeral joint motion, there should be 1 degree of scapulothoracic motion.

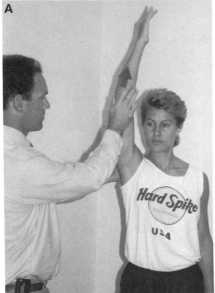

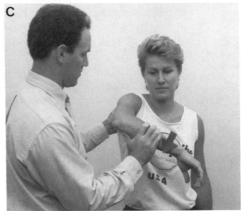

**FIGURE 5.** *A,* Impingement sign # 1; *B,* impingement sign # 2; *C,* impingement sign # 3.

2. **Impingement signs**
   a. #1—Extreme forward flexion of shoulder with forearm pronated (Fig. 5A).
   b. #2—Extreme horizontal adduction of arm. Also called the crossover test (Fig. 5B)
   c. #3—90 degrees of forward flexion and internal rotation of the shoulder (Fig. 5C).
   d. Pain with these maneuvers suggests inflammation or injury of the structures in the subacromial space.
3. **Clunk test**
   a. With patient supine, place one hand posterior to the humeral head while your other hand rotates the humerus. Keep the elbow flexed to 90 degrees. Bring the arm in to full overhead abduction while rotating the humerus through varying degrees of internal and external rotation. The sensation of a clunk, grind, or pop may indicate a labrum tear (Fig. 6).
   b. Compare with opposite side.
4. **Neurological examination**
   a. Deep tendon reflexes—quality and symmetry:
       i. Biceps—$C_5$ nerve root
       ii. Brachioradialis—$C_6$ nerve root
       iii. Triceps—$C_7$ nerve root.
   b. Sensation.
   c. Muscle strength of neck and arms against resistance. Compare with opposite side.

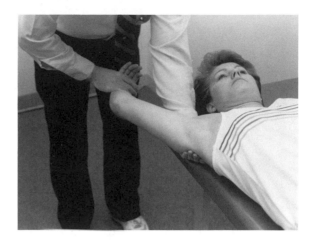

**FIGURE 6.**   Clunk test.

    d. Atlanto-occipital/axial compression test (Fig. 7).
        i. Pain or radicular symptoms may indicate C-spine fracture or nerve root compression.

## III. Specific Shoulder Injuries
### A. Glenohumeral instability
    1. **Anterior instability**—most common.
        a. **Description**
            i. Anterior capsule is stretched or torn from its attachment to the anterior glenoid.
            ii. Humeral head slips out of glenoid anteriorly to locate adjacent to the coracoid.
        b. **History**
            i. Patient may relate the problem to an injury in which arm was forced into extension, abduction, and external rotation, e.g., during open-arm tackle, arm may be forced into this position, or a fall on an abducted arm may also cause it.
            ii. Patient may describe blow to posterior or posterolateral shoulder, which forces humeral head forward, e.g., hit from behind or pile-up tackle on football field.

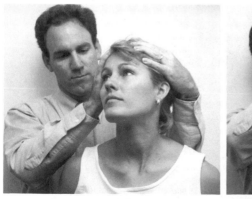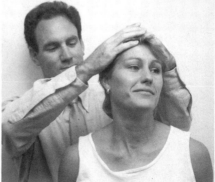

**FIGURE 7.**   Atlanto-occipital/axial compression test.

       iii. Acute injury
          (a) Intense pain with initial dislocation.
          (b) May have numbness and tingling in arm and hand.
       iv. Chronic injury
          (a) History of previous dislocations.
          (b) Requires progressively less trauma to cause dislocation, e.g., rolling over during sleep may eventually cause dislocations.
          (c) Poorly defined pain.
          (d) Vague feeling of instability or apprehension with overhead movement.
  c. **Examination**
      i. **Currently dislocated**
         (a) Presents with arm held by opposite hand in slight abduction and external rotation.
         (b) Sharp contour of affected shoulder when compared to smooth deltoid outline on uninjured side.
         (c) Prominent acromion.
         (d) Humeral head felt anterior to acromion and adjacent to coracoid.
         (e) Resistance to abduction and internal rotation.
      ii. **History of dislocation, but currently located**
         (a) Apprehension and laxity with anterior testing.
  d. **X-ray studies**
      i. Anterior displacement of humerus.
      ii. May show fracture such as an avulsion of the greater tuberosity.
     iii. West Point view (modified axillary) may show chip fracture off anterior-inferior rim of glenoid.
     iv. Hill-Sach's lesion—defect of humeral head caused by compression of head against glenoid as the humerus subluxes (Fig. 8).
      v. May need CT arthrotomogram to rule out rotator cuff tears; may show stretched-out joint capsule with arthrotomogram.
  e. **Differential diagnosis**
      i. Shoulder subluxation

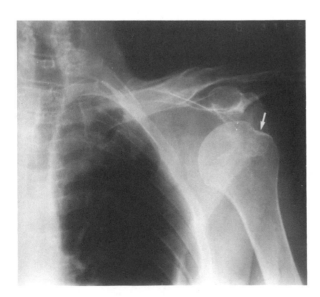

**FIGURE 8.** Hill Sach's lesion.

      ii. Glenoid labrum tear—will show up on CT arthrotomogram or MRI

      iii. Rotator cuff tear—will show tear on CT arthrotomogram or MRI

      iv. Avulsion of greater tuberosity

      v. Fracture of humeral head.

  f. **Treatment**

    i. **Initial or first dislocation**

      (a) Reduction—promptly

        (i) Athlete lies supine with arm held in 30–45 degree of abduction. Counter traction is maintained with sheet around upper thorax or unshod foot against upper chest wall. Apply gentle traction to arm in its longitudinal axis with increasing force exerted. Hold until arm slips back into glenoid fossa. Arm is then placed into internal rotation across chest.

      (b) Pre- (if possible) and postreduction x-rays are taken.

      (c) Shoulder immobilization across chest for 3 to 4 weeks.

      (d) Rehabilitation—ice, NSAIDs.

    ii. **Chronic recurrent dislocation**

      (a) Reduction—promptly (same technique as acute reduction).

      (b) Immobilization is not necessary.

      (c) Early rehabilitation—ice, NSAIDs.

      (d) Consider surgery.

2. **Inferior instability**

  a. **Description**

    i. Very similar to anterior instability except that humeral head also slips inferiorly to locate under the coracoid, thus stretching the inferior capsule and the inferior glenohumeral ligament.

  b. **Examination**

    i. Inferior laxity and apprehension on physical exam.

  c. **X-ray studies**

    i. X-ray films show inferior displacement of humerus.

  d. **Treatment**

    i. Treatment is similar to anterior dislocation.

3. **Posterior instability—uncommon**

  a. **Description**

    i. Posterior capsule is stretched or torn from posterior glenoid.

    ii. Humeral head slips posteriorly to rest under acromion.

  b. **History**

    i. Patient may relate an anterior blow to the upper extremity forcing the humeral head posteriorly. Most common position is with the shoulder flexed at 90 degrees and internally rotated. The force is usually transmitted up the humerus from a blow to an outstretched hand or flexed elbow.

    ii. Patient may relate to fall on outstretched arm with shoulder in internal rotation or adduction. Force may be translated up the arm, forcing the humeral head posteriorly.

    iii. Athlete may not realize the shoulder is dislocated.

    iv. May have pain radiating to tip of shoulder along axillary nerve distribution.

  c. **Examination**

    i. If currently dislocated:

      (a) Patient presents with arm across the chest with rigid internal rotation.

      (b) Flattening of the anterior shoulder when viewed from side.

       (c) Bulge posteriorly when viewed from above (may be masked by heavy deltoid musculature).

       (d) Prominent coracoid.

       (e) Cannot externally rotate or abduct arm.

    ii. History of dislocation, but currently reduced:

       (a) Apprehension and laxity with posterior testing.

### d. X-ray studies

    i. Posterior displacement of humeral head from glenoid. Best seen on axillary view.

    ii. May show avulsion fracture of subscapularis from the lesser tuberosity.

    iii. May show fracture of glenoid or proximal humerus.

### e. Differential diagnosis

    i. Subluxation

    ii. Humerus fracture.

    iii. Glenoid fracture.

### f. Treatment

    i. Reduction—prompt. Apply forward traction with the arm in forward flexion, internal rotation, and some adduction. Gradually elevate the arm. Apply pressure posteriorly to the humeral head with continued traction in elevation and internal rotation. If one or two trials are unsuccessful, open reduction is indicated.

    ii. Remaining treatment and immobilization are similar to anterior dislocation.

## 4. Multidirectional instability

### a. Description

    i. Generalized laxity of the shoulder capsule.

    ii. May involve a combination of anterior, posterior, or inferior laxity.

    iii. May be result of a connective tissue disorder such as Ehlers-Danlos syndrome.

    iv. Voluntary versus involuntary instabilities.

       (a) Voluntary instability—patient consciously and repetitively subluxates or dislocates shoulder.

### b. Mechanism of injury

    i. May result from many forms of trauma or overuse.

### c. History

    i. Pain and instability.

    ii. Often display bilateral pain but seldom symptomatic at the same time.

    iii. Onset:

       (a) One-third will give history of significant trauma to shoulder.

       (b) One-third will relate minor injury.

       (c) One-third will describe insidious onset of symptoms.

### d. Examination

    i. Positive apprehension tests in any direction.

    ii. Capsular laxity with joint play of the humerus.

    iii. Excessive external rotation at 90 degrees of abduction.

    iv. Positive sulcus sign (Fig. 9).

       (a) With inferior traction, a sulcus appears between the humeral head and acromion.

### e. X-ray studies

    i. May demonstrate Hill-Sach's lesion—defect in posterior aspect of humeral head caused as humeral head passes over glenoid rim during anterior dislocation.

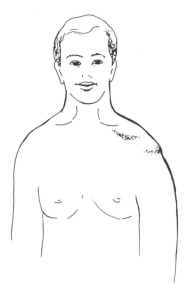

**FIGURE 9.** Sulcus sign.

    ii. May demonstrate Bankart lesion—glenoid labrum and capsule torn from the rim of the glenoid.

  f. **Differential diagnosis**

    i. Humeral fracture

    ii. Glenoid fracture

    iii. Glenoid labrum tear.

  g. **Treatment**

    i. **Voluntary instabilities—often due to related psychological overlay.** Often resistant to conservative and even surgical treatment.

    ii. Involuntary instabilities:

      (a) Dynamic strengthening of the shoulder musculature with emphasis on the areas of greatest instability.

      (b) Rehabilitation program often 6 to 12 months, with expectation of gradual improvement in symptoms.

      (c) Surgical management complicated by the occurrence of inferior instability and the complexity of other instabilities.

B. **Acromioclavicular sprains, separations, dislocations**

  1. **Description**

    a. Stretching and/or disruption of capsule and acromioclavicular ligament.

    b. May also disrupt coracoclavicular ligaments in Grade III sprains.

  2. **History**

    a. Patient may give a history of falling on outstretched arm. Force is transmitted up arm to AC joint.

    b. Patient may give history of a direct blow to lateral aspect of shoulder, e.g., falling with the lateral aspect of the shoulder impacting with the ground.

    c. Patient will complain of pain at the AC joint especially with arm movement.

  3. **Examination**

    a. Distal clavicle may ride above level of acromion.

    b. Pain and swelling at AC joint.

    c. Shoulder motion may induce a snapping sound at the AC joint.

    d. May be tender along the clavicle and at the trapezius and deltoid attachments.

    e. May be tender over coracoclavicular ligament.

    f. Pain with the crossover test (attempt to touch opposite shoulder with hand on injured side).

    g. Downward pressure on distal clavicle elicits pain.

4. **X-rays:** A/P view of the shoulders. May be augmented by a film with 5 to 10 lbs of weight held in hand of affected side and by comparing the opposite side.

    a. Grade I acromioclavicular sprain—normal x-rays.

    b. Grade II acromioclavicular sprain—slight elevation of the distal clavicle when compared to the opposite side.

    c. Grade III acromioclavicular sprain—greater than 1.3 cm between clavicle and coracoid or greater than 50% increase in same distance when compared to the opposite side (Fig. 10).

    d. May show fracture of clavicle, acromion, coracoid, or humerus.

    e. Alexander view shows posterior dislocation of clavicle.

5. **Differential diagnosis**

    a. Contusion to distal clavicle (shoulder pointer), which has no palpable tenderness at AC joint.

    b. Synovitis of the AC joint.

    c. Acromioclavicular degenerative arthritis aggravated by recent injury—look for joint spurring on x-ray.

    d. Fracture of distal clavicle.

6. **Treatment**

    a. Grade I and II

       i. Ice.

       ii. Sling or shoulder immobilizer for symptom control only.

       iii. Early rehabilitation when motion tolerated.

    b. Grade III

       i. If clavicle can be reduced and held in place, a sling or immobilizer can be used; and conservative treatment as in Grades I and II for 6–8 weeks is indicated.

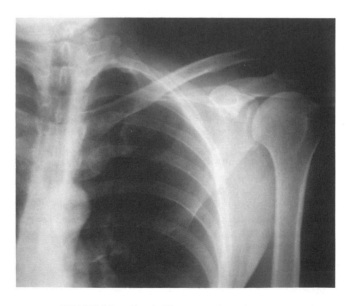

**FIGURE 10.** Grade III acromioclavicular sprain.

      ii. Surgical reduction and repair indicated for persistent pain or unsatisfactory reduction.

C. **Sternoclavicular dislocations**
1. Description
   a. Sprain or tear of costoclavicular and/or sternoclavicular ligaments present.
   b. Most commonly is anterior dislocation.
   c. Posterior dislocation is less common but has increased morbidity, with potential injury to the underlying vasculature, lung, trachea, and esophagus.
      i. Emergency referral warranted.
2. **History**
   a. Athlete may relate problem to injury in which he falls on one side with opposition force on top of other shoulder. This force drives the shoulder forward and inward. This force on the clavicle disrupts the costoclavicular and sternoclavicular ligaments. The proximal clavicle is forced medially, upward and forward.
   b. Less commonly, force drives proximal clavicle posteriorly.
   c. Patient will complain of sternoclavicular joint pain, especially with arm movement.
3. **Examination**
   a. Anterior dislocations
      i. Prominence of proximal clavicle
      ii. Tenderness and swelling over sternoclavicular joint.
   b. Posterior dislocation
      i. Proximal clavicle subluxed behind sternum
      ii. Hoarseness, dysphagia, and dyspnea
      iii. Discoloration, swelling, pulselessness in affected side arm
      iv. Subcutaneous emphysema.
4. **X-ray studies**
   a. Difficult to document sternoclavicular dislocation on routine A/P view.
   b. Rockwood view is best for both anterior and posterior dislocations.
   c. Tomogram or CT scan may be necessary.
5. **Differential diagnosis**
   a. Sternoclavicular joint sprain
   b. Fracture of the proximal clavicle.
6. **Treatment**
   a. Sling, possibly figure-of-eight bandage
   b. Ice and NSAIDs
   c. Spontaneous reduction in most cases
   d. Surgery if reduction is not maintained.

D. **Glenoid labrum tears**
1. Description
   a. Most are result of shoulder instability with forceful subluxation of humeral head over labrum.
   b. Also reported in stable shoulders, especially in throwing athletes.
2. **Mechanism of injury**
   a. During acceleration phase of throwing, horizontal adduction and internal rotation place grinding forces on anterior-superior labrum.
   b. Anterior force may damage labrum if posterior stabilizing muscles are weak.
3. **History**
   a. Common in throwing athletes.
   b. Patient may describe a painful clicking/snapping of the shoulder as arm goes into abduction with external rotation, e.g., during cocking phase of throwing.

      c. Patient may say that the release or follow-through phase of throwing is the most painful.

      d. Patient may note inability to throw ball as fast as preinjury.

  4. **Examination**

      a. Compare strengths and range of motion with opposite shoulder.

      b. Tenderness over anterior humeral joint is present.

      c. Positive "clunk" test.

  5. **X-ray studies**

      a. Routine x-rays generally normal.

      b. CT-arthrogram or MRI.

  6. **Differential diagnosis**

      a. Rotator cuff tear

         i. May occur concurrently with labrum tear.

      b. Glenohumeral instability.

      c. Impingement syndrome.

  7. **Treatment**

      a. **Rehabilitation**

         i. Treatment centers around flexibility and muscular strengthening, specifically the posterior rotator cuff muscles.

      b. Arthroscopic debridement of labrum tear if conservative treatment fails.

E. **Rotator cuff**

  1. **Rotator cuff tendinitis/impingement syndrome**

      a. **Description**

         i. Rotator cuff and biceps tendon impinged against acromion and coracoacromial ligament.

      b. **Mechanism of injury**

         i. Subacromial bursa and rotator cuff tendons become inflamed from friction against the coracoacromial ligament from overuse of the arm, compromising the space available under coracoacromial arch.

         ii. Trauma to acromion or acromioclavicular joint can also narrow the space under coracoacromial arch.

      c. **Predisposing factors**

         i. Any activity that requires repetitive motion of the shoulder above the horizontal plane puts the athlete at higher risk for developing this problem, e.g., swimming, throwing, tennis, and weight lifting.

         ii. Upper extremity inflexibility.

         iii. Mechanical or technique errors or changes in mechanics or technique of an activity.

         iv. Fatigue.

      d. **History**

         i. Typical mechanism as described above.

         ii. Pain (superolateral) with overhead movements.

         iii. Snapping feeling may occur with external to internal rotation or with abduction between 70 degrees and 120 degrees.

      e. **Examination**

         i. Positive impingement signs.

         ii. Rotator cuff and biceps weakness.

         iii. Positive supraspinatus test.

         iv. Pain with abduction from 70 degrees to 120 degrees (painful arc).

         v. May be atrophy of shoulder muscles—compare with opposite side.

         vi. May be tender over coracoacromial ligament.

f. **X-ray studies**
   i. May show subacromial spurring.
   ii. May show AC joint enlargement.
   iii. Enlarged coracoid which may impinge against the lesser tuberosity.
g. **Differential diagnosis**
   i. Rotator cuff tear
   ii. Thoracic outlet syndrome
   iii. Transient subluxation may mimic impingement syndrome.
h. **Treatment**
   i. Relieve aggravating motion (restricted activity). Restrict range of motion to below the horizontal.
   ii. Ice and NSAIDs.
   iii. Physical therapy—stretching especially in abduction and external rotation.
   iv. Corticosteroid injection to subacromial bursa.
   v. Surgical—decompression of subacromial space with resection of coracoacromial ligament and acromioplasty may be performed athroscopically or as an open procedure.

2. **Rotator cuff tear**
   a. **Description**—disruption of the fibers of the tendons that make up the rotator cuff. The most frequent site of injury is the supraspinatus tendon just proximal to the greater tuberosity of the humerus.
   b. **History**
      i. Acute—may result from indirect force on the abducted arm. Characterized by acute pain and weakness, especially with abduction.
      ii. Chronic—neglected rotator cuff tendinitis leads to cuff thinning, degeneration, and an ultimate rupture.
         (a) Usually seen in patients older than age 45.
         (b) Patient describes gradual loss of strength in abduction and external rotation.
         (c) Need not be single episode of giving way.
         (d) Persistent pain.
         (e) Nighttime pain.
   c. **Examination**
      i. Weakness and possibly atrophy of rotator cuff muscles and biceps.
      ii. Tenderness at insertion of supraspinatus tendon on the greater tuberosity of the humerus.
      iii. Painful range of motion on abduction between 70 degrees and 120 degrees.
      iv. Complete tear—may be unable to abduct arm against minimal resistance.
      v. May feel palpable defect in cuff over humeral head.
      vi. Differentiate limited range of motion due to pain versus limited range of motion due to cuff weakness.
         (a) Observe whether injection of local anesthetic into subacromial space eliminates pain and restores abduction.
   d. **X-ray studies**
      i. Plain films usually normal.
      ii. May show proximal migration of humeral head in chronic rotator cuff tears.
      iii. CT arthrotomogram will show dye leakage outside the joint.
      iv. MRI.
   e. **Differential diagnosis**
      i. Chronic tear may mimic impingement syndrome.

    f. **Treatment**
       i. Conservative (ice, NSAIDs, and rehabilitation) for small tear.
      ii. Surgery.

F. **Biceps tendon problems**
  1. **Biceps tendinitis**
    a. **Description**—tendinitis of the long head of the biceps tendon in the area of the bicipital grove.
    b. **History:** Patient generally presents with vague anterior shoulder pain or pain of variable duration.
       i. May be associated with underlying cuff disease or impingement syndrome.
    c. **Examination**
       i. Pain located along tendon and proximal humerus and shoulder joint.
      ii. Resistive supination aggravates pain.
    d. **X-ray studies**
       i. May show narrow bicipital groove.
      ii. May show calcific tendon.
    e. **Treatment**
       i. Rest, ice and NSAIDs.
      ii. Therapeutic exercise and stretching.
     iii. Phonophoresis/iontophoresis and cross-friction massage sometimes helpful.
     iv. Direct therapy toward underlying impingement or rotator cuff disease if indicated.
      v. Tennis-elbow strap placed on upper arm just proximal to biceps belly.
     vi. Do not inject with steroids.
        (a) Corticosteroid injections predispose to biceps tendon rupture.
  2. **Subluxation of the long head of biceps tendon**
    a. **Description**
       i. Tendon subluxes out of bicipital groove.
    b. **Mechanism of injury**
       i. May occur if tendinitis progresses to cause rupture of the transverse humeral ligament, which holds tendon in bicipital groove. This allows tendon to sublux with overhead movement.
      ii. Transverse ligament may also rupture with direct lateral blow to the proximal humerus.
    c. History: Patient will usually tell you that something is catching or snapping in the shoulder when moving through internal and external rotation.
       i. Usually have a long history of biceps tendinitis.
    d. **Examination**
       i. Same as biceps tendinitis.
      ii. May have snapping sensation with external rotation.
     iii. May have crepitus.
     iv. Tenderness over the bicipital groove.
      v. Palpate bicipital groove for instability of tendon while alternating internal and external rotation of the shoulder.
    e. **Differential diagnosis**
       i. Biceps tendinitis
      ii. Impingement syndrome
     iii. Rotator cuff disease.
    f. **Treatment**
       i. Conservative (ice, NSAIDs and rehabilitation).

ii. Surgery—remove long head from the glenoid and suture tendon to the bicipital groove.

3. **Biceps tendon rupture**
   a. **Description**
      i. Complete disruption of tendon at the distal or proximal attachment.
   b. **History**—usually a very dramatic injury as a result of forceful flexion of the arm, commonly against excessive resistance.
      i. May occur after prolonged tendinitis, making tendon vulnerable to forceful rupture.
      ii. May be associated with snapping sensation and pain at the time of rupture.
      iii. Corticosteroid injections weaken the tendon and predispose the tendon to rupture.
   c. **Examination**
      i. Ecchymosis.
      ii. Palpable and visible defect in muscle belly.
      iii. Muscle mass moves distally in cases of proximal long head rupture ("Popeye" appearance).
      iv. Partial ruptures associated with local pain and weakness and have only slight muscular deformity.
      v. Weakness with supination in proximal rupture.
      vi. Marked weakness with supination and elbow flexion with distal rupture.
   d. **X-ray studies**
      i. Usually normal.
      ii. May show avulsion fracture.
      iii. MRI and ultrasound may be helpful.
   e. **Differential diagnosis**
      i. Partial versus complete rupture.
      ii. Proximal versus distal rupture.
   f. **Treatment**
      i. Proximal rupture
         (a) Surgery in younger, more athletic patient.
         (b) Conservative management in older patient.
      ii. Distal rupture
         (a) Surgery in all patients.

G. **Shoulder contusion**
   1. **Description**
      a. Contusion to trapezius and/or deltoid muscles.
      b. Contusion of the exposed lateral portion of the clavicle or acromion, which results in bony bruising with associated periosteal reaction (shoulder pointer).
      c. If hemorrhages into muscle—may result in myositis ossificans or exostosis.
   2. **History**
      a. Typically results from blow to the shoulder: usually seen in contact or collision sports.
   3. **Examination**
      a. Tender over the contused area with pain on movement in surrounding tissues.
      b. Often swelling and rarely ecchymosis.
      c. Restriction of movement of affected arm.
   4. **X-ray studies**
      a. Normal with contusions.
      b. Ectopic bone formation with myositis ossificans and "tackler's" (blocker's) exostosis. Seen in upper lateral arms.
         i. Delayed findings 2 to 6 weeks postinjury.

5. **Differential diagnosis**
   a. Acromioclavicular separation
   b. Rotator cuff tear
   c. Glenohumeral subluxation/dislocation
   d. Clavicle fracture.
6. **Treatment**
   a. Rest, ice
   b. Gentle stretching and massage
   c. Pad and protect vulnerable areas
   d. Mature exostosis may be surgically removed.
      i. Often recurs postoperatively.

H. **Fractures of the clavicle**
   1. **Description**
      a. Most commonly fractured in the middle third.
   2. **History and mechanism of injury**
      a. Usually occurs from fall on outstretched arm or point of shoulder.
      b. Less commonly results from direct blow.
      c. Displacement due to muscle pull on bone fragments.
   3. **Examination**
      a. Visible and palpable deformity is present.
      b. Marked swelling, ecchymosis, and pain.
      c. Greenstick fracture in preadolescents may be without deformity.
      d. Pain may radiate to trapezius.
      e. Swelling and pain do not involve the AC joint.
      f. Auscultation to rule out pneumothorax.
      g. Neurovascular exam to rule out nerve and muscular injury.
   4. **X-ray studies**
      a. Will show disruption of clavicle.
      b. Need to see lung fields to rule out pneumothorax.
      c. Need to see scapula to rule out fracture.
      d. Check for subcutaneous emphysema.
      e. Oblique film to show degree of inferior displacement.
   5. **Differential diagnosis**
      a. Acromioclavicular separation
      b. Sternoclavicular separation
      c. Shoulder contusion.
   6. **Treatment**
      a. Usually figure-of-eight splint.
      b. Distal third fractures may be treated similar to Grade III acromioclavicular separations.
      c. Rarely needs surgical reduction.

I. **Fracture of the scapula**
   1. Fracture of body of scapula
      a. History
         i. Severe trauma.
      b. Examination
         i. May be associated with other fractures such as ribs, sternum, and spine.
         ii. May be associated with pneumothorax, subcutaneous emphysema, and brachial plexus injuries.
         iii. Local scapular pain with palpation.
         iv. Patient presents with arm close to body and avoids motion.

c. **X-ray studies**
i. Include lung fields.
ii. Oblique views to rule out angulation.

d. **Treatment**
i. Ice, NSAIDs, and rehabilitation.
ii. Shoulder immobilizer for unstable fractures and/or comfort.
iii. Surgery in rare cases when scapular fibrous tissue mass impinges on rib.

2. **Fracture of coracoid**
a. **Mechanism of injury**
i. Direct blow
ii. Sudden muscle pull of arm flexors
iii. Anterior shoulder dislocation.

b. **Examination**
i. Tenderness over coracoid
ii. Rule out anterior glenohumeral instability.

c. **X-ray studies**
i. Fracture of coracoid.

d. **Treatment**
i. Usually conservative—ice and NSAIDs.
ii. Occasional surgical reduction and/or excision and replacement of the tendons.

3. **Fracture of spine of scapula and acromion**
a. **Examination**
i. Tenderness over acromion
ii. May limit range of motion of humerus.

b. **X-ray studies**
i. Linear fracture of acromion may be mistaken for unfused acromial epiphysis. Compare to opposite side.

c. **Treatment**
i. Usually conservative.
ii. May require open reduction if fracture interferes with humeral head range of motion or if fracture is widely displaced.

4. **Fractures of the glenoid fossa and neck of scapula**
a. May be associated with shoulder dislocation.
b. Conservative treatment with stable shoulder.
c. Surgical reduction in unstable fractures.

5. **Fractures of the upper end of the humerus**
a. **Description**
i. Fractures of the upper humerus usually arise from violent force applied to the shoulder and should be considered in any athlete with acute traumatic shoulder injury.

b. **History**
i. Fall on upper arm.
ii. Fall on outstretched hand with the elbow extended.

c. **Examination**
i. Limited degree of motion secondary to pain.
ii. Swelling around the shoulder.
iii. Usually will want to hold arm against the body, to act as a splint for comfort.
iv. May have paresthesias around shoulder.

d. **X-ray studies**
i. A/P, lateral, and axillary views usually will demonstrate the fracture.

e. **Differential diagnosis**
  i. Glenohumeral dislocation
  ii. Acromioclavicular separation
  iii. Distal clavicle fracture
  iv. Shoulder contusion.
f. **Treatment**
  i. Fractures of surgical neck and anatomic neck (rare) often will not require reduction. Early range of motion is encouraged to lessen chance of loss of function. Generally 3 to 4 weeks of an immobilizer or sling, then initiating range of motion and pendulum exercises.
  ii. Fracture of lesser tuberosity should prompt consideration of possible posterior dislocation.
  iii. Fractures of the greater tuberosity require accurate reduction and assessment of rotator cuff function. Generally greater than 1 cm of displacement after reduction will require open reduction with internal fixation.
  iv. Fractures or fracture dislocations producing displacement of two or more anatomic parts will require open reduction and internal fixation.
  v. Early restoration of shoulder motion is important to restore the balance between deltoid and rotator cuff muscles and avoid muscle contractures. In most cases this can be achieved by deemphasizing bony injury and giving primary treatment to soft tissue injury.
J. **Effort thrombosis** (see Chapter 37).
  1. **Description**
    a. Common variant of thoracic outlet syndrome in which subclavian or axillary vein becomes acutely thrombosed.
  2. **Mechanism of injury**
    a. Thoracic outlet space is narrowed due to presence of cervical rib, abnormal first rib, or hypertrophy of scalenus muscles.
    b. Severe pressure is applied to underlying vasculature resulting in thrombosis.
K. **Adhesive capsulitis ("frozen shoulder")**
  1. **Description**
    a. Adhesions and capsular contracture causing restriction of motion and pain.
    b. Subgroup with stiff and painful shoulders without evidence of adhesive capsulitis.
  2. **Mechanism of injury**
    a. Common pattern—vicious circle:
      i. Pain → guarding → capsulitis → increased pain on motion → increased guarding → increased capsulitis.
    b. May be result of many disorders, e.g., dislocations, rotator cuff tendinitis, reflex dystrophy, coronary artery disease, fractures, and others.
  3. **History**
    a. Insidious onset.
    b. Increase in pain and decrease in motion.
    c. May or may not have had a preceding injury.
    d. Pain may extend down the arm.
  4. **Examination**
    a. Decreased motion, particularly internal and external rotation and abduction.
    b. Palpable mechanical block to motion that is not necessarily pain-related.
  5. **X-ray studies**
    a. Plain films usually normal.
    b. CT arthrotomogram demonstrates decrease in joint volume.

6. **Differential diagnosis**
   a. Impingement syndrome and rotator cuff tendinitis or tear.
   b. Fracture or dislocation about the shoulder
   c. Cervical radiculopathy
   d. Arthritis of the shoulder
   e. Thoracic outlet syndrome.

7. **Treatment**
   a. Exercise/rehabilitation program.
   b. NSAIDs.
   c. Steroid injections.
   d. Manipulation under anesthesia followed immediately by physical therapy.
   e. May resolve spontaneously following arthrogram as a result of forced distention of joint.
   f. Will often resolve on its own after 1 to 2 years.

L. **Trigger point spasms**
   1. **Description**
      a. Painful, persistent, localized muscle spasm.
      b. Location: any muscle
         i. **Most common site:** levator scapula muscle under upper one-third of trapezius
         ii. Other common sites:
            (a) Paraspinous musculature
            (b) Muscles originating on scapula.
         iii. Athlete may have multiple trigger points.
   2. **Etiology unknown**
      a. Often accompany another injury.
         i. May persist after other injury resolves.
      b. May be induced by stress.
   3. **Treatment**
      a. Deep muscle massage or acupressure (Fig. 11).
      b. Xylocaine injection
         i. Corticosteroids offer no additional benefit.
      c. Muscle relaxants generally ineffective.
      d. Adjuncts
         i. Ice
         ii. Non-narcotic analgesics.
   4. **Complications**
      a. Reversible thoracic outlet syndrome with severe trigger-point spasm in levator scapula.

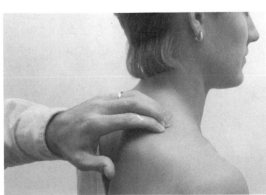

**FIGURE 11.** Deep muscle massage or acupressure for trigger-point spasm.

# Chapter 35: Elbow Injuries

THOMAS L. MEHLHOFF, MD
JAMES B. BENNETT, MD

I. **Diagnosis of Elbow Disorders in the Athlete**

A. **History**
1. Type of injury
2. Location of pain
3. Activities that aggravate symptoms
4. Activities that relieve symptoms
5. Recent changes in technique or training schedules
6. Results of previous treatment.

B. **Physical examination**
1. **Inspection**
   a. Visualize entire upper body
   b. Compare size (dominance, exercise hypertrophy)
   c. Swelling
   d. Carrying angle (cubitus valgus, cubitus varus).
2. **Manipulation** (painful movements last)
   a. Active and passive ROM (compared to uninjured elbow)
      i. Extension      (0°)
      ii. Flexion       (150°)
      iii. Pronation    (70°)
      iv. Supination    (90°)
   b. Resisted isometric movements
   c. Stability
      i. Valgus-varus stress
      ii. Anterior-posterior stress.
3. **Palpation**
   a. Identify areas of tenderness as anterior, posterior, medial or lateral
   b. Differential injection with local anesthetic may more precisely localize pain
      i. **Anterior elbow pain** (Fig. 1)
         (a) Biceps tendinitis
         (b) Biceps rupture
         (c) Anterior capsule tear
         (d) Median nerve compression syndrome.
      ii. **Posterior elbow pain** (Fig. 2)
         (a) Triceps tendinitis
         (b) Triceps rupture/olecranon fracture
         (c) Olecranon impingement syndrome
         (d) Olecranon bursitis.
      iii. **Medial elbow pain** (Fig. 3)
         (a) Medial epicondylitis
         (b) Flexor-pronator strain
         (c) Medial collateral ligament sprain
         (d) Ulnar nerve compression syndrome.

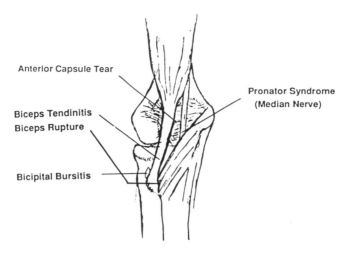

**FIGURE 1.** Anterior elbow pain.

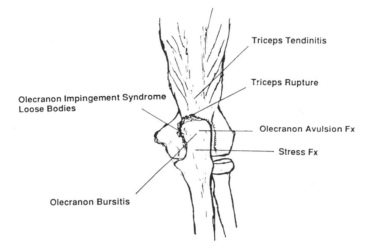

**FIGURE 2.** Posterior elbow pain.

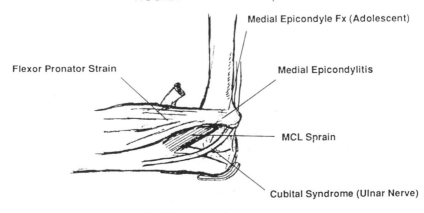

**FIGURE 3.** Medial elbow pain.

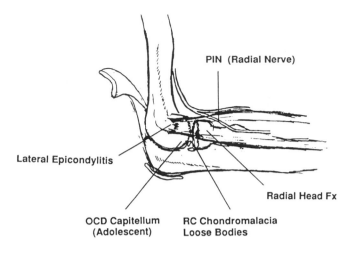

**FIGURE 4.** Lateral elbow pain.

iv. **Lateral elbow pain** (Fig. 4)
   (a) Lateral epicondylitis
   (b) Radiocapitellar chondromalacia
   (c) Osteochondritis dissecans capitellum
   (d) Radial head fracture
   (e) Posterior interosseous nerve compression syndrome.

C. **Ancillary tests**
   1. **X-ray**
      a. AP and lateral
      b. Special views
         i. Oblique views (radial head view)
         ii. Axial projections (olecranon fossa)
         iii. Gravity stress view.
   2. **Arthrogram/arthrotomogram**
      a. Articular incongruity
      b. Loose bodies.
   3. **Arthroscopy**
      a. Intra-articular inspection
      b. Loose bodies
      c. Joint debridement, synovectomy.

II. **Anterior Elbow Injuries**

A. **Biceps Tendinitis**
   1. Overuse syndrome due to repetitive overloading of biceps as a result of excessive elbow flexion and supination activities.
   2. Symptoms:
      a. Anterior elbow pain with flexion and supination
      b. Weakness secondary to pain.
   3. Signs:
      a. Tender biceps tendon to palpation
      b. Increased pain on resisted forearm supination
   4. X-rays: negative
   5. Differential diagnosis:

      a. Bicipital bursitis

      b. Biceps tendon rupture (partial or complete)

      c. Brachialis muscle tear

      d. Anterior capsule tear

      e. Lateral antebrachial cutaneous nerve compression syndrome.

   6. Management:

      a. Rest, ice or heat, NSAID

      b. Splint or cast

      c. Selected injection (complication: tendon rupture)

      d. Modification of training schedule or technique.

**B. Distal biceps rupture**

   1. 97% of biceps ruptures are proximal; only 3% of biceps ruptures occur at the elbow.

   2. Although a single traumatic event is usually recalled, pre-existing degenerative changes in the tendon make it vulnerable to rupture.

   3. Predisposing factors:

      a. Males

      b. Athletes over 30 years of age

      c. Steroid medication.

   4. Symptoms:

      a. Pain in the antecubital fossa

      b. Weakness of supination and flexion (decreased 40%).

   5. Signs:

      a. Tenderness, swelling, ecchymosis in antecubital fossa

      b. No palpable biceps tendon

      c. Deformity as muscle belly retracts proximally

      d. Can still flex (brachialis) and supinate (supinator), but these movements are weak when resisted.

   6. X-ray: unusual to see changes, but these may include:

      a. Avulsion fragment from the radial tuberosity, or

      b. Degenerative changes on volar aspect radial tuberosity.

   7. Management:

      a. Treatment of distal rupture is surgical.

      b. Goal is to restore full supination and flexion power.

      c. Repair biceps tendon to the radial tuberosity through two incision approach of Boyd and Anderson.

      d. Elbow is immobilized at 90° flexion with moderate forearm supination for 8 weeks, followed by gradual AROM and strengthening.

**C. Anterior capsule strain**

   1. Painful microtears of the anterior capsule resulting from a hyperextension injury, not sufficient to cause dislocation.

   2. Symptoms/signs:

      a. Anterior elbow pain poorly localized after traumatic event.

      b. Deep tenderness of anterior elbow joint to palpation.

   3. X-ray: usually normal, but may reveal:

      a. Capsular fleck avulsions from medial or lateral epicondyle

      b. Heterotopic ossification in capsule or collateral ligaments on later follow-up.

   4. Differential diagnosis:

      a. Dislocation (may have spontaneously reduced)

      b. Fracture-dislocation.

   5. Management:

      a. Document neurovascular examination and stability.

      b. Immobilize 3–5 days, then AROM as pain allows.

    c. Flexion contracture may result from fibrosis due to repeated injury (strain) of the capsule.

D. **Median nerve compression syndrome (pronator syndrome)**

  1. Entrapment neuropathy of the median nerve due to mechanical compression by hypertrophied muscle or aponeurotic fascia:

    a. Supracondylar process/ligament of Struthers

    b. Lacertus fibrosus

    c. Pronator teres

    d. Flexor digitorum superficialis arcade.

  2. Symptoms:

    a. Pain in anterior proximal forearm, sometimes cramping

    b. Aggravted by resisted pronation activities

    c. Numbness in volar forearm or radial $3\frac{1}{2}$ digits and thumb.

  3. Signs:

    a. Positive Tinel's sign proximal forearm

    b. Negative Tinel's, Phalen's sign at wrist

    c. May elicit symptoms for each site:

        i. Supracondylar process by elbow flexion 120–135°

        ii. Lacertus fibrosus by resisted forearm supination

        iii. Pronator teres by resisted forearm pronation

        iv. FDS arcade by resisted flexion long finger.

  4. X-ray: normal (supracondylar process present in 1% of limbs)

  5. Confirm with EMG/NCV test, although not always reliable.

  6. Management:

    a. Rest, modification of training

    b. Graduated flexibility and strengthening of forearm

    c. Surgical decompression in unrelieved cases.

III. **Posterior Elbow Injuries**

A. **Triceps tendinitis**

  1. Overuse syndrome due to overloading of triceps by repetitive extension of the elbow.

  2. Symptoms: Pain posterior elbow.

  3. Signs:

    a. Tenderness at or above the insertion of the triceps

    b. Increased pain with resisted extension of the elbow.

  4. X-rays: usually normal, but may reveal:

    a. Degenerative calcification

    b. Hypertrophy of the ulna

    c. Triceps traction spur.

  5. Differential diagnosis:

    a. Intratendinous or subtendinous bursitis

    b. Stress fracture of olecranon.

  6. Management:

    a. Rest, ice or heat, NSAID

    b. Injection (complication: rupture)

    c. Rehabilitation with graduated stretching and strengthening.

B. **Triceps rupture/olecranon avulsion**

  1. An uncoordinated triceps contracture during a fall or a direct blow to the elbow may cause tendon rupture or olecranon avulsion.

  2. Spontaneous rupture is associated with systemic disease or steroids.

3. Symptoms:
   a. Pain and swelling in the posterior elbow, usually severely acutely
   b. Weakness or loss of active elbow extension.
4. Signs:
   a. Tenderness at insertion of extensor mechanism
   b. Palpable defect in the triceps tendon or during step-off of olecranon
   c. If complete, no active extension of elbow
5. X-rays
   a. Flecks of avulsed bone (80% ruptures)
   b. Large olecranon fragment.
6. Management:
   a. Treatment is surgical
      i. Reattachment of avulsed triceps tendon to olecranon with nonabsorbable suture through drill holes.
      ii. Open reduction and internal fixation of fragment if sufficiently large, otherwise excision and repair of triceps to articular surface.
   b. Immobilize 45° flexion for 4 weeks, allow 0–45° flexion for 4 weeks, then graduated AROM and strengthening.

C. **Olecranon impingement syndrome**
   **(Olecranon hyperextension overload syndrome, olecranon fossitis, "boxer's elbow")**
   1. Overuse syndrome due to repetitive valgus extension overloading, which causes the olecranon process to be forced against the medial wall of the olecranon fossa.
   2. Symptoms:
      a. Insidious onset of pain while extending the elbow (especially throwing)
      b. Catching or locking of elbow in extension.
   3. Signs:
      a. Tenderness and swelling posteriorly
      b. Lack of full extension
      c. Pain on forced extension with valgus stress
      d. Palpable loose bodies.
   4. X-ray (recommend axial view in addition to AP and lateral):
      a. Hypertrophy of olecranon
      b. Spurring of olecranon tip and medial wall olecranon fossa
      c. Loose bodies.
   5. Management:
      a. Rest, NSAID
      b. Correction of poor throwing mechanics
      c. Surgical removal of olecranon tip, osteophytes, and loose bodies via arthroscopy or posterior arthrotomy.

D. **Olecranon bursitis ("miner's elbow," "student's elbow")**
   1. Repetitive trauma causes irritation to olecranon bursa.
   2. Symptoms: Relatively painless posterior swelling.
   3. Signs:
      a. Fluctuant bursa
      b. No cellulitis.
   4. X-rays: negative.
   5. Differential diagnosis:
      a. Septic bursitis.
   6. Management:
      a. Prevention with protective elbow pads
      b. Aspiration, ice, compression, NSAID, and splinting—useful although swelling will recur.

    c. Aspirate if septic bursitis is suspected.

    d. If chronic, surgical excision can be recommended, but there is risk of poor wound healing over the olecranon.

IV. **Medial Elbow Injuries**

  A. **Medial epicondylitis ("golfer's elbow")**

    1. Repetitive tension overloading of the wrist flexors causes microtears in the tendinous insertion at the epicondyle.

    2. Symptoms:

      a. Painful inflammation over the medial epicondyle

      b. Weakness secondary to pain.

    3. Signs:

      a. Tenderness at medial epicondyle

      b. Increased pain with resisted wrist flexion and forearm pronation

      c. Negative Tinel's sign at cubital tunnel.

    4. X-ray: usually negative, but small calcific deposits occasionally seen.

    5. Differential diagnosis:

      a. Flexor-pronator strain

      b. Medial collateral ligament sprain

      c. Ulnar neuritis.

    6. Management:

      a. Conservative management usually successful

        i. Rest

        ii. Splint (wrist in neutral)

        iii. NSAID

        iv. Steroid injection (limit to 3).

      b. Surgery for rare patient who does not improve

        i. Recession of flexor origin from medial epicondyle

        ii. 4 weeks' immobilization in splint followed by flexibility and strengthening for 12 weeks.

  B. **Flexor-pronator strain**

    1. Repetitive tensile stresses to a vulnerable flexor-pronator mass and may result in microruptures of the muscle, especially after inadequate warm-up or after fatigue.

    2. Symptoms:

      a. Medial elbow and proximal forearm pain

      b. Aggravated by wrist flexion (pitching curve balls, curling) and forearm pronation (golfing).

    3. Signs:

      a. Tender flexor-pronator muscle bellies distal to epicondyle.

    4. X-rays: negative.

    5. Management:

      a. Rest, ice, compression

      b. Modification of training schedule

      c. Proper warm-up activity

      d. Brief immobilization may be warranted in acute cases.

  C. **Medial collateral ligament sprain**

    1. Repetitive valgus stress (pitching, throwing, racquet sports) causes tensile loading of the MCL, resulting in microtears.

    2. Symptoms:

      a. Insidious medial elbow pain

      b. Provoked by valgus stress activities

      c. Relieved by rest.

3. Signs:
   a. Tenderness below the medial epicondyle over the humeroulnar joint (anterior oblique ligament)
   b. Pain increased by manual valgus stress
   c. Signs of ulnar neuritis may be associated since the MCL forms the floor of the cubital tunnel.
4. X-rays may reveal:
   a. Heterotopic ossification of the MCL
   b. Spurring at conoid tubercle of ulna
   c. Gravity stress view is negative unless MCL totally incompetent.
5. Management:
   a. Rest, NSAID
   b. Strengthening pronator-flexor group
   c. Complete MCL insufficiency in chronic cases will require surgical reconstruction with palmaris longus tendon.

D. **Medial epicondyle stress lesions ("Little Leaguer's elbow")**
   1. Since the closing growth plate of the medial epicondyle in adolescents is sensitive to tension stress, repetitive or a sudden muscular contraction may result in partial or complete avulsion of the medial epicondyle.
   2. Symptoms/signs:
      a. Acute pain medial elbow, usually severe
      b. Tenderness medial epicondyle with swelling, ecchymosis.
   3. X-rays:
      a. Widening of apophyseal line
      b. Partial or complete separation.
   4. Management:
      a. Medial epicondylar stress lesion
         i. Rest 2–3 weeks
         ii. No throwing allowed for 6–12 weeks.
      b. Medial epicondyle fracture
         i. May treat closed if minimally displaced ($<$ 5 mm)
         ii. Must treat open if:
            (a) Valgus instability is present ($>$ 10 mm displacement or positive gravity stress view)
            (b) Medial epicondyle is incarcerated within the elbow joint
            (c) Ulnar nerve symptoms are present.

E. **Ulnar nerve compression syndrome (cubital tunnel)**
   1. Entrapment neuropathy of ulnar nerve at the elbow, incited by trauma, cubitus valgus deformity, or subluxing ulnar nerve.
   2. Symptoms:
      a. Aching medial elbow pain, which may migrate proximally or distally
      b. Frequently accompanied by grip weakness
      c. Numbness and occasional shocking into ulnar 1½ digits
      d. No pain or limited ROM neck.
   3. Signs:
      a. Positive Tinel's cubital tunnel
      b. Pain increased with full-forced elbow flexion
      c. Weakness of thumb-index finger pinch
      d. Intrinsic muscle wasting uncommon unless problem long-term
      e. Negative foraminal compression testing for cervical radiculopathy.
   4. EMG/NCV: slowing of conduction velocity across the elbow.
   5. Differential diagnosis:

      a. Cervical radiculopathy

      b. Thoracic outlet syndrome

      c. Ulnar nerve compression at wrist (Guyon's canal)

   6. Management:

      a. Protection with elbow pad

      b. Rest, NSAID

      c. Modification of training

         i. Avoidance extreme flexion

        ii. Avoidance valgus stress.

      d. Surgical decompression necessary for increasing motor involvement, pain, sensory deficit, or chronic cases

      e. Anterior transposition reserved for neuropathy associated with elbow deformity (cubitus valgus) or subluxation of the ulnar nerve.

## V. Lateral Elbow Injuries

### A. Lateral epicondylitis ("tennis elbow")

   1. Painful degenerative tears in the extensor carpi radialis brevis due to repetitive tension overloading of the forearm and wrist extensors (hyperpronation greatly increases the overloading stresses).

   2. Lateral epicondylitis is 10 times more frequent than medial epicondylitis.

   3. Predisposing factors:

      a. Age 30–50 years

      b. Faulty mechanics ("leading" elbow; off-center hits in racquet sports)

      c. Poorly fitted equipment (handle too small, string too tight).

   4. Symptoms:

      a. Aching pain over lateral epicondyle radiating proximally into forearm extensors during and after activity

      b. Initially subsides but with repetition becomes more severe.

   5. Signs:

      a. Localized tenderness to lateral epicondyle

      b. Pain increased with resisted dorsiflexion of wrist

      c. "Coffee cup" test (Conrad)—pain is increased while picking up a full cup of coffee.

   6. X-rays: small calcific deposits in extensor aponeurosis (22% of cases).

   7. Differential diagnosis: posterior interosseous nerve compression (coexistent in 5% of cases).

   8. Management:

      a. Nonsurgical successful for most

         i. Rest

            (a) No grasping in pronation

            (b) Use supination when lifting

        ii. NSAID

       iii. Volar cock-up splint

       iv. Counterforce bracing

        v. Steroid injection (limit to 3)

       vi. Proper mechanics for the sport

      vii. Proper equipment

            (a) Larger racquet head

            (b) Correct grip size = midpalmar crease to tip of ring finger

            (c) Medium tension strings, 50–55 lb.

      b. Surgical treatment for refractory cases

         i. Debridement of ECRB with repair

    ii. Rehabilitation
       (a) Progressive strengthening, ROM below painful level
       (b) Daily warm-up
       (c) NSAID
       (d) Counterforce bracing 3 months
       (e) Return to sports 6 months.

B. **Radiocapitellar chondromalacia**
  1. Valgus stress of throwing and racquet sports imparts strong tensile forces to the medial collateral ligament and strong compressive forces to the lateral joint of the elbow.
  2. Repeated compressive forces can cause damage to the radial head, capitellum, or both (osteochondral fracture and even loose body may result).
  3. Symptoms:
    a. Lateral elbow pain with activity
    b. Catching or locking.
  4. Signs:
    a. Tender radiocapitallar joint, lateral swelling
    b. Crepitus with forearm pronation-supination.
  5. X-ray:
    a. Loss of radiocapitellar joint space
    b. Marginal osteophytes
    c. Loose bodies.
  6. Management:
    a. Difficult to treat once joint damage established
    b. Mild disorder
      i. Rest, NSAID
      ii. Graduated activity dictated by pain, swelling.
    c. Severe disorder
      i. Joint debridement through lateral arthrotomy with removal of marginal osteophytes and loose bodies
      ii. Prognosis is proportional to cartilage damage.

C. **Osteochondritis dissecans capitellum**
  1. Focal lesion in young athletes with open growth plates (age 10–15 years), attributed to lateral compressive forces.
  2. Symptoms:
    a. Pain with activity
    b. Pain improved with rest
    c. Occasionally clicking or locking of elbow.
  3. Signs:
    a. Tenderness radiocapitellar joint, swelling
    b. Grating with pronation—supination
    c. Lack of full extension.
  4. X-rays, tomograms or arthrotomograms:
    a. Irregularity or flattening of capitellum
    b. Crater with loose body.
  5. Differential diagnosis: Panner's osteochondrosis
  6. Management:
    a. Rest (6–18 months).
    b. If no loose body, no further treatment may be needed.
    c. If fragment is displaced, then recommend reattachment of the articular fragment if large, but otherwise excision.

D. **Radial head fracture**
1. Compressive axial loading force across the radiocapitellar joint during a fall onto outstretched arm may result in fracture of the radial head.
2. Mason describes types as:
   a. Type I—nondisplaced
   b. Type II—displaced (impaction > 3 mm, angulation > 30°,
   c. Type III—comminuted.
3. Symptoms: Severe lateral elbow pain.
4. Signs:
   a. Tenderness well localized to radial head
   b. Passive pronation-supination painful
   c. Crepitus may be present but examiner should not attempt to repeatedly demonstrate this
   d. May have associated valgus instability of the elbow or axial instability of the forearm (Essix-Lopresti lesion).
5. X-ray:
   a. Positive posterior fat-pad sign should suggest an intra-articular fracture.
   b. Nondisplaced fracture may be difficult to diagnose unless oblique views are taken.
   c. Check capitellum for osteochondral fracture.
6. Management:
   a. Type I—treatment is nonoperative, with early ROM.
   b. Type II—controversial but suggest ORIF for large fragments.
   c. Type III—usually requires excision radial head—beware of elbow or forearm instability.
E. **Posterior interosseous nerve (PIN) compression syndrome (radial tunnel syndrome)**
1. Entrapment neuropathy of the posterior interosseous branch of the radial nerve under the fibrous arch of supinator (arcade of Frosche) or more distally in the supinator muscle.
2. Symptoms:
   a. Aching lateral elbow pain radiating into dorsal forearm
   b. Aggravated by pronation-supination activities
   c. Extensor weakness of the wrist and fingers but no numbness.
3. Signs:
   a. Positive Tinel's sign 8 cm (4 fingerbreadths) distal to the lateral epicondyle
   b. Weakness of ECU and EDC
   c. No sensory loss.
4. X-rays: normal.
5. EMG/NCV rarely confirmatory for PIN compression.
6. Differential diagnosis:
   a. Lateral epicondylitis
   b. Extensor tendon rupture
   c. Extensor tendon dislocation (hood injury).
7. Management:
   a. Rest, modification of training schedule
   b. Surgical decompression in recalcitrant cases.

VI. **Dislocations and Fracture-dislocations**

1. Acute injury to the elbow following specific traumatic event, usually a fall into outstretched arm.
2. Symptoms: severe pain, often too painful to move.

3. Signs:
   a. Acute tenderness and swelling
   b. Deformity of the elbow
   c. Limited motion, possibly with crepitus
   d. Neurologic or vascular compromise
4. X-rays:
   a. Dislocation
   b. Dislocation with associated fracture
      i. Radial head
      ii. Coronoid process
      iii. Medial epicondyle.
   c. Monteggia fracture
   d. Supracondylar humerus fracture
   e. T-intercondylar humerus fracture.
5. Management:
   a. Document neurovascular examination
   b. Immobilize the injured extremity with splint
   c. Refer urgently to ER for X-ray evaluation and further treatment as indicated:
      i. Closed reduction
      ii. Open reduction and internal fixation.

## RECOMMENDED READING

1. Hoppenfield S: Physical Examination of the Spine and Extremities. Norwalk, CT, Appleton-Century-Crofts, 1976, pp 35–58.
2. Morrey F: The Elbow and Its Disorders. Philadelphia, WB Saunders, 1985.
3. Rockwood C, Green D: Fractures in Adults, Vol 1. Philadelphia, JP Lippincott, 1984, pp 559–652.
4. Zarins B, Andrews R, Carson WG Jr: Injuries to the Throwing Arm. Philadelphia, WB Saunders, 1985, pp 191 258.

# Chapter 36: Hand and Wrist Injuries

THOMAS P. FERLIC, MD

I. **History and Physical Examination:** An accurate history and physical examination must be done for each injury.

   A. Establish **mechanism of injury** historically.

   B. **Gentle examination**. Just because a structure is small does not mean that an accurate assessment cannot be done. Too often one tries to apply gross stresses and gross tenderness to smaller parts of the body, when actually, if one were very gentle and applied point tenderness, a great deal of information could be gleaned. This can be done with the tip of an eraser on a pencil. Precise location of tenderness will be of great help in determining the exact injury to the digit.

   1. **Comparison to the opposite side**—for physiologic laxity and for previous injury causing the same type of physical findings.

   C. **X-ray studies:** The subject of fractures is not included in this chapter. There are many good references available, some of which are noted in the references at the end of this chapter. Suffice it to say, however, that x-ray studies should be done whenever:

   1. An injury persists for more than a day or two.
   2. Swelling is present.
   3. Joint motion is limited.

II. **Distal Interphalangeal (DIP) Joint Injuries**

   A. **Mallet finger.** The term mallet finger implies that discontinuity of the extensor mechanism of the distal interphalangeal (DIP) joint is present. The extensor mechanism may be simply thinned or torn, or a small piece of bone may be avulsed from the proximal portion of the distal phalanx dorsally. A variant of this may include a fracture dislocation or fracture subluxation of the DIP joint.

   1. **Mechanism of injury:** The problem is usually caused by hyperflexion of the DIP joint. This is a common type of injury seen when a ball hits the tip of an extended finger and forces it into hyperflexion at the DIP joint, thereby either tearing or thinning the extensor mechanism.

   2. **Examination** shows lack of extension at the DIP joint. This may be full or may show only lack of the last 10 to 20 degrees of full extension.

   3. **X-rays** will indicate a joint that is held in flexion or may show a small fracture off the proximal portion of the distal phalanx (Fig. 1).

   4. **Therapy** consists of immobilization of the DIP joint in extension for 6 to 8 weeks full time. This implies that during this time the patient will not flex, actively or passively, the DIP joint.

      a. Several commercial splints are available for this immobilization. The proximal interphalangeal (PIP) joint does not need to be immobilized. Active rehabilitation should consist of movement of the metacarpophalangeal (MCP) and PIP joints while the DIP joint is immobilized. After the PIP immobilization is discontinued at 6 weeks, one should observe the patient serially to make sure that extension has been maintained after this injury.

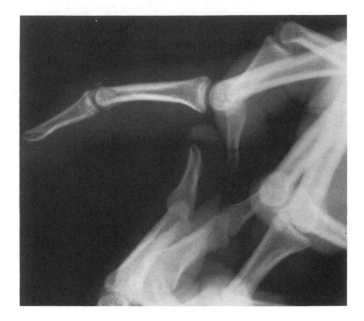

**FIGURE 1.** X-ray of a mallet finger. Note the flexed posture and the small fracture of the proximal dorsal portion of the distal phalanx.

5. **Differential diagnosis: A special note of caution should be made not to confuse a fracture dislocation with a mallet finger.** Generally, the rule is if the fragment is 10 to 15% or less at the joint space, there will generally not be a fracture dislocation. This commonly will be a mallet injury.

B. **Jersey finger** is a common term used for avulsion of the flexor tendon. This often happens to the fourth and fifth finger. Depending on the size and nature of the bony fragment, if one is present, the flexor tendon may be trapped in part of its sheath or may be retracted all the way to the palm.

1. **Mechanism of injury** is usually hyperextension on attempted flexion of the finger. This commonly happens to football safeties and line backers who attempt to stop a running back from behind, grab his jersey with their fingers flexed, and apply sudden and forceful power to the flexor tendon system. The flexor tendon may be avulsed from its bony bed.

2. **History:** The patient usually describes an attempt at severe flexion, followed by immediate pain.

3. **Examination** shows lack of flexion at the DIP joint. **In addition, the entire flexor tendon sheath will normally have a hematoma formation.** Tenderness may be felt over the middle portion of the middle phalanx—over the A-4 pulley, over the A-2 pulley area, or into the palm.

4. **X-ray films** will show either no abnormality or a small bony fragment caught either underneath the A-4 pulley, underneath the decussation in the flexor sublimis, or in the palm. It is often difficult to see the small bony fragment if it is in the palm, unless the examiner specifically is looking for it. If a bony fragment is present, often it is caught up underneath the A-4 pulley.

5. **Therapy includes operative intervention. No conservative treatment can be expected to bring the flexor tendon back to its normal length.** Surgery should be performed within the first few days of injury. Occasionally, this injury is missed, and, depending on the type and position of the flexor tendon, a later repair may be feasible.

6. **Rehabilitation** consists of partial immobilization with limited range of motion exercise under the supervision of a physical therapist for 5 weeks. After 5 weeks, normally immobilization may be removed, but caution has to be taken for up to 12 to 14 weeks to assure flexor tendon healing.

C. **Dislocation of the DIP joint**

    1. **Description:** Usually obvious, the patient presents with an obviously deformed joint with tenderness.

    2. **Mechanism of injury** includes any forceful blow or avulsion to the DIP joint.

    3. **Examination** shows tenderness over the DIP joint and inability to flex or extend the joint. The joint may be slightly lateral.

    4. **X-rays** will show a dislocation of the joint. **Caution:** at times an osteochondral fracture can be noted that initially might seem quite small to the examiner. These often involve a large amount of subchondral bone, not unlike a tibial plateau fracture. These should be treated aggressively if joint disruption is noted.

    5. **Treatment** consists of gentle **reduction.** The key to reducing joints is both pushing and pulling in a gentle manner. **Postreduction:** generally the DIP joint is stable without further mobilization. Caution must be noted once again: after the joint is reduced, **postreduction x-rays** are again reviewed to make sure no fractures are present.

III. **Proximal Interphalangeal Joint Injuries**

A. **Tear of volar plate**

    1. **Mechanism of injury** is a hyperextension of the PIP joint. This normally occurs when fingers are forcibly "bent back."

    2. **Examination** shows hyperextension of the joint. Comparison should be made to the opposite side, since many people are naturally hyperextensible at their PIP joints.

    3. **X-rays:** Since this injury is often painful to the patient because of hemarthrosis and swelling in the finger, it may be necessary to employ a **digital block** before stressing. The finger is then **gently stress by the examiner with an extension stress at the PIP joint,** holding pressure over the dorsum in attempting to gently rock the joint open on the volar aspect (Fig. 2). **Comparison radiographs may be needed.** X-rays may show no fracture or a very small fracture off of the proximal portion on the volar aspect of the middle phalanx. This finding is pathognomonic for a volar plate tear.

    4. **Differential diagnosis:** If the fracture fragment contains more than 10 to 15% of the volar surface, one must be concerned about a **fracture dislocation** that was spontaneously reduced. This is an entirely different injury.

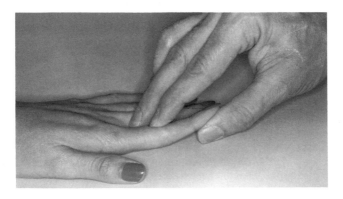

**FIGURE 2.** Stress applied to volar plate of the PIP by attempting to hyperextend it.

5. **Therapy:** Normally these are stable injuries. Treatment consists of splinting the affected digit at 15 to 30 degrees of flexion for 3 weeks, and then progressive motion with splinting is carried out for another 3 weeks to prevent hyperextension at the PIP joint. The PIP joint only should be immobilized. The DIP joint should not be immobilized.
   a. Dorsal block splint may be used.
   b. **Caution:** do not over-immobilize this injury, i.e., neither too much time nor in too much flexion, as either may cause a permanent flexion contracture.
   c. If at 6 weeks the patient is not able to extend the PIP joint fully, consideration should be given to having the patient see a therapist for use of a reverse knuckle bender.
   d. No splinting is necessary if, after reduction, the PIP joint is stable.
6. **Swan neck deformity:** If this injury is unrecognized and/or untreated and the joint goes on to permanent hyperextension, the DIP joint will naturally fall into flexion because of the positions of the lateral band. The so-called swan neck deformity will ensue.

B. **Tear of central slip**
   1. **Description:** This is a classic injury that ensues when the central slip of the extensor mechanism tears. If one visualizes the extensor mechanism, part of its duty is to extend the MCP joint. It does this by means of the sagittal bands, which do not really have a tendinous insertion on the proximal phalanx. It works more like a lasso pulling the phalanx up. The extensor mechanism's actual insertion is into the proximal portion of the middle phalanx, the so-called central slip of the extensor mechanism.

      If this amll area of tendinous insertion is torn, the lateral bands are free to sublux volarly. This is the mechanism of a boutonnière deformity—the joint "buttonholes" up through the extensor mechanism.
   2. **The mechanism of injury** may be a blow to the dorsum of or a volar dislocation of the middle phalanx that is spontaneously reduced.
   3. **Examination** is quite difficult.
      a. Point tenderness should be elicited over the middle phalanx proximally in the midline (Fig. 3). If one examines very closely, one might also note some tenderness over either collateral ligament, since a tear of the central slip may be accompanied by a tear or strain of one of the ligamentous structures.

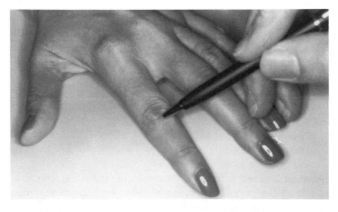

**FIGURE 3.** Pen pointing to insertion of central slip.

    b. The definitive sign of this injury is lack of extension of the middle phalanx. However, this is often quite difficult to identify, since initially one may see extension and over the following few weeks may see less and less ability to extend the finger.

    c. Also during this time, since the lateral bands are subluxed volarly, one will see progressive tightening in extension of the DIP joint. This is the classic differentiation between a central slip tear and a volar plate tear. In a volar plate tear, one may see tenderness over the volar aspect of the middle phalanx as well as scarring of the joint down into some flexion. However, usually the DIP joint will have a full range of motion and be unaffected.

    d. In a progressive boutonnière deformity, one will see loss of extension of the PIP joint with progressive tightening in extension of the DIP joint. This is a very difficult clinical diagnosis; and if one is unsure of the diagnosis, serial examinations are imperative over the first few weeks to make sure that the diagnosis is correct.

    e. Specific examination for this disorder includes flexing the wrist fully and flexing the MCP joints. This provides a **tenodesis** affect. If the finger is not actively extended in this position or cannot be extended to within about 20 degrees of neutral, one must suspect a central slip rupture.

4. **X-rays** generally will not show any particular bony abnormality. They may, however, show a very small avulsion from the dorsum of the middle phalanx proximally.

5. **Treatment** is directed at the PIP joint. The PIP joint should be treated in extension for 6 full weeks. During this time, active pull-through of the DIP joint is imperative.

    a. Consideration of realigning bony fragments must also be given. Although this is controversial, one might consider acute repair if a large bony fragment is present.

    b. After the 6 weeks of extension of the PIP joint have passed, one must direct the therapeutic program at gradual flexion of the PIP joint.

C. **Collateral ligament tear**

1. **Description:** Collateral ligament tear implies that the supporting structures for the medial or lateral side of the joint have been torn.

2. **Mechanism of injury** is usually a lateral blow or lateral tearing. Often, the patient may have had a dislocation that has spontaneously reduced or has been reduced.

3. **History** is usually that the finger was dislocated and pulled back into the joint or that the patient felt his finger hinge open and then shut.

4. **Examination** usually shows that the patient has tenderness over the specific site of tear. The tear may be in several locations but is more often found distally at the insertion on the middle phalanx rather than from the origin of ligament of the proximal phalanx. The midportion of the ligament may also be torn.

    a. Stress testing will show that, with lateral flexion at 0 degrees, a small amount of opening will be noted (Fig. 4). As the joint flexes down to 20 to 30 degrees of flexion, more opening will be noted.

5. **X-rays** will usually not show a great deal.

    a. A small fleck of bone may be noted on the AP, either median or laterally.

    b. Stress x-rays taken when a digital block has been given may show gross opening of the joint.

6. **Treatment** is aimed at reestablishment of the collateral ligament. Depending on surgical or nonsurgical preference of the examiner, one may consider operative repair verses buddy taping for 6 to 8 weeks. Obviously, the position of the finger may affect this decision.

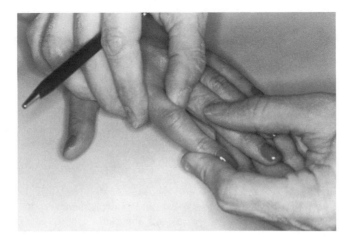

**FIGURE 4.** Stress applied to radial collateral ligament of index finger.

    a. **The radial ligament to the index finger** is obviously more important in pinch than the radial ligament of the fourth finger, and surgery may be a more likely choice when it is injured.

D. **Dislocation of the PIP joint**

    1. **Description:** The patient is unable to use the finger due to an obvious dislocation. The question follows whether this is a dorsal or a volar dislocation. The **type of dislocation** is determined by the position of the middle phalanx relative to the proximal phalanx. Hyperextension of the PIP joint would cause a volar disruption, i.e., volar tear, and the ultimate outcome would be a dorsal dislocation. Likewise, if the finger was hyperflexed or in some way pushed volarly, then the central slip would tear.

    2. Treatment of these injuries should be directed at the ligamentous disruption (See par. III.A. and B.).

IV. **Metacarpalphalangeal Joint**

A. Sprain of MCP joint

    1. **Description:** The patient may describe a hyperextension injury, such as falling on an outstretched hand and hyperextending the MCP joint(s).

    2. **Examination** shows some mild tenderness only. Usually the patient has a full range of motion.

    3. **Treatment:** No special treatment is needed.

B. **Dislocation**

    1. **Simple dislocation**

        a. **Examination:** Finger is hyperextended 60–80 degrees at the MCP joint.

           i. Rarely seen by physician, because the dislocation is usually reduced immediately by the patient or someone else at the scene of the injury.

        b. **Treatment:** Often reduced by a gentle pulling of the finger. No further treatment is necessary.

           i. The small finger may require some immobilization for 3 weeks to prevent abduction stresses.

    2. **Complex dislocation**

        a. **Description:** The patient presents with a finger that is extended at approximately 5 to 10 degrees of extension. It cannot be moved from this position.

b. **Examination** as above. Inability to flex or extend the MCP joint from its position. A skin dimple on the volar aspect of the joint is usually present.

c. **Radiographs** are often difficult to assess. AP and lateral radiographs will show overlap of the shadows. If an oblique x-ray is taken, at times an off-center MCP joint can be appreciated. This problem often requires clinical diagnosis.

d. **Treatment**

    i. A gentle attempt at manipulative reduction.

       (a) Often fails when the volar plate is trapped within the joint.

    ii. If one attempt at gentle reduction fails, operative reduction is indicated.

V. **Thumb**

  A. **Sprain of ulnar collateral ligament of the thumb MCP joint.**

    1. **Description: Tear of the ulnar collateral ligament (gamekeeper's thumb; skier's thumb).** The term gamekeeper's thumb implies the fact that the ulnar collateral ligament is torn at the level of the MCP joint.

    2. **Mechanism of injury:** usually a fall on an outstretched hand with the thumb caught in the position of abduction. The thumb is held at 90 degrees to the index finger in the plane of abduction and adduction. Hence, if the thumb is pulled away from the hand and away from the palm, this would cause ultimate stress on the ulnar aspect of the MCP joint.

    3. **Examination** shows point tenderness over the ulnar aspect of the joint. Specifically, point tenderness can almost always be elicited at the insertion of the collateral ligament at the volar aspect of the joint at the level of the proximal phalanx. When stress is applied by placing the examiner's finger over the radial aspect of the joint and applying a load to the ulnar aspect, a feeling of opening will be appreciated (Fig. 5). Often this examination is difficult to perform in acute painful injuries, and a digital block or regional block in the area must be given.

    4. **X-rays** will indicate, on occasion, a fragment of bone from the level of the MCP joint, which will be an interarticular fracture from the proximal phalanx (i.e., insertion of the ligament).

      a. Stress radiographs need to be taken at that point with the finger anesthetized. If it opens up 20 degrees more than the opposite side, there is good indication

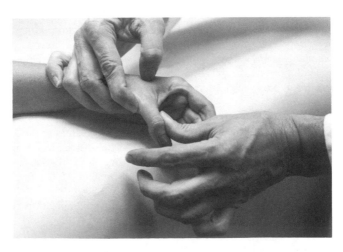

**FIGURE 5.** Stress applied to ulnar collateral ligament of the thumb.

that the ligament is ruptured. Although there is no definitive mechanisms to tell this, an arthrogram, may be helpful.

5. **Therapy** consists of surgical treatment if the ligament is fully torn. If not, a cast for 4 to 6 weeks, or a cone and cup (thumb spica) splint made by the occupational therapist, may be in order.

6. Rehabilitation consists of ongoing active motion and alleviating any web-space contracture between the index and thumb. A cone and cup (thumb spica) splint is also valuable if the athlete is sent back to competitive sports—to protect the joint against early reinjury.

B. **Metacarpophalangeal joint strain**

1. **Description:** In addition to the ulnar collateral ligament, the opposite or radial collateral ligament, as well as the volar plate and dorsal capsule of the MCP joint, can be injured.

2. **The mechanism of injury** is usually inappropriate directional stresses, either having the thumb hyperextended (bent backwards) or the volar plate hyperflexed, in the case of the dorsal structures, or deviated over the plane of the hand and adducted across the hand in the case of the radial collateral ligament.

   a. Volar plate tear or stretch injury—caused by forcible hyperextension.

   b. Dorsal capsule injury—usually caused by an abduction or adduction stress.

   c. Radial collateral ligament injury—caused by forcible adduction of the thumb above or below the palm.

3. **Examination** should be directed to finding the exact source of tenderness within the finger. Once again, gentle palpation should be performed with a small object, such as the eraser of a pencil, to elicit point of tenderness; and gentle stresses should be applied.

4. **X-rays** may be negative or may show small interarticular fractures.

5. **Therapy** includes appropriate splinting for volar plate and collateral ligament injuries.

   a. The volar plate injury should be treated like that of other joints, i.e., the joint should be held in a slight amount of flexion for 2 to 3 weeks and then allowed to regain extension. Caution must be taken not to **over-immobilize** this injury.

   b. The same is true for radial collateral injuries, which can be immobilized for 4 to 6 weeks, depending on their severity. An alternative is cone and cup splint to prevent stresses. These are available commercially or through an occupational therapist.

   c. Dorsal capsule injuries can be splinted in extension for 4 to 6 weeks.

VI. **Penetrating Injuries of the Hand: Guidelines for Evaluation and Management**

A. **Description:** One must establish an accurate history. The usual questions of when, where, how, and then what all need to be answered.

1. Certainly a penetrating injury that occurred 2 to 3 days previously on a football field is markedly different from one suffered from a clean, sharp object 20 minutes prior to examination.

2. Other appropriate elements of the history include the dominant type of sporting activity and constitutional factors that might predispose to complications, such as diabetes mellitus or sickle cell anemia.

B. **Examination** in the emergency room should be directed in a algorithmic manner. Many mistakes can be avoided if the examination and treatment are done in a systematic fashion. Several factors have to be addressed:

1. All jewelry needs to be removed in order to avoid complications of future swelling.

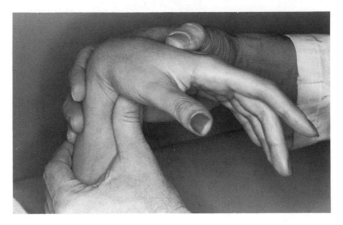

**FIGURE 6.** Wrist palmar flexed. Note extension of MCPs.

2. The patient has to be calm. The physician must question the patient to obtain an accurate assessment of the injury. It is obviously very difficult to examine a squirming patient who won't cooperate.
3. If the patient has already been bandaged by another individual, the dressing can be removed. Care must be taken to remove it gently to avoid disturbing either the patient or the wound. Often, a thorough washing with just normal saline will accomplish this.
4. **Inspection:** Inspection is directed at identifying the location and area that have been violated. If the object that lacerated the patient came in at an angle, one may be surprised to find other structures cut that are not underneath the entry wound, but some distance away under normal-appearing tissue.
   a. **Passive inspection:** After inspecting the area visually, the wrist is gently palmar-flexed (Fig. 6). When one does this, the extensor tendons naturally straighten the fingers into extension. If there is a laceration over the dorsum of the hand and one finger does not extend (and may actually appear to drop), it is obvious that there is some type of extensor tendon laceration. Likewise, with the wrist in dorsiflexion, the fingers normally flex (Fig. 7). If one finger fails to flex and stays in extension and the patient has a laceration on his palm, obviously a flexor tendon is lacerated. One may use the opposite wrist to determine the exact posturing for the affected wrist.

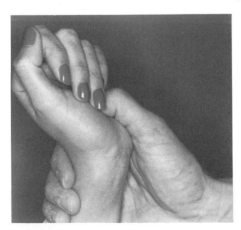

**FIGURE 7.** Wrist dorsiflexed. Note flexion of fingers.

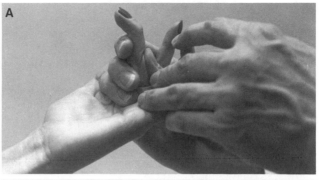

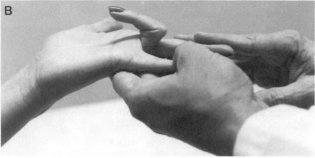

**FIGURE 8.** *A,* Testing of flexor profundus. *B,* Testing of flexor sublimis.

b. **Active inspection:** Examination in the active phase, requires patient cooperation. The flexor profundus to all fingers should be checked, including the thumb. This can be done by blocking the motion of the sublimis by holding the PIP of the affected finger in extension and having the patient flex the DIP joint (Fig. 8A). One should be careful to note any tenderness to resisted motion, as this is often the **hallmark of a partial tendon laceration.** Sublimis function may be noted by holding all the fingers in extension except for the finger to be tested (Fig. 8B). Extension is likewise checked by having the patient actively extend the DIP joint and the PIP joints separately.

    i. It is interesting to note that the intrinsic musculature as well as the extrinsics can extend these joints. Therefore, with a laceration of the extensor tendon over the dorsum of the hand, the patient will still be able to actively extend his PIP and DIP joints, depending on the position of the wrist and MCP joints.

5. **Sensation** should be checked carefully, remembering that there is a great deal of sensory nerve overlap in the hand.

a. One must be able to establish whether or not the patient has two-point discrimination. Often an easy test for this is simply to see if the patient can tell the difference between the serrated edge of a quarter and the smooth edge of a nickel. Blunt pins are also available for this test. One must be cautious not to use a hypodermic needle, as this often upsets the patient and destroys the already calm atmosphere.

b. The median nerve provides sensation to the volar aspect of the radial 3½ fingers, and the ulnar nerve provides sensation to the ulnar aspect of the ulnar 1½ fingers. Since there is a slight amount of cross innervation, it is important to note that the volar aspect of the index finger is always innervated by the median nerve and the small finger is always innervated by the ulnar nerve.

6. **Vascularity:** Temperature of the skin and nail-bed blanching can help determine vascularity. If one is unsure of the vascularity of the finger, it must be checked on several occasions to determine whether referral to a surgeon experienced in re-establishing circulation is necessary.

7. **Muscle strength testing of specific hand muscles, innervated by the median and ulnar nerve:**
   a. The median nerve can be checked by having the patient pull his thumb in to touch the tip of his fifth finger. If there is median nerve innervation, or if he or she has loss of innervation at the wrist rather than the forearm, the patient will bring across the thumb in the plane of the forearm rather than opposing it truly to the fifth finger.
   b. The ulnar nerve can be checked easily by having the patient cross his fingers. The index and long finger can be used for this. Also of value is checking the ability to abduct the small finger against resistance.
   c. **X-rays** should be taken in order to rule out a retained foreign body, underlying unsuspected fracture, or other findings that may have not been noted.

8. **Tetanus toxoid should be given with the guidelines of the U.S. Centers for Disease Control (CDC).**
   a. **Wound debridement** can only be done when there is good sterility, excellent light, assistance, instruments designed for hand surgery, and appropriate anesthesia. If all of these factors are present, then the following sequence of debridement and possible closure becomes possible:
      i. A tourniquet hemostasis is needed, and this can be done in the emergency room and may require that someone sustain a blood pressure cuff up to 250 mm of mercury over the proximal arm. The wound is then gently washed. If the appropriate anesthesia has been given, this will not bother the patient. The wound is gently sponged and then lavaged out with saline. The edges and necrotic area are then removed. Care must be taken to avoid the underlying tendons, nerve, and vascular structures. After this point, the hand is elevated, pressure is placed on the hand, and the tourniquet is released.
      ii. Gross hemostasis can be performed at this point. One must be cautioned, however, about trying to place a hemostat within a wound to "tie off a bleeder." Often, the vessel in question is running with the digital nerve, and iatrogenic injury to that nerve is a risk.
      iii. After hemostasis, the wound is ready to suture. Whether the wound should be closed or not depends on a variety of factors. If a wound is greater than 8 hours old, has any crush component, or if debridement is possibly inadequate, consideration must be given to secondary closure at a later date.
      iv. A sterile compressive dressing can be applied, and the wound should be inspected on a daily basis. If any tissue such as tendon or nerve is exposed, one must take care to keep the wound moist.
      v. Closure of the wounds is not necessarily as important as one may think. Late closure and healing by secondary intent is very effective in hand injuries.

VII. **Nerve Entrapments:** Entrapment syndromes are relatively rare in athletes but do occur.

   A. **Median nerve entrapments:** The median nerve may be entrapped at three major sites within the forearm and wrist. The median nerve functions as the chief innervation for the thenar musculature, as well as the flexor profundus to the index and long fingers, flexor of the thumb, and sublimis function to all fingers.

1. **Carpal tunnel**
   a. **Description:** Carpal tunnel syndrome is caused when the median nerve is entrapped at the level of the wrist joint. This is seen in athletes who use their hands repetitively and develop flexor tendon tenosynovitis within the distal forearm and hand. If a patient develops the tendinitis distally in the palm, a trigger finger will be noted. If the flexor tendon tenosynovitis develops in the wrist, however, the median nerve will be trapped within the confines of the carpal canal.
   b. **Symptoms** include tingling within the fingertips, especially those of the radial four fingers. One or all fingertips may be involved. The tingling may be intermittent. It is especially prevalent at night, at which time it will often awaken the patient and will cause him to shake his hand or to move his hand about to try and "get it awake." The pain may travel retrograde up the arm, and the patient may complain of pain as far as the shoulder or in the intrascapular areas. Proximal pain is a well-known phenomenon of distal entrapment syndromes of any nature.
   c. **Examination**
      i. **Early findings**
         (a) Night awakening, with wrist and hand pain and numbness.
         (b) Paresthesia with retrograde pain radiating into arm.
         (c) Sensory loss radial 3½ fingers.
         (d) Tinel's sign: percussion (tapping) the median nerve at the carpal tunnel reproduces the tingling sensation (Fig. 9).
         (e) Phalen's sign: Forced volar flexion of the wrist for 90 seconds reproduces the tingling sensation (Fig. 10).
         (f) Occasionally, Tinel's and Phalen's signs are present in people without carpal tunnel syndrome.
      ii. **Late findings**
         (a) Weakness of abductor pollicis brevis and opponens pollicis muscles.
         (b) Loss of 2-point discrimination in median nerve sensory areas of the hand.
   d. **Special tests:** Electromyography and nerve conduction velocity are generally diagnostic.
   e. **Therapy** is directed at reducing compression at the carpal tunnel.
      i. Splinting the wrist. Night splinting is particularly effective in reducing the tendon swelling that contributes to nerve compression. Twenty-four hour splinting may be necessary in some cases.

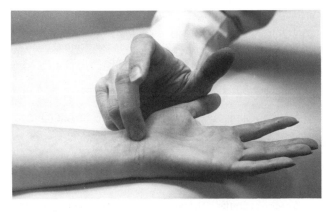

**FIGURE 9.** Tinel's sign for median nerve at the wrist.

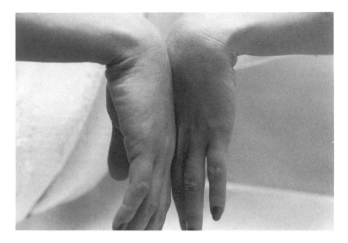

**FIGURE 10.** Phalen's test.

    ii. Nonsteroidal anti-inflammatory drugs help reduce inflammation and swelling.

    iii. Corticosteroid injections around tendons to relieve tenosynovitis are helpful.

       (a) **Caution:** Do not inject into median nerve or tendon bodies.

    iv. Surgical decompression if symptoms persist and there is EMG evidence of median nerve injury.

2. **Pronator teres entrapment** (a sensory syndrome)

   a. **Description:** The median nerve becomes trapped either between or just distal to the two heads of the pronator teres muscle. The patient generally experiences pain, paresthesias, and reduced sensation in the median nerve distribution. Impaired pronation and grip are rare. Manual muscle testing is normally negative.

   b. **Mechanism of injury:** Repetitive use of the forearm in pronation certainly can be implicated at times; at other times, no mechanism of injury can be noted. Anomalous anatomic situations may also be involved.

   c. **Examination** shows that the patient has numbness within the distribution of the median nerve; there is virtually no weakness associated with it. Forced pronation against resistance or isometric pronation may reproduce the symptoms. Likewise, resisted flexion of the elbow may also cause some difficulty. It is important to differentiate this from the more common carpal tunnel syndrome. Phalen's test is normally negative.

   d. **X-rays** are not indicated.

   e **Special tests** include EMGs. These may or may not be positive, as this is a difficult area to assess.

   f. **Therapy** should be addressed at relieving the offending motion and splinting for 3 to 6 weeks. If no improvement is noted, consideration may be given to operative intervention.

3. **Anterior interosseous syndrome** (a motor syndrome)

   a. **Description:** The anterior interosseous portion of the median nerve innervates the flexor profundus to the index finger, flexor pollicis longus, and the pronator quadratus. (The innervation of the long finger profundus is variable. It branches off the main trunk distal to the pronator teres.) Injury to this nerve may affect one or all of the above muscles. There is no sensory portion to the anterior interosseous nerve. Hence, the median sensation is unaffected.

b. **Mechanism of injury:** Presentation is usually in one of two ways: (1) an acute onset in which the patient suddenly loses use of his flexor pollicis longus, and the index finger profundus is isolated; (2) a very slow weakening of these muscles, in which the patient notes gradual weakness, progressive with heavy activity. The injury may come on after a set of very strenuous or repetitive elbow motion exercises.

c. **Examination** shows the patient has weakness or loss of flexion of the interphalangeal (IP) joint of the thumb and the DIP joint of the index finger. Characteristically, when attempting to make a circle or 0 (Fig. 11A) with the index and the thumb, the patient will not be able to get his thumb or the index finger flexed, therefore unable to make a circle (i.e., the distal joints of the thumb and index finger remain in extension) (Fig. 11B).

d. **X-rays** are of no benefit.

e. **Special test:** An EMG is certainly indicated after the injury has been present for at least 3 weeks. Prior to this time, the test may be false-negative. Conduction velocity will also be helpful.

f. **Therapy** consists of splinting the extremity and avoiding heavy activity during recovery. If after 6 weeks no return of function is noted, consideration may be given to exploration of the nerve.

B. **Entrapment of the ulnar nerve:** The ulnar nerve supplies the intrinsic musculature of the hand as well as the flexor profundus to the small and ring fingers. Normally it can be entrapped at two separate positions, the wrist and the elbow.

  1. **Ulnar nerve entrapment at the wrist (Guyon's canal;** can be a motor, sensory, or mixed syndrome)

    a. **Description:** Guyon's canal is an anatomic analogue of the carpal tunnel and lies just medial to it. It is sometimes called the pisohamate tunnel. Entrapment

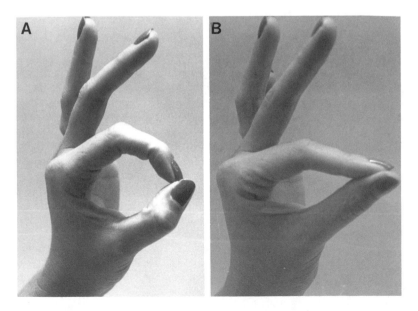

**FIGURE 11.** *A,* Test for anterior interosseus nerve; normal attempt at "making a circle." *B,* Abnormal test, with inability to flex the DIP of the index and IP of the thumb.

of the nerve in this area may cause some weakness of the intrinsic musculature as well as numbness in the ulnar 1½ fingers on their volar aspect.

  b. **Mechanism of injury:** Repetitive trauma or microtrauma to Guyon's canal related to athletic events such as bicycling or work situations such as operating a jack hammer.

  c. **Examination**

    i. Intrinsic muscle weakness:

      (a) Adductor pollicis.

      (b) 1st dorsal interosseous (may also be innervated by median nerve).

      (c) Adductor digitus quintus.

      (d) "Crossed fingers" test: Inability to cross index and middle fingers indicates intrinsic muscle weakness.

    ii. **Sensory loss: Small finger and ulnar half of ring finger.**

    iii. Point tenderness over Guyon's canal (palpable just lateral to pisiform and distal as far as the hook of the hamate).

  d. **X-rays** usually are of no benefit.

  e. **Special tests:** EMGs may or may not prove to be positive. One must be cautioned to wait at least 3 weeks before attempting EMG localization, since the false-negative may occur.

  f. **Therapy** consists of splinting, nonsteroidal anti-inflammatories, and the usual conservative regimen. If pain and weakness persist, an exploration of the area is indicated.

2. **Ulnar nerve entrapment at the elbow**

  a. **Mechanism of injury:** People who are engaged in repetitive flexion sports, especially those with any type of abnormal anatomy, may suffer an injury to this area.

    i. Fractures that occurred in childhood or adolescence may later give rise to a deformity that may cause stretching of the ulnar nerve at the elbow.

    ii. This injury can occur in throwing athletes.

  b. **Examination**

    i. Tenderness either above or below the elbow in the cubital tunnel ("ulnar groove").

    ii. Palpation in the area will generally reproduce the patient's paresthesias in the ulnar 1½ digits on the volar aspect. The patient may complain that this feels like you are "hitting his crazy bone."

    iii. Hyperflexion of the arm may reproduce the symptoms if held for a long period of time.

    iv. Weakness may be present in the intrinsic musculature of the hand. It is unusual to see weakness of the flexor profundus to the small and index finger unless the entrapment is quite profound.

    v. Numbness in the ulnar sensory path is usually noted, i.e., the ulnar 1½ fingers.

    vi. Patient may complain of lancinating pain in the volar medial forearm.

  c. **X-rays** will usually be of little benefit.

  d. **Special testing:** EMGs are indicated. This is a difficult area to apply EMGs. Occasionally the injury cannot be localized electrically.

  e. **Therapy** should be directed to relieving the pressure on the ulnar nerve.

    i. Avoid repetitive flexion activities.

    ii. Splinting in 20 degrees of flexion at night may benefit.

    iii. Nonsteroidal anti-inflammatories, when used judiciously, are also indicated.

iv. **Surgery:** This injury has a notorious poor prognosis once it has started, and conservative treatment often fails more often than it succeeds. Operative intervention is indicated if conservative treatment has failed. This will usually consist of transposition of the nerve itself anteriorly.

VIII. **Tendinitis**

A. **De Quervain's syndrome** is stenosing tenosynovitis of the first dorsal compartment of the wrist.

The abductor pollicis and extensor pollicis brevis traverse the top of the extensor muscles and then weave themselves around the first dorsal compartment in a sheath to allow the thumb to abduct and to extend at the MCP joint.

1. **Mechanism of injury** is usually repetitive use of the thumb for some activity. As tendonitis develops, the pain increases with more use. The patient usually can identify the activity. It may be as seemingly innocuous as typing.

2. **Examination**
   a. Tenderness, often marked, at and just proximal to the radial styloid.
   b. Finkelstein's test. With the patient tucking the thumb inside the other fingers, the examiner moves the fist into ulnar deviation. Pain in the tendons where they pass over the distal radius constitutes a positive test, suggesting stenosing tenosynovitis (Fig. 12).
   c. Swelling and inflammation of the first doral compartment is occasionally present.

3. **X-rays** are not indicated.

4. **Special tests:** None.

5. **Therapy**
   a. Thumb spica splint ≥ 1 week.
   b. Phonophoresis with 10% hydrocortisone gel.
   c. Corticosteroid injection.
   d. Musculoskeletal rehabilitation.
   e. Specific activity avoidance.
   f. Surgical correction occasionally necessary.

B. **Intersection syndrome**

1. **Description:** Tendinitis or friction tendinitis between the first and second dorsal compartments. On the dorsum of the forearm approximately 2 to 3

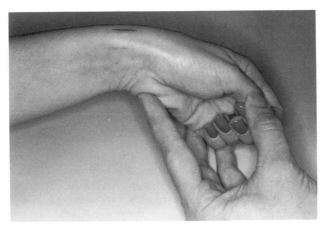

**FIGURE 12.** Finkelstein's test.

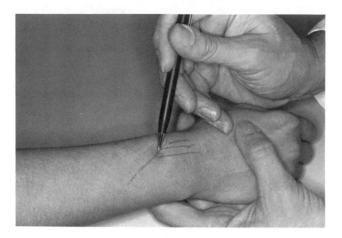

**FIGURE 13.**   Site of swelling and tenderness in intersection syndrome.

finger breadths proximal to the wrist joint, the muscle bellies of the first dorsal compartment transverse the second compartment at virtually a 60-degree angle. With overuse, there may be a friction tendinitis that develops between the tendons of the second compartment and the overlying or dorsal muscle bellies of the first compartment and their fascia.

2. **Examination** shows point tenderness in this area. This is approximately 2 to 3 finger breaths proximal to the wrist (Fig. 13). The patient will often complain that a squeaking or audible noise can be heard. The tendinitis in the area is often quite crepitant.

3. **Therapy**
    a. Wrist splint ≥ 1 week.
    b. Corticosteroid injection. Avoid bodies of tendons.
    c. Musculoskeletal rehabilitation.
    d. Specific activity avoidance.
    e. Surgical correction often necessary.

C. **Ganglion cysts**
    1. **Description:** Ganglion cysts are the common cysts seen on the dorsum of the wrist or over the radial artery. They represent a type of degenerative process from the scapholunate joint or interface. They can usually be traced back to this area surgically.
    2. **Mechanism of injury:** There is usually no specific injury associated with this problem. These cysts usually are spontaneous in onset.
    3. **Examination** shows a fusiform mass that is freely mobile and may transilluminate. This is normally over the dorsum of the wrist and the extensor tendons, but also may be seen over the radial artery. The mass may appear to be part of the radial artery. With auscultation, a radial artery aneurysm may be differentiated. At times, the patient will complain of tenderness directly over this area spontaneously and may not show a cystic mass that can be palpated. With careful historical documentation, the patient will note having had a mass there that has spontaneously abated. There are also very small ganglions that cannot be palpated, but that seem to cause some symptoms. These so-called "occult ganglions" may be the cause of obscure dorsal wrist pain.
    4. **X-rays** are not indicated.

5. **Therapy** consists of alleviating **symptomatic** ganglia. Since many ganglia are seen and are nonsymptomatic, they should obviously not be treated.
6. Differentiation for more significant types of tumors is normally quite easy because of their free mobility, transillumination, and characteristic location. If the ganglion is symptomatic, an injection with corticosteroids and aspiration of the ganglion may be indicated. This is sometimes, but not often, effective. Last, but not least, surgical intervention is warranted with continued pain and dysfunction. Splinting usually does not help.

D. **Wrist pain in gymnasts and weight lifters**
   1. **Description:** Gymnasts, especially those who do a high amount of floor exercises, often seem to have increasing pain over the dorsum of their wrists.
   2. **Mechanism of injury:** While the etiology of this pain is unclear, it appears to be from some type of injury in which the dorsal capsule is entrapped or repetitively traumatized by hyperdorsiflexion of the wrist. It is extremely difficult to treat, since normally the routines that gymnasts do involve gross dorsiflexion of the wrist.
   3. **Examination** shows diffuse dorsal tenderness. Tenderness may be more at the extremes of motion. One might evaluate the athlete's technique to make sure that the arm is being used solely as a functional unit, with the proper position of the hand, wrist, and forearm locked until transferring most of the pressure up into the shoulder girdle rather than with the arm unit in a highly flexed position at the elbow with the shoulder enclosed, giving abnormal stresses to the wrist.
   4. **Therapy:** Judicious rest, splinting, correction of technique, and nonsteroidal anti-inflammatories are the hallmarks of treatment in obscure wrist pain syndromes.
      a. Dorsal block splints may be made by taping a rectangle of closed cell foam to the dorsum of the wrists for practice and competition.
      b. Leather dorsal block splints are commercially available.
   5. **Diagnosis:** The differential diagnosis may be an obscure ganglion cyst that occasionally does cause pain over the dorsum and cannot be palpated, avascular necrosis of the carpal bone, and ligamentous injuries of the carpus. With appropriate radiologic studies, the latter two can usually be ruled out.

E. **Ligamentous injuries to the carpus**
   1. **Description:** The human wrist is an extremely complex organization of eight separate bones functioning as a unit. Any dorsiflexion or palmar flexion stress can cause a partial or total disruption of some of the ligaments within the carpus. It is outside the scope of this chapter to delineate all of the injuries of the carpus, but it is sufficient to say that if the athlete has swelling within the wrist and limitation of motion after an injury, a careful examination by an experienced physician should be undertaken. If one has a high enough suspicion that an x-ray is indicated, then the diagnosis of wrist ligament tear rather than fracture may be indicated. Since radiographically, wrist x-rays are often difficult to interpret, experience correlated with physical examination is a must.

## RECOMMENDED READING

1. American Academy of Orthopaedic Surgeons: Symposium on Upper Extremity Injuries in Athletes. Pettrone FA (ed). St. Louis, CV Mosby, 1988.
2. American Society for Surgery of the Hand: The Hand: Examination and Diagnosis, 2nd ed. New York, Churchill Livingstone, 1983.
3. American Society for Surgery of the Hand: The Hand: Primary Care for Common Problems. New York, Churchill Livingstone, 1985.
4. Barton N: Fractures of the Hand and Wrist. New York, Churchill Livingstone, 1988.

5. Brand PW: Clinical Mechanics of the Hand. St. Louis, CV Mosby, 1985.
6. Fess EE: Hand Splinting: Principles and Methods, 2nd ed. St. Louis, CV Mosby, 1987.
7. Green DP: Operative Hand Surgery, 2nd ed. New York, Churchill Livingstone, 1988.
8. Hoppenfeld S: Physical Examination of the Spine and Extremities. East Norwalk, CT, Appleton & Lange, 1976.
9. Hunter JM, Schneider LH, Mackin EJ, Callahan AD: Rehabilitation of the Hand, 3rd ed. St. Louis, CV Mosby, 1989.
10. Lichtman DM: The Wrist and Its Disorders. Philadelphia, WB Saunders, 1988.
11. Milford L: The Hand, 3rd ed. St. Louis, CV Mosby, 1988.
12. Morrey BF: The Elbow and Its Disorders. Philadelphia, WB Saunders, 1985.
13. Nicholas JA, Hershman EB, Posner MA: The Upper Extremity in Sports Medicine. St. Louis, CV Mosby, 1990.
14. Rockwood CA, Green DP: Fractures, 2nd ed. Philadelphia, JB Lippincott, 1984.
15. Spinner M: Injuries to the Major Branches of the Peripheral Nerves of the Forearm, 2nd ed. Philadelphia, WB Saunders, 1978.
16. Strickland JW: The Thumb. New York, Churchill Livingstone, 1989.

# Chapter 37: Athletic Injuries of the Thorax and Abdomen

## LARRY E. BRAGG, MD

I. **General Approaches**

  A. The thorax and abdomen can be conceptualized as a cylinder with an outer muscular/skeletal coat that protects the viscera within. The most common injuries consist of contusions to the outer muscular layer and are relatively unimportant. However, injuries involving fractures of the skeletal components with resultant injury to the underlying viscera, or direct visceral injuries can result in serious sequelae. The team physician should be alert to the early recognition of these injuries, since delays in diagnosis and treatment greatly increase the chance of serious complication or death.

  B. **Mechanisms of injury**

    1. The majority of athletic injuries result **from blunt forces, which can be categorized by four mechanisms:**

      a. Acceleration/deceleration

      b. Shearing

      c. Crushing

      d. Hydraulic.

    2. Penetrating injuries are extremely uncommon in athletics.

  C. **Initial evaluation and treatment**

    1. After the realization that a major injury has occurred, the principles of basic life support take priority.

      a. **Airway**

        i. Assure airway patency and adequate air exchange.

        ii. **Always** protect the cervical spine.

      b. **Breathing**

        i. Assess respiratory movement and quality of respiration.

        ii. Supply oxygen.

        iii. Assist ventilation if necessary.

      c. **Circulation**

        i. Assess pulse for quality, rate, and regularity,

        ii. Obtain blood pressure.

        iii. Observe skin color, temperature, and rate of capillary refill.

        iv. Control obvious external hemorrhage.

        v. Support blood pressure with the pneumatic antishock garment (MAST).

    2. If there is any suspicion of serious internal injury, the athlete must be transferred to a facility where definitive treatment can be administered.

    3. Field management of wounds

      a. Occlusive dressings to thoracic wounds

      b. Dry, sterile dressings for abdominal wounds

      c. Eviscerations

        i. **Do not** attempt to reduce.

        ii. Cover with **moist,** sterile dressings.

      d. Impaled objects—**do not** remove in the field.

II. **Thoracic Injuries**

A. **Injuries of the chest wall**

1. **Rib fractures**

a. **Nondisplaced** rib fractures are the most common and are generally benign. **Displaced** rib fractures may result in laceration of the lung or an associated intercostal artery.

b. Fractures usually involve the fifth to ninth ribs.

c. Tremendous forces are required to fracture the **first** and **second** ribs. Since they are well protected by the shoulder girdle, associated injuries must be strongly suspected.

d. Fractures of ribs **seven, eight,** and **nine** may be associated with injuries of the liver, spleen, or kidneys.

e. Symptoms

    i. Pain at site of fracture aggravated by coughing, breathing, movement

    ii. Dyspnea.

f. Physical findings

    i. Localized tenderness

    ii. Crepitation

    iii. Contusion.

g. Chest x-ray should be obtained to exclude an unsuspected pneumothorax.

h. Rib detail roentgenograms may be necessary to visualize fractures.

i. Treatment

    i. Rest.

    ii. Analgesics.

    iii. Intercostal nerve blocks may be required for severe pain.

    iv. Rib binders or adhesive strapping of the chest should not be used, since they contribute to development of atelectasis and pneumonia.

2. **Costochondral sprain and separation**

Blows to the anterolateral chest or twisting injuries may result in sprain of the costochondral junction or separation of the rib from the costocartilage that attaches it to the sternum.

a. Costochondral sprains are among the most common injuries that occur in contact sports.

    i. Symptoms include tenderness and pain of the involved joint.

b. Costochondral separation produces localized sharp pain followed by intermittent stabbing pain as the disrupted cartilage and bone override one another.

    i. Deformity due to displacement of the cartilage may be apparent on physical examination.

    ii. If chronic pain develops, excision of a segment of cartilage is curative.

c. Treatment is symptomatic with ice, analgesics, and rest.

3. **Sternal fractures**

Sternal fractures are uncommon and when they occur are related to high-impact injuries. Associated myocardial contusion is frequent and may be life-threatening.

a. Symptoms include localized pain directly over the sternum, aggravated by deep inspiration.

b. X-rays are diagnostic.

c. Treatment is directed at control of symptoms and monitoring for cardiac arrhythmias.

d. Displaced fractures may require open reduction and fixation.

4. **Sternoclavicular dislocation**

Sternoclavicular dislocations most commonly occur with falls on the acromioclavicular joint. The force of the fall is transmitted through the clavicle to the sternoclavicular joint. The proximal clavicle can displace anteriorally, superiorally, or posteriorly.

   a. Pain, swelling, and noticeable displacement of the sternoclavicular joint are the most frequent findings.

   b. Anterior dislocation of the clavicle is the most common.

   c. Posterior displacement is rare but can produce life-threatening impingement on the airway or great vessels.

   d. The athlete's arms should be supported against the chest, vital signs monitored, and the athlete transported to a medical facility.

5. **Rupture of the pectoralis major**

   a. The pectoralis major adducts, flexes, and rotates the shoulder internally.

   b. Excessive tension on the muscle may result in a tear of the muscle itself, at the musculotendinous junction, or an avulsion of the tendon from bone.

      i. Seen most often in athletes bench-pressing heavy weights.

   c. Symptoms

      i. Sudden sharp pain in the upper arm or chest

      ii. Ecchymosis

      iii. Weakened adduction, flexion, and internal rotation of arm

      iv. Bulging of the muscle belly on the chest.

   d. A defect may be evident in the anterior axillary fold with tendon avulsion.

   e. Chest x-ray may show an absent pectoralis major muscle shadow.

   f. Treatment

      i. Tears of the muscle are treated with ice, analgesics, and activity restriction.

      ii. Surgery is usually advised for athletes with disruption of the tendon.

6. **Breast injuries**

   a. **Runner's nipple:** Nipple chafing may occur as a result of friction from a runner's shirt. Wearing a proper brassiere may prevent this problem in women. Additional protection can be achieved by placing a piece of tape or a coating of Cramer's Skin Lube or Mueller's lubricant over the nipples.

   b. **Breast pain from jogging:** Breast motion during running can result in contusion of the breast tissue and straining of Cooper's ligaments, resulting in pain. A firm-fitting support brassier will help prevent excessive breast motion. In addition, large-breasted women can gain added support by wrapping a 4-inch elastic bandage over the brassiere.

   c. **Breast contusions:** Breast contusions are treated like contusions elsewhere, i.e., immediate ice and antiinflammatory medication followed later by heat and padding.

B. **Lung injuries**

1. **Simple pneumothorax**

   a. Classification

      i. Spontaneous, from rupture of pulmonary bleb.

      ii. Traumatic, most commonly from lung laceration or puncture by a fractured rib.

      iii. Described by extent of hemithorax occupied by free air (e.g., 25%, 50%, etc. . .).

   b. Symptoms

      i. Shortness of breath

      ii. Dyspnea

      iii. Chest pain.

   c. Physical findings

      i. Diminished breath sounds

      ii. Hyperresonance to percussion

      iii. Subcutaneous emphysema.

   d. Chest x-ray is diagnostic.

   e. Treatment depends on size and degree of symptoms.

      i. Small, stable and asymptomatic—observation, serial chest x-rays.

      ii. Large or symptomatic—tube thoracostomy.

2. **Tension pneumothorax**

   a. Progressive enlargement of pneumothorax with development of positive intrapleural pressure.

   b. The increasing pressure results in impairment of venous return, mediastinal shift, and further embarrassment of ventilation.

   c. If untreated, progressive hypoxia and hypotension lead to death.

   d. Presentation

      i. Acute respiratory distress

      ii. Hypotension

      iii. Tachycardia

      iv. Distended neck veins

      v. Absent breath sounds on involved side

      vi. Hyperresonance to percussion on involved side.

   e. Treatment should not be delayed for roentgenographic confirmation. If a tension pneumothorax is suspected clinically, treatment should be instituted.

      i. Immediate decompression can be achieved by placement of a large bore 14 to 16 gauge needle into the chest through the 2nd or 3rd intercostal space at the midclavicular line..

      ii. Tube thoracostomy through 5th intercostal space at anterior axillary line provides definitive treatment.

C. **Cardiac and great vessel injuries**

1. **Myocardial contusion**

   a. Myocardial contusion has been reported to occur after blunt chest trauma in as frequently as 60% of cases.

   b. A strong index of suspicion should be entertained when sternal contusions and sternal fractures are present.

   c. Diagnosis

      i. Electrocardiogram changes

      ii. Cardiac enzyme elevation

      iii. Echocardiogram.

   d. Cardiac dysrhythmias are the major risk, and patients suspected of having a myocardial contusion should be monitored.

2. **Cardiac tamponade**

   a. Unusual following blunt chest injury.

   b. Presentation

      i. Hypotension

      ii. Distended neck veins

      iii. Muffled heart tones.

   c. Treatment

      i. Pericardiocentesis

      ii. Emergency thoracotomy.

3. **Traumatic aortic rupture**

   a. Most often the result of a high speed deceleration injury.

   b. Most commonly occurs just distal to the left subclavian artery at ligamentum arteriosum.

   c. Ninety percent fatal at scene of accident.

      d. Associated chest roentgenograph findings:
         i. Widened mediastinum
        ii. Obscured aortic knob shadow
       iii. Deviation of trachea to right
       iv. Depression of left mainstem bronchus
        v. Left pleural effusion.
      e. Diagnosis is established by thoracic aortography or CT scan.
      f. Treatment is operative repair.

D. **Thoracic outlet syndrome**
   1. Caused by compression of brachial plexus or subclavian-axillary artery and/or vein in the region between the thoracic outlet and the insertion of the pectoralis minor into the coracoid process.
   2. Symptoms may range from neural, vascular, or combined neural and vascular compression.
   3. There are multiple sites and etiologies of compression.
      a. Interscalene triangle
      b. First rib
      c. Costocoracoid fascia
      d. Pectoralis minor tendon
      e. Cervical rib
      f. Long transverse process of C7
      g. Callus formation from first rib or clavicle fractures.
   4. Symptoms
      a. Ninety percent are neurologic.
         i. Pain, paresthesias, and numbness.
        ii. Symptoms are usually in ulnar distribution, but may occur anywhere in upper extremity.
       iii. Sensory loss, motor weakness, and atrophy are late neurologic defects.
      b. Symptoms of arterial compression
         i. Ischemic pain
        ii. Numbness
       iii. Fatigue
       iv. Paresthesias
        v. Coldness
       vi. Distal embolization.
      c. Symptoms of venous compression
         i. Pain
        ii. Edema
       iii. Cyanosis.
   5. Diagnosis
      a. Physical exam to detect evidence of neural, arterial and venous compression.
      b. Chest and neck roentgenograms.
      c. Myelograms, arteriograms, or venograms may be necessary.
   6. Treatment
      a. Nonoperative measures relieve symptoms in 50–70%.
         i. Weight reduction
        ii. Strengthening of shoulder girdle muscles
       iii. Avoiding hyperabduction of the shoulder.
      b. Operative management may be necessary for patients with major neurologic or vascular complications and those that do not respond to a trial of nonoperative management.

E. **Primary thrombosis of the subclavian and axillary veins—"effort thrombosis"**
  1. Thrombosis of the subclavian and axillary veins most commonly occurs after activities associated with hyperabduction and external rotation of the arm.
     a. Throwing a baseball or football
     b. Playing handball or tennis
     c. Rowing.
  2. Symptoms almost always start within 24 to 72 hours of activity.
     a. Arm edema
     b. Distention of superficial arm veins
     c. Reddish blue discoloration of skin
     d. Arm pain.
  3. Diagnostic tests
     a. Noninvasive venous studies
     b. Venography.
  4. Treatment
     a. **Elevation** and **anticoagulation** are the time honored standard methods of treatment.
     b. **Thrombolytic agents** have also been effective.
     c. **Thrombectomy** and **first rib resection** are occasionally undertaken in those patients with external compression.
     d. There is a high incidence of late morbidity (swelling, pain, fatigability, numbness) with most forms of treatment.

III. **Abdominal Injuries**

  A. **Injuries of the abdominal wall**
    1. **Contusion of abdominal muscles**
       a. Treatment is the same as for contusions elsewhere (i.e., analgesics and anti-inflammatory medication), and after 48 hours, local heat.
       b. **Rectus sheath hematoma** may occur with rupture of the deep epigastric vessels.
          i. Self-tamponading usually occurs.
          ii. Enlarging hematomas may require evacuation and ligation of epigastric vessels.
       c. Recurrent contusion or hematomas in the young athlete should prompt an evaluation for an underlying blood dyscrasia.
    2. **Iliac apophysitis**
       a. Adolescent athletes participating in athletics that involve repetitive contractions by the oblique abdominals, gluteus medius, and tensor fascia lata may develop an inflammatory response of the iliac apophysis. This occurs primarily in runners with crossover arm swings.
       b. Symptoms—local pain over the anterior iliac crest during activity.
       c. Diagnosis
          i. Tenderness at the origin of the tensor fascia lata, the gluteus medius, and the abdominal obliques.
          ii. X-ray may show a discontinuity between the anterior one-third and posterior two-thirds of the apophysis.
       d. Treatment
          i. Abdominal wall, quadriceps, hamstring, and iliotibial band stretching
          ii. 4 to 6 weeks of rest
             (a) Relative vs. absolute rest
          iii. Training resumes with less mileage, and care to avoid arm swings across the body.

B. **Inguinal hernias in athletes**
  1. **General principles**
     a. **Indirect** hernias are the most common type.
     b. **Direct** hernias occur with greater frequency in performance athletes than would normally be expected for the age group under consideration.
     c. Clinically apparent hernias, symptomatic or not, should be repaired electively.
     d. Complications of hernias
        i. Pain
        ii. Incarceration
        iii. Strangulation
        iv. Bowel obstruction
        v. Testicular infarction
        vi. Traumatic visceral injury.
  2. **Groin pain in the athlete**
     a. Differential diagnosis
        i. Occult hernia
        ii. "Groin pull"
        iii. Hydrocele
        iv. Varicocele
        v. Prostatitis
        vi. Iliopectineal bursitis (see below)
        vii. Osteochondritis of pubis.
     b. **Herniography** may be a useful diagnostic measure in patients with groin pain and a normal musculoskeletal and hernia exam.
        i. Herniography is performed by injecting water soluble contrast into the peritoneal cavity under fluoroscopic guidance.
        ii. Identifies occult hernia sacs.
        iii. **Symptomatic** hernias identified by herniography may improve with operation.
        iv. **Asymptomatic** hernias identified by herniography may not need to be repaired.
     c. **Iliopectineal bursitis** (iliopsoas or iliofemoral bursitis)
        i. Presents as insidious onset of groin pain in the runner or the athlete that uses repetitive hip flexion.
        ii. Pain reproduced by passive hip flexion.
        iii. Results from inflammation of the bursa between the pectineus muscle and psoas muscle.
        iv. Treated by relative rest, local heat, and anti-inflammatory medications.
C. **Injuries to the abdominal viscera**
  1. **General features**
     a. Early signs of visceral injury are often subtle, and a high index of suspicion should be present to avoid overlooking such injuries.
     b. The most important determination to be made is whether or not a significant injury exists, requiring treatment, rather than the diagnosis of a **specific** organ injury.
     c. Careful physical examination, with repeated exams to detect changes, is the key to detecting intra-abdominal injury.
     d. Intra-abdominal injuries produce pain, guarding, rebound tenderness, and loss of bowel sounds.
     e. There may be a long symptom-free interval after injury, especially with retroperitoneal injuries.

      f. Physical examination of the patient with blunt abdominal trauma is frequently equivocal, and adjunctive maneuvers, such as peritoneal lavage or abdominal CT scanning, are often employed.

  2. **Patterns of injury**

      a. Solid organs (liver, spleen, pancreas, adrenals, kidneys)

         i. All have an excellent blood supply.

         ii. Injuries are manifested mainly by **hemorrhage.**

      b. Hollow organs (GI, GU, and biliary tracts)

         i. Injuries are manifested by peritonitis, which may be **chemical** or **bacterial.**

         ii. Chemical peritonitis develops immediately and results from irritation by gastric acid, bile, or urine.

         iii. Bacterial peritonitis develops slowly, over several hours, usually from fecal contamination.

      c. Vascular injuries are manifested by

         i. Hemorrhage

         ii. Loss of distal pulses

         iii. Development of bruits.

  3. **Splenic injury**

      a. Splenic rupture is the most common intra-abdominal injury caused by blunt trauma.

      b. The majority of patients rapidly develop hypovolemic shock and signs of peritoneal irritation.

      c. Referred pain to the left shoulder (Kehr's sign) from diaphragmatic irritation may be present.

      d. Infectious mononucleosis and splenic injury (see Chapter 21).

         i. Mononucleosis may result in splenic enlargement and weakening of the capsule and pulp.

         ii. These changes result in a predisposition to splenic rupture, which may persist for several weeks after disappearance of symptoms.

         iii. Noncontact sports may resume 3 weeks following onset of illness if symptoms and splenic enlargement have resolved.

         iv. Contact sports may resume in 4 weeks if the above conditions are met.

## IV. **Genitourinary Injuries**

  1. **Renal injuries**

      a. Flank pain, tenderness, and hematuria are the most frequent findings with renal injury.

      b. If renal injury is suspected, intravenous pyelography (IVP) or contrasted CT should be performed to evaluate kidney function and exclude urinary extravasation.

      c. The majority of kidney injuries are intracapsular and heal without serious complications.

  2. **Ureter injuries**

      a. Rarely occur as isolated injuries following blunt abdominal trauma.

      b. May be associated with pelvic fractures.

      c. IVP is diagnostic.

      d. Genitourinary referral is necessary.

  3. **Bladder injuries**

      a. Lower abdominal blunt trauma and pelvic fractures may result in contusion or rupture of the urinary bladder.

      b. Cystography will establish the diagnosis of bladder rupture.

4. **Urethral injuries**
   a. The membranous and prostatic urethra in the male are susceptible to blunt injury, especially with pelvic fractures and straddle injuries.
   b. In the athlete with lower abdominal blunt trauma or pelvic fracture, the presence of hematuria, blood at the urethral meatus, scrotal hematoma, or high riding prostate, retrograde urethography should be performed under the guidance of a genitourinary surgeon.
   c. Urethral injuries are uncommon in the female athlete.
5. **Injuries of the scrotum and its contents**
   a. Protective equipment should be used in all contact sports.
   b. Contusion is the most common injury and is treated by ice and elevation.
   c. A **hematocele** can form when blood accumulates in the tunica vaginalis.
      i. Hematoceles do not transilluminate.
      ii. Treatment consists of ice, elevation and bedrest.
      iii. Rapidly expanding hematomas may require surgical exploration.

# Chapter 38: Thoracic and Lumbosacral Spine

JOHN WILHITE, MD
WALTER W. HUURMAN, MD

I. **Anatomy**

  A. **Bony** (Fig. 1)

    1. **Lumbar vertebra**

      a. Composed of:

         i. Vertebral body: a large anterior weight-bearing structure of each lumbar vertebra.

         ii. Vertebral arch: a horseshoe-shaped structure surrounding the vertebral foramen (through which the spinal cord runs), which is composed of:

            (a) Pedicles: two short, stout, rounded structures projecting from the body, one on each side.

            (b) Lamina: broad, flat structures that meet in the midline posteriorly where they are continuous with the posteriorly directed spinous process.

         iii. Where each pedicle and lamina meet there is a mass of bone from which three processes arise:

            (a) Transverse process-projects laterally

            (b) Superior articular process—projects cranially (cephalad)

            (c) Inferior articular process—projects caudally.

         iv. Pars interarticularis: the area between the superior and inferior articular processes on each vertebra.

            (a) This area is particularly susceptible to sheering forces and stress fracture.

      b. Lumbar vertebrae articulate with each other by intervertebral discs and superior and inferior articular processes forming the facet joints.

         i. The facet joints have a synovial lining and capsule.

  B. **Soft tissues**

    1. **Disc** (Fig. 1)

      a. Annulus fibrosus: the outer layer of fibers that functions to hold the nucleus pulposus and limit its displacement during flexion, extension, and load-bearing.

      b. Nucleus pulposus: the gelatinous structure occupying an eccentric position within the annulus fibrosus.

    2. **Ligaments** (Fig. 1)

      a. Anterior longitudinal ligament:

         i. Runs entire length of spine along the anterior surface of the vertebral bodies.

         ii. A broad, strong band of fibrous tissue.

      b. Posterior longitudinal ligament:

         i. Runs along the posterior surface of the vertebral bodies (anterior surface of spinal canal).

         ii. Slightly weaker and narrower than the anterior longitudinal ligament.

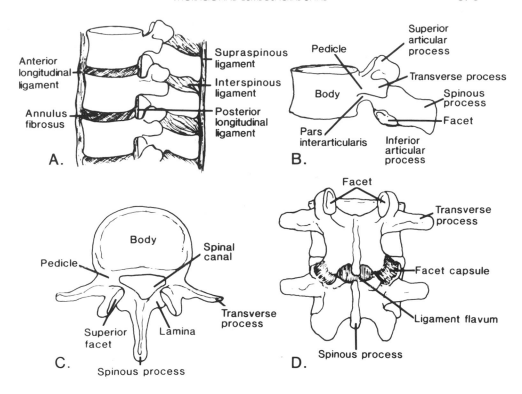

**FIGURE 1.** Normal lumbar vertebrae anatomy. *A,* Lateral view of three lumbar vertebrae with surrounding ligaments. *B,* Lateral view of one lumbar vertebra. *C,* Looking from above. *D,* Posterior view indicating facet joint and capsule.

    c. Interspinous ligament:
       i. Runs between the posterior spinous processes.
    d. Supraspinous ligament:
       i. Connects the spinous processes.
    e. Facet capsule.
  3. **Fascia and muscles**
    a. Thoracolumbar fascia
       i. Represents fascia and fused aponeuroses of several muscles.
       ii. Lies over the muscles of lower back.
    b. Paraspinal muscles are composed of three layers of muscles of which only the superficial layer is palpable—the sacrospinalis.
    c. Abdominal wall muscles
       i. Provide approximately 30% of the lumbar spine support via hydrostatic column effect.
       ii. Weakness results in abnormal increase in lumbar lordosis with concomitant stress on soft tissue supporting structures.

II. **Function**
  A. Soft tissues act as "guy wires" to maintain alignment and affect the strong, coordinated torso movements.
  B. Bony structures and discs provide mobility, support, and protection.
  C. Both provide longitudinal support for the abdomen and thorax.

D. Spinal structures permit "universal joint" motion.

E. The spine provides protection for the very delicate neurological structures of the spinal column.

III. **Diagnosis**

A. **History**

1. **Pain**

a. **Potential pain-producing structures:** Supraspinous ligament, interspinous ligament, longitudinal ligaments, ligamentum flavum, facet joint capsules, peripheral fibers of annulus fibrosis, and back muscles.

b. **Pain—local, radicular or referred?**

c. **Onset**—traumatic or gradual?

d. **Exacerbating factors:**

i. Discogenic: worse with prolonged standing or sitting and increased with Valsalva maneuvers (coughing, sneezing, or straining on defecation).

ii. Spondylolysis: worse with hyperextension (i.e., walkovers, tennis serve, golf stroke follow-through).

iii. Spinal stenosis: "Pseudoclaudication"—worse with ambulation.

e. **Relieving factors:**

i. Discogenic: lying with knees flexed improves (by increasing foraminal space).

ii. Spinal stenosis: sitting will improve. The room in the lumbar canal enlarges with the spine in flexion, thus decreasing the pain.

f. **Worrisome factors:**

i. Fever may indicate infection (osteomyelitis or disc space infection).

ii. Weight loss and anorexia may indicate malignancy.

iii. Bladder, bowel, or sexual disturbances may indicate cauda equina syndromes or central midline disc herniation.

iv. Pain at rest—suspicious for tumor.

g. **Referred pain** may come from abdominal or pelvic disorders (abdominal aortic aneurysm, pelvic tumors or infections, renal disorders, or prostate disease).

2. **Work and social history:**

a. Underlying secondary gain?

i. Financial

ii. Frustration with job or family.

B. **Physical examination**

1. **Inspection**

a. **Stance**

i. Listing seen in nerve root compression.

ii. Flattening of lumbar lordosis seen in spondylolisthesis.

b. **Gait**

i. A peculiar short-stride, forward-flexed, rigid gait is seen in disc space infections.

2. **Range of motion**

a. **Flexion**

i. Look for reversal of normal lordosis.

ii. Schober test (for spinal flexibility) (Fig. 2)

(a) Performed by aligning a tape measure vertically along the spine beginning 10 cm above an imaginary line that joins the "dimples of Venus" (small hollows located on either side of the lumbosacral spine).

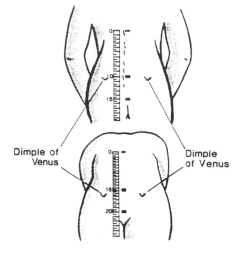

**FIGURE 2.** Schober test.

Dimple of Venus

Dimple of Venus

    (b) Marks are made at 0, 10, and 15 cm, with the tape measure held in place.

    (c) Patient is asked to touch his/her toes and the amount of flexibility is measured (normal is 5 cm, that is, an increase in the total distance from 15 cm to a total of 20 cm between initial reference points).

    (d) A good way to follow patients with ankylosing spondylitis.

  b. **Extension.**

  c. **Lateral flexion** to right and left.

    i. Unilaterally limited in painful disc.

  d. **Rotation.**

  e. Measure **chest expansion.**

    i. Normally approximately 3 inches.

    ii. Significant when reduced to 2 inches and may reveal underlying ankylosing spondylitis.

3. **Palpation**

  a. Muscle spasm

    i. Paraspinal muscles seem prominent and feel more rigid.

  b. Trigger points.

  c. Deformities.

    i. Step-off deformity in spondylolisthesis.

  d. Tenderness.

    i. In disc herniation with radicular pain, frequently able to elicit tenderness in sciatic notch (midway between ischial tuberosity and greater trochanter).

  e. Palpation of iliac crest levels to check for pelvic obliquity.

4. **Percussion over spine**

  a. Almost always elicits tenderness in nerve root impingement, tumors, or infections.

5. **Neurologic** (deep tendon reflexes, strength, and sensation)

  a. Common nerve root findings (Table 1)

  b. Dermatomes (Fig. 3)

6. **Specific maneuvers:**

  a. **Straight leg raising test (SLR):**

    Aggravates radicular-type pain. Indicative of nerve root impingement or irritation along course of sciatic nerve.

**TABLE 1.** Common Nerve Root Findings

| Root | Reflexes | Strength | Sensation |
|------|----------|----------|-----------|
| L4 | Patellar | Anterior tibialis | Medial leg & foot |
| L5 | None | Extensor hallucis longus | Lateral leg and dorsum of foot |
| S1 | Achilles | Peroneus longus and brevis | Lateral foot |

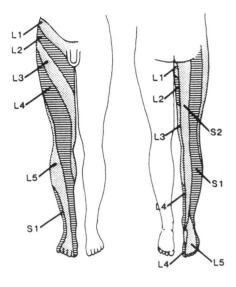

**FIGURE 3.** Dermatomes of lower extremities.

b. **SLR** with dorsiflexion of the foot **(Lasegue's test)** (Fig. 4):
Creates additional sciatic stretch and when pain is increased on this maneuver is indicative of nerve root compression or involvement of sciatic nerve along its course.

c. **Crossed SLR:**
Considered by some to be pathognomonic of herniated disc. With the patient supine, the examiner lifts the unaffected leg and, in the presence of a herniated disc, this maneuver will exacerbate the pain in the affected leg.

d. **SLR while sitting (sitting root test):**
Is positive when extending the knee causes radicular pain, or causes the patient to sit back in an effort to relax tension on the sciatic nerve. Useful test

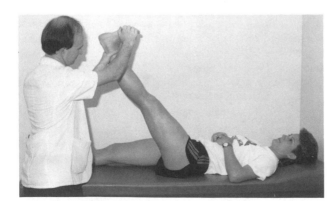

**FIGURE 4.** Straight leg raising with dorsiflexion of the foot (Lasegue's test) creates additional sciatic stretch, and, when pain is increased on this maneuver, is indicative of nerve-root compression or involvement of sciatic nerve along its course.

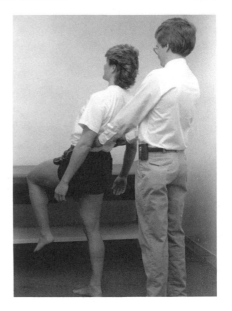

**FIGURE 5.** One-legged standing hyperextension test aggravates discomfort in presence of spondylolysis.

in helping to differentiate malingerer. If patient allows SLR while seated but will not permit it in supine position, he is malingering.

    e. **One-legged standing hyperextension test** (Fig. 5):
      Causes low back pain and is suggestive of spondylolysis.

    f. **Patrick's or FABER test** (Flexion, ABduction, and External Rotation of hip):
      If painful, is indicative of sacroiliac joint disorder.

  7. Examination should include abdominal, pelvic and rectal (to evaluate anal sphincter tone), and peripheral vascular exams to exclude referred cause of pain.

C. **Radiological studies**

  1. **Plain films**

    a. **Usually unnecessary in acute phase, but collision and strength sports may necessitate earlier x-ray evaluation.**

    b. There are many who argue that x-rays are indicated only when there is

        i. History of serious trauma (fracture)

       ii. Known cancer (pathological fracture)

      iii. Pain at rest (tumor)

      iv. Unexplained weight loss (malignancy)

       v. Drug or alcohol abuse (disc space infection)

      vi. Treatment with corticosteroids (pathological fracture)

     vii. Temperature $> 38°C$ (infection)

    viii. Suspicion of ankylosing spondylitis by history, or if physical exam demonstrates a neuromotor deficit

      ix. Unremitting pain of 2 to 4 weeks duration

       x. Suspicion of pars defect (spondylolysis, spondylolisthesis).

    c. **Provide no information about the presence or location of disc herniation, even when narrowed disc space is observed.**

    d. **Plain films may reveal:**

        i. Spondylolysis = a defect in the pars interarticularis (Fig. 6).

       ii. Spondylolisthesis = forward displacement of a superior vertebral body in relation to an inferior vertebral body (Fig. 7).

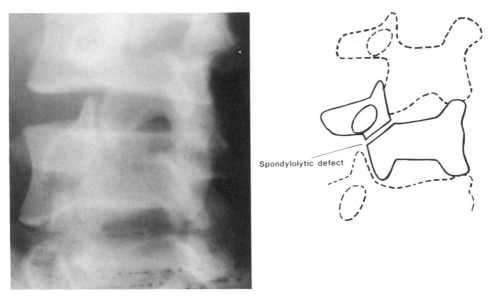

**FIGURE 6.**   The spondylolytic defect is seen as a collar on the Scotty dog's neck (pars interarticularis) on an oblique x-ray of lumbar spine.

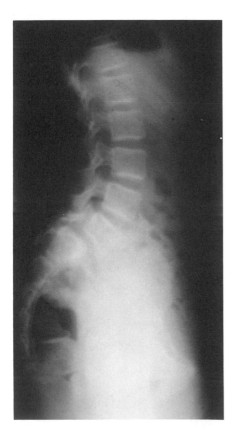

**FIGURE 7.**   Lateral x-ray of lumbosacral spine revealing spondylolisthesis.

      iii. Evidence of disc space infection consisting of narrowing of intervertebral disc space, irregularities and sclerosis of vertebral end plates.

      iv. Degenerative changes evidenced by disc space narrowing and osteophyte formation.

2. **Bone scans**
   a. Useful when locating a lesion that is symptomatic but not yet visible on plain film x-rays (i.e., stress fracture of pars interarticularis).
   b. When positive, a scan is indicative of increased bone metabolic activity, which could represent fracture, infection, tumor, or arthritis.
   c. Three-phase study (all bone scans should be performed in three phases):
      i. When positive in early phase, indicative of soft tissue inflammation.
      ii. When positive in second and late phases, indicative of bone disease.

3. **Tomography, CT scanning, MRI, and myelography** are expensive but are of great help in making or confirming a diagnosis and therefore should be used judiciously.
   a. **Tomography of the spine** is helpful in delineating congenital anomalies, fractures, and infections.
   b. **CT scan** is used in evaluating the bony spine for fractures and spondylotic defects, herniated discs, extra-spinal soft tissue abnormalities (i.e., hematoma or myositis ossificans), and infections and neoplasms of the spine.
   c. **MRI** is particularly helpful in detection of herniated disc, intrinsic spinal cord lesions, spinal cord and nerve root compression, as well as benign or malignant bony lesions.
   d. **Myelography** remains valuable in evaluation of intrinsic spinal cord and nerve root lesions and compression.
   e. CT scan is most helpful in instances of bone disease (especially cortical bone), whereas MRI is most helpful with soft tissue problems and in bone disease involving marrow.
   f. **Because 30–40% of CT scans and myelograms show abnormalities in asymptomatic subjects, a positive study is not diagnostic unless it conforms to the clinical picture.**[8]
      i. A CT scan not parallel to the disc may give an erroneous impression of disc herniation.
   g. The sensitivity of CT, myelography, and electromyography (EMG)/nerve conduction velocity (NCV) studies in diagnosing a *herniated disc* is each around 90%. The specificities of CT and myelography are around 88%; however, the specificity of EMG/NCV studies in diagnosing a herniated disc is much less at 38%.[8]

4. **Neurologic study—EMG/NCV.**
   a. It takes 14–21 days for denervation changes to occur to the degree that they can be picked up on EMG study.
   b. Helpful in localizing herniated disc syndromes.

## IV. Thoracic Spine

### A. Postural (flexible) roundback

1. Most commonly seen in older adolescents.
2. **Presents** with roundback deformity in the form of a long, graceful curve and may or may not have back pain.
3. **Characterized** by the patient's ability to voluntarily assume a properly erect position (in Scheuermann's disease, the patient cannot correct the kyphosis).

4. **Radiologic exam:**
   a. **Lateral** view—the kyphosis measured between the inferior margin of T12 and an upper thoracic vertebra exceeds 40°; there are no structural abnormalities of the vertebral bodies.
   b. A **supine** hyperextension film (with bolster under the thoracic spine) will show correction of the kyphosis to measurably normal degrees.
5. **Treatment:**
   a. Postural exercises.
   b. When severe, treatment is similar to that offered for Scheuermann's disease (see next section).

B. **Scheuermann's disease**
1. Most commonly seen in older adolescents.
2. Typically **presents** with round-shouldered appearance and may or may not have back pain.
3. **Etiology** is unknown but suspected to be secondary to inflammatory reaction in the vertebral bodies' ring apophyses.
4. **Physical exam:** The patient cannot voluntarily correct the kyphosis (as in postural roundback) and on forward-bending the kyphosis is accentuated, showing an area of acute, sharp angulation usually around T7 (whereas postural roundback will show a smooth symmetrical contour).
5. **Radiological exam:** Lateral view must show three successive thoracic vertebral bodies, each anteriorly wedged more than 5°, slight irregularity of the vertebral endplates, and Schmorl's nodes (herniations of the disc into the vertebral endplates).
6. **Treatment**
   a. Milwaukee brace (Fig. 8) and supervised exercise program usually give excellent results.
   b. Surgical treatment rarely necessary.

C. **Vertebral apophysitis ("ring apophysitis")**
1. **Presents** with symptoms or findings ranging from vague pain to point tenderness along the spine in adolescents.
2. **Symptoms** are aggravated by activity and relieved with rest.
3. Often seen in athletic individuals (i.e., gymnasts) and felt to be **due to repetitive micro-fractures of the vertebral endplates.**
4. **Radiological exam:** Changes of vertebral endplate irregularity at one or more anterior vertebral bodies without kyphotic deformity distinguish this from Scheuermann's disease.
5. Treatment consists of decreased activity, stretching, and strengthening exercises.

D. **Scoliosis**
1. **Definition:** Lateral curvature of the spine.
2. Present to a minor degree in up to 8–10% of population.
3. Most common form of scoliosis is **idiopathic** and begins in adolescence.
4. **Relatively unrestricted physical activity is desirable for almost all adolescents with scoliosis.**
   a. Participation improves strength, flexibility, overall fitness, and self-esteem.
5. Decisions regarding appropriate sports and levels of participation require knowledge about the natural history of scoliosis as well as the particular sport. Each case should be evaluated individually; a routine prohibition from participation is inappropriate.
   a. In general, an otherwise healthy patient with mild-to-moderate scoliosis, even if under treatment with bracing, can safely participate in most levels of sport activity.

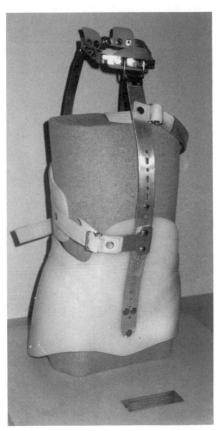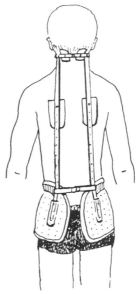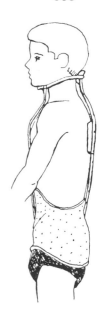

**FIGURE 8.** *Left,* Milwaukee brace used in treatment of Scheuermann's disease. (From Labelle H, Dansereau J: Orthopedic treatment of pediatric spinal disorders and diseases. Spine State Art Rev 4(1):242, 1990, with permission.) *Right,* Note the pelvic bucket extends low enough posteriorly over the buttocks and holds the patient in a slightly flexed attitude. This helps control the lumbar lordosis so that the dorsal pads can correct the kyphosis. (From Drummond DS: Kyphosis in the growing child. Spine State Art Rev 1(2):347, 1987, with permission.)

      i. Patients with vertebral abnormalities in the cervical spine (or at the cervicothoracic junction) should be counseled against contact or collision sports. (The American Academy of Pediatrics has published useful guidelines on classification of sports by degree of contact and intensity of exertion. *Pediatrics* 81(5):737–739, 1988.)

     ii. **Patients who have had spinal fusion for scoliosis** should be counseled against participating in collision sports and should be warned that even strenuous noncontact sports may increase the risk of degenerative disease in the segments above and below the fusion.

6. **Physical exam:** Look for asymmetry of the back and presence of a rib hump noted when patient bends forward (Adam's test).

7. **Radiological exam:** Should include standing PA and lateral views of the thoracolumbar spine, carefully measuring the curvature.

8. **Treatment of idiopathic adolescent-onset scoliosis:**

    a. If curvature is mild (less than 20°) when first detected, reassessment every 3 to 4 months during adolescence and until skeletally mature is the usual

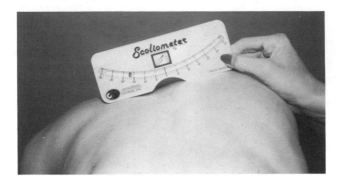

**FIGURE 9.** Scoliometer. A patient is placed in the forward-bending position and the Scoliometer is placed on the patient's back. The mid-portion of the Scoliometer is located directly over the mid-line of the spine. The Scoliometer is placed over the maximum rib prominence. Note the deflection of the ball within the level. (From Green NE: Adolescent idiopathic scoliosis. Spine State Art Rev 4(1):213, 1990, with permission).

        course of follow-up. Active treatment is not required so long as the curve is nonprogressive.

    b. If the rib deformity is mild (less than 10°), the individual may be followed by scoliometric measurement (Fig. 9), with x-rays only when rotational deformity is progressive.

    c. If skeletally immature and the curve is moderate (between 20–45°) when first detected and is documented to be progressive, bracing is the mainstay of therapy. The goal of bracing is to arrest progression (not effect correction of the curve).

       i. In many instances, the treatment regimen may safely permit enough time out of the brace for daily participation in sport activity; each case must be individualized and this decision made by a scoliosis specialist.

    d. Severe curvature may require surgery (fusion with spinal instrumentation) and discussion is beyond the scope of this text. These patients should be followed by a scoliosis specialist and their activity level adjusted according to the treating physician's established guidelines.

## V. Lumbosacral Spine

A. **Acute lumbar strain**

1. May be **defined** as low back pain which is nonradiating and is associated with mechanical stress to the lumbar spine and its supporting structures.

2. The **cause** is not always evident.

    a. It may be related to a specific traumatic episode.

    b. Some feel that it is more often related to prolonged poor posture, poor physical conditioning, and anterior migration of the center of gravity.

3. **Poor sitting posture** may predispose one to develop low back pain.

    a. Relaxed sitting for any length of time will usually result in the lumbar spine assuming a fully flexed position, becoming painful due to stretching of the posterior muscles and ligaments.

    b. In sitting, the intradiscal pressure increases as the spine assumes a forward-flexed position and decreases as one moves into lordosis.

4. **Improper lifting** may precipitate an episode of low back pain.

    a. Lifting with the back flexed and knees straight significantly increases the intra-discal pressure as compared to a lift with flexed hips and knees, back straight.[19]

5. **Physical exam**
   a. Local tenderness may be found over the involved areas and at times muscle spasm may be present.
   b. Usually will find a limited range of motion (forward and lateral flexion and rotation).
   c. Neurologic exam is entirely normal.
6. **Radiographic evaluation**
   a. In acute low back strain, x-rays are usually not necessary on the initial visit.
   b. Should consider x-rays if no improvement occurs within 2 to 4 weeks.
7. **Treatment**
   a. **Rehabilitation program** consisting of strengthening and flexibility exercises is most important:
      i. Knee to chest exercises—performed in supine position.
      ii. Hamstring stretching—performed while patient lies comfortably on his/her back.
      iii. Abdominal strengthening exercises—partial sit ups, partial sit ups with rotation, and pelvic tilt exercises.
      iv. Chair flexion exercises (Fig. 10).
      v. Extension exercises while prone with two pillows under patient's abdomen (Fig. 11) and push-up extension exercises while prone (Fig. 12).
      vi. Rotational stretch exercises while sitting.
   b. NSAIDs are helpful in relieving acute pain.
   c. Muscle relaxants are useful only in patients with palpable muscle spasm.
   d. The use of narcotic analgesics should generally be avoided.
   e. Ice packs or ice massage alternating with heat may decrease pain and spasm.
   f. Use of a TENS unit is often helpful in those unresponsive to the above measures.
   g. Patient education
      i. Sitting
         (a) When in acute pain, patient should sit as little as possible (to avoid lumbar flexion) and when sitting, only for short periods.
         (b) When sitting one should maintain a normal lumbar lordosis with muscle control or use of a lumbar roll.
         (c) Sitting in a high, straight-back chair is much better than a low, soft couch (to avoid increased lumbar flexion).

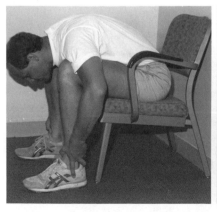
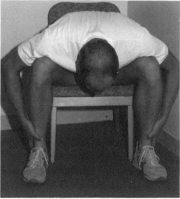

**FIGURE 10.** Chair flexion exercises.

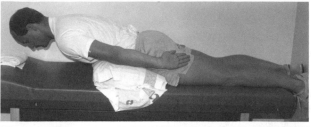

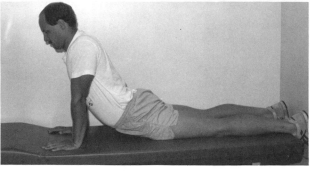

**FIGURE 11** *(above).*   Extension exercise while prone with two pillows under abdomen.

**FIGURE 12** *(below).*   Push-up extension exercise while prone.

      ii. Lifting
         (a) When in acute pain, one should avoid lifting altogether.
         (b) After the acute phase subsides, one should lift with legs keeping the back straight and avoid lifting over 20 to 30 lb.
     iii. Lying
         (a) Using a firm mattress and/or putting a $\geq 5/8$ inch plywood bed board between the mattress and springs is advisable.
         (b) Using a supportive roll around the waist, such as a rolled-up towel tied in front, is helpful in maintaining lumbar lordosis.
         (c) Lying with knees slightly flexed (supported by a pillow) is helpful.
  8. **Prognosis**
    a. The usual course is one of gradual improvement over a 2-week period.
    b. 90% are well within 2 months.
 B. **Spondylolysis**
  1. Vertebral lysis (Gr.—a loosening). Actually a melting away of a portion of the vertebral bony complex.
  2. Occurs in the **"pars interarticularis"**—that portion of the posterior vertebral elements located between the superior and inferior facet (Figs. 1 and 13).
  3. **Pathophysiology**—in the athletic population, spondylolysis is felt to be one of the "overuse syndromes." Repeated shear placed upon this thin, inherently weaker portion of the bony vertebral column results in an attempt at osseous remodeling and frequently stress fracture.
  4. **Etiology:** Repeated longitudinal loading of the vertebral column as seen in upright weight lifting, dismounts from gymnastic equipment, contact while in three-point stance position of the football lineman, tennis players with hard overhead service motion, etc.

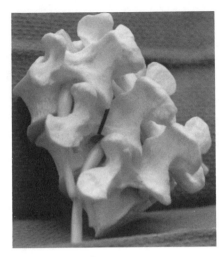

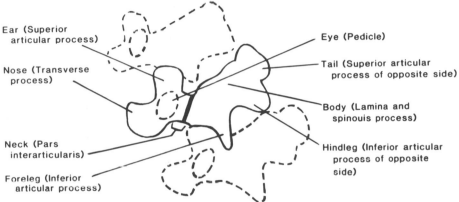

**FIGURE 13.** "Scotty dog" outline as seen on the oblique view of lumbar spine. The black line on the neck or pars interarticularis is where the spondylolytic defect occurs and on x-ray is seen as a "collar" on the Scotty dog's neck.

5. **Clinical presentation:**
   a. History of low back pain, with a specific activity relationship, relieved by rest. May have acute or gradual onset.
   b. Usually nonradicular, occasionally with radiation to buttock on side of involvement.
   c. Age: Onset common in teenage athletes. Not a common initial diagnosis over 40 years of age.
6. **Physical examination:**
   a. Gait normal, occasional slight list to the side due to *b* (below).
   b. Muscle spasm and tenderness, paravertebrally at level of vertebral defect and surrounding segments.
   c. Pain on forward flexion, rotation away from side of the lesion, and lateral bending toward lesion.
   d. Pain on spinal extension when standing on single leg on side of lesion (positive one-legged hyperextension test) (Fig. 5).
   e. Pain with spinal extension while standing on both legs when lesion is bilateral.

f. Straight leg raise, Laseque's test, FABER test—usually negative.

g. Neurological exam normal.

7. **Radiographic examination:**

a. Lumbar spine series to include anteroposterior, lateral, and oblique views. At least **the lateral must be taken in upright (standing) position.**

b. Defect best seen in neck of the "Scotty dog" outline, noted on the oblique view (Fig. 13).

c. Occasionally visible as lytic line on the lateral view.

d. If not well visualized, but suspicion is high, tomograms or CT scan may be of benefit.

8. **Nuclear imaging:**

a. Technetium[99] (Te[99]) bone scan of value in identifying occult lesion (negative x-ray, positive bone scan).

b. Te[99] bone scan of value in determining age and/or healing potential of radiographically identifiable lesion—negative ("cold") scan indicates lack of healing effort and likely failure of conservative measures; positive scan (Fig. 14) mirrors effort on part of bone to heal the defect.

9. **Treatment:** Proceed with treatment depending on characteristics of fracture healing.

a. **Acute lesion:**

i. Rest alone may be sufficient for lesion with positive bone scan without radiographic defect (stress response of bone that has not proceeded to fracture). Rest to include avoidance of all physical activity placing loading force on spine for 8 to 12 weeks.

ii. If full relief of symptoms with everyday activity, not experienced within 2 to 3 weeks, consider a body cast.

b. **Semi-acute lesion (positive bone scan, positive x-ray):**

i. Immobilization, as in any fracture, will promote healing.

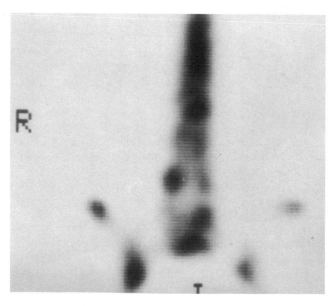

**FIGURE 14.** Technetium-99 bone scan demonstrates increased uptake in lumbar vertebrae as seen in acute or semiacute spondylolysis.

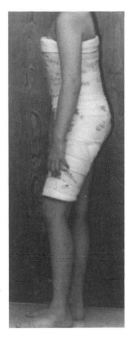

**FIGURE 15.** Single leg, pantaloon, body cast used in treatment of spondylolysis—acute or semiacute lesions.

  ii. Due to usual location of lesion (lumbar 5), pelvis must be immobilized (joint above and joint below fracture).
  iii. Body cast that includes one thigh (pantaloon) adequate (Fig. 15).
  iv. Athlete may be ambulatory in cast.
  v. Cast must be worn for 12 weeks.
  vi. Slow return to activity following cast removal; begin with flexibility enhancing, low vertebra stress functions, gradually increase over 3 months.
  vii. Avoid upright weight training (squats, dead lifts, snatch and jerk, etc.) permanently.
  viii. Micheli and associates report success in use of the anti-lordotic Boston brace.[17] Some athletes are able to continue participation to some degree in their sport activity while under treatment. Micheli suggests immobilization for at least 12 weeks.
     (a) Patient must be symptom-free in the brace before resuming activity and must remain symptom-free during graduated return to full participation.
     (b) Beware of the risk that a noncompliant patient may discard the brace early because of symptom relief.
  c. **Chronic lesion (positive x-ray, negative bone scan):**
     i. Immobilization will not result in healing of this established nonunion.
     ii. If symptomatic and athlete does not wish to give up aggravating activity, operative fusion of two or three involved segments necessary.
     iii. Return to full activity permissible one year after successful fusion.
     iv. Probably wise not to return to upright weight lifting activities, as noted above.
  C. **Spondylolisthesis**
     1. Vertebral *olisthanein* (Gr.—a slip). Forward slippage of one vertebra upon the one below.

2. **Pathophysiology:** Made possible by loss of continuity between anterior and posterior elements at one level of the vertebral column.
   a. **Defect in pars interarticularis (spondylolysis) most common predisposing abnormality; subsequent loss of soft tissue stability results in slip.**
3. **Classification**
   a. **Pathologic anatomy classification**
      i. **Dysplastic spondylolisthesis:** Congenital deficiency of superior sacral or inferior fifth lumbar facets (or both) with gradual slipping of fifth lumbar vertebra.
      ii. **Isthmic (spondylolytic) spondylolisthesis:** The lesion occurs in the pars interarticularis permitting slipping of the vertebra. **Three subtypes:**
         (a) **Lytic (fatigue fracture of the pars interarticularis):** Results from stress with repeated microfractures rather than from one acute traumatic episode. Most common form in athletes.
         (b) **Elongated but intact pars interarticularis:** Results from repeated fatigue microfractures which heal in somewhat elongated position. Also common in athletes.
         (c) **Acute fractures of pars interarticularis.**
      iii. **Degenerative spondylolisthesis:** Stability between segments of vertebral column mildly compromised due to loss of intervertebral disc space and narrowing of facet joint cartilage.
      iv. **Traumatic spondylolisthesis:** Acute fractures of the bony hook other than the pars interarticularis (pedicle, lamina, or facets) and disruption of soft tissue continuity due to trauma (seat-belt injuries).
      v. **Pathologic spondylolisthesis:** Attenuation of pedicle secondarily to structural weakness of bone (i.e., osteogenesis imperfecta).
   b. **Degree of slip classification:**
      Determined by dividing distance superior vertebra displaced upon inferior by anterior-posterior dimension of inferior vertebral body.
      i. 0–25%—first degree
      ii. 25–50%—second degree
      iii. 50–75%—third degree
      iv. > 75%—fourth degree.
4. **Clinical presentation:**
   a. History of low back pain, occasionally severe.
      i. Generally improved but not totally relieved by rest.
   b. May be radicular, not uncommonly into both lower extremities.
   c. Degree of slip usually not progressive after skeletal maturity.
5. **Physical examination:**
   a. In stance, depending upon degree of slip, one may find:
      i. Flattening of lumbar lordosis
      ii. Palpable step-off at level of defect
      iii. Shortening of trunk with ribs approximating pelvis anteriorly
      iv. Transverse abdominal crease.
   b. Forward flexion markedly limited—individual often unable to bring fingertips below mid-thigh.
   c. Neurologic examination usually normal.
   d. Straight leg raising; limited due to hamstring tightness.
   e. FABER test usually normal.
6. **Radiographic examination:**
   a. *Standing* views of the lumbar spine are mandatory in anteroposterior and lateral projections. Oblique views may be taken with patient lying on x-ray table.

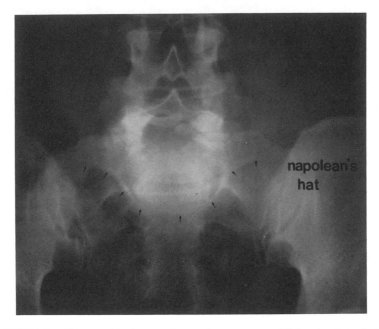

napolean's hat

**FIGURE 16.** AP view of lumbosacral spine showing inverted "Napoleon's hat" sign.

b. In anteroposterior view, superior slipped vertebra may overlie inferior vertebra, creating "Napoleon's hat" illusion (Fig. 16).

c. In lateral view, forward-slipping and tilting of superior (usually L5) vertebra on inferior (usually S1). Rounding and remodelling of superior portion of the sacrum.

d. Spondylolytic defect best seen on oblique views.

e. CT and MRI imaging not usually necessary unless visualization of spinal canal contents desired.

   i. Useful for evaluation of associated spinal stenosis or nerve-root compression.

f. Annual radiographic study with standing lateral view generally adequate until skeletal maturity is recommended to detect progression.

7. **Nuclear imaging**—not indicated for diagnosis of spondylolisthesis.

8. **Treatment:**

a. Loss of support provided by skeletal elements puts excessive stress on soft tissues.

b. Exercise program to strengthen muscle-tendon units and stretch hamstrings helpful.

c. If symptoms not well controlled, surgery and fusion tailored to patient's needs necessary.

9. **Complication**

a. The slippage of the vertebral body may cause a constriction in the size of the spinal canal **(spinal stenosis).**

   i. Outstanding feature of spinal stenosis is **neurogenic claudication ("pseudoclaudication").**

      (a) **Pain** is evoked or accentuated by walking.

      (b) Pain is **relieved** by sitting.

      (c) Neurogenic claudication is due to bony constriction of the neural structures (spinal cord, cauda equina, or individual nerve roots).1

(d) Neurogenic claudication can be distinguished from peripheral arterial claudication by:
(i) Failure of standing still to provide relief.
(ii) Relief with sitting.
(iii) Presence of good peripheral pulses and absence of trophic changes in the skin.
(e) Ability to ride a bicycle without problems but inability to walk for comparable length of time.
ii. **Neurologic examination** is frequently normal.
iii. The **history** rather than the objective findings is the decisive factor in the diagnosis.
iv. **CT scanning, MRI, and myelogram** are used to determine the degree and site of stenosis.
v. **Treatment**
(a) In most cases of significant stenosis, conservative measures are unsuccessful.
(b) Surgical fusion is needed for high-degree slips that cause spinal stenosis.

D. **Disc disease and herniation**
1. Anatomic abnormality present in annulus fibrosus, which is thinnest posterolaterally. Annulus may sustain traumatic or degenerative tear, allowing intervertebral disc material to bulge or escape through this restraining structure.
2. Commonly seen in athlete between 20 and 35 years of age; less common in teenage athlete.
3. L5–S1 disease most common; in younger individuals L4–5 problems occur and more rarely L3–4.
4. **Etiology:** Increased pressure within disc space may occur with flexion-rotation motion. With this posture, nucleus pulposus migrates posteriorly and laterally. Repeated activity of this nature may cause gradual compromise and rupture of annulus fibrosus posterolaterally—anatomically its thinnest area—with herniation of disc material.
5. **Clinical presentation:**
a. History of gradually worsening lower back pain with muscle spasm.
i. Aggravated by motion.
ii. Relieved by lying with hips and knees flexed.
b. Leg pain and paresthesias in dermatomal distribution.
c. Symptoms increased with Valsalva maneuvers, which increase intra-abdominal (and intradiscal) pressure.
i. Example: coughing, sneezing, or straining on bowel movement.
d. With more severe nerve root compromise, patient may note weakness in foot "push-off" (S1 root) or ankle-foot dorsiflexion (L5 root).
e. Central herniation may cause bladder and rectal sphincter dysfunction due to pressure in the cauda equinus.
6. **Physical examination:**
a. Individual stands and walks with some spine flexion and list:
i. List to side away from disorder if disc herniation is lateral to nerve root.
ii. List to side of disorder if disc herniation is medial to nerve root.
b. Forward flexion limited due to muscle spasm.
c. Straight leg raise positive; sciatic stretch testing (Lasegue's test) positive.
d. Manual testing of extensor hallucis (L5) and tibialis anterior (L5) strength may reveal weakness.

e. Functionally testing the extensor hallucis longus and extensor digitorum longus and brevis (L5) by having the patient walk on his heel may reveal weakness.

f. Functionally testing the gastrocnemius-soleus muscles (S1, S2) by having the patient walk on his toes may reveal weakness.

g. Deep tendon reflexes; tendo-achilles (S1) or patellar tendon (L4) may be decreased or absent. (Hyperactive reflexes signify an upper motor neuron lesion.)

h. Sensation to pin prick or light touch may be diminished in appropriate dermatomal distribution (see Fig. 3).

7. **Radiologic studies:**

a. **Plain x-ray:**

 i. May be normal, especially in young athlete.

 ii. May reveal narrowed intervertebral disc space at involved level in more chronic situation.

b. **Imaging studies:**

 i. MRI visualizes soft tissues well and reveals nerve root compression and/or edema nicely (Fig. 17).

 ii. CT scan helpful, most specific for bony pathology, although disc may be noted to be bulging (Fig. 18); free fragments difficult to identify.

8. **Neurologic studies:**

a. EMG: May show alteration in specifically innervated muscle due to nerve root irritability.

b. Nerve conduction may be slowed and signal amplitude altered.

9. **Treatment:**

a. Initial treatment should be conservative, with the use of relative rest, and analgesic and muscle relaxant medication. This will allow nerve root edema to subside and permit root to accommodate to narrowed confines. **Bed rest is contraindicated in all but severe disc disease in athletes because of deconditioning effects.**

b. Early initiation of therapeutic exercise program is basis of therapy.

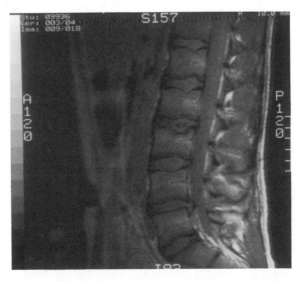

**FIGURE 17.** MRI of lumbosacral spine (lateral view) shows herniated disc at L4–L5 level.

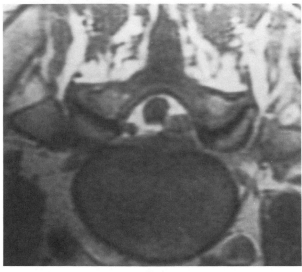

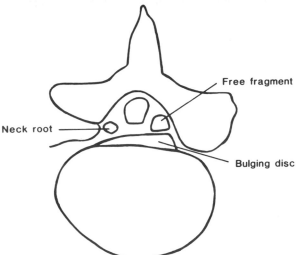

**FIGURE 18.**   CT scan of lumbar spine showing bulging disc and a free fragment.

    i. Extension exercises may dramatically improve symptoms.
   c. Long-term treatment includes life-style alteration to decrease incidence of exacerbation of symptoms.
   d. Ultimate course of treatment may include surgical excision of disc material for those unresponsive to conservative care.
   e. Successfully treated disc herniation athletes often may be able to return to vigorous athletic activity.
 E. **Sacroiliac sprain syndrome**
   1. The sacroiliac (SI) joints are among the strongest joints in the body.
    a. Possess a synovial membrane.
    b. Lined by strong anterior and posterior ligaments.
    c. Very little movement is permitted.
   2. SI joints are a commonly overlooked source of low back pain.

3. **History:**
   a. May be a history of trauma.
   b. Pain is usually felt over the SI joint.
   c. Pain may also be felt in the leg, suggesting a radiculopathy.
      i. Thus, many patients may have already been worked up with negative CT scans and myelograms.
      ii. A spur or inflamed SI joint could irritate the sciatic nerve due to the close approximation of the sciatic nerve over the lower SI joint.
   d. Pain is usually unilateral.
4. **Physical examination:**
   a. Tenderness over SI joint, posterior superior iliac spine, or buttock.
   b. Painful knee-to-chest maneuver (Fig. 19).
      i. Produces rotatory stress on SI joint increasing pain in SI joint disorder.
      ii. A traditional therapeutic exercise given to many back pain patients that may aggravate symptoms.
   c. Sacroiliac compression test produces pain in majority of patients.
      i. Patient lies on side and downward pressure is exerted on lateral pelvis.
   d. Gaenslen's extension test produces pain.
      i. Patient positions leg of affected side overhanging the side of table and the examiner presses down on thigh to hyperextend the hip while performing knee-to-chest maneuver to unaffected side (Fig. 20).
   e. FABER test may elicit pain.
   f. Neurological exam is normal.

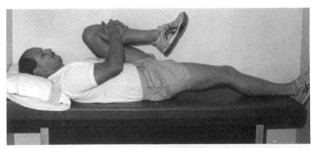

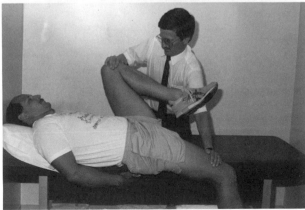

**FIGURE 19.** *(top).* Knee-to-chest maneuver causes pain in sacroiliac sprain syndrome.

**FIGURE 20** *(bottom).* Gaenslen's extension test produces pain in sacroiliac sprain syndrome.

5. **Radiological evaluation:**
  a. Usually is normal.
  b. Assists in ruling out other disorders such as ankylosing spondylitis.
6. **Treatment:**
  a. SI joint mobilization exercises and manipulation.
  b. NSAIDs are useful.
  c. X-ray–guided SI joint injection with corticosteroid.
F. **Facet syndrome**
  1. Radicular pain due to impingement upon the nerve root by the anterior lip of the facet joint.
  2. Most common in degenerative disc disease.
  3. **Pathophysiology:** With collapse of disc space anteriorly, facet joint sublux posteriorly, narrowing the intervertebral foramen and impinging on the nerve root. In the athlete, facet fracture and mal/nonunion may be causative.
  4. **Clinical presentation:**
    a. All complaints present in disc herniation are also present in facet syndrome.
    b. Patients may suffer from more back pain than the individual with isolated herniated disc material.
  5. **Physical examination:**
    a. Findings essentially the same as with other nerve root impingement.
    b. Increased muscle spasm palpable in the perivertebral musculature.
  6. **Radiographic examination:**
    a. Routine oblique x-rays may reveal foraminal encroachment.
    b. CT scan to visualize narrowed foramen.
  7. **Treatment:**
    a. Activity limitation and nonsteroidal anti-inflammatory medications to reduce nerve root edema.
    b. Exercise programs not usually of benefit.
    c. Fluoroscopically controlled intra-articular facet corticosteroid injection may relieve pain in some patients.
    d. Surgical decompression (foraminotomy) with or without spinal fusion may be necessary.
G. **Ankylosing spondylitis**
  1. Clinically oversimplified approach is to think of ankylosing spondylitis as the presence of symptomatic sacroiliitis (low back pain and radiologic evidence of sacroilitis).
  2. **Etiology** is unknown but thought to be in the rheumatoid family of autoimmune diseases.
  3. **Prevalence** appears to be around 1%.
  4. **Clinical presentation:** age 15–35 years, insidious onset, symptoms persisting longer than 3 months, morning stiffness, and improvement of pain with exercise.
  5. **Skeletal involvement:**
    a. **Spine**—back pain.
    b. **Extraspinal**—20% peripheral joint disease.
    c. **Insertional tendinitis (enthesopathy):**
      i. Plantar fasciitis
      ii. Achilles tendinitis
      iii. Costochondritis.
  6. May have **extraskeletal involvement** in eyes, lungs and heart.
  7. **Radiographic evaluation:**
    a. Sacroiliac joints frequently first involved.

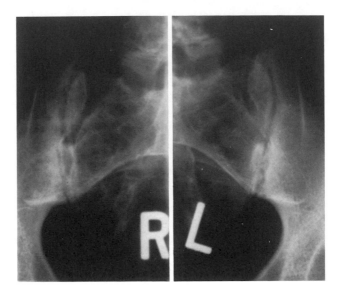

**FIGURE 21.** Sacroiliac views reveal sclerosis, irregular erosions, and narrowing of the sacroiliac joints in ankylosing spondylitis.

       i. SI joints show blurring of joint margins, irregular erosions, patchy sclerosis, and narrowing (Fig. 21).

      ii. Usually bilateral.

  b. Spine

       i. Initially straightening of lumbar spine and "squaring" of vertebral bodies due to erosion at the corners of the vertebrae where the annulus fibrosus inserts.

      ii. With progression of disease, syndesmophytes appear along lateral and anterior surfaces of discs bridging adjacent vertebrae.

        (a) Syndesmophytes extend vertically from vertebrae along outer aspect of the disc, differing from osteophytes, which project horizontally before curving to form a bridge.

        (b) In advanced disease, the widespread formation of syndesmophytes produces the "bamboo" spine.

  8. **Treatment**

    a. Maintaining normal posture and activity key to decreasing progressive deformity (kyphosis).

    b. NSAIDs relieve inflammation and pain.

    c. Surgery may be helpful in correcting extreme flexion deformities.

H. **Piriformis syndrome**

  1. **Definition:** Irritation of the sciatic nerve as it passes underneath or through the piriformis muscle producing a deep localized pain in the posterior aspect of the hip (near the sciatic notch) that often radiates down into the leg.

  2. **Etiology** is thought to be piriformis muscle spasm or hypertrophy irritating the adjacent sciatic nerve.

    a. A history of trauma can only be elicited in approximately half the cases, and the nature of the trauma is seldom dramatic.

Piriformis Syndrome = Compression of sciatic
nerve by tight piriformis muscle

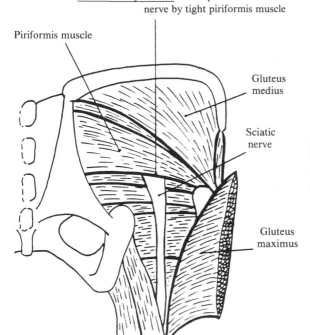

**FIGURE 22.** Illustration indicating the site of compression irritation of the sciatic nerve by piriformis muscle spasm or hypertrophy.

3. **Anatomy:** The piriformis muscle arises from the anterior surface of the sacrum near the sacroiliac joint, then runs laterally through the sciatic notch and inserts as a tendon on the greater trochanter of the femur.
   a. In the majority of cases the sciatic nerve passes underneath the piriformis muscle (Fig. 22).
4. **Function of the piriformis muscle:** External rotation of the hip.
5. **Additional historical clue:** Dyspareunia in females.
   a. Piriformis syndrome occurs about 6 times more frequently in women than in men.
6. **Physical exam**
   a. May find excellent ROM of lumbar spine despite severity of symptoms.
   b. Almost invariably there will be sciatic notch tenderness.
   c. Often have positive straight leg raising test indicative of sciatic nerve irritation.
   d. **Most significant finding:** both active external rotation of the hip against resistance and a passive stretch into internal rotation will produce pain.
   e. On pelvic and/or rectal exam, there is often a distinct tender trigger point proximal to the ischial spine; during palpation the patient will experience pain and often exclaim that this is the first time someone has found "my pain."
7. There are no laboratory or radiological findings in this syndrome.
8. **EMG/NCV studies** show normal activity in the gluteus medius and tensor fascia lata muscles (innervated by the superior gluteal nerve, which arises above the piriformis muscle); however, abnormalities are present below this level.
9. **Differential diagnosis:**
   a. It is difficult to diagnose with any certainty and may be a diagnosis of exclusion.

b. Most likely to be confused with herniated intervertebral disc.

   i. In herniated disc with sciatica, the pain is usually increased on coughing, sneezing, or straining on defecation, indicating epidural involvement not noted in piriformis syndrome.

   ii. Pain is not aggravated with passive internal rotation of the hip, as it is in piriformis syndrome.

10. **Treatment:**

    a. Initially conservative with rest, anti-inflammatory agents, muscle relaxants, and physical therapy consisting of good stretching, ROM, and isometric exercises to help relieve spasm and pain.

    b. Local injection of the muscle belly with lidocaine and corticosteroid by those skilled enough to inject the specific location without injuring the sciatic nerve (can be both diagnostic and therapeutic), but this is not recommended for those occasionally making the diagnosis.

    c. If these measures fail, then in rare instances operative dissection of the compressive portion of the piriformis muscle may be necessary.

I. **Infections**

1. **Disc space infection** and **vertebral osteomyelitis** should be included in the differential diagnosis of back pain.

2. Usually **present** with back pain aggravated by motion, localized tenderness, limited range of motion, and paravertebral muscle spasm.

3. **Pathophysiology:**

   a. Hematogenous migration from distant focus via venous plexus.

   b. Secondary introduction of bacteria to region (surgery, lumbar puncture) also can be a source of inoculation.

4. **Temperature** may be normal or mildly to moderately elevated.

5. **Blood culture** possitive in $< 50\%$ of cases.

6. **Sedimentation rate** is usually elevated to 40 mm/hr or more and the **white blood cell count may be** normal or mildly elevated, with normal differential or slight left shift.

7. **Radiologic evaluation**

   a. **Disc space infections:**

      i. **Plain films:** Intervertebral disc space narrowing and irregularity of adjacent vertebral endplates, which may not be visualized for 10–14 days.

      ii. **Technetium[99] bone scan** helpful in confirming or localizing diagnosis (Te[99] bone scans are positive in both infection and tumor.)

      iii. **Gallium/indium-labeled white cell scans** are more specific for infection and are helpful in differentiating other processes such as tumors from infection.

   b. **Vertebral osteomyelitis**

      i. Early on, findings on **plain films** same as in disc space infection. Later followed by erosion through the vertebral endplate, and destructive and sclerotic changes involving the vertebral bodies.

      ii. Te[99] bone scan and gallium/indium-labeled white cell scan as above in disc space infection.

      iii. **CT scan** can detect early involvement of vertebral body.

J. **Referred pain**

1. **Pelvic disorders** may involve the sacral plexus or its branches, producing low back pain and/or sciatica.

   a. Upon examination, may find positive straight leg raise but careful pelvic and rectal exam will usually reveal underlying pelvic disease (i.e., uterine fibroids, ovarian tumors, pelvic inflammatory disease).

2. **Prostatitis** may present with low back pain.
   a. Rectal exam reveals enlarged, tender, boggy prostate.
3. **Renal disorders** such as nephrolithiasis, pyelonephritis, or perinephric abscess may present with back pain.
   a. Thorough abdominal exam, urinalysis, and appropriate radiologic studies will reveal these renal disorders.

## REFERENCES AND RECOMMENDED READING

1. Akbarnia BA, Keppler L: Spinal deformities. In Principles of Orthopaedic Practice, Vol 2. New York, McGraw-Hill, 1989, pp 889–991.
2. Aprin H, Dee R: Infections of the spine. In Principles of Orthopaedic Practice, Vol 2. New York, McGraw-Hill, 1989, pp 941–955.
3. Benson DR: The back: Thoracic and lumbar spine. In D'Ambrosia RD: Musculoskeletal Disorders, 2nd ed. Philadelphia, JB Lippincott, 1986, pp 287–365.
4. Calin A: Ankylosing spondylitis. In Kelley WN, et al: Textbook of Rheumatology, 2nd ed. Philadelphia, WB Saunders, 1985, pp 993–1007.
5. DeGowin EL, DeGowin RL: Bedside Diagnostic Examination, 4th ed. New York, Macmillan, 1981, p 728.
6. Destouet JM, Murphy WA: Lumbar facet block indications and technique. Orthop Rev 14(5):57–65, 1985.
7. Epstein JA, Epstein NE: Lumbar spondylosis and spinal stenosis. In Wilkins RH, Rengachary SS (eds): Neurosurgery, Vol 3. New York, McGraw-Hill 1985, pp 2272–2278.
8. Frymoyer JW: Back pain and sciatica. N Engl J Med 318:291–300, 1988.
9. Gaines RW, Humphreys WG: Spondylolisthesis. In Chapman MW, Madison M (eds): Operative Orthopaedics, Vol 3. Philadelphia, JB Lippincott, 1988, pp 2005–2014.
10. Gould JA, Davies GJ: Orthopaedic and Sports Physical Therapy. St. Louis, CV Mosby, 1985, pp 404–406.
11. Hoppenfeld S: Orthopaedic Neurology. Philadelphia, JB Lippincott, 1977, pp 51–74.
12. Hoppenfeld S: Physical Examination of the Spine and Extremities. East Norwalk, CT, Appleton-Century-Crofts, 1976, pp 237–263.
13. Huurman WW: Spine in sports. In Mellion MB: Office Management of Sports Injuries and Athletic Problems. Philadelphia, Hanley & Belfus, 1988, pp 199–212.
14. Jackson DW, Ciullo JV: Injuries of the spine in the skeletally immature athlete. In Nicholas JA, Hershman EB (eds): The Lower Extremity and Spine in Sports Medicine. St. Louis, CV Mosby, 1986, pp 1350–1352.
15. Lipson SJ: Low back pain. In Kelley WN, et al: Textbook of Rheumatology, 2nd ed. Philadelphia, WB Saunders, 1985, pp 448–465.
16. Micheli LJ, Marotta JJ: Scoliosis and sports. Your Patient and Fitness 2(2):5–11, 1989.
17. Micheli LJ, et al: Use of modified Boston brace for back injuries in athletes. Am J Sports Med 8:351–356, 1980.
18. Morris JM: Spinal stenosis. In Operative Orthopaedics, Vol 3. Philadelphia, JB Lippincott, 1988, pp 2065–2075.
19. Nachemson A: Towards a better understanding of low back pain: A review of the mechanics of the lumbar disc. Rheumatol Rehabil 14:129–142, 1975.
20. Nakano KK: Sciatic nerve entrapment: The piriformis syndrome. J Musculoskel Med 33–37, 1987.
21. O'Neill DB, Micheli LJ: Recognizing and preventing overuse injuries in young athletes. J Musculoskel Med 106–125, 1989.
22. Pace JB, Nagle D: Piriformis syndrome. West J Med 124:435–439, 1976.
23. Schuchmann JA, Cannon CL: Sacroiliac strain syndrome: Diagnosis and treatment. Texas Med 33–36, 1986.
24. Wiltse LL, Widell EH, Jackson DW: Fatigue fracture: The basic lesion in isthmic spondylolisthesis. J Bone Joint Surg 57A:17–22, 1975.
25. Winter RB: Spinal problems in pediatric orthopaedics. In Pediatric Orthopaedics, 2nd ed. Philadelphia, JB Lippincott, 1986, pp 619–631.

# Chapter 39: Pelvis, Hip and Thigh Injuries

### PAUL W. ESPOSITO, MD

This chapter is about an anatomical region where injuries result from torsional, tensile, and direct traumatic forces. These injuries may become chronic, may prevent participation, and, on some occasions, may even threaten the life or the long-term function of the athlete. The keys to treatment of problems in this anatomic area are primarily prevention, recognition, protection, and appropriate, graded rehabilitation.

I. **The Physical Examination—Special Considerations**
   A. **General alignment of spine and pelvis to lower extremities**
      1. Leg length can be best judged by palpating and visualizing the iliac crests of the patient standing with legs straight.
      2. Check for malrotation of pelvis and spine.
      3. Note skin lesions, dimples, nevi.
   B. **Motor exam and flexibility**
      1. Hamstring tightness
         a. May indicate spinal pathology (Figs. 1–3).
         b. Lack of flexibility may lead to hamstring tears and patellar problems.
   C. **Bursae**
      1. Examine iliopsoas, greater trochanter, and ischium.
   D. **Sensory exam**
      1. Obturator nerve innervates hips as well as medial thigh and knee.
         a. Medial thigh pain may frequently indicate hip problems.
   E. **Specific tests for tightness**
      1. Thomas test—iliopsoas contracture (Fig. 4)
         a. Flex both hips to flatten lordosis, then slowly extend one hip at a time. Contracture won't allow full extension.
            i. May be cause of iliopsoas bursitis and "snapping hip" syndrome.
      2. Iliotibial band contracture (see Chap. 30, Fig. 8).
      3. Hip flexion test (Fig. 5)
         a. Spontaneous external rotation of the hip while flexing the hip, especially in the adolescent or immature athlete, can indicate either slipped capital femoral epiphysis or a significant joint incongruity.
      4. Joint motion symmetry
         a. Asymmetrical loss of motion may indicate hip disorder.
      5. Log roll test (Fig. 6)
         a. Gentle to and fro motion in extension—exquisite pain.
            i. Infection, fracture, or synovitis.
         b. Pain only with extreme internal rotation.
            i. Low grade synovitis
      6. Leg externally rotates and appears to shorten when hip is flexed in patient with slipped capital femoral epiphysis (Fig. 7).
      7. Flexion, abduction, external rotation test (Patrick test; Fig. 8)
         a. Pain in sacroiliac (SI) joint when this joint is involved.
   F. Radiographs
      1. Taken except with obvious contusions and muscle pulls.
         a. Detect fractures, stress fractures, avulsion fractures, bony problems.
         b. Reveal pelvic, spine, lower extremity malalignment.
         c. Risk of long-term disability and loss of competition if appropriate, timely x-ray studies are not obtained.

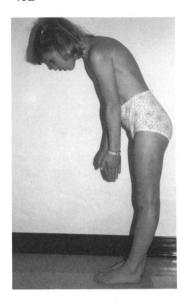

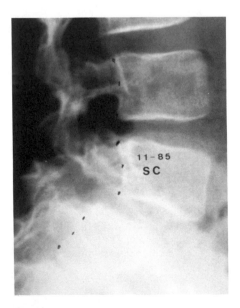

FIGURE 1.   Child with acute spondylolisthesis. Note loss of lumbar lordosis and tight hamstrings.

FIGURE 2.   More severe listhesis. Note step-off when upper lumbar segments have slipped forward on lower lumbar segments, as well as tight hamstrings. There is total loss of lumbar lordosis.

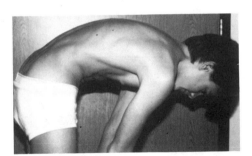

FIGURE 3.   Radiograph demonstrating spondylolisthesis in child in Figure 1.

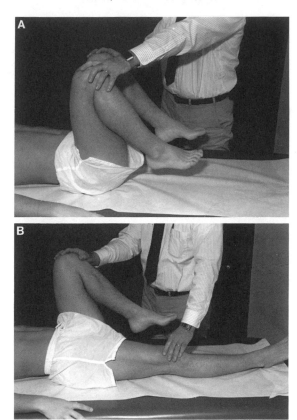

**FIGURE 4.**   Thomas test. *A,* Flexion of both hips to flatten lumbar lordosis, *B,* then extend one hip—measures hip flexion contracture and tightness in the iliopsoas.

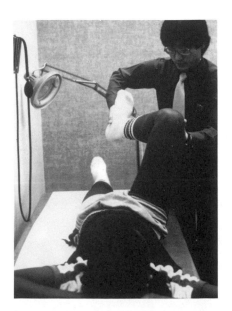

**FIGURE 5.**   Hip flexion test. With slipped capital femoral epiphysis, spontaneous external rotation occurs with hip flexion.

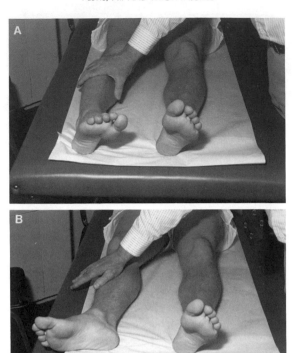

**FIGURE 6.** Log roll test. *A,* Gently rolling the leg internally and *B,* externally with the hip extended is the most sensitive indicator of inflammatory arthritis or traumatic hemarthrosis in the hip.

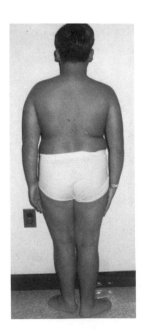

**FIGURE 7.** External rotation posture and shortening noted with slipped capital femoral epiphysis. Note that this patient is standing on his left toes with his heels off the ground to equalize his leg lengths. Also note the asymmetrical truncal skin folds.

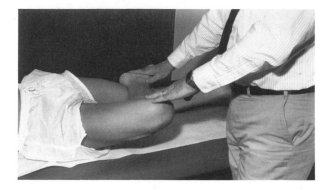

**FIGURE 8.** Patrick test (also known as FABER for Flexion, ABduction, External Rotation test). Used for sacroiliac joint evaluation and for *subtle* pelvic trauma.

    G. Bone scan
        1. Positive in stress fractures long before the fracture is revealed on plain x-ray studies—more sensitive than radiographs in stress reaction.
        2. Extremely helpful in seronegative arthrography (SI arthritis).

II. **Specific Injuries and Problems**

    A. **The sacroiliac joint**
        1. **Seronegative arthropathy** (ankylosing spondylitis and Reiter's syndrome) (Fig. 9)
            a. Often confused with sports injuries and overuse.
            b. Diagnosed by x-ray, bone scan, and decreased chest wall expansion.
                i. Generally HLA-B27 positive.
            c. May be accompanied by heel pain, urethritis, or other joint and spine involvement.
        2. SI joint sprain or contracture
            a. Pelvic rotation

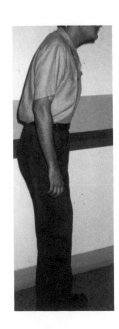

**FIGURE 9.** Clinical photograph of a young adult male with sacroiliitis (Reiter's syndrome). Note stiff, forward flexion posture).

b. Asymmetrical stride or stroke

c. Leg length inequality.

3. SI fracture or dislocation

    a. Usually only with major, high-energy, pelvic trauma.

4. Treatment:

    a. Anti-inflammatory agents, shoe lift, stretching, rest.

B. **Avulsion injuries**

  1. **Mechanism**

    a. Injuries follow acute muscular contraction against a fixed resistance.

    b. A result of inadequate stretching or conditioning.

    c. Frequent in sprinters, hurdlers, or others who rely on sudden, very forceful acceleration.

       i. Especially during maximum growth period of puberty, when the physeal plate is thick.

  2. **Diagnosis**

    a. **Palpation of bony prominence/x-ray**

       i. **Anterior superior iliac spine**

          (a) Sartorius avulsion

          (b) Swelling, tenderness, immediate pain

          (c) Exacerbated with flexion of hip against resistance.

       ii. **Anterior inferior iliac spine** (Fig. 10)

          (a) Rectus femoris.

          (b) Pain, swelling in groin, directly over hip capsule just distal to mid-point inquinal ligament.

          (c) Follows forceful quadriceps contraction.

          (d) Pain increased with flexion of hip against resistance.

      iii. **Ischium**

          (a) Hamstring origin avulsion (Fig. 11)

             (i) Especially common in adolescent apophyseal avulsion.

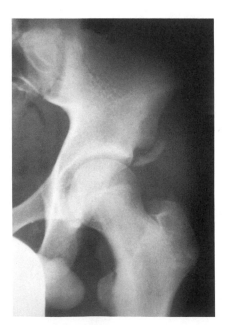

**FIGURE 10.** Anterior, inferior iliac spine avulsion by rectus femoris.

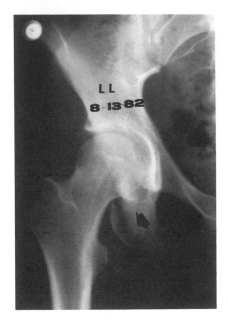

**FIGURE 11.**   Ischial spine avulsion by hamstrings.

        (ii) May require open reduction and fixation to avoid large, reactive fracture callus—may lead to pain when sitting.
    iv. **Piriformis**
       (a) Local tenderness over greater trochanter.
    v. **Iliopsoas**
       (a) Tender, medial groin over lesser trochanter.
       (b) Pain with flexion/extension/rotation of hip against resistance.
  3. **Treatment**
    a. Emphasize prevention
      i. Adequate stretching, conditioning.
    b. Sartorius (anterior superior iliac spine [ASIS]) rectus iliopsoas/pyriformis.
      i. Ice, rest, crutches with touch-down weight bearing for up to 4–6 weeks.
       (a) Too quick a return to vigorous activity may result in formation of bony prominences at the site of the avulsion.
      ii. Surgical reduction if displaced, large cartilaginous or bony fragment exists.
      iii. May require late surgical excision if large bony fragment is present.
      iv. Repeat x-ray studies to assess healing.
    c. Ischium/hamstring avulsion
      i. If significantly displaced, surgically repair.
      ii. Undisplaced—use ice, crutches for 4–6 weeks.
C. **Muscle tears and strains**
  1. Mechanism: Similar to avulsion injuries.
    a. Inadequate stretching, warm-up, and conditioning.
  2. Diagnosis: Common in quadriceps, hamstrings, adductors.
    a. Localized tenderness, swelling, ecchymosis.
    b. Palpable gap in muscle.
    c. Pain with gentle passive stretch.
  3. Treatment
    a. Acute—compression from toe to groin with elastic bandage.

    b. Compression around thigh only may lead to venous thrombosis and/or distal edema.

    c. Ice, rest, elevation, 48–72 hrs for major strains.

    d. Crutches, touch-down weight bearing.

       i. Symptom-guided return to ambulation. May take several days to several weeks.

4. **Treatment principles**

    a. Gentle, progressive stretching

    b. Gradual strengthening and reconditioning

    c. Burst type activities should be done last.

5. **Complications**

    a. **If tear occurs near musculotendinous junction, surgical repair may be indicated** (especially quadriceps tendon).

    b. **Retear**—if inadequate rehabilitation, stretching, or premature return to competition.

    c. **Myositis ossificans** (Fig. 12)

       i. Mechanism

          (a) Most commonly direct blow/tear to muscle.

          (b) Metaplasia of muscle to bone.

          (c) More frequent with repetitive trauma.

          (d) Very common in quadriceps.

       ii. Diagnosis

          (a) Firm mass in muscle after acute hematoma phase.

          (b) Progressive contracture of muscle.

          (c) May see decreased passive knee flexion with quadriceps involvement.

          (d) X-ray findings—early fluctuant calcification in soft tissues later becoming mature, woven bone.

       iii. Treatment

          (a) Avoid reinjury

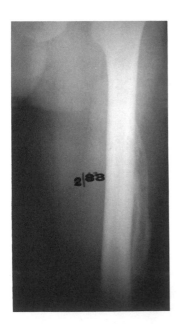

**FIGURE 12.** Myositis ossificans after football helmet blunt trauma several months previously. Note mature looking bone in muscular region, superficial to periosteum.

(i) If significant swelling, muscle tenderness, pain with passive stretch after contusion—stay out of competition until pain-free, nontender with normal motion.

(b) Physical therapy

(i) Gentle stretching to maintain muscle length and avoid joint contracture (especially knee).

(c) Crutch ambulation.

(d) Late treatment

(i) Not always compatible with return to participation.

(ii) Surgical release considered only after myositis is very mature (determined by x-ray, clinical exam, and bone scan).

d. **Contusions**

i. Mechanism: direct blow.

(a) Bleeding/swelling into muscle, periosteum or nerve.

ii. Diagnosis

(a) Localized tenderness, swelling and occasionally ecchymosis.

(b) Specific patterns

(i) Anterior thigh contusion

(ii) Hip pointer

• Direct blow to anterior, superior iliac spine.

(iii) Sciatic nerve involvement

• Rarely may be involved with direct blow to buttocks.

• Look for appropriate sensory and motor findings.

iii. Treatment

(a) Toe to groin compression with elastic dressing.

(b) Ice, elevation.

(c) Maintain muscle length with **gentle** stretching.

(d) Avoid premature return to competition and re-injury.

(e) Failure to treat appropriately may lead to myositis ossificans (see above).

D. **Stress fractures**

1. **Mechanism**

a. Excessive and precipitous increase in activity. Osteoblasts are unable to lay down new bone fast enough to completely remodel.

2. **Common sites**

a. Femoral neck and pubis.

i. Common in distance runners, especially females.

b. Supracondylar femur region.

3. **Diagnosis**

a. Condition is worse before and after activity.

b. Localized bone tenderness is present.

c. Persistent, increasing pain.

d. X-rays are normal for many weeks. Bone scan is extremely sensitive even early—benchmark of diagnostic tests.

e. X-rays late will show periosteal new bone and potentially a faint fracture line.

4. **Treatment**

a. No alternative to rest. When diagnosis is made, no participation in running competition until complete healing, then a gradual resumption of activity.

b. Femoral neck—usually requires prophylactic pin fixation or, at a minimum, prolonged touch-down weight bearing with crutches for many months. Completion of this fracture due to persistent physical activity or inadequate treatment may lead to avascular necrosis of the femoral head with catastrophic results.

      c. Ischium and pubis. Crutch walking, symptom guided, followed by 2–3 months of rest.

      d. Supracondylar femur: Crutches and/or casting to prevent completion of fracture. There is no place for limited treatment and continued activity in stress fractures in this region.

E. **Osteitis pubis**
  1. **Mechanism**
     a. Mechanical inflammatory process of symphysis pubis.
  2. **Diagnosis**
     a. Tenderness in the symphysis pubis with lysis on both sides of the synchondrosis on plain x-ray.
     b. Bone scan may be positive.
       i. Often an incidental finding.
  3. **Treatment**
     a. Only when symptomatic.
     b. Usually responds to rest and anti-inflammatory medications.

F. **Bursitis**
  1. **Mechanism**
     a. Caused by friction where a tendon passes over bony prominence.
     b. Potential space that becomes inflamed and fills with fluid in response to this friction.
     c. Usually caused by excessive activity and insufficient stretching of the involved muscle.
  2. **Diagnosis**
     a. Greater trochanter
       i. Tenderness just posterior to the greater trochanter.
       ii. Aggravated by contraction of the tensor fascia lata with the hip abducted against resistance and with patient on his/her side (Fig. 13).
     b. Iliopsoas
       i. Tenderness over lesser trochanter.
       ii. Medial groin pain, sometimes pain with flexion, abduction, external rotation against resistance.
     c. Ischial
       i. Tenderness over the ischium.
       ii. Aggravated by sitting and contraction of hamstrings.

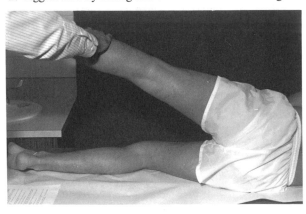

**FIGURE 13.** Abduction against resistance. Pain seen in trochanteric bursitis and iliotibial band syndrome.

     d. **CAUTION: Bursitis is a diagnosis of exclusion.**
        i. Bone scan is indicated unless diagnosis is very clear cut.
        ii. Femoral neck and ischial stress fractures may mimic bursitis symptoms exactly.
        iii. X-ray studies are almost universally required to exclude underlying bony pathology, such as tumor, as the cause of symptoms.
3. **Treatment**
     a. Identifying and developing a stretching and strengthening program for the contracted muscle.
     b. Anti-inflammatory medications.
     c. Corticosteroid therapy in resistant bursitis.
        i. By injection, iontophoresis, or phoresis.
        ii. Ice and deep friction massage may be of some benefit.

G. **Snapping hip syndrome**
1. **Mechanism**
     a. Occasionally a communication between the hip joint and the iliopsoas bursa. Usually secondary to tightness in the iliopsoas muscle.
2. **Diagnosis**
     a. Patient complains of snapping in medial groin with flexion of hip.
3. **Treatment**
     a. Frequently requires only reassurance.
     b. Sometimes will respond to stretching of the hip flexion contracture.
     c. May respond to anti-inflammatory agents if persistent and painful.

H. **Hernias**
1. **Mechanism**
     a. Musculofascial hernia follows a tear in overlying fascia with herniation of underlying muscle through hole.
     b. May strangulate if fascial opening is small or constricting.
2. **Common sites**
     a. Inguinal
     b. Femoral.
3. **Treatment:** See Chapter 37.

I. **The immature athlete:**
1. Immature athletes are prone to injuries peculiar to their anatomy, especially those related to their physis. There are also specific diseases and disorders peculiar to specific age groups that may mimic athletic injuries.
2. **Hip**
     a. Obturator nerve innervates both hip and medial thigh.
        i. Children with knee and medial thigh pain should be closely evaluated for hip disorders.
3. **Legg-Calve-Perthes disease** (Fig. 14)
     a. Present with irritable hips and medial thigh pain.
     b. Most common in 3–8 year age group.
     c. Early x-ray studies are normal.
     d. Bone scan or MRI positive.
     e. Suspicion with positive log roll, limp, or limited motion in the hip.
4. **Toxic synovitis**
     a. Transient inflammatory process of the hip.
     b. X-rays universally normal.
     c. Diagnosed by irritable hip (positive log roll)—see Figure 6.
        i. Must be differentiated from septic arthritis.

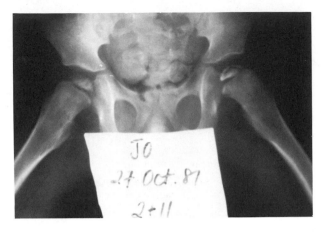

**FIGURE 14.** Legg-Calve-Perthes disease. AP pelvis x-rays demonstrating subchondral collapse on left (crescent sign) and sclerosis on right.

    d. **Treatment**
        i. Rest is key.
       ii. Traction for prompt resolution and avoidance of prolonged course.
  5. **Slipped capital femoral epiphysis**
    a. Usually age 12–15.
    b. Present with medial thigh, knee, or groin pain.
    c. Limp and limited internal rotation/increased external rotation.
    d. Flexion rotation test positive (leg externally rotates with flexion).
    e. AP and frog lateral pelvic x-rays mandatory in all hip disease.
  6. Severe pelvic, hip, and thigh pain requires immediate radiographic evaluation. Additionally, any child with leg, medial thigh, or knee pain that does not resolve in 1 week requires, at a minimum, radiographic evaluation and preferably orthopedic consultation to avoid missing diagnoses that may cause lifelong problems and disability. Persistent, unexplained complaints may necessitate extraordinary diagnostic measures before the child can safely return to athletic activity. If a slipped epiphysis is detected, immediate hospitalization, bed rest, and surgical fixation is indicated. Radiographs are mandatory in these children also to exclude tumors, bone cysts (which may present with pathologic fractures after activities), and underlying osteochondromas, which may well cause mechanical symptoms similar to bursitis.
J. **Fractures and dislocations**
  1. **Mechanism**
    a. Rarely occur in contact sports.
    b. More common in high-energy motor vehicle, skiing or equestrian sports.
    c. Typically severe, direct blows.
  2. **Diagnosis**
    a. Localized tenderness with direct pressure or pelvic compression.
    b. Radiographs are mandatory.
    c. Minimal linear fractures may lead to exsanguination. Must be treated aggressively in hospital.
    d. Frequent associated visceral injuries and urinary tract injuries.
  3. **Dislocations**
    a. **Anterior**
        i. Occur with direct blow with hips abducted.

    ii. Prominence in anterior pelvis with hip lying in abduction.

    iii. Frequent associated femoral nerve injury.

    iv. Rare arterial injury.

    v. Risk of avascular necrosis.

      (a) Risk increases with length of time prior to reduction.

  b. **Posterior**

    i. Usually follows direct blow to knee with hip and knee flexed.

    ii. Hip adducted with palpable femoral head in buttocks.

    iii. Often posterior acetabular hip fracture associated.

    iv. Mandatory in any hip dislocation to obtain x-rays of entire femur as well as pelvis to exclude associated high energy injuries.

III. **Summary.** In summary, the best treatment for pelvic and thigh injuries is prevention. An emphasis on adequate conditioning and adequate stretching before participation will prevent many of the injuries to this region. Gentle, protected rehabilitation is vital after adequate assessment of bony and muscular involvement is completed.

# Chapter 40: Knee Injuries

## W. MICHAEL WALSH, MD

I. **Physical Examination**

  A. **Observation and measurement**

    1. **Standing**

      a. **Alignment** of lower extremities: View patient from front, side, and back. Look for:

        i. **Angular and rotational deformities**—excessive valgus; varus; recurvatum; flexion contracture; femoral or tibial torsion.

        ii. **Foot alignment and mechanics**—excessive cavus or pes planus. Heels should invert and arches increase on toe rising.

        iii. **Leg length inequality**—best judged by pelvic levelness on standing.

      b. **Other observations**

        i. **Difference in size** of legs—atrophy of one limb vs. hypertrophy of the opposite limb.

        ii. **Popliteal masses**—may be seen better in prone position.

    2. **Sitting**

      a. **Patellar position**—with knees flexed 90°, look from side to judge high or low position. Anterior patellar surface will normally face wall in front of patient sitting with legs over side of exam table. View from front to judge lateral posture. Patella should appear centered in soft tissue outline of knee.

      b. **Osgood-Schlatter's** changes—enlarged and/or tender tibial tuberosity.

      c. **Vastus medialis obliquus (VMO)/vastus lateralis (VL) relationship**—knees held actively at 45° of flexion. Distal one-third of vastus medialis normally should present as substantial muscle from adductor tubercle inserting into upper one-third to one-half of medial patella. Dysplastic VMO appears as hollow in this normal muscular location (Fig. 1). Also observe for apparent hypertrophy of vastus lateralis.

      d. **Patellar tracking**—observe on active flexion and extension. Watch for excessive displacement of patella.

    3. **Lying**

      a. **Supine**

        i. **Range of motion**—both active and passive. Compare injured with uninjured side.

        ii. **Muscle bulk**—thigh and calf. Can measure circumferences, but simple observation may be just as helpful.

        iii. **Quadriceps (Q) angle**—with quadriceps **contracted,** angle between the line from anterior superior iliac spine to midpoint of patella, and the line from midpoint of patella to tibial tuberosity (Fig. 2). Normal in males is 10° or less; in females, 15° or less.

        iv. Hamstring and heelcord tightness—see Chapter 29.

      b. **Prone**

        i. **Range of motion**—lack of full knee flexion may show quadriceps tightness.

        ii. **Popliteal masses**—compare contours with those of opposite knee.

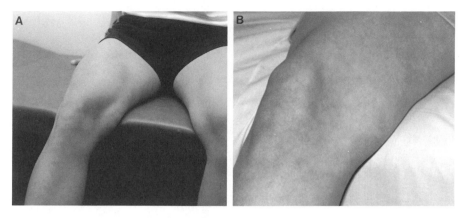

**FIGURE 1.** *Vastus medialis obliquus (VMO) muscle. A,* With patient holding knee at 45° of flexion, normal VMO bulk is seen. *B,* Patient with marked VMO dysplasia. This is probably most important predisposition to all extensor mechanism syndromes.

4. **Walking/running**
    a. **Mechanics of gait**—Stance and swing phase from side to side is even. Look for limp, other asymmetry, excessive limb rotation, limb malalignment.
    b. **Patellofemoral tracking**—observe patella closely from front view.
B. **Palpation**
    1. **Joint effusion**—with knee extended, milk fluid from suprapatellar pouch and palpate along medial and lateral sides of patella. Try to distinguish intra-articular effusion that can be moved about from extra-articular swelling that feels more like thick, soft tissues and is not movable.
    2. **Tenderness**—significant areas of tenderness (Fig. 3) include:
        a. **Menisci**—medial and lateral joint lines.
        b. **Ligament attachments**—medial femoral epicondyle, adductor tubercle, lateral femoral epicondyle, proximal medial tibia.

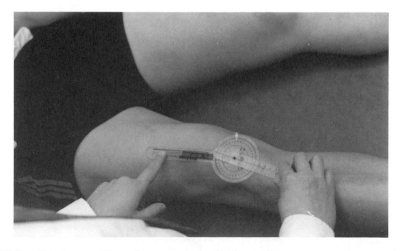

**FIGURE 2.** *Quadriceps (Q) angle measurement.* With quadriceps contracted, proximal arm of goniometer is directed toward anterior superior iliac spine, pivot point of goniometer is placed over center of patella, and distal arm of goniometer is placed on tibial tuberosity. Normal in males up to 10°, females 15°.

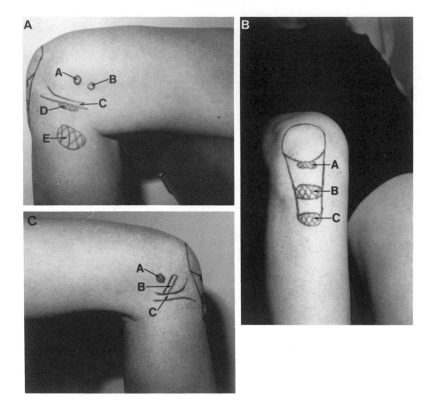

**FIGURE 3.** *Topographical anatomy of knee. A,* shows medial aspect, with medial epicondyle (A), adductor tubercle (B), medial joint line (C), tibial collateral ligament bursa (D), pes anserinus bursa (E). *B,* Shows anterior aspect, with areas of tenderness in patellar tendonitis (A), deep infrapatellar bursitis (B), Osgood-Schlatter's disease (C). *C,* Shows lateral aspect, with iliotibial band friction area (A), popliteus tendon (B), lateral joint line (C).

    c. **Tendons**—patellar tendon, quadriceps tendon, popliteus tendon, hamstrings.

    d. **Bursae**—prepatellar, pes anserinus, tibial collateral ligament, deep infrapatellar.

    e. **Other**—patellar facets, extensor retinaculum.

  3. **Crepitation**

    a. **During range of motion**—from any rough joint surface (especially patello-femoral joint), fractures, or soft tissue thickness.

    b. **Patellofemoral compression**—longitudinal and/or transverse compression of patella against femur (Fig. 4). Feel for crepitation or ask about elicited pain.

  4. **Muscle tone**—overall turgor of muscle tissue. May be decreased early after injury, even if bulk still measures normal.

C. **Specific tests—perform all tests on uninjured knee first to establish "normal" for that patient.**

  1. **Ligaments**

    a. **Medial**

      i. **Abduction stress test at 30° and 0°** (Fig. 5): Patient is supine and relaxed, thigh supported on table. Examiner applies valgus force at foot, while using other hand as fulcrum along lateral side of joint. Watch and feel for medial joint line opening. Perform first with knee flexed 30°, then with maximum possible extension or hyperextension.

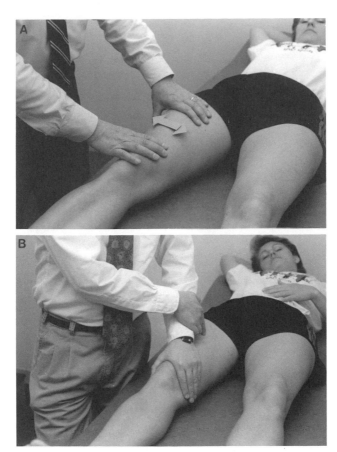

**FIGURE 4.** *Patellofemoral compression. A,* Compression of patella in transverse direction. Check for crepitation and/or tenderness. *B,* Longitudinal compression of patellofemoral joint. Trap patella distally with hand, then ask patient to maximally contract quadriceps. Check for crepitation and/or tenderness.

ii. **Anterior drawer test with external rotation of tibia** (Fig. 6): Patient is supine and relaxed, hip flexed to 45° and knee to 90°. Externally rotate foot 30°, then pin foot to table with examiner's thigh. Grasp proximal tibia with both hands and pull toward examiner. Positive test is excessive anterior rotation of medial tibial condyle.

b. **Lateral**

i. **Adduction stress test at 30° and 0°** (Fig. 7): Patient is in same position as for abduction stress test (C.1.a.i., above). Reverse hand position so that one hand applies varus stress, while opposite hand acts as fulcrum along medial side of joint. Watch and feel for lateral joint line opening. Perform at 30° of flexion and then at full possible extension or hyperextension.

ii. **External rotation recurvatum test** (Fig. 8): Patient is supine and relaxed. Lift entire lower extremity by first toe. Observe for excessive recurvatum and external rotation of proximal tibia (tibial tuberosity) and apparent varus deformity of knee. Indicates posterolateral corner injury.

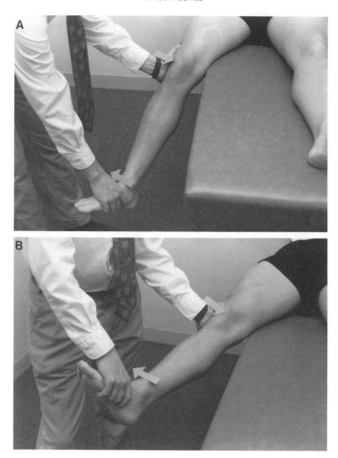

**FIGURE 5.** *Abduction stress test. A,* Test done at 30° of flexion for medial ligament injury. *B,* Test done in full extension for associated acute posterior cruciate injury.

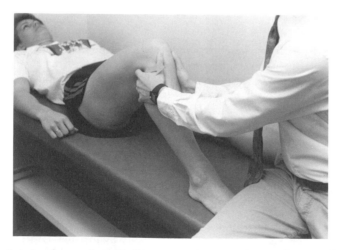

**FIGURE 6.** *Anterior drawer sign with tibia in neutral rotation.* Anterior force applied to proximal tibia while index fingers ensure that hamstrings are relaxed. May also be done with external rotation and internal rotation of foot and tibia.

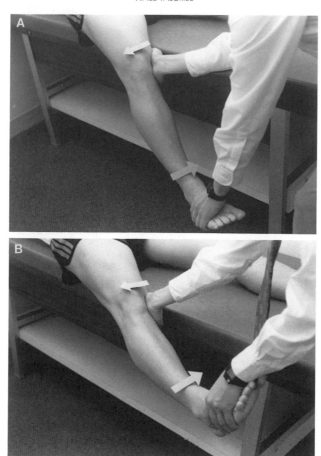

**FIGURE 7.** *Adduction stress test for lateral compartment injury. A,* shows test done at 30° of flexion for lateral compartment rupture. Most knees will have mild instability with this test normally. *B,* Test done in full extension for acute posterior cruciate ligament injury associated with lateral compartment injury.

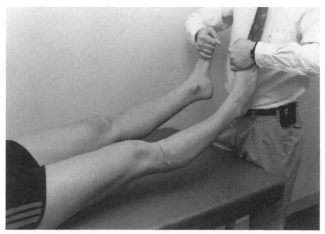

**FIGURE 8.** *External rotation recurvatum test.* Both lower limbs are lifted by great toes. Positive test is excessive recurvatum, external tibial rotation proximally, and development of apparent varus at knee. Indicates posterolateral corner injury.

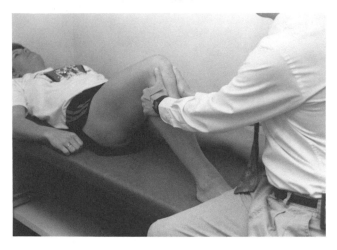

**FIGURE 9.**  *Posterior drawer sign.* Same position as for anterior drawer sign, but force on proximal tibia is posterior instead of anterior.

          iii. **Posterolateral drawer test** (Fig. 9): Same position as for anterior drawer test with external rotation of tibia (C.1.a.ii., above). Examiner's hands push posteriorly on proximal tibia. Positive test is excessive posterior rotation of lateral tibial condyle.

          iv. **Reverse pivot shift test:** See pivot shift test (C.1.c.iii., below). Performed with tibia in external rotation rather than internal rotation. With knee flexed 90°, lateral tibial condyle is subluxed posteriorly. With further knee extension, tibia reduces with detectable "clunk."

    c. **Anterior cruciate ligament (ACL)**

          i. **Lachman test** (Fig. 10): Patient is supine and relaxed. Examiner grasps distal femur with one hand, while other hand grasps proximal tibia. Knee flexed to approximately 15°–20°. Apply anterior force to proximal tibia. Positive test is excessive anterior translation of tibia beneath femur and lack of firm end-point.

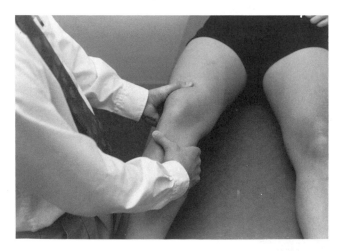

**FIGURE 10.**  *Lachman test.* Distal femur is stabilized while proximal tibia is pulled anteriorly. Positive test is increased anterior translation of proximal tibia beneath distal femur.

ii. **Anterior drawer test in neutral rotation** (see Fig. 5). Same position as for anterior drawer with external rotation of tibia (C.1.a.ii., above), except that foot and tibia are in neutral rotation. Anterior pull is applied to proximal tibia. Positive test is anterior translation of both tibial condyles from beneath femur.

NOTE: This *test is influenced by structures other than the anterior cruciate ligament. DO NOT rely on this test for diagnosis of ACL tear.*

iii. **Pivot shift test, jerk test** (Fig. 11): Patient is supine and relaxed. Begin with knee fully extended (pivot shift) or flexed to 90° (jerk test). Foot and tibia internally rotated. Valgus applied at knee. Knee progressively flexed (pivot shift) or extended (jerk test). At approximately 30°, watch and feel for anterior subluxation of lateral tibial condyle. Tibia suddenly reduces with further flexion (pivot shift) or extension (jerk test).

d. **Posterior cruciate ligament (PCL)**

i. **Posterior drawer test** (Fig. 9): Same position as for anterior drawer test in neutral rotation (C.1.c.ii., above). Posterior force is applied to proximal tibia. Positive test is straight posterior displacement of both tibial condyles.

CAUTION: *Make sure of neutral position as starting point. Compare position of tibia relative to femur with normal knee. It is easy to start from posteriorly displaced position and interpret reduction to neutral as positive <u>anterior</u> drawer sign rather than starting at neutral and interpreting as positive <u>posterior</u> drawer sign.*

ii. **Gravity or sag test** (Fig. 12): Patient is supine and relaxed. Flex hips to 45° and knees to 90° with feet flat on table. With quadriceps relaxed, observe from lateral side for posterior displacement of one tibial tuberosity compared to the other. Then flex hips to 90° and support both legs by ankles and feet. With quadriceps relaxed, observe for posterior displacement of one tibial tuberosity compared to the other.

iii. **Abduction or adduction stress test at 0°**—as described for abduction and adduction stress tests at 30° and 0° (C.1.a.i. and C.1.b.i., above). Positive test in full extension in acute case is often due to posterior cruciate ligament rupture.

2. **Menisci**

a. **McMurray's test** (Fig. 13): Patient is supine and relaxed. Flex knee maximally with external tibial rotation (medial meniscus) or internal tibial rotation (lateral meniscus). While maintaining rotation, bring knee into full extension. Positive test is painful pop occurring over medial joint line (medial meniscus) or lateral joint line (lateral meniscus).

b. **Apley's compression test** (Fig. 14): Patient is in prone position. Knee flexed to 90° with external tibial rotation (medial meniscus) or internal tibial rotation (lateral meniscus). Apply axial compression to tibia while flexing and extending knee. Positive test is painful pop over medial joint line (medial meniscus) or lateral joint line (lateral meniscus).

3. **Patella**

a. **Hypermobility/apprehension test** (Fig. 15): Patient is supine and relaxed. Examiner sits on edge of table with patient's knee flexed approximately 30°–45° across examiner's thigh. With quadriceps relaxed, examiner uses both thumbs to forcefully displace patella over lateral femoral condyle. Positive test is increased lateral mobility of patella compared to opposite knee or other patients. More important is discomfort or extreme apprehension that patella is going to dislocate due to lateral displacement.

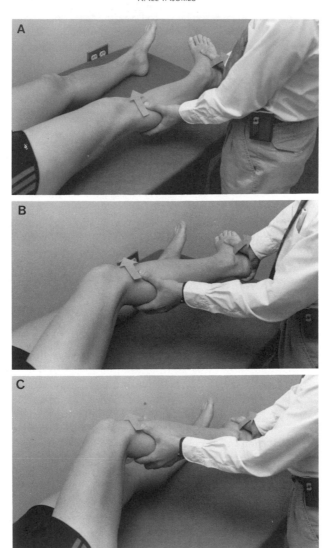

**FIGURE 11.** *Pivot shift/jerk test. A,* Starting position for pivot shift test. Foot internally rotated and pulled somewhat laterally, creating valgus of knee. Anterior force applied at fibular head. *B,* Position at which anterior subluxation of lateral tibial condyle is seen in positive test. *C,* Ending position for pivot shift test in which reduction of proximal tibia takes place. Jerk test would be reverse of pivot shift, starting at 90° of flexion and ending in full extension.

       b. **Plica tests** (Fig. 16): Patient is supine and relaxed. With tibia internally rotated, examiner passively flexes and extends knee from 30°–100° of flexion. Examining fingers laid along medial patellofemoral joint may feel tender pop of a pathologic plica.

III. **Knee Ligament Injuries**

    A. **Medial ligaments**

      1. **Description:** Injury to medial (tibial) collateral ligament and/or medial capsular ligament.

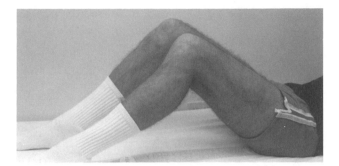

**FIGURE 12.** *Posterior cruciate ligament rupture.* Left knee shows positive gravity test with posterior sag of left tibia.

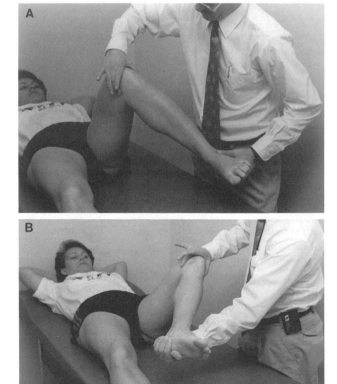

**FIGURE 13.** *McMurray test.* A, Position for lateral meniscus. With foot in internal rotation, knee is brought from full flexion to extension while fingers palpate lateral joint line. *B,* Position for medial meniscus. With external tibial rotation, knee is brought from full flexion to extension while fingers palpate medial joint line.

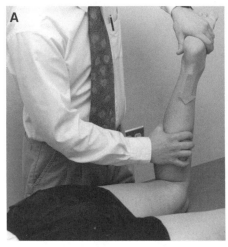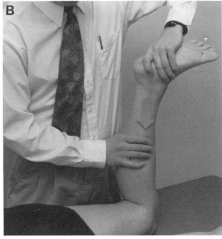

**FIGURE 14.** *Apley compression test. A,* Position for medial meniscus. With pressure on sole of foot, tibia is externally rotated while knee is flexed and extended. *B,* For lateral meniscus, foot is internally rotated while knee is flexed and extended.

2. **Mechanism of injury:** Valgus force applied to knee with external tibial rotation. May be noncontact twist or a blow to lateral side of joint.
3. **History**
   a. Typical mechanism as described above.
   b. Initial pain on medial side of knee.
   c. If complete tear, complaints of knee giving way into valgus.
4. **Examination:** Positive abduction stress test at 30° flexion. Compare with opposite knee. If posterior cruciate ligament is intact, will be stable in fullest possible extension or hyperextension. Frequently, but not always, will be a positive anterior drawer sign with tibia in external rotation. Medial tibial condyle rotates anteriorly.
5. **X-rays:** Abduction stress film may be used to distinguish ligament injury from epiphyseal fracture in skeletally immature. Fracture opens at growth plate. Ligament tear opens at joint line. Do in 20°–30° of flexion.
6. **Differential diagnosis**
   a. In the young, epiphyseal fracture of distal femur or proximal tibia.
   b. Patellar dislocation (may be associated with medial ligament tear).
   c. Medial meniscus tear (may be associated with medial ligament tear).
7. **Treatment**
   a. Grades I and II sprain: PRICES (see Chapter 30), crutches, rehabilitation.
   b. Grade III sprain (complete ligament tear)
      i. Surgery, especially with other associated injuries.
      ii. Immobilization has been shown to be effective treatment in **isolated** medial ligament tear.
      iii. Mild instability may be treated by PRICES and functional rehabilitation.

B. **Lateral ligaments**
   1. **Description**
      a. Sprain or tear of lateral (fibular) collateral ligament and/or lateral capsular ligament.

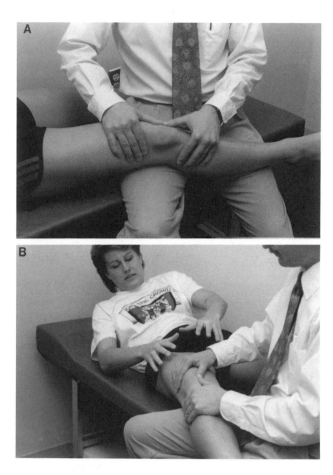

**FIGURE 15.** *Patellar hypermobility/apprehension test.* A, With knee flexed across examiner's thigh, patella is firmly displaced over lateral edge of femoral trochlea, checking for hypermobility. B, Extreme apprehension is created as patient senses impending dislocation or subluxation of patella.

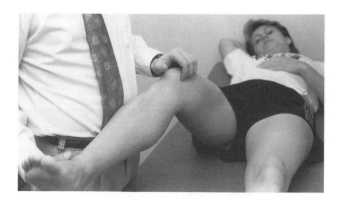

**FIGURE 16.** *Palpation for plica.* With tibia internally rotated, knee is passively flexed and extended. Fingers along medial patellofemoral joint feel for tender pop of pathologic synovial plica.

        b. May be associated injuries to popliteus tendon, iliotibial band, peroneal nerve.

  2. **Mechanism of injury**

        a. Varus or twisting injury.

        b. May be contact or noncontact.

        c. Posterolateral ligaments often injured by hyperextension mechanism, frequently with blow to anteromedial tibia.

  3. **History**

        a. Typical mechanism, as above.

        b. Pain is present over the lateral ligament complex.

        c. Giving way of the knee on twisting, cutting, or pivoting.

        d. In chronic case, posterolateral corner injury gives a feeling of giving way into hyperextension when standing, walking, or running backwards.

  4. **Examination**

        a. Compare with opposite knee.

        b. In acute case, **may** be increased adduction stress test at 30° flexion and positive posterolateral drawer sign.

        c. In chronic case, shows positive reverse pivot shift test and external rotation recurvatum test.

        d. External rotation recurvatum may also be apparent on standing, giving an increased varus appearance to the knee.

  5. **X-rays**

        a. Lateral capsular sign shows avulsion of midportion of lateral capsular ligament with small fragment of proximal lateral tibia. Associated with a high incidence of anterior cruciate tear and indicates anterolateral instability.

        b. Arcuate sign shows avulsion of proximal fibula with posterolateral ligament complex. Indicates posterolateral instability.

  6. **Differential diagnosis**

        a. Chronic posterolateral injury may be confused with medial compartment arthritis due to progressive varus appearance. Also difficult to differentiate from posterior cruciate injury.

        b. Acute lateral ligament injury may be confused with lateral meniscus tear.

        c. Injury to middle third of lateral capsular ligament, as shown by lateral capsular sign on x-ray, usually associated with anterior cruciate ligament injury.

  7. **Treatment**

        a. Grade I and II: PRICES (see Chapter 30), crutches, rehabilitation.

        b. Grade III sprain (complete ligament tear)

            i. Surgical repair is usually preferable.

           ii. Immobilization is not really useful by itself.

          iii. Mild instability may be treated by PRICES and functional rehabilitation.

C. **Anterior cruciate ligament (ACL)**

  1. **Description**

        a. Tear of part or all of two major bundles (posterolateral, anteromedial) of anterior cruciate ligament.

        b. May be associated with tears of the middle one-third of lateral capsular ligament.

        c. Anterior cruciate ligament is torn from the femur or tibia, or torn in its midportion.

        d. May avulse the tibial spine in young patients.

  2. **Mechanism of injury**

        a. May be multiple mechanisms of ACL injury.

    b. Hyperextension, varus/internal rotation, and extremes of valgus and external rotation are all possible causes.

3. **History**
   a. Usually a loud pop occurs.
   b. May be followed by autonomic symptoms of dizziness, sweating, faintness, slight nausea.
   c. Large swelling usually occurs within the first 2 hours following acute injury (hemarthrosis). Conversely, majority of acute hemarthroses (85%+) will be anterior cruciate tears.
   d. In chronic cases, complaints of giving way on twisting, pivoting, cutting.

4. **Examination**
   a. **Acute**
      i. Finding of a large hemarthrosis
      ii. Positive Lachman test.
   b. **Chronic**
      i. Positive Lachman test
      ii. Positive pivot shift or jerk test
      iii. **Perhaps** positive anterior drawer sign, but not reliable. DO NOT rely on anterior drawer sign.

5. **X-rays**
   a. Lateral capsular sign (see above).
   b. Avulsion of tibial spine may be seen in young patients.
   c. MRI becoming more useful in diagnosis as techniques improve.

6. **Differential diagnosis**
   a. Acute: differentiate from other causes of hemarthrosis (e.g., osteochondral fracture, peripheral meniscus tear, patellar dislocation).
   b. Chronic: differentiate from other types of ligamentous laxity and/or meniscal tears.

7. **Treatment**
   a. **Acute**
      i. Most important to delineate degree of injury.
      ii. May require examination under anesthesia and arthroscopy.
      iii. For mild laxity with firm end-point (partial ACL injury), may treat with PRICES, functional rehabilitation, and protective bracing.
   b. **Chronic**
      i. May attempt functional stabilization through rehabilitation and bracing.
      ii. Often requires surgical reconstruction.

D. **Posterior cruciate ligament (PCL)**
   1. **Description:** tear of part or all of two major bundles of the posterior cruciate ligament (posteromedial and anterolateral).
   2. **Mechanism of injury**
      a. Valgus/varus in full extension
      b. Rarely a severe twist
      c. Direct blow to anterior proximal tibia, as in a fall on artificial turf or other hard playing surface.
   3. **History**
      a. Usually less swelling than with anterior cruciate ligament.
      b. Otherwise, in acute stage, nothing particularly distinguishing.
      c. Chronically, a feeling of femur sliding anteriorly off the tibia, especially when rapidly decelerating or descending slopes or stairs.
   4. **Examination**
      a. **Acute**

i. If produced by varus or valgus mechanism, may find abduction or adduction stress test positive in full extension.
ii. If produced by blow to anterior tibia, posterior drawer sign may be positive.
   b. **Chronic:** rely on posterior drawer sign and gravity test (see C.1.d.i. and C.1.d.ii., above)
5. **X-rays**
   a. Cross-table lateral view may show sag of tibia compared to opposite side.
   b. May accentuate by doing posterior drawer sign while taking cross-table lateral view.
   c. May see bony avulsion with tibial attachment of the posterior cruciate ligament.
   d. MRI shows posterior cruciate well and may help in difficult case.
6. **Differential diagnosis**
   a. Most difficult is distinguishing posterior cruciate injury from posterolateral corner injury (see above).
   b. Posterior drawer sign and posterolateral drawer sign may appear the same.
   c. Both injuries may exist in the same knee.
7. **Treatment**
   a. **Acute**
      i. It is most important to delineate degree of injury.
      ii. May require examination under anesthesia and arthroscopy.
      iii. For mild laxity (partial PCL tear), may treat with PRICES, function rehabilitation, and protective bracing.
      iv. For moderate or severe laxity, surgical repair/reconstruction is usually required.
   b. **Chronic**
      i. May attempt functional stabilization through rehabilitation and bracing.
      ii. Often requires surgical reconstruction.

IV. **Meniscal Injuries**

A. **Medial meniscus**
   1. **Description**
      a. Disruption of medial semilunar cartilage of the knee.
      b. May be from single traumatic episode, degenerative processes, or a combination.
      c. Tears take different forms, such as radial, longitudinal, horizontal, etc.
      d. Most important surgical factor is whether tear is peripheral, in vascular zone, or more central, in nonvascular zone.
   2. **Mechanism of injury**
      a. Twisting or squatting
      b. May be in association with ligament injuries due to any of their precipitating mechanisms.
   3. **History**
      a. Usually mild swelling and joint line pain.
      b. In acute setting, important to know whether knee lacked full extension from the time of injury (locked knee from displaced fragment), or knee lacked full extension the next day (pseudolocking from hamstring spasm).
      c. In chronic setting, recurrent locking is typical.
      d. Otherwise, symptoms may include slipping or catching over the joint line.
   4. **Examination**
      a. Positive McMurray's test.

    b. Positive Apley's test.

    c. Results of these tests may vary considerably from one examination session to the next.

    d. Joint line tenderness may be present, as may mild effusion.

    e. Chronically, there is commonly quadriceps atrophy.

    f. With a peripheral meniscus detachment and a positive anterior drawer test, a loud "clunk" may be elicited as the meniscus displaces during anterior drawer testing.

5. **X-rays**

    a. Plain films usually normal, unless the meniscal tear has been present for a significant time.

    b. After that time, they may show joint line spurring.

    c. Arthrograms were commonly done in the past but are now being supplanted by magnetic resonance imaging (MRI), which is noninvasive and has at least the same diagnostic accuracy, if not better.

6. **Differential diagnosis**

    a. Ligamentous injury, causing pain in the same area.

    b. Patellar problems, which might cause anteromedial joint pain that is confused with pain from a medial meniscus injury.

    c. Pathologic synovial plicas, which can cause pain, swelling, catching and popping, also may be confused with medial meniscus injuries.

    d. Loose bodies may cause locking.

    e. Medial compartment arthritis may cause medial joint pain similar to that from torn meniscus.

7. **Treatment**

    a. A suspected meniscus tear with no ligamentous instability may be managed initially through symptomatic treatment and functional rehabilitation.

    b. If no improvement, or if time constraints do not allow initial conservative treatment, diagnostic arthroscopy is the most certain way of diagnosing and treating meniscal injury.

    c. Most meniscal tears still require arthroscopic partial meniscectomy.

    d. Vertical tears in the peripheral vascular zone are now routinely treated by meniscal repair rather than removal of the meniscus.

    e. An MRI may help decide whether to proceed with surgical treatment or continue with nonsurgical care.

B. **Lateral meniscus**

1. **Description**

    a. Disruption of lateral semilunar cartilage of the knee.

    b. May be from single traumatic episode, degenerative processes, or a combination.

    c. With lateral meniscus injury, may also encounter injuries of congenital discoid meniscus.

    d. Tears take different forms, such as radial, longitudinal, horizontal, etc.

    e. Most important surgical factor is whether tear is peripheral, in vascular zone, or more central, in nonvascular zone.

2. **Mechanism of injury** is the same as for medial meniscus injury.

3. **History**

    a. Same as for medial meniscus injury, though often more pain and fewer mechanical symptoms than with medial meniscus tears.

    b. May give history of cystic lesion directly over lateral joint line.

4. **Examination**

    a. Is much the same as for medial meniscus injury.

    b. May palpate localized puffiness or distinct cystic lesion over lateral joint line.

5. **X-rays**
   a. Same findings as for medial meniscus injury.
   b. In child with congenital discoid lateral meniscus, may see **widening** of lateral joint space.
6. **Differential diagnosis**
   a. Lateral ligamentous injury
   b. Loose bodies
   c. Degenerative arthritis of the lateral compartment
   d. Popliteus tendonitis
   e. Iliotibial band friction syndrome.
7. **Treatment**
   a. Same as for medial meniscus injury.
   b. Special consideration in youngsters with lateral discoid meniscus is whether to remove or repair, how much meniscus to remove, etc.

V. **Extensor Mechanism Problems**

   A. **Instability syndromes**
      1. **Dislocation**
         a. **Description:** complete, usually lateral displacement of patella from femoral trochlea that persists until reduced, usually by extending knee.
         b. **Mechanism of injury:** valgus and/or twisting with strong quadriceps contraction.
         c. **Predisposing factors:** all of the stigmata indicating congenital **extensor mechanism malalignment,** including vastus medialis obliquus dysplasia, vastus lateralis hypertrophy, high and lateral patellar posture, increased Q-angle, bony deformity, etc. Usually more easily seen in acute case on opposite uninjured side.
         d. **History**
            i. May or may not be previous symptoms of instability or patellofemoral pain.
            ii. Feeling of patellar dislocation when injury occurred.
            iii. Report of lying on ground with knee flexed.
            iv. Report of "something coming out" medially, which usually represents uncovered medial femoral condyle rather than the patella going medially.
            v. Report of something "going back into place" when knee extended.
            vi. Swelling that occurs within the first 2 hours.
         e. **Examination** will depend on whether patella is still dislocated or has been reduced.
            i. Predisposing physical findings seen on opposite knee. If patella is still dislocated, will be located over lateral femoral condyle with prominence of uncovered medial femoral condyle.
            ii. If patella has been reduced, there may be large hemarthrosis with hypermobilty and marked apprehension on hypermobility testing.
            iii. May also find associated medial ligamentous instability.
         f. **X-ray studies**
            i. Unusual to find patella still dislocated on x-ray, since positioning on x-ray table usually reduces dislocation.
            ii. Infrapatellar view may show avulsion of medial edge of patella.
            iii. Large osteochondral fracture may be visible.
            iv. Important to take infrapatellar view with knee flexed only 30°–45°, rather than traditional "sunrise" or "skyline" view with knee flexed beyond 90°.
            v. Patella alta can be measured objectively on lateral view.

g. **Differential diagnosis**
   i. In acute case, differentiate from ligamentous tears.
   ii. In chronic recurrent case, distinguish from meniscus disorders.
h. **Treatment**
   i. If patella is still dislocated, knee extension and gentle pressure along lateral patellar edge will usually reduce it easily and without anesthesia.
   ii. Aspiration may be indicated for comfort or to search for fat in blood secondary to osteochondral fracture.
   iii. In first-time dislocation, immobilize in full extension with foam pad over vastus medialis obliquus (VMO) and lateral buttress holding patella medially.
   iv. Immobilize acute case for 6 weeks, followed by extensive rehabilitation program and functional patellar bracing.
   v. An obvious disruption of VMO insertion into medial patellar edge does best with early surgical repair.
   vi. If recurrent dislocation, treat symptomatically with temporary immobilization and crutches, followed by functional rehabilitation and bracing.

2. **Subluxation**
   a. **Description**
      i. Transient partial displacement of patella from femoral trochlea.
      ii. May occur acutely, as in patellar dislocation, or may be intermittent.
      iii. There is spontaneous reduction of displacement.
   b. **Mechanism of injury**
      i. Same as for patellar dislocation.
      ii. May occur with less severe force or in normal everyday activity.
   c. **Predisposing factors:** same as for patellar dislocation.
   d. **History**
      i. May or may not be past history of complete dislocation or patellofemoral pain.
      ii. Feeling of slipping when cutting, twisting, or pivoting.
      iii. Mild recurrent swelling.
   e. **Examination**
      i. Predisposing physical findings seen in both knees, but may be more obvious on asymptomatic side, especially if there has been an acute injury on symptomatic side.
      ii. Mild effusion.
      iii. Positive hypermobility and apprehension test.
   f. **X-rays**
      i. Infrapatellar view must be done with proper technique and knee flexed only 30°–45°.
      ii. Infrapatellar views may show lateral tilt and/or lateral subluxation.
      iii. X-rays may all be **normal** in appearance.
      iv. Patellofemoral indices (Merchant, Laurin, Brattstrom) show tendency to patellofemoral problems, but do not give specific diagnosis.
   g. **Differential diagnosis:** chronic knee ligament instability, causing giving-way of knee.
   h. **Treatment**
      i. In acute subluxation, use temporary symptomatic immobilization, followed by functional rehabilitation and bracing of the patella.
      ii. If no acute episode, treat with functional rehabilitation, bracing, and nonsteroidal anti-inflammatory medication.

         iii. If patient is disabled by subluxation, may require arthroscopic lateral release or open extensor mechanism reconstruction.

B. **Painful syndromes**
  1. **Patellofemoral pain syndrome (PFPS)**
    a. **Description**
      i. Any of a variety of syndromes characterized by anterior knee pain as major symptom.
      ii. An **imprecise** term in which pain is not explained by a more readily definable cause, such as those discussed below.
      iii. Often referred to as "chondromalacia patella," a term that should be reserved for articular cartilage damage actually observed.
    b. **Mechanism of injury**
      i. May result from extensor mechanism malalignment, with or without an instability syndrome.
      ii. May occur as overuse injury with extreme and/or repetitive loading of patellofemoral joint (e.g., knee flexion, running, jumping, etc.).
    c. **Predisposing factors:** same as for instability syndromes, above.
    d. **History**
      i. Anterior knee pain, often worse with sitting in tight space with knee flexed.
      ii. Pain worse on descending stairs or slopes.
      iii. Mild swelling (may be bilateral).
      iv. May be snapping and popping around patella.
    e. **Examination**
      i. Findings predisposing to extensor mechanism problems seen in both legs.
      ii. Pain on patellofemoral compression test.
      iii. Crepitation about patella on range of motion.
      iv. May be mild effusion.
      v. Tenderness to palpation around patella.
      vi. Foot malalignment or leg length inequality may aggravate symptoms.
    f. **X-rays**
      i. Same as for subluxation.
      ii. **May be normal.**
    g. **Differential diagnosis**
      i. In preadolescent and young adolescent, consider referred pain from hip disorder (e.g., Legg-Calve-Perthes disease, slipped capital femoral epiphysis).
      ii. Osteochondritis dissecans of femur or patella.
      iii. Bone tumor, especially in case of unilateral symptoms.
      iv. In older patient, osteoarthritis or some other inflammatory joint disease.
    h. **Treatment**
      i. Functional rehabilitation program, nonsteroidal anti-inflammatory medication, functional bracing of patella, orthotics for foot malalignment.
      ii. If other treatments unsuccessful, surgical treatment may be considered, either lateral release or extensor mechanism reconstruction.
      iii. Should always look for other more specific cause of anterior knee pain, such as those listed below.
  2. **Patellar tendonitis ("jumper's knee")**
    a. **Description:** Inflammation of patellar tendon, usually at its attachment to inferior pole of patella.

b. **Mechanism of injury**
   i. Usually excessive jumping or bounding activity or other high patello-femoral stress activity.
   ii. Less commonly from running.
c. **Predisposing factors**
   i. Same as for other extensor mechanism disorders.
   ii. Possibly ankle dorsiflexor muscle weakness, perhaps secondary to ankle injury.
d. **History**
   i. Participation in activity typically associated with this problem, such as a jumping sport.
   ii. Complaint of infrapatellar pain, originally after exercise, later during exercise and while at rest.
e. **Examination**
   i. Tenderness present at inferior pole of patella.
   ii. Less commonly, tenderness over body of patellar tendon.
   iii. Other findings of extensor mechanism malalignment.
   iv. Weakness of ankle dorsiflexors.
   v. Hamstring, heelcord, and/or quadriceps muscle tightness.
f. **X-rays**
   i. Occasionally see irregularity at inferior pole of patella.
   ii. May be findings of extensor mechanism malalignment, including patella alta.
   iii. MRI may demonstrate degenerative changes in tendon.
g. **Differential diagnosis**
   i. Usually firm diagnosis not difficult with this entity.
   ii. May consider some other soft tissue lesion of patellar tendon or fat pad, such as a tumor.
   iii. Otherwise, could be any of the other causes of patellofemoral pain.
h. **Treatment**
   i. Rehabilitative exercise program, concentrating on hamstring, heelcord, and quadriceps flexibility, as well as quadriceps strength.
   ii. Eccentric strengthening exercises for ankle dorsiflexors are important.
   iii. Anti-inflammatory medication.
   iv. Ultrasound, utilizing hydrocortisone phonophoresis.
   v. Iontophoresis.
   vi. Questionable benefit from infrapatellar strap.
3. **Synovial plica**
   a. **Description**
      i. Structurally, a remnant of the embryologic walls that divide the knee into medial, lateral, and suprapatellar pouches.
      ii. Appears as a fold of synovium attached to the periphery of the joint and to the underside of quadriceps tendon (suprapatellar plica).
      iii. May also present as a free edge along the medial patellofemoral joint (medial plica), or may be in both locations.
      iv. Rarely seen in other configurations.
      v. Edge protruding into joint may be of various sizes.
   b. **Mechanism of injury**
      i. Overuse with repetitive flexion and extension, e.g., running.
      ii. Direct blow to medial patellofemoral joint, e.g., falling on turf or dashboard injury.

    c. **Predisposing factors**
        i. Congenital presence of plica.
        ii. Other extensor mechanism malalignment predispositions may increase likelihood of symptoms due to plica.
    d. **History**
        i. Overuse or direct trauma.
        ii. Complaints of anterior knee pain.
        iii. Pain over suprapatellar or medial peripatellar regions with long periods of knee flexion, especially when accompanied by distinct snap or pop when knee is extended.
        iv. Painful catching episodes over medial patellofemoral joint.
    e. **Examination**
        i. Often difficult to palpate plica. Best done with passive flexion and extension with tibia held internally rotated. Fingers should lie over medial patellofemoral joint.
        ii. May see other extensor mechanism malalignment stigmata.
        iii. Heelcord tightness and hamstring tightness aggravate significantly.
    f. **X-ray studies:** None is helpful.
    g. **Differential diagnosis**
        i. Other painful patellofemoral conditions.
        ii. Possibly medial meniscus injury or loose body.
        iii. Patients often dismissed as "neurotic" because of lack of findings in face of significant symptoms.
    h. **Treatment**
        i. If inflammatory process in synovium is still reversible:
            (a) May improve with hamstring stretching, heelcord stretching, VMO exercises (if VMO is dysplastic).
            (b) NSAIDs, ice, activity modification.
            (c) Simple external patellar support may help.
            (d) Phonophoresis to plica area may also be beneficial.
        ii. If inflammatory process is not reversible and plica is fibrotic, persistent symptoms require arthroscopic removal of plica. Promises good relief of symptoms and good future function.

4. **Osgood-Schlatter's "disease"**
    a. **Description**
        i. Painful enlargement of tibial tuberosity at patellar tendon insertion.
        ii. Rather than being a "disease," condition is due to mechanical stress and excessive tension on growing tibial tuberosity apophysis.
        iii. Occurs in preadolescence and early adolescence, usually during rapid growth period.
    b. **Mechanism of injury**
        i. Overuse in normal childhood activities, including sports.
        ii. Rarely, acute onset of popping and pain over tibial tuberosity.
    c. **Predisposing factors**
        i. Patella alta
        ii. Other evidence of extensor mechanism malalignment and altered extensor mechanics
        iii. Tight hamstrings, heelcords, quadriceps muscles predispose to symptoms.
    d. **History:** complaints of painful enlargement of tibial tuberosity.
    e. **Examination**
        i. Enlarged, tender tibial tuberosity

      ii. Stigmata of extensor mechanism malalignment, especially patella alta

      iii. Tight hamstrings, heelcords, and quadriceps muscles.

  f. **X-rays**

      i. Enlarged tibial tuberosity

      ii. Irregularity of tibial tuberosity

      iii. Loose ossicle separated from tuberosity

      iv. Patella alta.

  g. **Differential diagnosis**

      i. Other forms of patellar tendinitis

      ii. In acute episode, avulsion fracture of tibial tuberosity

      iii. Tumorous processes of the tibial tuberosity.

  h. **Treatment**

      i. Hamstring stretching, heelcord stretching, and quadriceps stretching exercises

      ii. VMO strengthening exercises

      iii. Activity modification as necessitated by symptoms

      iv. Simple modalities

      v. Local padding.

5. **Quadriceps tendonitis** (including vastus lateralis tendonitis and VMO tendonitis)

  a. **Description**

      i. Inflammation of quadriceps tendon at its insertion into superior edge of patella.

      ii. May involve only vastus lateralis insertion into superolateral pole of patella, or vastus medialis obliquus insertion into superomedial pole of patella.

  b. **Mechanism of injury:** same as for patellar tendonitis (B.2., above).

  c. **Predisposing factors:** extensor mechanism malalignment.

  d. **History**

      i. Involvement in activity consistent with causing this entity.

      ii. Complaints of suprapatellar pain.

  e. **Examination**

      i. Tenderness at superior pole of patella.

      ii. May be over central rectus femoris insertion, superolateral vastus lateralis insertion, or superomedial vastus medialis obliquus insertion.

      iii. Other findings of extensor mechanism malalignment.

      iv. Hamstring, heelcord, and quadriceps muscle tightness.

  f. **X-rays:** Usually there are no findings on x-ray studies.

  g. **Differential diagnosis**

      i. Suprapatellar pain from synovial plica

      ii. Bone tumor of distal femur.

  h. **Treatment:** same as for patellar tendinitis (B.2., above).

## VI. **Miscellaneous Knee Conditions**

  A. **Bursitis**

    1. **Description**

      a. Inflammation of any of various bursae around the knee, evidenced by swelling and/or pain.

      b. Typically prepatellar bursa, pes anserinus bursa, tibial collateral ligament bursa, deep infrapatellar bursa.

    2. **Mechanism of injury**

      a. Usually overuse

      b. May be secondary to direct blow with bleeding into bursa.

3. **Predisposing factors**
   a. For pes anserinus bursitis, tight hamstrings seem to predispose.
4. **History**
   a. Direct blow
   b. Overuse
   c. Complaints of swelling (if prepatellar bursa)
   d. Compliants of pain in prepatellar region (for prepatellar bursitis), in distal patellar tendon region (for deep infrapatellar bursitis), in proximal medial tibia (for pes anserinus bursitis), or over medial joint line (for tibial collateral ligament bursitis).
5. **Examination**
   a. For prepatellar bursa, look for localized swelling and tenderness.
   b. For others, tenderness over described areas.
6. **X-rays** are not helpful in diagnosis.
7. **Differential diagnosis**
   a. For deep infrapatellar bursitis, other causes of patellar tendon pain.
   b. For tibial collateral ligament bursitis, medial meniscus tear.
   c. For prepatellar bursitis, usually no differntial.
   d. For pes anserinus bursitis, pain from pes anserinus tendons, tumors, other causes of proximal medial tibial pain.
8. **Treatment**
   a. Acute prepatellar bursitis: ice, compression, possible aspiration, padding.
   b. Chronic prepatellar bursitis: NSAIDs, compression, hamstring stretching, ultrasound, possible aspiration and corticosteroid injection.
   c. Pes anserinus bursitis: hamstring stretching, ultrasound, NSAIDs, corticosteroid injection.
   d. Tibial collateral ligament bursitis: injection, both as a diagnostic test as well as treatment.
   e. Deep infrapatellar bursitis: hamstring stretching, possible injection **behind** patellar tendon.

B. **Other tendinitis**
  1. **Description**
     a. Inflammation of any of the other tendinous structures about the knee, typically the semimembranosus, popliteus, or biceps femoris tendons.
     b. Rarely, inflammation of the gastrocnemius tendon.
  2. **Mechanism of injury**
     a. Usually overuse.
     b. Much less commonly, a single episode of strain is the cause.
     c. Popliteus tendonitis is usually a running injury.
  3. **Predisposing factors:** for semimembranosus, pes anserinus, or biceps femoris tendinitis, hamstring tightness predisposes.
  4. **History**
     a. Overuse activity
     b. Occasionally, acute strain
     c. Complaints of pain over the appropriate tendon area
     d. For popliteus tendonitis, lateral knee pain, especially while running downhill.
  5. **Examination**
     a. Tenderness over appropriate tendon
     b. Tight hamstrings
     c. For popliteus tendinitis, painful resisted internal rotation of tibia with knee flexed
     d. For all, initially pain on stretching tendon, later pain on active contraction of tendon.

6. **X-rays:** usually not helpful.
7. **Differential diagnosis**
    a. Hamstring tendinitis occasionally to be differentiated from sciatica.
    b. Semimembranosus tendinitis may be confused with medial meniscus disorders.
    c. For popliteus tendinitis, lateral meniscus injury, iliotibial band friction syndrome.
8. **Treatment**
    a. Usual anti-inflammatory methods
    b. Hamstring stretching exercises
    c. May require corticosteroid injection.

C. **Neuromas**
1. **Description**
    a. Non-neoplastic enlargement of nerve, usually from direct trauma.
    b. Typically involves various portions of saphenous nerve around the knee.
2. **Mechanism of injury**
    a. Direct blow
    b. Previous surgery.
3. **Predisposing factors:** previous surgical incisions.
4. **History**
    a. Direct blow
    b. Previous surgery
    c. Pain, particularly nerve-like quality, i.e., paresthesias, burning, other alterations of sensation.
5. **Examination**
    a. Tenderness over neuroma
    b. Positive Tinel's sign
    c. Objective changes in sensation in appropriate distribution.
6. **X-rays:** not helpful.
7. **Differential diagnosis:** more central sources of nerve compression.
8. **Treatment**
    a. Injection
    b. Surgical excision.

D. **Loose bodies** ("joint mouse," chondral fracture, osteochondral fracture, osteochondritis dissecans).
1. **Description**
    a. Cartilaginous or osteocartilaginous fragments usually free-floating within knee joint (though may be attached to synovium more or less firmly).
2. **Mechanism of injury**
    a. Dislocation of patella (see V.A.1., above).
    b. Other trauma to joint surface.
    c. May be result of preexisting osteochondritis dissecans.
    d. Rarely due to synovial osteochondromatosis.
3. **Predisposing factors**
    a. Predisposition to patellar dislocation (see above).
    b. Preexisting osteochondritis dissecans.
4. **History**
    a. Consistent with previous patellar instability (see above).
    b. Other twisting or direct blow injury.
    c. Locking episodes.
    d. Subcutaneous mass that comes and goes and may be felt in various locations about the knee.

5. **Examination**
   a. Patellar findings (see above).
   b. May feel movable mass, usually around patellofemoral joint, though it may be at anteromedial or anterolateral joint line.
6. **X-rays**
   a. Purely cartilaginous fragments are not visible.
   b. Very small bony loose bodies may be obscured.
   c. Most loose bodies of significance containing bone are visible.
   d. Source (e.g., osteochondritis dissecans) may be seen.
   e. Tomogram, CT scan, or arthrogram may help in delineation.
7. **Differential diagnosis:** meniscal tears as source of locking.
8. **Treatment**
   a. Symptomatic loose bodies require surgical removal, usually arthroscopically.
   b. A few loose bodies may require replacement and internal fixation.
   c. Patellofemoral instability may require treatment.
   d. Osteochondritis dissecans may require other treatment.
   e. Large chondral or osteochondral fracture may require surgical debridement of joint surface and prolonged protected weight-bearing.

E. **Cysts** (popliteal cyst, popliteal ganglion, Baker's cyst, meniscus cyst).
   1. **Description:** fluid-filled lesion about the knee arising usually as an extension of the synovial space, either into a normal bursal structure or into soft tissue surrounding the knee.
   2. **Mechanism of injury:** normally, no specific injury involved.
   3. **Predisposing factors:** none.
   4. **History:** localized swelling in popliteal space or over meniscus.
   5. **Examination:** cystic swelling in medial popliteal space or over mid-joint line, usually lateral joint line.
   6. **X-rays**
      a. Plain films are no help.
      b. Arthrogram may show dye extension into cyst.
      c. MRI very helpful in delineating cysts.
   7. **Differential diagnosis:** other tumorous lesions about the knee.
   8. **Treatment**
      a. May try aspiration and injection with corticosteroid; however, not very likely to give permanent cure.
      b. Surgical excision is usually curative.
      c. **Most important** is to understand that presence of cyst is usually secondary to another process in the knee that leads to excessive synovial fluid, in turn causing the cyst. Most likely: a meniscal tear causing a popliteal cyst, or lateral meniscus tear causing a lateral mensicus cyst. **Underlying disorders must be treated.**

F. **Iliotibial band friction syndrome**
   1. **Description**
      a. Chronic inflammatory process involving soft tissues adjacent to the lateral femoral epicondyle.
      b. Presumably due to chronic "friction" of iliotibial band rubbing over bony prominence of this area.
   2. **Mechanism of injury**
      a. Overuse mechanism
      b. Majority of cases due to running.
   3. **Predisposing factors**
      a. Varus alignment of knee
      b. Running on sloped surfaces.

4. **History**
   a. Lateral knee pain on activity
   b. Occasional popping.
5. **Examination**
   a. Tenderness over lateral femoral epicondyle
   b. Tight iliotibial band
   c. Absence of intra-articular findings.
6. **X-ray:** no help.
7. **Differential diagnosis**
   a. Other causes of lateral knee pain, especially popliteus tendinitis
   b. Lateral meniscus disorders
   c. Lateral patellofemoral joint sources such as vastus lateralis tendinitis.
8. **Treatment**
   a. Iliotibial band stretching exercises
   b. Anti-inflammatory treatment
   c. Ultrasound to lateral femoral epicondyle
   d. Corticosteroid injection
   e. Rarely, surgery to release area of tightness.

# Chapter 41: Ankle and Leg Injuries

DAVID E. BROWN, MD

I. **Physical Examination**

  A. **Inspection:** The goal is to localize the patient's symptoms to a particular anatomic structure. Check for localized swelling, abrasions, ecchymosis, or deformity.

  B. **Palpation:** Carefully locate specific structures that are tender or swollen. Is it bone or soft tissue, localized or diffuse, intra-articular or extra-articular? Gross crepitus indicates a fracture, whereas fine crepitus can be due to tenosynovitis. Check for hypertrophic spurs over the ankle, thickening of the Achilles tendon. Are all tendons in continuity? Are the compartments of the calf tight?

  C. **Ankle range of motion:** Assess the total arc of ankle motion in dorsiflexion, plantarflexion, inversion and eversion. Compare to the opposite side. Marked muscle guarding is usually due to a severe ligament injury, fracture, or sepsis. Determine if active, passive or resisted motion causes pain.

  D. **Neurovascular assessment:** Test both manual muscle strength and sensation. Check the dorsalis pedis and posterior tibialis pulses.

  E. **Specific tests**

   1. **Anterior drawer test:** Use to assess anterior-posterior translation of the ankle. Stabilize the distal tibia and grasp the heel with your dominant hand and apply an anterior force (Fig. 1). Perform this test with the ankle in neutral position and plantarflexion. Compare to the opposite side. Significant excursion indicates laxity of the anterior talofibular ligament. Grinding or clicking during translation may indicate irregularity or degeneration of the articular surfaces.

   2. **Talar tilt:** Position your hands as in the drawer test. Apply an inversion stress to the heel and ankle (Fig. 2). Excessive excursion occurs with injury to the calcaneofibular ligament.

   3. **Thompson squeeze test:** Place the injured player prone with the feet over the end of the table. Squeezing the calf should cause passive plantarflexion of the ankle (Fig. 3). Absence of plantarflexion is due to a completely torn Achilles tendon.

   4. **Syndesmosis squeeze test:** Squeeze the distal fibular shaft toward the tibia (Fig. 4). Localized pain usually indicates a fibular fracture or disruption of either the interosseous membrane or the distal tibiofibular syndesmosis.

   5. **Compartment pressure measurements:** Intracompartmental pressures in all four leg compartments (anterior, lateral, superficial posterior, and deep posterior [Fig. 5]) are determined using either a slit catheter or the solid-state intracompartment catheter (STIC$^R$). Measurements are made at rest. The patient is then exercised until symptoms occur. Pressure measurements are made postexercise until they return to normal. In normal legs, resting pressures are below 12 mm Hg, rise quickly with exercise to levels as high as 80 mm Hg, and return to the resting level within 5 minutes. Values greater than the above are suspicious for a chronic compartment syndrome, with the most important finding being a failure to return to the resting pressure level within 5 minutes after cessation of exercise.

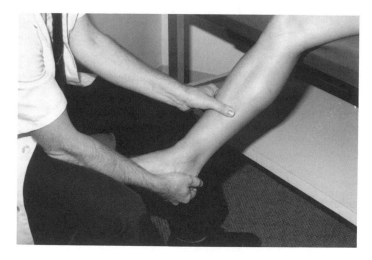

**FIGURE 1.** Anterior drawer test.

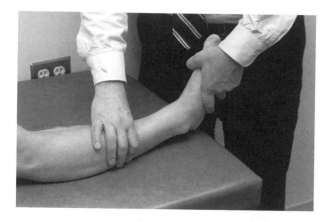

**FIGURE 2.** Talar tilt stress test.

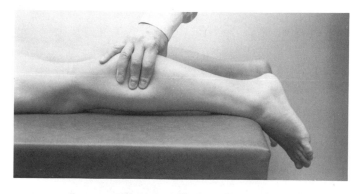

**FIGURE 3.** Normal Thompson test.

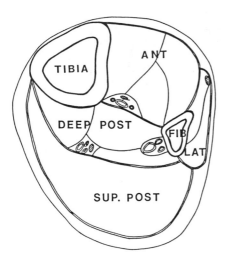

FIGURE 4.   The four compartments of the leg.

F. **Radiographic tests**
   1. **Plain x-rays:** At least an AP and lateral of the injured segment should be obtained. The joint above and below must be visualized. If the ankle is involved, a mortise view is also obtained.
   2. **Stress x-rays:** These allow documentation of the degree of ankle instability.
      a. **Anterior drawer:** A lateral radiograph is made while the examiner manually performs the anterior drawer test. More than 8 mm of anterior displacement of the talus (compared to the unstressed lateral x-ray) indicates an incompetent anterior talofibular ligament (Fig. 6).
      b. **Talar tilt:** A mortise radiograph is made while the examiner performs the talar tilt test. The test is performed on both the injured and the normal ankles. The angle between the tibial plafond and the talar dome is measured. If the injured ankle has a tilt of 25 degrees or is 10 degrees greater than the normal side the calcaneofibular ligament is incompetent.
   3. **Technetium bone scan:** The bone scan will detect stress fractures as early as 1–2 days after the onset of symptoms (plain x-rays commonly are negative for the first 2 weeks of symptoms). Since the scan is also more sensitive than plain x-rays, it can be used for earlier detection of infections or degenerative arthritis.
   4. **Tomograms and computed tomography (CT):** Useful for evaluating the size and position of talar dome osteochondral lesions.

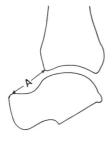
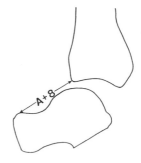

**FIGURE 5.**   Anterior drawer sign is positive if there is greater than 8 mm displacement between the two fixed points.

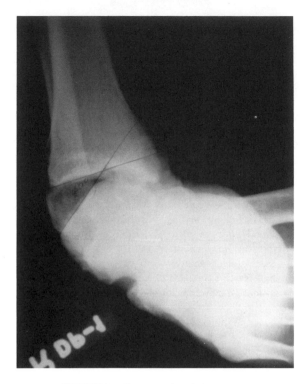

**FIGURE 6.**   Positive talar tilt stress x-ray.

5. **Magnetic resonance imaging (MRI):** Very sensitive in evaluating soft tissue disorders (partial tears of muscle and tendon, periosteal avulsion from the tibia, and soft tissue masses).

## II. Specific Clinical Conditions

### A. Traumatic fractures of the leg and ankle

1. **Tibial shaft fractures**
   a. **Description:** A fracture of the tibia below the tibial plateau and above malleoli. Does not involve the articular surfaces.
   b. **Mechanism of injury:** Results from direct impact or severe rotation on a fixed foot. Usually the result of high energy transmitted to the leg. Most common in skiers and soccer players.
   c. **History:** The athlete recalls a sudden severe pain after the injury, is unable to bear weight, and often "heard the bone crack."
   d. **Examination:** Determine if the fracture is **OPEN!** Even the smallest laceration or puncture site near the fracture should arouse concern for an open fracture. Always note the distal neurovascular status prior to moving or manipulating the patient. Check for deformity, gross bone motion at the suspected fracture site, crepitus, extreme bone tenderness, immediate swelling. Examine the joints above and below the fracture site for additional injuries.
   e. **X-ray studies:** AP, lateral, and obliques of the whole tibia are necessary. If there is any concern for the nearby joints, obtain additional x-ray films.
   f. **Treatment:**
      i. Immediate splinting using air, plaster, or preformed metal splints. Immobilize the joints above and below the injury.

ii. Open fractures require irrigation and debridement in the operating room and antibiotic coverage.

iii. Stable fractures with less than 5 degrees of varus/valgus angulation may be treated in a long leg cast, with partial weight-bearing for 2 to 4 weeks. This is followed by a fracture brace (which allows knee and ankle motion) until the fracture is completely healed.

iv. If there is more than 5 degrees malalignment, fracture reduction is indicated.

v. Comminuted or oblique fractures require longer periods of protection from weight-bearing. Distal fractures with an intact fibula tend to heal in varus and internal rotation. Therefore, the first cast should be applied with the fracture in mild valgus and external rotation. As the fracture heals, it will become more stable, allowing use of a fracture brace.

vi. Intramedullary nailing generally allows earlier weight-bearing and rehabilitation of unstable fractures, but involves higher morbidity. However, intramedullary nailing should be strongly considered for the very unstable fracture.

2. **Fibular shaft fracture (intact tibia and ankle)**
   a. **Description:** Usually appears as a transverse or short oblique fracture in mid-shaft.
   b. **Mechanism of injury:** Direct blow to the side of the calf.
   c. **History:** The athlete can usually walk or even run, but may note moderate pain over the fracture site.
   d. **Examination:** Reveals tenderness and mild crepitus over the shaft of the fibula. The ankle is normal.
   e. **Treatment:** Protection from activities that cause pain. May need crutches for several days to 2 weeks. Rarely requires a cast.

3. **Ankle fractures**
   a. **Description:** Fractures of one or both malleoli, or any spiral fracture of the fibula regardless of its position.
   b. **Mechanism of injury:** Usually involves external rotation of the foot, combined with either pronation or supination.
   c. **History:** The athlete is unable to bear weight on the injured extremity, often heard a "crack," and is in considerable pain.
   d. **Examination:** Reveals tenderness and crepitus over the involved bone. There may be gross instability or deformity of the ankle. **Check the neurovascular status** distally. Determine if the fracture is **OPEN.**
   e. **X-rays:** Confirm the fracture location and displacement. Carefully assess the mortise view. If the distance between the medial malleolus and the medial talus is greater than the distance between the superior talar dome and the tibial plafond, suspect a torn deltoid ligament. Although a widened mortise is most commonly seen with distal fibular fractures, widening may also occur without a fibular fracture or with high fibular fractures.
   f. **Treatment:**
      i. Splint immediately (see tibial fractures).
      ii. Open fractures require urgent, thorough irrigation and debridement in the operating room followed by antibiotic coverage.
      iii. **Nondisplaced fractures** with an intact mortise can be treated with cast immobilization for 4 to 6 weeks followed by a functional brace until completely healed.
      iv. **Displaced fractures** are best treated with anatomic open reduction and internal fixation.

4. **Transchondral talar dome fractures**
   a. **Description:** A fracture of the superior dome of the talus.
   b. **Mechanism of injury:** Inversion or eversion of the ankle.
   c. **Predisposing factors:** Often seen with displaced ankle fractures or ankle ligament instability.
   d. **History:**Usually noted acutely, but may present as chronic pain after an ankle "sprain."
   e. **Examination** There is usually an ankle effusion and tenderness directly over the corner of the talus where the lesion is located. Mild crepitus may be present. Assess for ligament instability.
   f. **X-rays:** AP, lateral, mortise, or plantarflexed mortise may reveal the lesion. An example is shown in Fig. 7. Tomograms or CT scans are frequently needed to confirm and better define the extent of the lesion.
   g. **Treatment:**
      i. **Acute, nondisplaced:** Immobilize for 6 weeks in cast or rigid brace. Once healed, rehab as for ankle sprain.
      ii. **Acute or chronic, displaced:** Surgical excision with curettage of the base of the lesion or replacement of the lesion and internal fixation
      iii. **Chronic, nondisplaced:** Splint or cast for 4 weeks and re-assess x-rays and clinical symptoms. Persistent symptoms require surgical drilling or excision of the lesion.
      iv. In chronic cases always assess for concomitant ligament instability. This may require ligament reconstruction at the time of excision of the fragment.
5. **Posterior process fractures of talus, dorsal avulsion fractures of the talus, and anterior process fractures of the calcaneus**
   a. **Mechanism of injury:** Posterior process fractures (Fig. 8) occur with inversion and extreme plantarflexion, whereas the latter two result from inversion only.
   b. **Examination:** A careful exam is essential to make the diagnosis. The athlete will not be point-tender over the lateral ligaments. Instead, tenderness will be localized to the posterior ankle just anterior to the Achilles (posterior process of talus), over the dorsal surface of the talus, or 2 to 3 cm distal and anterior to the lateral malleolus (anterior process of the calcaneus).
   c. **X-rays:** Lateral views of the ankle should reveal the talus fractures, whereas the calcaneus fracture is best seen on an oblique foot view.

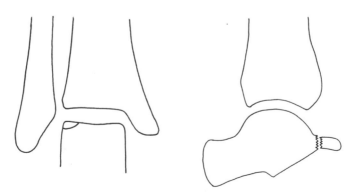

**FIGURE 7 *(left)*.**   Transchondral lateral talar dome fracture.

**FIGURE 8 *(right)*.**   Posterior process talus fracture.

   d. **Treatment**
      i. **Posterior process of talus**
         (a) Acute. Short leg nonweight-bearing cast for 6 weeks.
         (b) Chronic, symptomatic. Excision.
      ii. **Dorsal avulsion fracture of talus**
         (a) Short leg weightbearing cast for 3 to 4 weeks.
      iii. **Anterior process calcaneus fracture**
         (a) Acute. Short leg nonweight-bearing cast for 6 weeks.
         (b) Chronic. Injection of corticosteroid using fluoroscopy. Continued symptoms warrant excision.
B. **Stress fractures of the tibia and fibula**
   1. **Description:** Tibial stress fractures occur most commonly at the junction of the mid and distal thirds of the tibia, the posterior medial tibial plateau, or just distal to the tuberosity. Fibular stress fractures usually occur in the distal meta-diaphyseal region.
   2. **Mechanism of injury:** Repetitive overload of the bone, usually due to a change in training habits (increased intensity, duration or type of workout, a change in running surface or style of shoe) causes microfracture at area of excessive bone resorption.
   3. **History:** Pain increases during the run, decreases or stops after completion. Often will have a precipitous onset of pain.
   4. **Examination:** There is localized bone tenderness. Ultrasound will increase the pain when applied over the fracture site.
   5. **X-rays:** Rarely positive until 2 weeks after onset of symptoms. The earliest finding is periosteal thickening or layering.
   6. **Special consideration: Beware of the anterior tibial cortical stress fracture.** These frequently have delayed union, nonunion, and fracture completion.
   7. **Treatment**
      a. Positive x-ray: Use the following stress fracture protocol:
         i. Rest until all bone tenderness subsides.
         ii. Allow pain-free activities only. This may require crutches for a short time.
         iii. Start a flexibility and strength program.
         iv. Cross-training: Swim, bike, "run" in pool with flotation vest. Ice after workout.
         v. Begin the following running schedule when pain free (usually 4–8 weeks):
            (a) **Week 1:** Run every other day, half the usual training distance, 1 minute per mile slower than usual training pace.
            (b) **Week 2:** Normal training frequency, 3/4 usual training distance, same pace as week 1.
            (c) **Week 3:** 3/4 usual training distance, 30 seconds per mile slower than usual training pace.
            (d) **Week 4:** Resume usual distance, 30 seconds per mile slower than usual training pace. After completing this week, if no pain, may resume full training schedule.
      b. Negative x-ray, but suspicious clinical picture: Begin using the stress fracture protocol, repeat x-ray in 2–3 weeks. If you must know immediately or the athlete refuses to follow the protocol, obtain a bone scan to confirm the diagnosis.
      c. The long Aircast[R] may allow earlier return to activity for competitive athletes. This device probably disperses forces over a greater area, resulting in decreased stress at the fracture site. Use must be pain free!

C. **Acute shin splints (overuse myositis of the posterior tibialis, anterior tibialis, or peroneal muscles)**
   1. **History:** Usually occurs early in season in inexperienced athletes. Symptoms are similar to periostitis but located over muscle-tendon units instead of along the tibial ridge.
   2. **Treatment**
      a. Rest—begin with several weeks of relative rest.
      b. Ice, stretch, and careful warm-up.
      c. Correct anatomical variations with a semi-rigid foot orthosis.
      d. Wear a running shoe that provides both shock absorption and a firm heel counter.
      e. Anti-inflammatory medication.
D. **Chronic shin splints (medial tibial stress syndrome)**
   1. **Description:** The periosteum is inflamed or avulsed from the posteromedial distal tibia. If avulsed, fibrofatty tissue fills the defect.
   2. **History:** May be associated with the same training errors as stress fractures, but more likely to have an anatomical variation (heavy runner, cavus foot, overpronation) or poor running technique (increased leg rotation, leg crossover). Most of these patients have had symptoms for a long time. Pain may eventually occur with minimal exertion or shortly after the onset of exercise.
   3. **Examination:** Pain and tenderness is localized to the area immediately posterior to the tibial ridge and extending for 6–10 cm. Obtain compartment pressure measurements, since many of these patients have a concomitant deep posterior compartment syndrome.
   4. **X-rays:** In chronic cases there may be mild thickening or undulation of the posterior distal tibia. The bone scan is normal or shows a mild diffuse uptake along the painful area.
   5. **Treatment**
      a. Nonsurgical treatment is the same as in acute shin splints. However, many chronic cases may require many months of rest to alleviate the symptoms
      b. Resistant cases may require surgical cauterization of the tibial ridge with excision of the fibro-fatty tissue.
E. **Acute compartment syndrome**
   1. **Description:** Acute increase in tissue pressure within an enclosed anatomic space → increased local venous pressure → decrease in arteriovenous gradient → decrease in blood flow.
   2. **History:** Recent history of trauma (blunt blow to the leg by a helmet in football), sudden increase in exercise (forced, prolonged run in an untrained athlete), vascular injury, or prolonged, externally applied pressure (prolonged application of "temporary" air splint for a leg fracture). The athlete will have severe pain out of proportion to the apparent injury situation.
   3. **Examination**
      a. Weakness of muscles in the compartment.
      b. Pain with passive stretch of these muscles.
      c. Tenderness and tightness of compartment.
      d. Hypesthesia of nerve traversing the compartment.
      e. Compartment pressure measurements (at rest):
         i. 0–10 mm Hg = normal.
         ii. 10–30 mm Hg = elevated, but not dangerous.
         iii. 30–40 mm Hg = watch very closely, correlate with the clinical picture, perform repeated pressure measurements until symptoms resolve.
         iv. 40–60 mm Hg = usually dangerous, requiring compartment release.
         v. > 60 mm Hg = consistently dangerous, requires urgent release.

4. **Treatment**
    a. Remove circular dressings.
    b. Position leg at level of the heart.
    c. Decompress compartment if there is not **prompt** resolution of symptoms.
    d. Delayed skin closure.
F. **Chronic exertional compartment syndrome**
    1. **Description:** Intermittant excessive pressure within an enclosed leg fascial compartment, causing reduction in blood flow to that compartment. The increase in pressure occurs during exercise only and decreases after cessation of exercise to a normal level.
    2. **History:** These athletes typically have pain that begins at a consistent time into the exercise session. Symptoms then subside slowly after termination of the exercise. Pain is rarely present before exercise. There may be numbness on the dorsum of the foot with weakness of ankle dorsiflexion.
    3. **Examination:** The involved compartment may be tense when the athlete is symptomatic. The rest of the exam is usually normal. Compartment pressure measurements are the key in making the diagnosis. See par. I.E.5.
    4. **Treatment:** Surgical release of the offending compartment provides good results.
G. **Achilles tendon ruptures**
    1. **Description:** Complete disruption of the tendinous portion of the gastrocsoleus complex.
    2. **History:** Athlete feels "pop" and sensation of being kicked or cut in the heel. Commonly seen in a 30–50-year-old athlete.
    3. **Examination:** There is weak ankle plantarflexion and a palpable defect in tendon. The Thompson test demonstrates no plantarflexion of the ankle with calf squeeze.
    4. **Treatment**
        a. May be either surgical repair or cast immobilization. The options must be discussed with athlete, who should then decide which method is preferable.
        b. Surgical repair is usually recommended in athletes, as this provides better push-off strength and lower risk of rerupture. A cast is needed following repair. There is a risk of infection or skin breakdown with surgery.
        c. Nonoperative treatment is usually reserved for sedentary individuals or athletes who are unwilling to accept the risks of surgery. This method requires cast immobilization for 8–12 weeks.
            i. Long-leg cast in equinus with flexed knee for 4–6 weeks.
            ii. Short-leg cast in partial equinus for 4–6 weeks.
        d. Follow with heel lift for 3 months.
        e. Stretching and strengthening program to achieve full motion and maximum strength by 6 months after injury.
H. **Acute partial gastrocnemius tears**
    1. **Description:** Partial disruption in medial head of the gastrocnemius muscle at the musculotendinous junction.
    2. **History:** Acute event while hill running, jumping, or other activity that requires forceful push-off.
    3. **Examination:** No defect and negative Thompson test (plantarflexion occurs when the calf is squeezed).
    4. **Treatment**
        a. ½ inch heel lift, calf sleeve.
        b. Avoid running, jumping, push-off.
        c. Ice until pain and swelling subside.

    d. Isometric calf contractions in plantarflexion followed by gentle stretching.

    e. 3–6 weeks to full recovery.

I. **Achilles tendinitis**

1. **History:** Athletes with tight heel cords, overpronation, a recent change in shoes, or recent increase in training are most susceptible. Chronic cases are probably due to a partial tear of the tendon.

2. **Examination:** Tenderness, thickening, and fine crepitation are present over the middle of the tendon.

3. **X-rays:** MRI or diagnostic ultrasound will demonstrate a partially torn tendon.

4. **Treatment**

    a. Correct anatomic variations.

    b. Heel lift and decreased training acutely.

    c. Ice, anti-inflammatory medication and phonophoresis to control inflammation.

    d. Chronic symptoms may require surgical release of the peritenon with debridement of degenerative or partially torn tendon.

J. **Retrocalcaneal bursitis**

1. **Description:** Bursal inflammation immediately anterior to the insertion of the Achilles tendon.

2. **History:** Aching pain with exercise. The athlete's heel counter may be too constrictive causing friction in this area.

3. **Examination:** Tenderness and swelling are localized anterior to the insertion of the Achilles tendon.

4. **X-rays:** May demonstrate a prominent superior projection of the calcaneus or obliteration of the normal radio-opaque space anterior to the tendon.

5. **Treatment**

    a. Nonsurgical treatment is similar to Achilles tendinitis.

    b. Resistant symptoms deserve debridement of the bursa and excision of the superior projection of the calcaneus.

K. **Acute ankle sprains**

1. **Description:** Complete or partial disruption of the talofibular, calcaneofibular, deltoid or tibiofibular ligaments. There may be associated tearing of the interosseous membrane.

2. **Associated injuries:** Fractures of the fibula, talus, calcaneus, or metatarsals. Very commonly there are tendon strains or subluxations and neuropraxia of the sensory nerves of the foot.

3. **History:** Acute inversion or eversion of the ankle. The amount of acute swelling is a good guide to the severity of the injury. **Persistent pain after a sprain has been rehabilitated** requires a work-up for chronic instability; DJD; loose body, talar dome, or anterior process of calcaneus fractures; intra-articular meniscoid lesion.

4. **Examination:** Localize the tenderness to a specific anatomic structure. Pain with the syndesmosis squeeze test is rare but indicates a fibular fracture or disruption of the syndesmosis. Determine the degree of ligament laxity with anterior drawer and talar tilt tests.

5. **X-rays:** Should be obtained in any significant injury. Look for associated fractures. **Carefully assess the mortise view for widening.** Beware of the high fibular fracture or tibia-fibula diastasis.

6. **Grade the injury**

    a. Grade I—no laxity, minimal pain, weight-bears without pain.

    b. Grade II—mild laxity and swelling.

    c. Grade III—complete ligament disruption resulting in significant laxity and swelling, may be unable to bear weight.

7. **Treatment of Grade I–II**
    a. **Acute Phase**
        i. Ice for 20 minutes, at least QID until all swelling is gone.
        ii. Compression (wrapping the ankle with a "U" of orthopedic felt surrounding the involved malleolus to prevent swelling; taping).
        iii. Elevation (48–72 hours).
        iv. Nonsteroidal anti-inflammatory medication.
        v. Use crutches if the athlete is unable to weight bear or walks with any significant limp. Advance weight-bearing as tolerated by pain, swelling, and the elimination of the limp.
    b. **Rehabilitation phase**
        i. Support (tape, Aircast, lace-up ankle brace).
        ii. ROM—plantarflexion and dorsiflexion.
        iii. Strengthen with resistive exercises.
        iv. Later, add inversion and eversion, proprioception retraining.
        v. Before return to sport, add agility drills.
8. **Treatment of Grade III:** Because of pain, swelling, and instability, this injury needs additional protection (short-leg cast, Aircast or other rigid support) for 1–3 weeks. Some surgeons feel surgical repair is needed when there is gross instability.
9. **Treatment of syndesmosis sprains:** In addition to the above methods, these need prolonged support (consider high Aircast). They will often have pain for several months after injury.
10. **Treatment of tibia-fibula diastasis:** Open reduction and internal fixation with a syndesmosis screw.

L. **Chronic lateral ankle ligament instability**
    1. **History:** Recurrent ankle ligament sprains, often requiring several weeks to return to sport. The athlete feels his ankle is unstable on hills or uneven ground. Swelling occurs with activity.
    2. **Examination:** There is a positive anterior drawer and/or talar tilt test.
    3. **X-rays:** Stress x-rays must be obtained and are diagnostic.
        a. Talar tilt stress x-ray is positive if 10 degrees more than the normal side.
        b. Anterior drawer stress x-ray is positive if shift of 8 mm from a fixed point on talus to tibia.
    4. **Treatment**
        a. Rehab—strength, ROM, proprioception.
        b. Ankle support (tape, lacer, Aircast).
        c. Surgical reconstruction if above measures fail and athlete remains symptomatic.

M. **Intra-articular meniscoid lesion**
    1. **Description:** A localized fibrotic synovitis in the lateral ankle that may occur after inversion sprains.
    2. **History:** Persistent pain, swelling, catching in the anterolateral aspect of the ankle many months after a severe ankle injury.
    3. **Examination:** Mild swelling with tenderness localized to the anterolateral ankle may be the only abnormalities.
    4. **Treatment:** Arthroscopic debridement provides good relief.

N. **Posterior tibial tendinitis**
    1. **History:** Diffuse pain and swelling posterior to medial malleolus or at its insertion into navicular. May be a sequelae of an ankle sprain. Athletes at risk have planovalgus foot; play sports with sudden start-stop or push-off actions.
    2. **Examination:** Tenderness is localized to posterior tibialis tendon. There is pain with passive pronation and active supination.

3. **Treatment**
   a. Rest, ice, anti-inflammatory medication.
   b. Acute—support strapping or cast if severe.
   c. Chronic—medial posted orthosis.
   d. Persistent—debride partial tears and proliferative synovium, decompress sheath, possibly add Kidner procedure.
   e. Complete rupture—reconstruct with contiguous long flexor tendons.

O. **Flexor hallucis longus tendinitis**
   1. **History:** Pain and swelling posterior to medial malleolus; runners may have pain at sesamoids. Dancers or athletes involved in repetitive stop-start or push-off activities are susceptible.
   2. **Examination:** Pain with hallux ROM.
   3. **Treatment**
      a. Rest, ice, anti-inflammatory medication.
      b. Rigid shoe plus a heel lift.
      c. Persistent—treat as for posterior tibialis.

P. **Anterior tibialis tendinitis**
   1. **History:** Pain over dorsum of the foot. Runners doing hill work and skiers (due to direct irritation from boots) are most prone.
   2. **Examination:** Tenderness and swelling localized to the anterior tibialis tendon. Pain increased by resisted ankle dorsiflexion.
   3. **X-rays:** Look for osteophytes on anterior distal tibia.
   4. **Treatment**
      a. Rest, ice, anti-inflammatory medication, physical therapy modalities.
      b. Persistent symptoms—excise osteophytes, debride peritenon.

Q. **Peroneal tendon subluxation**
   1. **Description:** The peroneal retinaculum is detached from its normal insertion on the posterior border of the fibula to the lateral surface of the fibula. This occurs during an acute dorsiflexion and inversion stress injury while the peroneal muscles are contracting forcefully.
   2. **History:** Prior history of an ankle "sprain." Athlete may sense the tendons subluxating with ankle range of motion. Most common in skiing, basketball.
   3. **Examination:** Subluxation of the peroneal tendons with active dorsiflexion and eversion. If the patient can relax, the tendons may be subluxated manually by the examiner. Mild, chronic swelling may be present.
   4. **X-ray:** May reveal a fracture of the lateral ridge of fibula. In the habitual dislocator, some authors recommend a CT to evaluate the depth of groove on the posterior aspect of fibula. A shallow groove may predispose the patient to tendon subluxation.
   5. **Treatment**
      a. Acute—Primary repair of retinaculum; reconstruct retinaculum if inadequate.
      b. Habitual—Reconstruct retinaculum with periosteal flap or autogenous tendon graft. Deepen groove if determined to be shallow. A sliding slot graft on the distal fibula is needed if the soft tissue reconstruction is deemed inadequate due to the poor quality of the local tissue.
      c. Apply short-leg cast for 6 weeks.

# Chapter 42: Foot Problems

STEPHEN C. HUNTER, MD
WILLIAM L. CAPPIELLO, MD
GREGORY P. HESS, MD
DANIEL JOYCE, MD

I. **Normal Anatomy** (Figs. 1 and 2)

II. **Anatomical Variants** (Table 1)

III. **Foot Problems**

A. **Skin and nail problems** (Table 2)

B. **Tendinitis** (Table 3)

1. **Etiology:** Stress causes macrotears (acute trauma) or microtears (chronic overuse) with resultant inflammation.

2. **Common types:** posterior tibialis, peroneal, Achilles.

3. **Radiographic assessment**

a. Plain films usually not helpful—do not show tendon damage.

b. Occasionally see associated bony changes (e.g., avulsion of base of fifth metatarsal at peroneus brevis insertion, calcification or erosion at Achilles tendon insertion).

c. CT or MRI may help detect complete tendon tear.

C. **Plantar fasciitis** (Fig. 5A)

1. **Etiology:** Excessive tightness of gastrocsoleus complex pulling into heelcord (Achilles) causes overload at plantar fascia origin on calcaneus during weight-bearing activities; microtears and inflammation ensue.

2. **Symptoms/signs:** Point tenderness/pain (particularly on first arising in morning).

a. Specifically along medial tubercle of calcaneus.

b. Sometimes relieved with activity, returning at rest.

3. **Radiographic assessment:** Traction spurs off calcaneus may be seen (secondary findings and usually **not** a cause of pain).

4. **Differential diagnosis**

a. Entrapment of medial calcaneal branch of tibial nerve (calcaneal branch neurodynia—thought by some to be a component of plantar fasciitis syndrome).

b. Plantar arch strain: pain located directly under arch.

c. Tarsal tunnel syndrome (see below).

d. Calcaneal stress fracture (see below).

5. **Treatment**

a. Heelcord stretching.

b. NSAIDs.

c. Shock-absorbing heel pad and/or soft plantar arch orthotic (Fig. 5B, 5C).

d. Decrease weight-bearing activities initially with graduated return.

e. Maintenance of aerobic, well-leg, and upper-body fitness.

f. Corticosteroid injection.

g. Surgical release: only with failure of conservative measures.

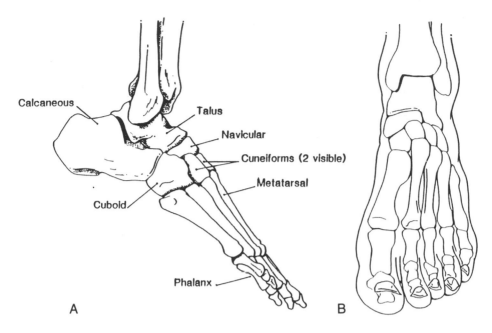

**FIGURE 1.**   *A,* Normal lateral anatomy of the foot. *B,* Normal dorsal anatomy of the foot.

**TABLE 1.**   Anatomical Variants of the Foot

| Variants | Description | Etiology | Functional Consequence |
|---|---|---|---|
| Hyperpronated foot | A flat foot that is excessively dorsiflexed, abducted, and everted at subtalar joint | Structural abnormality. Compensation for tibia vara, Achilles tendon inflexibility, heel or forefoot varus | Excessive subtalar motion, stress overloading |
| Tarsal coalition | Bony or cartilaginous bar between bones of hindfoot and midfoot | Congenital | Limits eversion/inversion. Clinically may appear as rigid flat foot |
| Pes planus | Flat foot (Fig. 3A) | Structural (e.g., tarsal coalition or neurologic disorder) | Abnormal stress loading (often associated with hyperpronation) |
| Pes cavus | High-arched foot, usually rigid (Fig. 3B) | Structural or neurological disorder | Less shock absorption; abnormal stress loading leads to overuse syndromes |
| Metatarsus primus adductus | Adduction of first ray | Structural abnormality | Difficulty fitting shoes; blister, callus, or bunion formation often complicated by claw or hammer toes (Fig. 4) |
| Morton's toe | Elongated second metatarsal compared to first | Congenital | Excessively mobile first metatarsal; abnormal stress-loading from great toe to second toe; pain and callus formation; functional overuse syndromes |

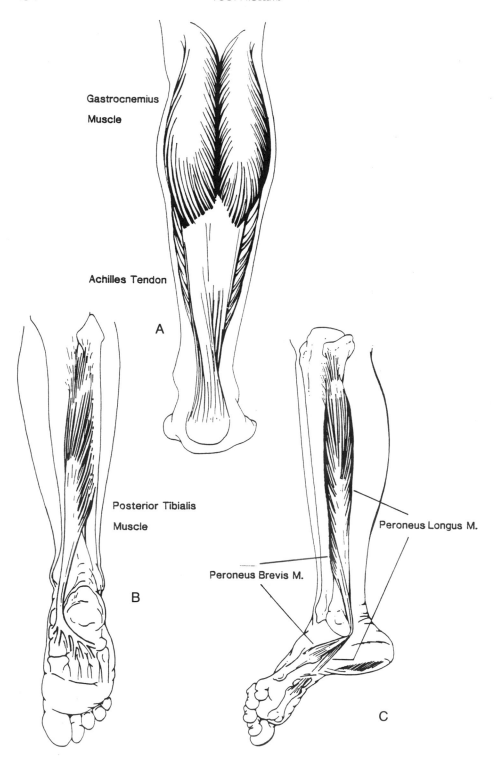

Gastrocnemius
Muscle

Achilles Tendon

A

Posterior Tibialis
Muscle

B

Peroneus Longus M.

Peroneus Brevis M.

C

**FIGURE 2.**   *A–C,* Normal lower leg muscles and tendons.

Pes Planus (Valgus)

Pes Cavus (Varus)

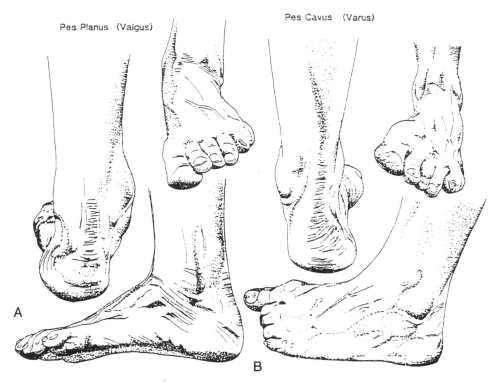

A

B

**FIGURE 3.**   *A,* Pes planus (flat foot). *B,* Pes cavus (high-arched foot).

D. **Turf toe**
  1. **Etiology**
     a. Hyperextension of the metatarsophalangeal (MTP) joint of the great toe leads to ligament sprain, possible tearing of flexor tendon.
     b. Often occurs in football linemen pushing off on artificial turf.
  2. **Symptoms/signs**
     a. Pain, tenderness, and swelling at great toe MTP joint.
     b. Persistent symptoms with continued activity may lead to hallux rigidus.
  3. **Radiographic assessment**
     a. Usually normal.
     b. May show degenerative changes of first MTP joint (chronic).
     c. May have associated sesamoid fracture (**note:** normally two sesamoid bones beneath MTP joint of great toe).
  4. **Differential diagnosis**
     a. Classic joint for presentation of gout.
     b. Phalangeal or metatarsal fracture.
  5. **Treatment:** Rest and protection are key.
     a. Ice/NSAIDs acutely.
     b. Taping to limit motion of MTP joint may assist in return to activity (Fig. 6).
     c. Metatarsal pad to unload first metatarsal may be helpful.
     d. Rigid shoe or rigid metal or plastic forefoot plate provides forefoot support and limits MTP hyperextension.
E. **Fractures** (Fig. 7A)
  1. **Talus**
     a. **Etiology**

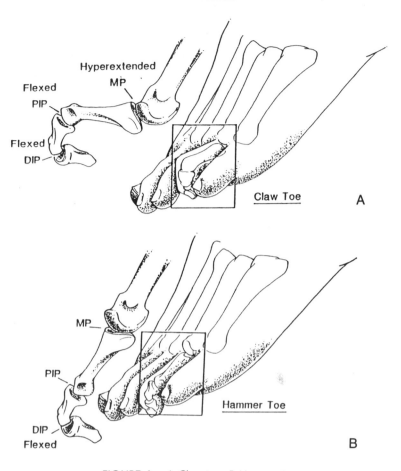

**FIGURE 4.** *A*, Claw toe. *B*, Hammer toe.

    i. Acute trauma: rare in sports, usually surgical emergency; after radiographic confirmation, orthopedic referral mandatory; talar neck fractures are associated with severe foot dislocation (**note:** osteochondral fractures of the talar dome may occur with ankle sprains).

    ii. Stress fractures: also rare.

      (a) Symptoms—functional diffuse midfoot pain.

      (b) Signs—anterior ankle tenderness on palpation, resistance to active and passive motion of subtalar joint (**note:** subtalar joint allows eversion/inversion).

  b. **Radiographic assessment—gives definitive diagnosis.**

    i. Subtle or stress fractures usually require bone scan or CT.

    ii. Aseptic necrosis of talar head may occur after stress or traumatic fractures.

  c. **Treatment** of stress fractures of talus

    i. Modified rest/cessation of weight-bearing activity; cast or support shoe, crutches; healing process may take up to 6 months (repeat radiographs should document healing).

    ii. Progressive return to weight-bearing activity with confirmation of healing; initial limitation of ankle and subtalar motion on return to activities (e.g., ankle brace) is helpful.

**TABLE 2.** Skin and Nail Problems

| Type | Cause | Signs and Symptoms | Treatment |
|------|-------|--------------------|-----------|
| Calluses and corns (calluses of the toes) | Excessive localized friction or pressure from, e.g., tight shoes or structural abnormalities of the feet, such as claw or hammer toes | Pain; thickening and hardening of the skin (kept soft by moisture when between the toes) | Proper shoe fitting, padding (e.g., doughnut pad), debridement, bony resection |
| Blisters | Friction, pressure Epidermal/dermal separation by serous fluid | Painful vescicles | Unruptured: sterile drainage (if painful), dressing. Ruptured: sterile cleansing, dressing (consider antibiotics for diabetic patient, or for signs of secondary infection in any patient) |
| Warts | Virus (papilloma) | Pain at site; skin thickening with a central core; flat or raised | Trichloracetic acid or salicylic acid or other debridement, e.g., liquid nitrogen |
| Tinea pedis (athlete's foot) | Fungus | Dry or vesicular lesions; scaling, peeling, and cracking fissures in skin; deformed nails; hyphae and buds on KOH wet mount; iridescence by Wood's light | Dry: miconazole nitrate, clotrimazole, salicylic acid, tolnaftate, tar compounds. Vesicular: wet dressings with potassium permanganate or Burow's solution. Erythema or other signs of infection: consider antibiotics |
| Paronychia (ingrown toenail) | Fungal/bacterial infection | Inflamed nail margin with or without drainage | Antibiotics acutely (e.g., erythromycin); partial nail resection; proper nail cutting techniques |
| Subungual hematoma | Trauma | Dark blood under nail: pain/pressure at site | Drainage (insert no. 18 needle through nail or burn hole in nail with the tip of a heated paper clip) |

**TABLE 3.** Tendinitis

| Type | Signs and Symptoms | Treatment |
|------|--------------------|-----------|
| Posterior tibialis | Medial pain, swelling, pain with active inversion (hyperpronation could be a sign of complete posterior tibialis rupture) | Initial: rest, ice, NSAIDs,* plantar arch orthotic. Rehab: plantar flexion and inversion strengthening exercises, heelcord flexibility |
| Peroneal | Lateral pain, swelling, pain with active eversion; may complain of snapping sensation in cases of subluxation of tendon(s) | Initial: rest, ice, NSAIDs.[†] Rehab: resistive eversion foot exercises. Surgery may be required for subluxation |
| Achilles | Decreased gastrocsoleus flexibility Pain, tenderness, swelling, and crepitus at site; pain with active plantar flexion | Initial: rest, ice, NSAIDs,* orthotic to correct hyperpronation or heel pad to decrease tension on tendon. Rehab: heelcord stretching and strengthening exercises. Possible surgical repair in chronic cases or with complete tendon rupture |

* Rehab includes maintenance of aerobic, well-leg, and upper-body fitness in all three types of tendinitis. Physical therapy modalities such as phonophoresis may also be useful.
[†] NSAIDs = nonsteroidal anti-inflammatory drugs.

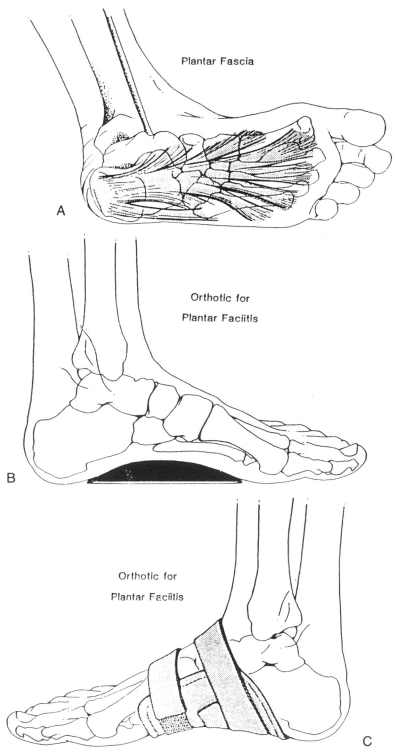

Plantar Fascia

A

Orthotic for
Plantar Faciitis

B

Orthotic for
Plantar Faciitis

C

**FIGURE 5.**   *A,* Plantar fascia. *B,C,* Orthoses for plantar fasciitis.

Turf Toe Taping

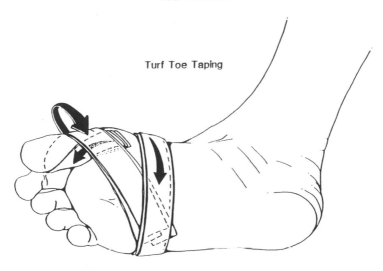

**FIGURE 6.** Taping to limit motion of MTP joint in treating turf toe.

2. **Calcaneus** (see Fig. 7A)
   a. **Etiology**
      i. Traumatic: rare; orthopedic emergency.
      ii. Stress: more common; usually related to endurance sports.
   b. **Symptoms/signs**
      i. Localized pain in heel, accentuated by weight-bearing.
      ii. Mild swelling.
      iii. Pain with medial-lateral compression of calcaneus.
   c. **Radiographic assessment:** definitive
      i. Plain film; Bohler's angle may be < 28° in traumatic fractures.
      ii. If negative, bone scan or CT.
   d. **Treatment** of stress fractures of calcaneus
      i. Modified rest and cessation of weight-bearing activities; cast or support shoe with crutches may be appropriate.
      ii. Gradual return to activity when clinical symptoms abate and serial radiographic assessment documents healing; full healing usually within 3 months; ankle support to prevent subtalar motion and/or hindfoot shock-absorbing orthotic helpful on return to activity.
3. **Midfoot** (Fig. 7B)
   a. **Etiology**
      i. Major trauma: again, orthopedic emergency; Lisfranc fracture/dislocation (tarsometatarsal fracture/dislocation)—if left untreated, permanent deformity/disability results.
      ii. Stress fractures: usually in tarsal navicular bone (common in jumpers, ballet dancers, equestrians).
   b. **Symptoms/signs** of navicular stress fracture
      i. Localized pain, swelling over navicular.
      ii. Limited midfoot motion.
   c. **Radiographic assessment**
      i. Plain films often negative.
      ii. Bone scanning and/or CT are typically necessary with tarsal navicular fractures.

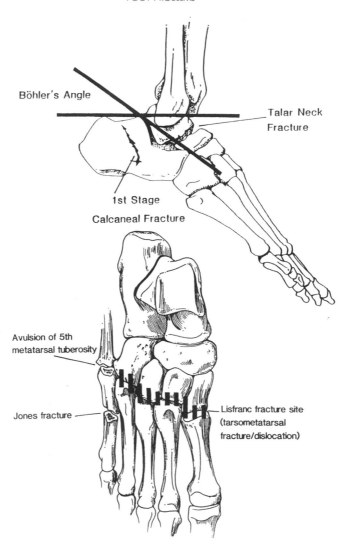

Böhler's Angle

Talar Neck
Fracture

1st Stage
Calcaneal Fracture

Avulsion of 5th
metatarsal tuberosity

Jones fracture

Lisfranc fracture site
(tarsometatarsal
fracture/dislocation)

**FIGURE 7.**    Fractures of the foot.

    d. **Treatment**
      i. Rest, cessation of weight-bearing activities, casting.
      ii. Complications: high incidence of nonunion with tarsal navicular fractures; persistent symptoms and delayed union on x-ray studies beyond 3 months may indicate need for surgery.
      iii. Surgery: usually bone grafting with internal fixation when indicated; recovery may be up to 1 year.
4. **Metatarsal fractures**
    a. **Etiology**
      i. Trauma: rare.
      ii. Stress: common; seen in endurance running and jumping sports (e.g., in hurdlers and cross-country runners).
    b. **Symptoms/signs:** localized pain with weight-bearing, swelling, tenderness.

    c. **Radiographic assessment**
       i. Plain films are usually diagnostic.
      ii. Bone scan may be necessary to detect early lesions.
    d. **Treatment**
       i. Second through fourth metatarsal stress fractures: conservative treatment (first metatarsal stress fracture rarely seen); modified rest with cessation of weight-bearing activities (immobilization in cast or splint may be used, especially for pain control); graduated return to activity when symptoms subside.
      ii. Avulsion at attachment of peroneus brevis tendon at the base of the fifth metatarsal (see Fig. 7B) (common with ankle sprains): also conservative treatment.
     iii. Jones fracture (see Fig. 7B): stress fracture of proximal fifth metatarsal shaft seen in sprinters and jumpers.
        (a) Often have prolonged symptoms and delayed or nonunion with conservative treatment.
        (b) Surgery: bone grafting and internal fixation indicated for motivated athlete with delayed or nonunion.

  5. **Phalangeal fractures**
    a. **Etiology:** trauma such as crush injuries or jamming.
    b. **Symptoms/signs:** pain, deformity, swelling, ecchymosis.
    c. **Radiographic assessment:** plain films confirmatory.
    d. **Treatment:** conservative unless open fracture.
       i. Undisplaced: buddy taping to adjacent toe; protection in stiff shoe; symptoms dictate activity restrictions.
      ii. Displaced: reduced by manipulation; subsequent buddy-taping/splinting.
     iii. Complications: intra-articular fractures can result in joint stiffness and arthritis; if resistant to closed manipulation, refer to orthopedist.

## F. Dislocations
  1. **Subtalar/pantalar dislocations**
    a. Etiology: severe trauma; orthopedic emergency.
    b. Immediate care indicated to avoid neurovascular damage.
  2. **Metatarsophalangeal/interphalangeal dislocations:** relatively common.
    a. **Etiology:** trauma.
    b. **Symptoms/signs:** pain, dysfunction, gross deformity of toes.
    c. **Radiographic assessment:** done to rule out associated fracture.
    d. **Treatment**
       i. Reduction with steady traction; if dislocation persists, orthopedic referral to rule out tendon entrapment, which may require surgical treatment.
      ii. Splint/buddy taping after reduction.
     iii. Functional toe can usually be expected.

## G. Neurologic injury
  1. **Tarsal tunnel syndrome** (Fig. 8): impingement of posterior tibial nerve beneath flexor retinaculum behind medial malleolus.
    a. **Etiology:** Hyperpronation that leads to stress/traction on nerve with impingement is a correctable cause.
    b. **Symptoms/signs**
       i. Aching pain at medial foot; aggravated by weight-bearing.
      ii. Trigger-point usually detectable by palpation at site of impingement (positive Tinel's sign: tapping over trigger point causes radiating pain along medial or lateral plantar nerve distribution).

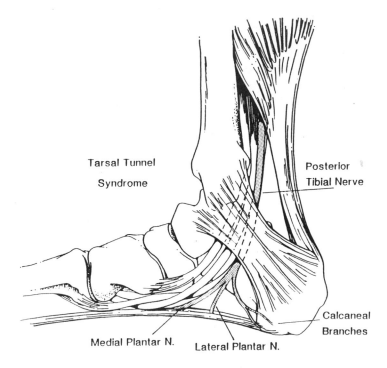

**FIGURE 8.** Tarsal tunnel syndrome.

  c. **Diagnostic measures**
    i. Radiographs not helpful.
    ii. Electromyographic (EMG) studies show fibrillation potentials in muscles in the foot innervated by the nerve (e.g., abductor hallucis, abductor digiti quinti).
    iii. Nerve conduction studies (chronic cases).
  d. **Treatment**
    i. Rest, NSAIDs, graduated return to activity.
    ii. Orthotic with support, especially with hyperpronation or other contributory structural deformities.
    iii. Surgical decompression for intractable cases.
2. **Differential diagnosis**
  a. Posterior tibialis tendinitis
  b. Calcaneal stress fracture
  c. Gout.
3. **Morton's neuroma:** impingement of interdigital nerves as they bifurcate at metatarsal heads
  a. **Etiology**
    i. Trauma or repetitive stress leads to irritation of nerves as they cross under transverse metatarsal ligament to toes.
    ii. Swelling results, and a vicious cycle of swelling causing more pain and irritation causing more swelling occurs; "tumor" or inflammatory neuroma forms in chronic stages.
  b. **Symptoms/signs**
    i. Pain: typically, burning neuralgia, worse with standing.

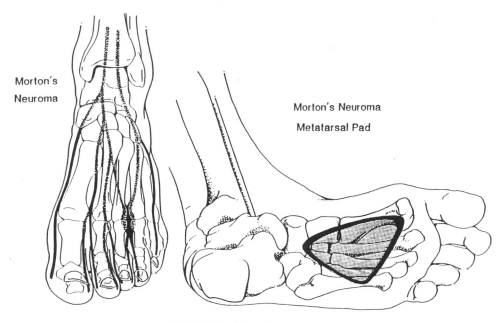

Morton's Neuroma

Morton's Neuroma

Metatarsal Pad

**FIGURE 9.** Morton's neuroma.

    ii. Trigger-point, tender to palpation between metatarsal heads; classically located between third and fourth MTs but can also occur between second and third (Fig. 9A).

    iii. Compressing the metatarsals on either side of the neuroma together manually causes pain.

  c. **Differential diagnosis**

    i. Metatarsalgia

    ii. Metatarsal stress fractures.

  d. Radiographic assessment: not helpful.

  e. Treatment

    i. Initial: NSAIDs; metatarsal pads to lift and spread metatarsal heads (Fig. 9B); sometimes corticosteroid injection.

    ii. Chronic: surgical excision; patient left with permanent anesthesia between involved toes, but no functional deficits.

    iii. Use of metatarsal pad on return to sports.

# Chapter 43: Taping and Bracing

RONNIE D. HALD, PT, ATC
DENISE FANDEL, MS, ATC

I. **Team Physician's Role in Taping and Bracing**

   A. **Determine appropriateness** of taping/bracing.
   B. **Facilitate selection** process.
   1. **Identify** available options.
   2. **Communicate** with treatment team (athletic trainer, coach, and athlete).
   C. **Evaluate effectiveness** of selected support.

II. **Selection Considerations**

   A. **Diagnosis of injury**
   1. **Location.** Taping/bracing restricts undesired motion. Contraindicated when restriction of motion may lead to decreased function or other problems.
   2. **Nature of injury**
      a. Taping/bracing provides support to acutely injured tissues.
      b. Taping/bracing decreases the effect of repetitive biomechanical forces resulting in chronic injuries.
   3. **Severity.** More severe injuries require more aggressive treatment.
   B. **Goals of taping/bracing**
   1. **Prophylactic:** To reduce the incidence or severity of injury to uninjured normal anatomy or fully rehabilitated injuries.
   2. **Rehabilitative:** To provide protection of healing injuries during their rehabilitation. **TAPING/BRACING DOES NOT SUBSTITUTE FOR OR REPLACE THE NEED FOR COMPLETE REHABILITATION.** Taping/bracing is only an adjunct to rehabilitation.
   3. **Functional:** To protect against reinjury following rehabilitation and/or surgical reconstruction.
   C. **Resources available**
   1. Taping
      a. Supplies are usually available.
      b. Requires application by an athletic trainer or other skilled individual.
      c. Repeated applications may become costly.
   2. Braces
      a. Over-the-counter (OTC) braces are instantly available.
      b. Custom-made braces require time for fabrication.
      c. Once instructed, athlete can self-apply the brace.
      d. Initially costly, but may be cost-effective over time.
         i. Need to consult coaches and parents.
   3. **Recommendation: If taping or bracing cannot provide any additional benefit, it is probably best to do without it.**
   D. **Sport and position of the athlete**
   1. **Physical requirements.** Taping often tailored to the allow the athlete to perform his/her skills.
   2. **Equipment,** including footwear, may need modification.

3. **Environment** may affect choices.
   a. Temperature
   b. Humidity
   c. Aquatic.
4. **Rules.** Must use materials that do not endanger other participants.

E. **Athlete's acceptance**
   1. Taping and bracing must not be uncomfortable or decrease performance.
   2. Involve the athlete in the decision-making process. Provide choices when possible.
   3. Realize the positive psychological effect of taping/bracing. Assists the athlete's confidence upon returning to competition.

F. **Research findings**
   1. Few studies are available.
   2. Many articles are supported only by clinical experience or tradition.
   3. New products should be viewed with an open but critical mind.

G. **Personal preferences.** Most physicians and athletic trainers develop a list of favorite techniques and devices, but they should view each case individually.

III. **Implementation**

A. **Communication**
   1. Selection process, decision, and plan involves many individuals.
      a. Physician          e. Sports physical therapist
      b. Athlete            f. Orthotist
      c. Coach              g. Parent(s) or guardian(s).
      d. Athletic trainer

B. **Education**
   1. **Taping**
      a. Teaching the trainer or coach the desired technique.
      b. Prevention of skin problems (see below).
   2. **Bracing**
      a. Instruction in the correct application of the brace.
      b. Provide written instructions on application and care.
   3. **Promote the concept of "earning the taping/brace" by insisting on complete rehabilitation prior to resumption of sport.**

C. **Follow-up**
   1. Usually occurs at the conclusion of the athlete's season.
      a. Reassess the injured area; encourage "prehabilitation" of deficits before the next season.
      b. Re-evaluate the effectiveness of the method of support.
      c. May need to provide other alternatives for multi-sport athletes.
   2. Provides opportunity to collect data for greatly needed research.

IV. **Taping**

A. **Principles of taping**
   1. **Prepare** to tape.
      a. Decide on appropriate technique.
      b. Gather needed tape supplies.
      c. Position athlete's body part.
         i. Position of function and/or protection
         ii. Appropriate table height to optimize taper's body mechanics.
   2. **Tape selection**
      a. Qualities of a good athletic tape:
         i. Good adherence to the athlete's skin.

    ii. Adequate tensile strength to provide the necessary support.

    iii. Allows perspiration to escape.

    iv. Easily unwinds and tears from the roll.

  b. Size of the body part determines the appropriate width.

  c. Elasticity allows increased ease of application and desired movement, yet provides adequate injury protection.

    i. More expensive.

    ii. Many elastic tapes do not tear and require cutting with scissors.

### 3. Skin care

  a. **Preventive measures**

    i. **Shave hair.**

      (a) Increases adhesion of the tape.

      (b) Reduces irritation.

      (c) Reduces build up of residue.

    ii. **Apply a taping base** (e.g., tincture of benzoin).

      (a) Increases adhesion of the tape.

      (b) Provides a protective layer between the tape and skin.

    iii. **Apply a tape underwrap,** e.g., thin polyester urethane foam.

      (a) Decreases skin problems.

      (b) Increases the athlete's comfort.[8]

      (c) May not be appropriate for all uses.

    iv. **Apply a lubricant to possible areas of irritation,** e.g., lace and heel areas of the ankle.

  b. **Proper tape removal**

    i. Use scissors or cutters with a blunt tip.

    ii. Teach athlete proper removal technique

    iii. Cleanse skin to remove tape residue

    iv. Treat skin irritations and wounds promptly; these problems can prevent further taping.

  c. **Allergic reactions to tape materials**

    i. Recognize and treat problems

    ii. Alternative tape supplies may provide a solution.

    iii. May need to abandon taping in favor of some other form of support and protection.

### 4. Application

  a. **Requires a skilled individual—proficiency results from practice.**

  b. **Elements of proper taping technique**

    i. Tearing tape is a basic skill; tape must be torn often.

    ii. Every piece of tape should have a distinct purpose.

    iii. Place anchor strips proximal and distal to the injured area directly to the skin.

    iv. Bridge across the injury, duplicating the anatomy needing support.

    v. Weave the strips to add strength, overlapping by at least one-half the width of the tape.

    vi. Adapt the two-dimensional tape to a three-dimensional body part.

    vii. Limit pressure around bony prominences, especially when vascular and neural structures are superficial.

    viii. Use elastic materials over muscle bellies to allow normal muscle expansion.

    ix. Inspect for and tape over any gaps in the taping to prevent blisters and tape cuts.

    x. Restrict undesired motion, yet allow wanted motion.

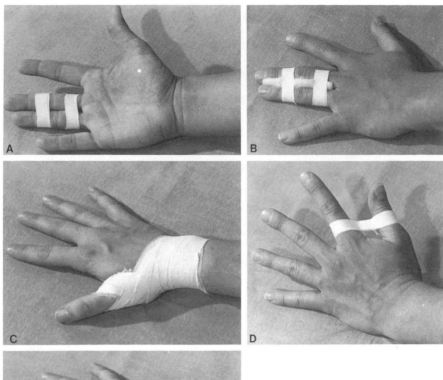

**FIGURE 1.** *A,* Buddy taping. *B,* Buddy taping with felt/foam insert. *C,* Thumb figure-of-eight. *D,* Thumb checkrein. *E,* Wrist taping.

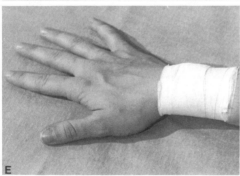

c. **Avoid common problems that restrict circulation.**
   i. Applying too much tape.
   ii. Continuous application of repeated circumferential strips without tearing between turns about the body part.
   iii. Forcing the tape to go in a desired direction.
   iv. Do not tape acute injuries; swelling will cause taping to become too tight.

V. **Selected Taping Procedures**
   A. **Buddy taping** (Fig. 1A, B)
      1. Common indications: finger sprains, minor fractures of proximal interphalangeal joint.
      2. Materials: ¼ inch tape, felt or foam strip (optional).
      3. Athlete position: felt or foam strip placed between injured and adjoining finger; avoid using the index or little finger as a splint.
      4. Technique: circular strips placed proximal and distal to injured joint; restrict varus/valgus forces.

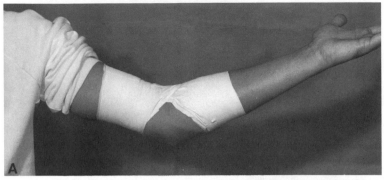

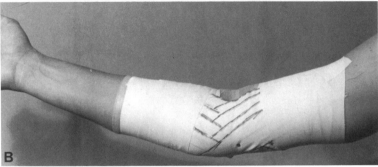

**FIGURE 2.** *A,* Elbow hyperextension taping. *B,* Medial elbow taping.

B. **Thumb figure-of-eight** (Fig. 1C)
   1. Common indications: hyperflexion injuries to the metacarpophalangeal (MCP) joint of the thumb.
   2. Materials: ½ inch tape, cloth or elastic.
   3. Athlete position: thumb abducted, wrist in slight extension.
   4. Technique: encircle the wrist and thumb in a figure-of-eight pattern, repeat as necessary.
C. **Thumb checkrein** (Fig. 1D)
   1. Common indications: hyperextension or hyperabduction injuries to the MCP joint of the thumb; can result in injuries to the MCP joint of the index finger.[24]
   2. Materials: ¼ inch and/or ½ inch tape.
   3. Athlete position: thumb slightly abducted.
   4. Technique
      a. Encircle proximal phalanx of the thumb and proximal phalanx of the index finger.
      b. Press together adhesive surfaces between the thumb and index finger.
      c. Anchor by taping around the checkrein.
D. **Wrist taping** (Fig. 1E)
   1. Common indication: wrist sprains, dorsal impingement.
   2. Materials: 1 inch or 1½ inch tape, foam pad (for dorsal impingement).
   3. Athlete position: wrist slightly extended, pad on dorsum of wrist if needed to act as a "block" to extension range of motion.
   4. Technique: circumferential strips about the wrist.
E. **Elbow taping**
   1. Common indications: elbow hyperextension, varus/valgus injuries.

2. Materials: 1½ inch cloth tape or 2 inch elastic tape.
3. Athlete position: slight flexion of elbow.
4. **Technique for hyperextension injuries** (Fig. 2A)
   a. Place anchor strips about the mid-upper arm and mid-forearm.
   b. Criss-cross strips in an "X" pattern, creating a fan across the anterior aspect of the elbow.
   c. Repeat anchors to close, taking care to not restrict circulation.
5. **Technique for varus/valgus injuries:** modified to provide medial (Fig. 2B) or lateral support.

F. **Shoulder taping**
   1. Restriction of motion required to provide adequate support decreases function.
   2. Suggest time and effort is probably better spent on rehabilitation.

G. **Hip, hamstring, and groin taping**
   1. Restriction of motion required to provide adequate support decreases function.
   2. Recommend use of elastic wraps in a figure-of-eight pattern about the waist and upper thigh or neoprene thigh sleeves.

H. **Medial or lateral knee taping**
   1. Common indications: collateral ligament sprain.
   2. Materials: 1½ inch or 2 inch cloth tape, or 3 inch elastic tape.
   3. Athlete position: standing with knee flexed about 15° by placing 1½ inch to 2 inch block under athlete's heel.
   4. **Technique for medial knee injuries** (Fig. 3):
      a. Place anchor strips about the mid-thigh and mid-calf.
      b. Criss-cross strips in an "X" pattern, creating a fan across the medial aspect of the knee.
      c. Repeat anchors to close, taking care to not restrict circulation.
      d. Cut the area posteriorly over the calf and close the gap.
   5. **Technique for lateral knee injuries:** modified to provide lateral support.

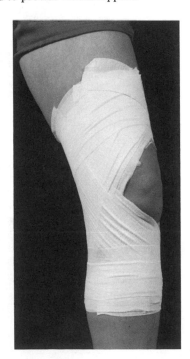

**FIGURE 3.** Medial knee taping.

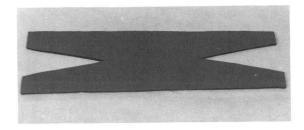

**FIGURE 4.** Neoprene support for ACL taping.

I. **Anterior cruciate ligament (ACL) knee taping**[32]
   1. Common indications: ACL sprains, functional support following reconstructive surgery.
   2. Materials: 3 inch elastic tape, 1½ inch cloth tape, four-tailed neoprene rubber support (15 inch × 6 inch with 5 inch × 3 inch cutouts [Fig. 4])

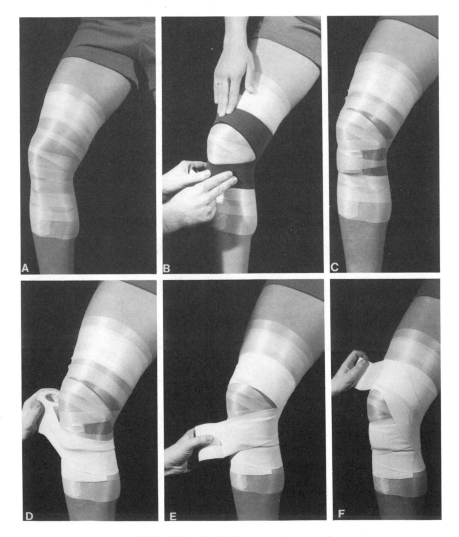

**FIGURE 5.** *A–F,* ACL taping *(continued).*

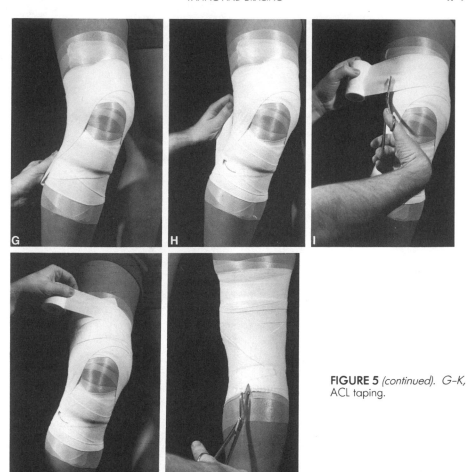

**FIGURE 5** (continued). G–K, ACL taping.

3. Athlete position: same as medial knee taping.
4. Technique based on "Duke Simpson" knee strapping[31]; limits hyperextension (Fig. 5).[26]
   a. Shave skin, apply tape adherent, and underwrap (Fig. 5A).
   b. Place neoprene support in the popliteal space (Fig. 5B).
   c. Neoprene support covered by underwrap (Fig. 5C).
   d. Apply circumferential anchor about the calf, revolving laterally, then upward across the lateral joint line (Fig. 5D).
   e. Apply circumferential anchor about the thigh, then downward across the medial joint line (Fig. 5E).
   f. Revolve about the calf, then upward across the medial joint line again, forming a medial "X" and covering the neoprene support (Fig. 5F).
   g. Revolve about the thigh, then downward across the lateral joint line, completing a lateral "X" (Fig. 5G).
   h. Revolve about the calf, then upward and posteriorly, enclosing the popliteal space (Fig. 5H); circulation is not compromised due to padding provided by the neoprene support.

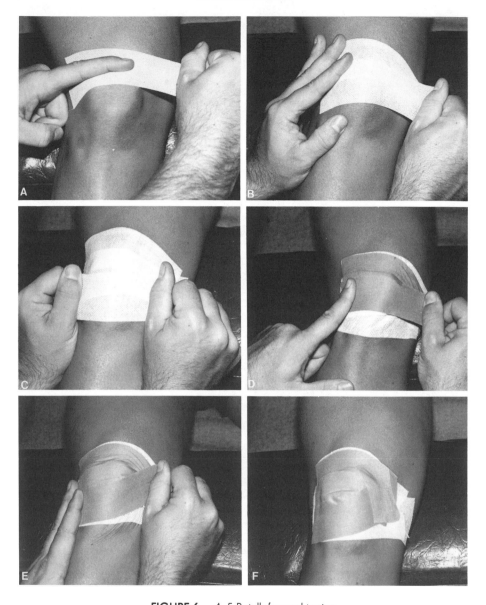

**FIGURE 6.**   *A–F,* Patellofemoral taping.

    i.  Apply circumferential anchor about the thigh and cut the tape (Fig. 5I).

    j.  Apply cloth tape anchors about the thigh and calf (Fig. 5J).

    k.  Cut the area posteriorly over the calf and close the gap with cloth tape (Fig. 5K).

    l.  Neoprene support may be reused by removing the taping strip by strip

 J.  **Patellofemoral taping**[19] (Fig. 6).

    1.  Common indications: patellofemoral pain syndromes, patellar tendinitis.

    2.  Materials: Hypafix,* Sports Tape,* Skin-prep wipes.

---

\* Hypafix (2″ roll, #4209) and Sports Tape (1½″ roll, #1853A) available from Don Joy Co., 5966 LaPlace Court, Carlsbad, CA, 92008, 1-800-228-4421.

3. Athlete position: knee slightly flexed, may vary depending on athlete's symptoms.
4. Technique
   a. Shave hair from anterior aspect of knee, clean with Skin-prep.
   b. Apply three strips of Hypafix.
      i. Starting laterally, place first strip over proximal half of patella, pushing knee cap distally, pulling medially and puckering the skin (Fig. 6A).
      ii. Starting more laterally, place second strip over middle of patella, pulling patella medially and tilting medial edge downward, again puckering the skin (Fig. 6B).
      iii. Apply third strip over distal half of patella (Fig. 6C).
   c. Apply three strips of Sports Tape
      i. First and second strips are applied similarly as Hypafix strips (Fig. 6D).
      ii. Starting laterally, place third strip over inferior pole of patella, rotating it medially and superiorly (Fig. 6E).
      iii. Apply optional anchor strip over all three previous strips, again pulling medially (Fig. 6F).
K. **Ankle taping** (Fig. 7)
   1. **Most researched taping procedure.**[20]
      a. Restricts extreme ranges of motion.
      b. Does not increase the incidence of knee injuries or affect athletic performance.
      c. Protective effect of taping due to increased proprioceptive input.
      d. Prevents reinjury to ankles previously injured.
      e. Some benefit provided by reusable cloth ankle wrapping[12] or high-top shoes.[17]
   2. Common indications: prevention or treatment of ankle sprains; subluxing peroneal tendons and dorsal impingement by using appropriate padding.
   3. Materials: 1½ inch or 2 inch cloth tape, foam/felt as needed.
   4. Athlete position: sitting on table, knee extended, ankle at a right angle of plantarflexion/dorsiflexion and neutral inversion/eversion.
   5. Technique: specific application can be adapted by the experienced taper to achieve goal.
      a. Shave skin and apply lubricated heel and lace pads (Fig. 7A).
      b. Place foam or felt padding for specific purposes.
         i. "J" pad posterior and distal to the lateral malleolus for subluxation of the peroneal tendons (Fig. 7B)
         ii. In cases of anterior ankle impingement, use a square "dorsal block" pad on the lace area to restrict dorsiflexion in cases of anterior impingement (Fig. 7C)
         iii. "Horseshoe," "U," or "donut" pad about malleolus to place compression to the swelling of subacute injuries (Fig. 7D).
      c. Apply tape adherent and underwrap (Fig. 7E); underwrap may be omitted to provide additional support, especially to more acute injuries, but special care of the skin is required.
      d. Closed basketweave, basic to most applications.
         i. Apply anchor strips around the calf at the level of the musculotendinous junction of the gastrocsoleus and around the arch proximal to the base of the fifth metatarsal (Fig. 7F).
         ii. Apply a "stirrup" strip, starting medially on the calf anchor medially, passing beneath the heel posterior to the malleoli, pulling laterally to the other side of the calf anchor (Fig. 7G); in eversion sprains, the stirrup is placed with equal tension medially and laterally.

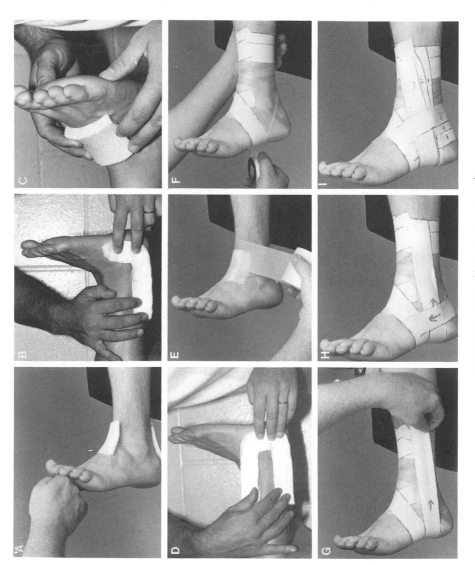

**FIGURE 7.** *A-I,* Ankle taping *(continued).*

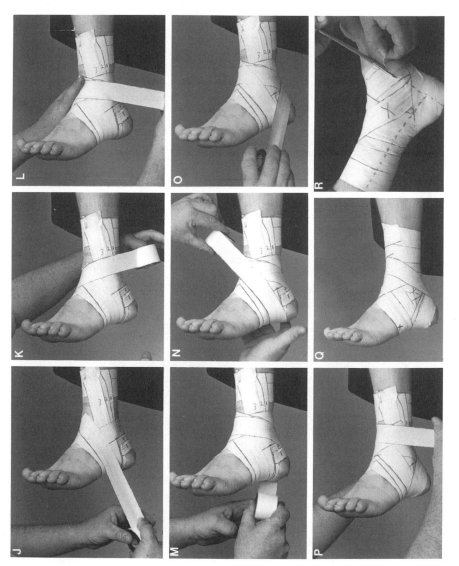

**FIGURE 7** *(continued).* *J-R,* Ankle taping.

       iii. Apply a "horseshoe" perpendicular to the stirrup, distal to the malleoli, starting and finishing on the arch anchor (Fig. 7H).

       iv. Repeat stirrups and horseshoes twice more, overlapping the previous strip by one-half, completing the "basketweave" (Fig. 7I).

    e. "Figure-of-eight" to restrict plantarflexion

       i. Apply tape on outside of the foot and angle under the foot (Fig. 7J).

       ii. Cross over the lace area and encircle the leg (Fig. 7K).

    f. "Heel locks" to restrict inversion/eversion.

       i. Medial heel lock restricts inversion.

         (a) Apply tape on lace area (Fig. 7L).

         (b) Angling behind and across the medial aspect of the heel (Fig. 7M).

         (c) Continue under the heel and return to the lace area (Fig. 7N).

       ii. Lateral heel lock restricts eversion.

         (a) applied in the opposite direction, angling across the lateral aspect of the heel (Fig. 7O).

       iii. Heel locks repeated to obtain desired support.

       iv. Circular strips are placed about the lower leg, overlapping distal to proximal, to cover remaining open spaces (Fig. 7P).

    g. Repeat anchors to close (Fig. 7Q).

    h. Taping removed by cutting along the medial aspect, posterior to the medial malleolus (Fig. 7R).

L. **Arch figure-of-eight** (Fig. 8)

  1. Common indications: arch sprains, conditions resulting from excessive pronation.

  2. Materials: 1 inch or 1½ inch tape.

  3. Athlete position: Same as ankle taping.

  4. Technique

    a. Perspiration of the soles of the feet requires elimination of the use of underwrap.

    b. Apply anchor strip loosely around the metatarsal heads (Fig. 8A); allow for expansion of the foot upon weightbearing.

    c. Apply a half figure-of-eight, starting at the base of the great toe, angling across the longitudinal arch, around the heel, and returning to the base of the great toe (Fig. 8B).

    d. Apply the other half figure-of-eight, starting at the base of the little toe, angling across the longitudinal arch, around the heel, and returning to the base of the little toe (Fig. 8C).

    e. Repeat steps c. and d. once or twice more (Fig. 8D).

    f. Apply horizontal strips, pulling medially, from the heel to the ball of the foot (Fig. 8E).

    g. Apply a "low dye" strip[33] starting at the base of the little toe, passing behind the heel, and ending at the base of the great toe (Fig. 8F).

    h. Close by applying a half anchor dorsum of the foot over the original anchor (Fig. 8G).

M. **Achilles tendon taping** (Fig. 9)

  1. Common indications: strain of the gastrocsoleus/Achilles tendon, Achilles tendinitis.

  2. Materials: 3 inch elastic tape, 1½ inch or 2 inch cloth tape (optional).

  3. Athlete position: prone with ankle plantarflexion.

  4. Technique

    a. Apply anchors around the arch of the foot and the calf (Fig. 9A).

    b. Apply support strips, repeat as needed; may use any of the following alternatives:

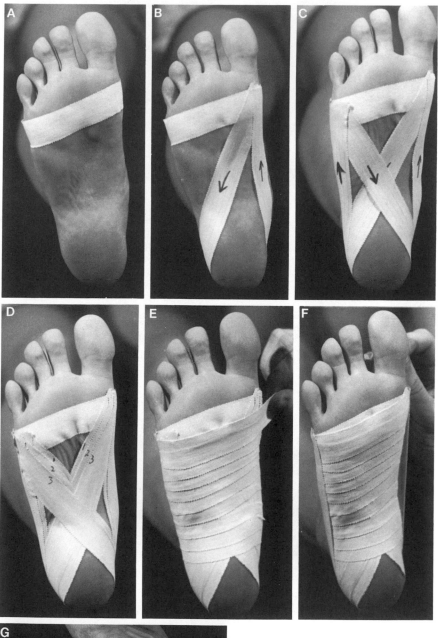

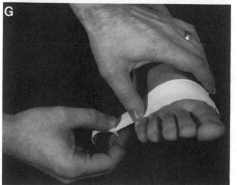

**FIGURE 8.** *A–G,* Arch figure-of-eight.

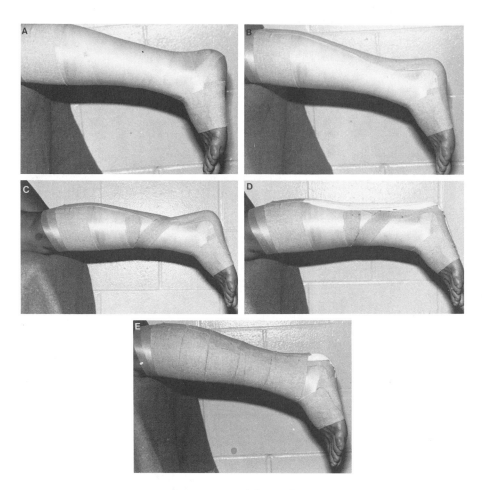

**FIGURE 9.** *A–E,* Achilles tendon taping.

      i. Start from the foot anchor, pull proximally to end at the calf anchor (Fig. 9B).

      ii. Start from the foot anchor, pull proximally, split tape in half to achieve better attachment to the anchors (Fig. 9C).

      iii. Using cloth tape, fan strips from the calcaneus to achieve greater support (Fig. 9D).

    c. Close applying circular strips about the foot and calf (Fig. 9E).

N. **Turf-toe taping** (Fig. 10)

    1. Common indications: sprains of the first metatarsophalangeal joint and sesamoiditis, using appropriate padding.

    2. Materials: 1 inch tape, felt/foam (optional).

    3. Athlete position: same as ankle taping, positioning great toe in direction opposite of injury.

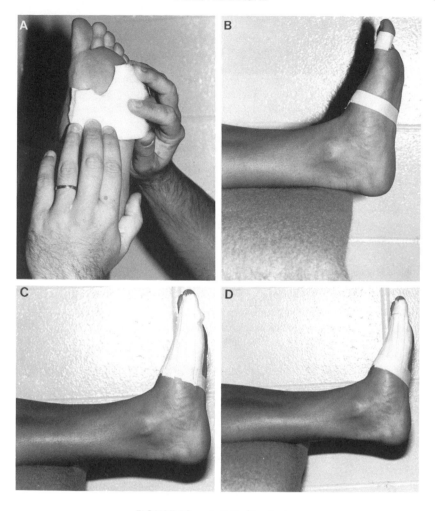

**FIGURE 10.** *A–D,* Turf-toe taping.

4. Technique.
   a. Place metatarsal pad with cut-out for base of first metatarsal for sesamoiditis (Fig. 10A).
   b. Apply anchor strips about the mid-arch of the foot and about the proximal phalanx of the great toe (Fig. 10B).
   c. Apply support strips from the distal anchor to the proximal; dorsal strips restrict flexion, ventral strips restrict extension (Fig. 10C).
   d. Repeat anchors to close (Fig. 10 D).

VI. **Bracing**

   A. **Comparisons of bracing to taping**
      1. **Advantages of bracing**
         a. Braces do not require a skilled individual to be applied.
         b. Sometimes more cost effective.
         c. Increased convenience.
         d. Unique means of support not provided by taping.

2. Disadvantages of bracing
   a. Migration of braces during active use.
      i. Failure to provide support.
      ii. May lead to decreased performance.
      iii. Migration may be reduced by use of tape adherent, or specially designed straps or undergarments.
   b. Athletes commonly complain about the weight of some braces required to provide adequate protection.
   c. Brace parts wear out or may break, requiring untimely replacement.
   d. Athlete may be between sizes of OTC braces.
   e. Custom-made braces are more expensive and require time to be fabricated.

B. **Considerations of brace prescription**
   1. **Brace market full of unsubstantiated claims and disclaimers of liability.**
   2. **Need to be knowledgeable about and critically evaluate new devices.**
   3. **Often need to evaluate a currently used or "borrowed" device.**
   4. **Brace-related problems** (e.g., skin irritation, altered function) need appropriate attention.
   5. **Discuss options with treatment team.**

VII. **Selected Braces**

A. **Tennis elbow "counter-force" strap** (Fig. 11)
   1. Common indications: lateral epicondylitis, medial epicondylitis (less often).
   2. Description: OTC Velcro and elastic strap placed on proximal forearm, designed to reduce contractile force of wrist and finger extensors.[21]
   3. Application and usage: worn during activities (sport or nonsport) that aggravate condition.

B. **Silicone rubber wrist/hand cast** (Fig. 12)
   1. Common indications: hand and wrist injuries requiring immobilization to participate in contact or collision sports, e.g., moderate sprains, healing nondisplaced or internally fixated fractures. Physician decides if injury can be adequately supported by silicone casting.
   2. Description: custom-made.[5,9]
   3. Application and usage: Splint is univalved and secured by tape; bivalved cast maintains immobilization when not actively participating in sport.

C. **Lateral prophylactic knee braces** (Fig. 13)
   1. Common indications: decrease incidence and severity of valgus force injuries to the knee; most commonly used in football.
   2. Description: OTC hinged single lateral upright or hinged double upright device taped or otherwise strapped to the knee.

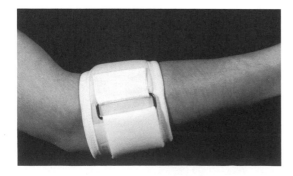

**FIGURE 11.** Tennis-elbow counter-force brace.

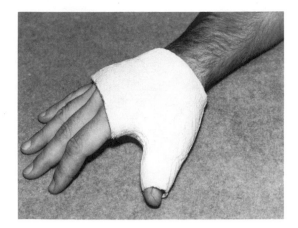

**FIGURE 12.** Silicone rubber wrist/hand cast.

   3. Application and usage
     a. Brace migration prevention
       i. Shave the skin, as for taping.
       ii. Use tape adherent.
     b. Maximal effectiveness requires team approach.
       i. Use of audio-visual aids (i.e., video tapes, posters) supplied by manufacturers to teach players proper application and daily reminders.
       ii. Daily check of positioning by coaches and trainers.
       iii. Weekly check on upkeep by the coaches, parents, equipment managers, trainers, and players.
     c. **Effectiveness debatable.**[1,2,7,10,11,13–15,22,25,27,30]

D. **Functional knee braces** (Fig. 14)
   1. Common indications: mild/moderate instability or post-reconstructive surgery of moderate/severe instability.
   2. Description: various designs utilizing hinged double uprights with range-of-motion stops, straps, and/or fitted cuffs or shells; some OTCs, but most are custom-fitted; many utilize a neoprene sleeve undergarment.
   3. Application and usage
     a. Migration and fit can be a problem (see lateral prophylactic knee braces).
     b. Exposed metal must be covered in contact-sport applications.
     c. Some studies have investigated the relative effectiveness of these braces.[4,10]

E. **Knee sleeves** (Fig. 15)
   1. Common indications: conservative management of many knee-pain complaints resulting from acute or chronic inflammation, including strains, cartilage tears, and patellofemoral problems; may be used postoperatively for effusion control.
   2. Description: OTC elastic or neoprene pull-over sleeve.
   3. Application and usage
     a. Easily acquired and accepted.
     b. Neoprene support increases sense of warmth and comfort.
     c. Athletes with patellofemoral problems usually require use of sleeve with a patellar cut out.
     d. Report of increased stability probably due to increased proprioceptive input.
     e. Similar braces with hinges rarely provide additional support.
     f. **Similar devices available for other areas of the body—forearm, wrist, calf, thigh.**

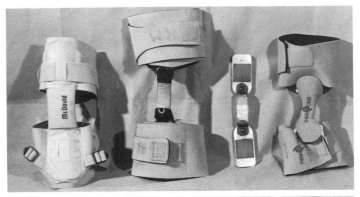

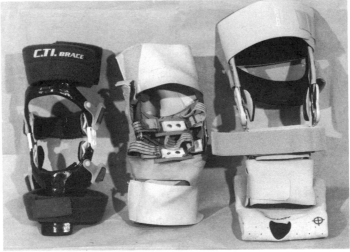

**FIGURE 13.** *(top)*  Examples of lateral prophylactic knee braces.

**FIGURE 14** *(bottom)*.   Examples of functional knee braces.

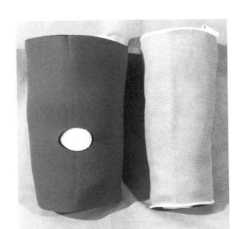

**FIGURE 15.**  Knee sleeves, neoprene (left) and elastic (right).

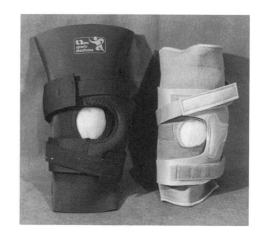

**FIGURE 16.** Palumbo braces, neoprene (left) and elastic (right).

F. **Palumbo lateral patella stabilizing brace** (Fig. 16)
1. Common indications: conservative or postoperative management of patellofemoral joint problems.
2. Description: OTC elastic or neoprene knee sleeve with patellar cut out and a "Y"-shaped lateral buttress strap to dynamically decrease excessive lateral patellar tracking.[18,22]
3. Application and usage
   a. Usually place counterbalancing strap superiorly.
   b. Cases of infrapatellar tendinitis may be aided by inferior placement of the counterbalancing strap.
   c. Cases of medial patellar subluxation (rare) may be aided by medial positioning of the buttress strap.
G. **Ankle braces**
1. Common indications: healed/healing ankle sprains or fractures; tendinitis about the ankle.
2. Description, application, and usage
   a. **Slip-on elastic support** (Fig. 17) provides even compression to decrease edema; not a prophylactic support.[16]
   b. **Slip-on Spandex sleeve with elastic and Velcro straps** to restrict inversion/eversion (Fig. 18); good prophylactic support.

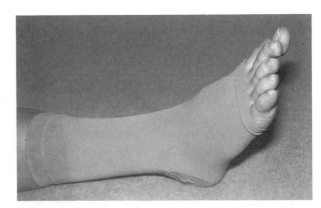

**FIGURE 17.** Slip-on elastic support.

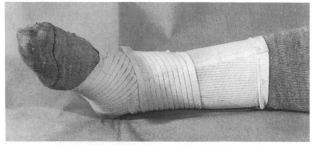

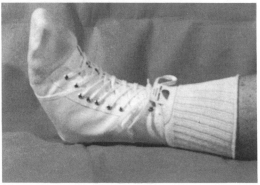

**FIGURE 18** *(top)*.   Slip-on Spandex sleeve with elastic and Velcro straps.

**FIGURE 19** *(bottom)*.   Lace-up ankle support.

   c. **Lace-up ankle support** (Fig. 19) uses medial and lateral stays to restrict inversion/eversion; best alternative to ankle taping[6]; may be used as a prophylactic or functional support.

   d. **Stirrup splints**—based on semirigid orthosis[28]; use Velcro straps to hold in place; designed for rehabilitative and functional uses.

      i. **Air Cast** (Fig. 20) uses adjustable air pressure linings to improve individual fit, decrease edema, and prevent excessive inversion/eversion.[29]

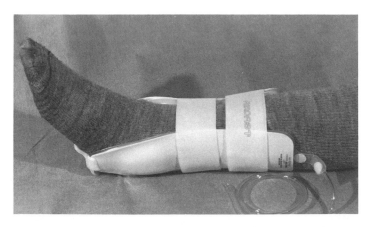

**FIGURE 20.**   Air cast with pressure adjustment tube attached.

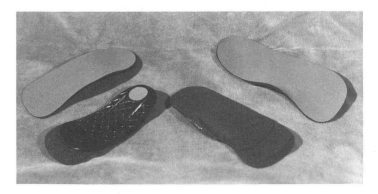

**FIGURE 21.** Spenco arch supports, rigid (left) and semi-rigid (right).

    ii. **Gel Cast** uses gel-filled linings to improve individual fit; can be placed in freezer to be used as one form of cryotherapy; holds in body heat for increased comfort with functional use.

    iii. Other devices use foam rubber linings or other materials; may be OTC or custom-made.

H. **Orthotics—devices placed in athlete's shoe to balance the foot during activity**

    1. Common indications: lower extremity kinetic chain conditions resulting from excessive pronation, cavus foot, or other foot dysfunctions.

    2. Description, application and usage

        a. **Soft orthotics** provide OTC and cheaper solution; easy break-in.

        b. **Hard orthotics** provide customized solution for road runners not involved in agility activities.

        c. **Semi-rigid orthotics** (Fig. 21) provide support of hard orthotics for athletes involved in agility sports.

        d. **Sorbothane viscoelastic insoles** (Fig. 22) reduce impact loading forces.

        e. **Heel cups** (e.g., Tuli's, Fig. 23) decrease impact and improve the shock absorption capabilities of the calcaneal fat pad.

        f. **Metatarsal arch pads** (Fig. 24) provide symptomatic relief of painful foot conditions; may be held in place with tape or glue or may be self-adhesive to the shoe.

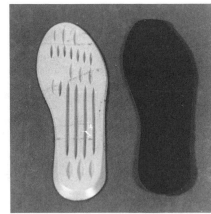

**FIGURE 22.** Sorbathane insoles.

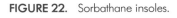

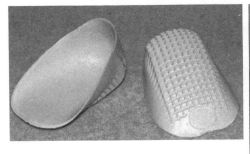

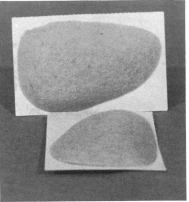

**FIGURE 23** *(left).* Tuli's heel cups.

**FIGURE 24.** *(right).* Metatarsal arch pads.

    g. **Longitudinal arch pads** (Fig. 25) provide symptomatic relief of painful foot conditions; may be held in place with tape or glue or may be self-adhesive to the shoe.

    h. **Steel shoe inserts** (Fig. 26) provide support to metatarsal fractures and "turf toe."

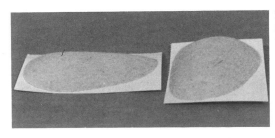

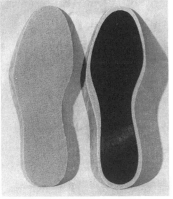

**FIGURE 25** *(left).* Longitudinal arch pads.

**FIGURE 26.** *(right).* Steel shoe inserts.

## REFERENCES

1. American Academy of Orthopaedic Surgeons Committee on the Knee: Prophylactic Knee Braces. Park Ridge, IL, AAOS, October 19, 1987.
2. Baker BE, VanHanswyk E, Bogosian S IV, et al: A biomechanical study of the static stabilizing effect of knee braces on medial stability. Am J Sports Med 15:556, 1987.
3. Bassett FH, Malone T, Gilcrist RA: A protective splint of rubber. Am J Sports Med 7:358, 1979.
4. Beck C, Drez D, Young J, et al: Instrumented testing of functional knee braces. Am J Sports Med 14:253, 1986.
5. Bradley JA: The modified rubber playing cast. Phys Sportsmed 10(11):168, 1982.
6. Bunch RP, Bednarski K, Holland D, Macinanti R: Ankle joint support: A comparison of reuseable lace-on braces with taping and bracing. Phys Sportsmed 13(5):59, 1985.
7. Cowell HR: College football: To brace or not to brace (editorial). J Bone Joint Surg 69A:1, 1987.
8. Distefano V, Nixon JE: An improved method taping. J Sports Med 2:209, 1974.
9. Doughtie M: The use of RTV-11 silicone rubber for a carpal navicular fracture. Athletic Training 14:146, 1979.
10. France EP, Paulos LE, Jayaraman G, et al: The biomechanics of knee bracing. Part II: Impact response of the braced knee. Am J Sports Med 15:430, 1987.

11. Functional knee braces help stabilize medial collateral ligament. Orthopedics Today 6(8):1, 1986.
12. Garrick JG, Requa RK: Role of external support in the prevention of ankle sprains. Med Sci Sports 5:200, 1973.
13. Grace TG, Skipper BJ, Newberry JC, et al: Prophylactic knee braces and injury to the lower extremity. J Bone Joint Surg 70A:422, 1988.
14. Hewson GF, Mendini RA, Wang JB: Prophylactic knee bracing in college football. Am J Sports Med 14:262, 1986.
15. Knee braces to prevent injuries in football: A round table. Phys Sportsmed 14(4):108, 1986.
16. Laughman RK, Carr TA, Chao EY, et al: Three-dimensional kinematics of the taped ankle before and after exercise. Am J Sports Med 8:425, 1980.
17. Libera D: Ankle taping, wrapping, and injury prevention. Athletic Training 7:73, 1972.
18. Lysholm J, Nordin M, Ekstrand J, Gilquist J: The effects of a patella brace on performance in knee extension strength test in patients with patellar pain. Am J Sports Med 12:110, 1984.
19. McConnell JS: The management of chondromalacia patellae: A long-term solution. Aust J Physiotherapy 32:215–223, 1986.
20. Metcalf GR, Denegar CR: A critical review of ankle taping. Athletic Training 18:121, 1983.
21. Nirschl RP: The etiology and treatment of tennis elbow. J Sports Med 2:308, 1974.
22. Palumbo PM: Dynamic patellar brace: A new orthosis in the management of patello-femoral disorders. A preliminary report. Am J Sports Med 9:45, 1981.
23. Paulos LE, France EP, Rosenbergy TD, et al: The biomechanics of knee bracing. Part I: Response of the valgus strains to loading. Am J Sports Med 15:419, 1987.
24. Peppard A: Thumb taping. Phys Sportsmed 10(4):139, 1982.
25. Prentice WE, Toriscelli T: The effects of lateral knee stabilizing braces on running speed and agility. Athletic Training 21:113, 1986.
26. Ross SE: The supportive effect of modified Duke Simpson strapping. Athletic Training 13:206, 1978.
27. Rovere GD, Haupt HA, Yates CS: Prophylactic knee bracing in college football. Am J Sports Med 15:111, 1987.
28. Stover C: A functional semirigid support system for ankle injuries. Phys Sportsmed 7(5):71, 1979.
29. Stover CN: Air stirrup management of ankle injuries in the athlete. Am J Sports Med 8:360, 1980.
30. Teitz CC, Hermanson BK, Kronmal RA, et al: Evaluation of the use of braces to prevent injury to the knee in collegiate football players. J Bone Joint Surg 69A:2, 1987.
31. Thorndike A: Athletic Injuries: Prevention, Diagnosis and Treatment. Philadelphia, Lea & Febiger, 1948.
32. Weber JE: Personal communication, 1987.
33. Whitesel J, Newell SG: Modified low-dye strapping. Phys Sportsmed 8(9):129, 1980.

# PART IV

# SPECIFIC SPORTS

## Chapter 44: Football

PATRICK E. CLARE, MD

*From the opening of college in September, in all sections of the country, to its close in June, football is the most potent factor in the moulding of spirit, in the making of men, and in the bringing them together in the democracy of a common cause in the collegiate life.*

– Fielding H. Yost, 1905

*Football is properly described as a contact sport but it can equally be described as a collision sport. I must remind you of the formula most of us learned in high school physics—$E = \frac{1}{2}M \times V^2$, in which E is the energy expended, M is mass or weight, and V is the velocity. We could conclude from this that the bigger athlete who moves faster must create more energy and thus hit harder—and in doing so may inflict or sustain injury in this delivery of energy.*

– O. Charles Olson, 1962

Football is a sport with a special role in American life. As early as 1905 Yost realized that its importance far exceeded the playing field experience of the athletes.[7] By 1962, Olson observed that bigger, faster, stronger athletes would "inflict or sustain" more injuries than those who had played before them.[2] With increasing television coverage in the last three decades, football has become a popular form of entertainment in most American homes. Playing football brings psychological, social, and, occasionally, economic rewards that often surpass the joy of participating in a team sport.

During the same time span, strength, speed, and agility-training techniques have improved; sports nutrition has become a recognized discipline; and athletes have discovered a variety of ergogenic aids, including anabolic steroids and growth hormone. Consequently, football players have become bigger, stronger, faster, and more frequently injured. Americans accept this pattern to be as natural as morning sunrise.

I. **Risk of Injury**

  A. **High school**
    1. Over 30,000 high schools field organized teams consisting of approximately 1.5 million athletes.
    2. Per-season injury estimates derived from existing studies range from 11% to 81%. "This represents nationally a minimum of 165,000 and more likely 300,000 to 1,215,000 young men sustaining football injuries each year—an epidemic that recurs each fall."[5]

  B. **College**
    1. National Collegiate Athletic Association (NCAA) Injury Surveillance System Data (Table 1):[3]
      a. Rated in terms of injuries/1000 athlete-exposures (AEs).

489

**TABLE 1.**   1988–1989 NCAA Total Injury Rates Per 1,000 Athlete Exposures*

| Sport | Years Sampled | Practice | Game | Combined Practice and Game |
|---|---|---|---|---|
| Spring football | 1 | 10.01 | 35.41 | 10.58 |
| Wrestling | 4 | 7.27 | 31.92 | 9.91 |
| Women's gymnastics | 4 | 7.11 | 20.62 | 8.27 |
| Women's soccer | 3 | 5.43 | 16.46 | 8.13 |
| Men's soccer | 3 | 4.35 | 19.31 | 7.63 |
| Football | 5 | 3.94 | 34.68 | 6.37 |
| Men's lacrosse | 4 | 3.87 | 15.38 | 5.99 |
| Men's ice hockey | 3 | 2.49 | 15.94 | 5.70 |
| Women's basketball | 1 | 4.56 | 9.35 | 5.62 |
| Men's gymnastics | 3 | 4.87 | 16.06 | 5.52 |
| Women's field hockey | 3 | 4.07 | 8.67 | 5.21 |
| Men's baskketball | 1 | 3.95 | 8.77 | 4.94 |
| Women's volleyball | 5 | 4.60 | 5.25 | 4.84 |
| Women's softball | 3 | 3.76 | 5.33 | 4.37 |
| Women's lacrosse | 3 | 3.62 | 6.82 | 4.28 |
| Baseball | 4 | 2.08 | 5.49 | 3.23 |

* Adapted from Dick RW: Football: 1989–90 NCAA Injury Surveillance System. Mission, KS, National Collegiate Athletic Association, 1990.

    b. Based on 551,684 athlete exposures at a cross-section of 82 schools distributed proportionally through all three divisions of college football.

    c. **Regular seasons:**
        i. Practice       3.94/1000
        ii. Games       34.68/1000
        iii. Combined   6.37/1000

    d. **Spring football:**
        i. Practice       10.01/1000
        ii. Spring games  35.41/1000
        iii. Combined   10.58/1000

    e. The spring practice injury rate is 2½ times greater than the regular season rate. Consequently, the NCAA shortened spring practice for Division I and II and eliminated contact for Division II starting in 1990. Division III doesn't hold spring practice.

    f. Injuries are considerably more frequent per athlete-exposure in preseason practices and scrimmages than in regular season and postseason practice and competition (Table 2). This observation indicates that special attention to proper warmup, stretching and athletic technique is warranted in the preseason.

**TABLE 2.**   Preseason, Regular Season and Post-Season NCAA Football Injury Rate Summary, 1988–89 and 1989–90*

| Period of Play | Exposures | Injuries | Injuries per 1000 Athlete-exposures |
|---|---|---|---|
| Preseason | 357,051 | 2,934 | 8.22 |
| Regular season | 791,729 | 4,865 | 6.14 |
| Post-season | 10,799 | 59 | 5.46 |
| | 1,159,579 | 7,858 | 6.78 |

* Adapted from Dick RW: Football: 1989–90 NCAA Injury Surveillance System. Mission, KS, National Collegiate Athletic Association, 1990.

**TABLE 3.**   NCAA Injuries by Body Parts*

| Part | Injuries in 551,684 Athlete-exposures | Injuries per Athlete-exposure |
|------|---------------------------------------|-------------------------------|
| Knee | 755 | 1.37 |
| Ankle | 546 | .99 |
| Upper leg | 418 | .76 |
| Shoulder | 410 | .74 |
| Pelvis, hips, groin | 222 | .40 |
| Neck | 190 | .34 |
| Head | 170 | .31 |
| Lower back | 162 | .29 |
| Lower leg | 154 | .28 |
| Ribs | 69 | .13 |
| Fingers | 57 | .10 |
| Elbow | 55 | .10 |

* Adapted from Dick RW: Football: 1989–90 NCAA Injury Surveillance System. Mission, KS, National Collegiate Athletic Association, 1990.

    g. The knee, ankle, upper leg, and shoulder are the most frequently injured body parts (Table 3).

    h. The offense has a higher injury rate than the defense. Running backs, flanker/wide receivers, and tight ends are most likely to be injured on offense; and linebackers and cornerbacks on defense.[4]

    i. 8–9% of injuries are season-ending.

    j. The injury rate on natural playing surfaces is lower than on artificial turf (Table 4).

## II. Head Injuries (See also Chaps. 25, 26 and 31)

    A. **Cerebral concussion**—characterized by transient impairment of the level of consciousness. Usually associated with blurred vision, and loss of equilibrium and memory.

        1. **First-degree concussion**

            a. Presents with slight disorientation and dizziness without loss of consciousness, equilibrium, or memory.

            b. Athlete not to return to competition until fully alert without headache or dizziness.

**TABLE 4.**   NCAA Injury Rates by Playing Surface 1984–85 Thru 1989–90 Seasons*

| Surface | Exposures | Injuries | Injuries per 1000 Athlete-exposures |
|---------|-----------|----------|-------------------------------------|
| Combined practice and games: | | | |
| Natural | 2,383,797 | 14,560 | 6.11 |
| Artificial | 598,054 | 4,723 | 7.90 |
| Totals | 2,981,851 | 19,283 | 6.47 |
| Game only: | | | |
| Natural | 169,176 | 5,772 | 34.12 |
| Artificial | 61,825 | 2,416 | 39.08 |
| Totals | 231,001 | 8,188 | 35.45 |

* Adapted from Dick RW: Football: 1989–90 NCAA Injury Surveillance System. Mission, KS, National Collegiate Athletic Association, 1990.

2. **Second-degree concussion**
   a. Presents with loss of consciousness from 20 seconds to 1–2 minutes followed by some disorientation and mild amnesia.
   b. These players forget football plays and signals.
   c. These players usually do not return to competition the day of the injury.
   d. Neurological consultation is reasonable here before returning to play.
3. **Third-degree concussion**
   a. These players exhibit prolonged loss of consciousness and disorientation, and a severe brain injury must be ruled out.
   b. Should be observed closely and if any question or change occurs, neurological evaluation is necessary.
   c. Repeated episodes are grounds for removing the athlete from football permanently.
   d. Neurological evaluation is mandatory before resuming sports participation after the initial recovery.

B. **Cerebral contusion and intracranial hemorrhage** From the early 1960s to the mid-1970s the incidence of severe head injuries declined as the protective capabilities of the modern football helmet improved. However, the head is still a very commonly injured body part in NCAA football.
   1. These are severe brain injuries and require hospitalization and observation.
   2. Prolonged unconsciousness is common.
   3. Temporary confusion and amnesia are common, plus personality and intellectual changes may occur.
   4. These are medical emergencies characterized by neurological deterioration; therefore, speedy neurological evaluation is necessary.
   5. Emergency resuscitation measures are often necessary, since they can be career-ending and life-threatening injuries.

C. **Summary**
   1. Treat all head injuries in football as serious.
   2. Observe closely for any sign of brain dysfunction or deterioration.
   3. Establish and maintain an airway if necessary.
   4. Rule out spine or other regional injury.
   5. Seek medical attention if there is any evidence of cerebral deterioration.
   6. Evaluate football helmets for defects regularly.

III. **Cervical Spine Injuries** (See also Chaps. 17 and 31)

Helmet improvements that led to a decrease in head injuries also led to the ". . . development of playing techniques that used the top of the crown of the helmet as the initial point of contact and . . . [t]hese head-first techniques placed the cervical spine at risk for serious injury."[6] By 1976 the negative effects of these techniques led the NCAA and the National Federation of High School Athletic Associations (NFHSAA) to adopt rules prohibiting players from using the top of the helmet to strike another player. Thus, the practices of butting, ramming and "spearing" (using the helmet deliberately to punish an opponent) were banned.[1,6]

A rule is only as good as the officials, coaches, and players make it. To reduce cervical spine injuries, officials must enforce the rule against head-first contact, coaches must teach safe playing techniques, and players must be smart enough to avoid butting, ramming, and spearing. During the 1989–90 NCAA football season, 14% of injuries reported were described as a direct result of impact from a helmet.[4]

A. **Cervical strain (nonradicular)**
   1. Results in mechanical overload from a force greater than the neck can withstand, with tearing of cervical musculature.

2. Characterized by pain, tenderness, decreased range of motion, and spasm.
3. Treatment includes rest, heat, anti-inflammatory agents and physical therapy.

B. **Cervical strain (radicular).** Common in linemen and linebackers.

1. Usually secondary to a blow to the side of head; places muscles and plexus structures on stretch.
2. Brachial plexus or nerve root stretching injury, also known as "burner" or "stinger," may lead to upper extremity symptoms including numbness to transient paralysis.
3. Rehabilitation includes rest, immobilization, anti-inflammatories, muscle relaxants, plus therapy modes.
4. Cervical collar and support to prevent extremes of cervical motion can help.
5. In the off-season, neck strengthening is important.
6. Football players should be taught not to spear or head butt.
7. Avoid any devices on the equipment that flexes the cervical spine.

C. **Return-to-play after cervical injury**

1. Little or no pain with full active range of motion.
2. Absence of paresthesias or tingling in the extremities.
3. Normal neurological status in the extremities.
4. Normal cervical spine x-rays.

D. **Fractures and/or dislocations of the cervical spine**

1. These are more serious injuries because of the increase in spinal instability and chance of nerve or spinal cord injury.
2. Usually the result of compression in slight flexion and to a lesser degree compression and extension of the cervical spine.
3. Each patient must be assessed for neurological deficit or sign of cervical instability.
4. Appropriate measures must be taken to stabilize the spine and patient until full assessment is accomplished, including indicated x-rays.
5. Leave the football helmet on until the neck can be supported and protected before removing it.
6. A Philadelphia collar or like device is useful to protect the cervical spine at this stage.
7. It is important to teach tacklers, blockers, and ball carriers not to flex or duck their head upon contact and to avoid spearing and butting.

IV. **Shoulder Injuries** (See also Chap. 34)

A. **Clavicle fractures**

1. Common fracture secondary to a direct blow to the clavicle.
2. More common in younger athletes.
3. Basically treated by nonoperative means with a figure-of-eight strap and requires 6 to 8 weeks to heal.
4. Surgical treatment is rarely indicated.
5. Special padding under shoulder pads on return to play.

B. **Sternoclavicular separation**

1. Separation of the clavicle/sternal junction in varying degrees of severity and direction. More dangerous if clavicle is dislocated posteriorly.
2. Usually a closed reduction with sling and rest time will suffice.
3. Operative treatment rarely indicated and then in chronic, symptomatic, unstable cases.

C. **Acromioclavicular separation**

1. Separation of the clavicle from the acromion and in varying degrees of severity.
2. Local tenderness at the acromioclavicular joint with variable deformity.
3. X-rays with and without weights are helpful for a more definitive diagnosis.

4. Treatment ranges from sling and rest for the lesser grade injury to surgical repair for the more severe separation.
5. There are varying opinions on surgical indications, procedures, and timing.
6. Acromioclavicular pad should be worn under shoulder pads after an A-C joint injury (see Fig. 4).

D. **Glenohumeral subluxation and dislocations**
1. Common joint instability, with over 95% involving the anterior direction.
2. Initial injury requires reduction of the dislocation, whereas a subluxation (partial dislocation) reduces spontaneously.
3. Primary injuries are treated with immobilization and then rehabilitation and strengthening before returning to sporting activities.
4. Recurrence of either is extremely high in those under 20 years of age and surgical repair is then necessary.
5. Strengthening measures have had some success in preventing recurrences.
6. Reduction of a dislocation requires some experience and should not be done until neurovascular evaluation is completed.
7. As a rule, 3 weeks of immobilization is reasonable time with an initial injury, during which the arm is internally rotated and strapped across the abdomen chest.
8. Limitation straps are available to wear when playing and help prevent dislocation but also restrict effectiveness of the arm.
9. Surgical repair is successful without recurrence in over 97% of cases.
10. Surgical repair of this injury in a thrower (passer, pitcher) is risky and can markedly restrict his ability to throw permanently.

E. **Rotator cuff injuries**
1. Biceps tendinitis and rotator cuff impingement occur in football players, especially associated with weight training, throwing, and local injury.
2. Glenohumeral instability is also a contributing factor.
3. Symptoms include local tenderness, painful range of motion, especially abduction, plus a catching sensation with shoulder movement.
4. Treatment includes rest, anti-inflammatory medications, and rehabilitative exercises.
5. Unresponsive cases require more extensive evaluation, including arthrograms or MRI studies. Arthroscopy is a helpful tool, during which one can remove torn tissue, loose fragments, and decompress chronic impingement in this fashion.

F. **Blocker's exostosis *(myositis ossificans)*** (See also Chap. 29)
1. Local pain and tenderness at the lateral aspect of the arm (humerus) secondary to a local blow to an unprotected area.
2. X-rays confirm the bony prominence on the humerus.
3. Local padding is usually sufficient, but occasionally surgical excision is necessary.
4. The recurrence rate is high.

V. **Elbow Injuries** (See also Chap. 35)

A. **Hyperextension injuries**
1. Usually involves a fall on the outstretched elbow-arm or another player landing on the extended elbow.
2. Range of motion may be limited initially and x-rays necessary to rule out fracture.
3. Rest and ice followed by range of motion exercises are usually sufficient.
4. Bracing or supports to restrict hyperextension are helpful.

B. **Dislocation**
1. Dislocation of the radial ulnar joint posteriorly on the humerus is most common.
2. Fractures and neurovascular injury may be associated, so x-ray and clinical evaluation of the hand and forearm are important.

3. Closed reduction with forward or anterior pull of the forearm on the flexed elbow is usually successful.
4. Immbolization in flexion for 2 to 3 weeks before resuming rehabilitative measures.
5. Return of full extension can take several weeks but will usually respond to active stretching and strengthening.

C. **Fractures other than strains and sprains**
1. X-rays of the elbow are indicated.
2. Displaced fractures including intra-articular fractures, epicondylar fractures, and fractures of the radial head usually require surgical fixation.
3. Undisplaced fractures are splinted or casted appropriately and require considerable lost playing time.

D. **Loose bodies**
1. The result of fragmentation of the articular (joint) cartilage or bone that becomes free bodies in the joint.
2. The player notes pain, catching, and locking of the joint.
3. Treatment usually requires surgical removal, and this can usually be done by arthroscopic means.

E. **Ulnar nerve palsy**
1. Ulnar nerve injury in football can be secondary to a local blow or strain or a throwing injury.
2. Symptoms include elbow pain medially to numbness/weakness over the ulnar nerve distribution of the hand (ring/little finger).
3. Treatment includes rest, splinting, oral anti-inflammatories, and occasionally corticosteroid injection.
4. If conservative care fails, then surgical transposition of the ulnar nerve is indicated.

VI. **Wrist Injuries** (See also Chap. 36)

A. **Sprains**
1. A ligament injury in which a fracture cannot be diagnosed even after repeat x-ray evaluation.
2. Treatment includes immobilization, ice, rest, and anti-inflammatories.

B. **Fractures**
1. **Scaphoid**
   a. **Acute fracture**
      i. Usually a hyperextension injury of the wrist characterized by radial pain and tenderness.
      ii. Diagnosis confirmed by x-ray.
      iii. Treatment by cast immobilization, including incorporation of the thumb in the cast plus a long-arm cast for the first 4–6 weeks, then a shorter thumb-spica cast until healed.
      iv. If initial x-rays are negative for fracture, treat the wrist injury as a fracture of the scaphoid and repeat the x-rays in 10–14 days before ruling out the fracture.
   b. **Nonunion of fracture**
      i. Result of nondiagnosis or nontreatment of an acute injury (fracture) or failure to heal.
      ii. Symptoms include chronic pain in the wrist, with local tenderness and decreased wrist range of motion.
      iii. Treatment is surgical, with autogenous bone grafting to the nonunion plus immobilization.
2. **Carpal avulsion fractures**
   a. Usually hyperextension injury with dorsal wrist pain, tenderness, and swelling.

      b. X-rays will reveal a bony fragment on the dorsum of the carpals.

      c. Treatment includes casting/splinting, and little playing time is lost.

  3. **Other carpal fracture-dislocations**

      a. These rare injuries include lunate, paralunate, and scaphoid fracture dislocations and are diagnosed by wrist deformity, limitation, and x-ray.

      b. These require reduction and frequently internal fixation.

      c. These are serious injuries that require considerable healing time.

VII. **Hand—Finger Injuries** (See also Chap. 36)

  A. **Tendon injuries**

    1. **Extensor injuries**

      a. **Distal joint**

         i. Avulsion of the extensor tendon from the distal phalanx with and without fracture results in a "mallet" or "drop" finger.

        ii. Distal phalanx is flexed and lacks active extension and may reveal a fracture fragment.

       iii. Continued splinting of the distal finger joint in extension for at least 6 weeks is necessary unless the fracture fragment involves a large portion of the articular surface of the joint, in which instance intervention is necessary.

      b. **Proximal joint**

         i. Avulsion of the central slip to the middle phalanx results in flexion deformity and can result in a boutonniere defect.

        ii. Splinting the finger proximal joint in extension for 6 weeks is necessary. Occasional surgical repair and reconstruction are required.

    1. **Flexor tendon injuries**

      a. **Distal joint**

         i. Avulsion of the profundus tendon of the distal phalanx of the finger or "Jersey finger."

        ii. Ring finger is most commonly involved and usually injured while tackling.

       iii. Surgical reattachment of the tendon is the treatment of choice.

       iv. Some athletes (college, professional) have chosen not to have surgery, since it would end their season, and defer to a later arthrodesis of the joint or no treatment at all.

  B. **Ligament injuries**

    1. **Metacarpophalangeal joint (thumb)**

      a. Ulnar collateral ligament is most commonly injured.

      b. Evaluation includes comparing collateral stability of the normal thumb, plus x-rays to rule out avulsion fracture from the proximal phalanx.

      c. Treatment ranges from cast immobilization to surgical repair, depending on the degree of laxity and ligament damage.

    2. **Interphalangeal joints**

      a. Dislocations are common and mostly in the dorsal direction, and deformity is obvious.

      b. X-rays are necessary to rule out fractures.

      c. Usually easily reduced and splinted for 3 weeks, with little playing time lost.

      d. Continuous buddy taping for support while playing.

  C. **Fractures**

    1. **Metacarpals**

      a. Local pain, swelling, tenderness, and deformity are usual, and fractures confirmed by x-ray evaluation.

b. A single metacarpal fracture can be splinted or casted, unless it is malrotated or shortened, for which internal fixation is necessary.

c. Two or more metacarpals are usually treated surgically unless undisplaced and stable.

2. **Phalanges**

a. Proximal phalangeal fractures require good reduction and frequently surgical fixation, especially if the joint is involved.

b. Middle phalanx requires less need for surgery unless joint is involved.

c. Distal phalangeal fractures, usually crush or tuft fractures, will heal by splinting. A hematoma beneath the finger nail may have to be relieved by placing a hole in the nail.

3. **Thumb**

a. Intra-articular fractures of the base of the thumb (Bennett's) require reduction, frequently internal fixation, and casting.

VIII. **Spine Injuries (Lumbar)** (See also Chap. 38)

A. **Low back strain**

1. Can be acute or chronic recurrent low back pain secondary to physical efforts.

2. Usually related to soft tissue tightness and muscle weakness.

3. Physical exam reveals spasm and tenderness in the lumbar spine with decreased flexibility.

4. X-rays are usually normal.

5. Treatment includes rest, analgesics, muscle relaxants, ice early and heat later, stretching, strengthening, and physical therapy.

B. **Low back pain with herniated nucleus pulposus**

1. A rare condition but must be considered when low back pain is associated with leg pain and/or paresthesias.

2. Exam may include some neurological changes (motor, sensory, or reflexes), plus abnormal straight leg raising.

3. Repeat conservative measures for low back strain, and if poor response, then further diagnostic investigation is warranted.

C. **Spondylolysis/spondylolisthesis**

1. A defect in the pars interarticularis of a vertebral body related to trauma in some form, including athletic trauma.

2. Usually local pain, unilateral, and without leg symptoms.

3. X-rays of the spine (oblique films) reveal a defect, and a lateral film may reveal displacement of one vertebrae on the other.

4. Bone scans are helpful after an injury to reveal acute or chronic abnormalities.

5. Spondylolisthesis or slippage of the vertebral body at the point of the defect can be of varying degree.

6. These young men may participate in sports if they are without pain.

7. Skeletally immature teens must be observed closely for progression of the slippage.

8. Conservative treatment of rest, physical therapy, stretching, and exercises may help.

9. Spinal fusion is the ultimate treatment if slippage progresses and/or the pain persists.

IX. **Chest and Upper Back** (See also Chap. 37)

A. **Rib fractures**

1. Local pain and tenderness after a blow to the chest; athlete may experience shortness of breath.

2. X-rays to confirm the diagnosis and rule out any lung involvement (pneumothorax).

3. If the x-ray is negative, then treatment with rest; protective flak jacket necessary for football.

B. **Scoliosis and kyphosis**
  1. These familial or congenital defects are usually treated in the adolescent teen years to correct spinal deformity.
  2. These conditions are not a contraindication to football and, in fact, some athletes can remove their braces for practice and playing time.
  3. Individuals who have undergone spinal fusion with internal fixation are disqualified to play football.

X. **Hip and Pelvis** (See also Chap. 39)

A. **Contusions and strains**
  1. **Hip pointer**
    a. The result of a direct blow to the anterior crest of the ilium producing soft tissue bleeding with secondary local pain and swelling.
    b. Marked local tenderness and restricted motion in the hip.
    c. Treatment includes immediate pressure, ice, rest. Occasionally, injecting a corticosteroid preparation may help, and then therapy to reinstitute motion and strength.
    d. This may be a slow-healing injury.
  2. **Osteitis pubis**
    a. Groin to lower abdominal pain that can radiate into the adductor region.
    b. Commonly secondary to heavy squats in the weight room.
    c. Exam reveals tenderness over the symphysis pubis and resists abduction of the hips.
    d. X-rays may reveal widening and irregularity of the symphysis pubis.
    e. Treatment includes rest, anti-inflammatory medications, corticosteroid injections, plus stretching and strengthening exercises.

B. **Avulsion fractures**
  1. **Anterior/superior iliac spine avulsion**
    a. Sudden onset of pain with sprinting, cutting, or kicking can detach actual bone fragment from the anterior superior iliac spine by sudden muscle contracture. Most common during peak of growth spurt.
    b. X-rays reveal abnormality of the normal apophysis or displacement fragment of bone.
    c. Treatment includes rest and gradual increase in activities as symptoms lessen. Occasionally surgical repair is done for a large fragment.
  2. **Ischial tuberosity fracture**
    a. Sudden movement or stretching of the hamstrings can lead to an ischial tuberosity pain with local tenderness over the ischial tuberosity.
    b. X-rays reveal avulsion of the bony fragment in that area.
    c. Treatment ranges from protection of movements in minimal cases to rarely reported surgical repair in grossly displaced fragments.

C. **Stress fractures**
  1. Usually secondary to increased activity and overuse.
  2. Usually occurs distal to the hip in the proximal femur.
  3. Symptoms include pain with weight-bearing and range of motion, especially rotation.
  4. X-rays usually negative early, and a bone scan can be most helpful in diagnosis at that stage.
  5. Treatment includes rest to crutches until asymptomatic and then the x-rays are clear.

6. Do not allow these patients to run, jump, or stress the involved area if painful for fear of complete fracture.

D. **Dislocation of the hip**

1. A rare but serious injury that can risk the blood supply to the femoral head.
2. Posterior dislocation is more common than anterior dislocation.
3. Early reduction is important after assessing neurovascular status of the lower extremity.
4. Treatment includes immediate reduction, short-term light leg traction and partial weight-bearing for 6 weeks, and then rehabilitation.
5. Anterior dislocation is rare and the reduction can be difficult.

E. **Thigh injuries**

1. **Hamstring strain or "pull"**
   a. Sudden stretching of a tight hamstring muscle/tendon complex.
   b. Imbalance of hamstrings to quadriceps muscle ratio is usually a factor, as hamstring strength deficit is contributory.
   c. Exam reveals local pain and tenderness, with swelling acutely and even ecchymosis.
   d. Treatment includes crutches, ice and compression, with gentle stretching and strengthening of the hamstring muscles, including eccentric then isometric maneuvers.
   e. Return to competition after normal flexibility and normal quadriceps-hamstring ratio, bilateral strength, and power.

2. **Myositis ossificans**
   a. Secondary to deep contusion to the quadriceps from a local blow.
   b. Local swelling, tenderness, and x-ray evidence of calcification to ossification in the anterior thigh.
   c. Acutely apply ice, pressure with some gentle stretching but avoid massage, heat, ultrasound, corticosteroid injections, or vigorous active stretching of the quadriceps.
   d. Protect weight-bearing until full range of motion in the knee, especially flexion.
   e. After full, relatively painless range of motion, athlete can resume running and football but should protect the anterior thigh with adequate padding.

XI. **Leg and Knee Injuries** (See also Chaps. 40 and 41)

A. **Meniscal injuries**

1. Meniscal injuries occur secondary to twisting or rotation of the knee, but also deep flexion and hyperextension plus varus or valgus stresses can contribute.
2. Symptoms include pain, catching, recurrent effusions, clicking, and locking, with associated limited range of motion plus giving way.
3. Exam typically reveals a joint effusion, tenderness at the joint line, limited range of motion, and tenderness on attempted deep flexion, plus the inability to squat and a palpable click.
4. Regular x-rays are usually normal, whereas an MRI scan can be diagnostic, though can be over interpreted. Arthrograms can assist in the diagnosis, especially medially, though lateral views are less helpful.
5. Treatment includes initial rest, pressure, ice, anti-inflammatories, analgesics, and rehabilitation. If improvement is not occurring, then arthroscopy should be considered.
6. Repairable meniscal tears should be repaired, especially in younger patients.
7. Operative arthroscopy is usually done as an outpatient, with recovery in 3–4 weeks, depending on the type and extent of tear.

B. **Ligament injuries**
   1. **Medial collateral ligament sprains**
      a. Typically due to a lateral blow to the fixed leg and knee.
      b. The player frequently hears a pop and notes medial knee pain and a feeling of laxity.
      c. Exam reveals swelling, medial tenderness especially at the adductor tubercle and the joint line, plus laxity to valgus stress with the knee in a slightly flexed position.
      d. The knee is usually stable in full extension to valgus stress if the cruciate ligaments are intact.
      e. With the knee flexed 15–20 degrees, valgus stress will reveal displacement in varying gradations.
      f. If the knee reveals valgus laxity in full extension, then more severe damage is present, including cruciate ligament incompetence.
      g. Treatment includes aspiration, pressure wrap, ice, and immobilization to bracing. These injuries are usually successfully treated conservatively, though occasionally surgery may be indicated in the more severe laxities.
      h. Rehabilitation including range of motion, and strengthening is usually necessary to return a patient to football; I favor a double functional brace rather than a lateral stabilizer only.
   2. **Lateral collateral ligament sprains**
      a. Usually due to a medial blow to the knee, giving a varus sprain.
      b. Much less common than medial collateral ligament sprains.
      c. Patients complain of lateral pain and laxity.
      d. Evaluate the knee in full extension, then slight flexion, and note lateral laxity of varying degrees to the varus stress.
      e. Severe varus injuries can include can include peroneal nerve injuries that can be devastating.
      f. Treatment is similar to medial collateral ligament sprains.

---

**Points to Remember**

1. In evaluating ligament injuries, always compare the injured knee to the normal opposite knee.
2. X-rays are necessary to rule out epiphyseal fractures and osteochondral fractures, especially in the younger patient.
3. Always evaluate the neurovascular status of the leg and foot.
4. In the extremely unstable knee, beware of a knee dislocation.
5. Knee braces, while popular, have not proven to be effective in preventing knee ligament injuries.

---

   3. **Anterior cruciate ligament injuries**
      a. Typically a noncontact injury, whereby the player suddenly stops (decelerates) or cuts, notes a pop in the knee, a feeling of giving way, and subsequent onset of effusion.
      b. Exam indicates a moderate-to-severe effusion plus evidence of forward displacement of the tibia on the femur (Lachman's, anterior drawer tests).
      c. Lachman's test is done at 20 degrees of flexion and is more accurate than the anterior drawer test because of hamstring spasm restricting the latter.
      d. One may be able to demonstrate a pivot shift maneuver or tibial femoral subluxation that is definite evidence of anterior cruciate ligament deficiency.

    e. Approximately 50% of these knees are associated with meniscal damage.

    f. In the active, athletic, physically demanding individual, anterior cruciate ligament reconstructive surgery is indicated, whereas the more sedentary individual my be treated by nonsurgical means (rehabilitation and bracing).

    g. Repeated episodes of pivot shifting of the knee with the anterior cruciate ligament deficiency lead to secondary stabilizer laxity and further knee deterioration.

4. **Posterior cruciate ligament injuries**

    a. A less common injury and usually secondary to falling directly on the flexed knee or hyperextension injury.

    b. Pain, effusions, and meniscal injuries frequently associated.

    c. Not as common as anterior cruciate ligament injuries. Frequently can function athletically with the deficit.

    d. Generally with an isolated posterior cruciate ligament tear surgical treatment is unnecessary, whereas greater associated instability and laxity may require reconstructive procedure.

5. **Combined injuries**

    a. One may see more than one ligament injured and usually a more severe trauma is responsible.

    b. Thorough evaluation of joint instability is always required to assess ligament stability.

    c. Assessment commonly reveals anterior cruciate ligament deficiency with a collateral ligament injury and occasionally a posterior cruciate ligament-collateral ligament combination.

    d. These combination injuries almost always require surgical correction.

C. **Patella**

1. **Subluxation**

    a. Players experience episodes of pain, catching, giving way, with symptoms centering around the patella.

    b. Examination reveals local swelling, tenderness, hypermobility of the patella, plus varying degrees of malalignment, with apprehension to stressing of the patella.

    c. X-rays reveal varying degrees of patellar malposition and tilt.

    d. Conservative management includes patellar support or bracing plus quadriceps exercises and strengthening. If this does not suffice, then surgical treatment ranges from a lateral patellar release to surgical realignment of the patella.

2. **Dislocation**

    a. Complete displacement of the patella, to the lateral side of the knee, which requires reduction.

    b. Examination ranges from patellar hypermobility to lateral instability and apprehension. Acute dislocations reveal lateral patellar displacement.

    c. X-rays confirm obvious patellar displacement laterally or a normally positioned patella (reduced) with an effusion present, plus an osteochondral fracture fragment.

    d. Treatment includes immobilization in extension, plus strengthening and bracing. Recurrent dislocations require surgical stabilization.

3. **Anterior knee pain with chondromalacia of the patella**

    a. Patellar and parapatellar pain of a chronic nature.

    b. May experience additional symptoms of catching, giving way, and effusions.

    c. Symptoms are worsened with squatting, cramped sitting, and stairs.

    d. Examination reveals patellar tenderness and guarding, with crepitation on range of motion and positive apprehension.

     e. X-rays usually are negative or reveal mild patellar tilt.

     f. Treatment includes quadricep strengthening exercises, patellar sleeve support, anti-inflammatories, and appropriate ice and pressure after activities. Surgery may be necessary if symptoms persist.

  **4. Infrapatellar tendinitis (jumper's knee)**

     a. Complains of pain along the inferior pole or tip of the patella associated with physical activity.

     b. Tender locally at the inferior tip of the patella.

     c. X-rays are usually negative, though occasionally one may note bony reaction or calcifications along the tip of the patella inferiorly.

     d. Treatment includes local ice massage, rehabilitation, patellar supports, and anti-inflammatories.

**D. Femur—tibia (See also Chap. 41)**

  **1. Osteochondritis dissecans**

     a. Abnormality of blood supply secondary to trauma leading to a specific bony lesion, typically in the medial femoral condyle. If it does not heal, it can separate and eventually become a loose body.

     b. The majority of the cases involve the nonweight-bearing surface of the medial femoral condyle.

     c. The athlete is usually an adolescent and will complain of vague pain and occasionally catching.

     d. Examination reveals local tenderness to palpation and with deep flexion, plus effusions.

     e. X-rays, especially notch or tunnel view and lateral view, will reveal a characteristic bony defect in the medial femoral condyle and, in more advanced cases, a loose body.

     f. Treatment ranges from nonweight-bearing with crutches in adolescents to various surgical techniques to promote healing of the defect. These range from drilling a fixed defect to internal fixation to removal of a loose fragment.

  **2. Osgood-Schlatter disease**

     a. A condition of gradual, partial, and painful separation of the tibial tuberosity apophysis that is common in active adolescents and teenagers.

     b. These youngsters complain of anterior tibial tuberosity pain associated with sporting activities including football.

     c. Examination reveals a characteristic "bump" or prominence in the tibial tuberosity that is locally painful.

     d. X-rays confirm varying degrees of anterior displacement of the tibial tuberosity apophysis.

     e. Treatment is symptomatic and ranges from hamstring stretching and local pressure wraps plus padding. Surgery may be warranted when there are loose bodies or in older, skeletally mature patients..

     f. Cast and immobilizers are unnecessary and the youngster may continue to participate in athletics, with activity modification in extreme cases.

**E. Synovium**

  **1. Plica**

     a. A synovial fold present in 70–80% of individuals.

     b. A normal structure that can become symptomatic, including symptoms of pain, catching, and locking.

     c. Examination will frequently reveal local tenderness over the involved plica, which is usually to the medial side of the knee and above the joint line.

     d. Treatment ranges from rest and anti-inflammatory medications to arthroscopic excision of the abnormal symptomatic fold.

2. **Baker's cyst**
   a. A cystic swelling, fluid-filled in the popliteal region and to the medial side.
   b. May fluctuate in size, depending on an athlete's activity level.
   c. In over 50% of the cases, it is reflective of an abnormality within the joint that leads to increased fluid production, i.e., meniscal tear.
   d. Treatment ranges from rest, pressure, and ice to arthrogram investigation and arthroscopy of the knee joint.
   e. Cyst excision has recurrence rates of 15–20%, so one must be sure that nothing is abnormal intra-articularly. In juveniles and adolescents, cysts will usually resolve without excision.

F. **Leg**
1. **Shin splints (posterior tibial tendinitis)**
   a. Athletically associated medial leg pain in the distal one-half of the leg that is common in the early season; overuse and poor conditioning are common factors.
   b. Can be related to individuals with severe flat feet or pronation. These athletes will respond to orthotics, which balance the foot and relieve the soft tissue stresses on the medial aspect of the foot and leg.
   c. Examination reveals tenderness along the course of the posterior tibial muscle and tendon with normal neurovascular status.
   d. Treatment includes rest, anti-inflammatories, local ice, plus support to the medial foot and ankle.
   e. Must rule out a compartment syndrome or stress fracture if no improvement.

2. **Stress fracture**
   a. A cause of leg pain in any running athlete.
   b. Pain can be vague and fluctuates but is directly related to running and physical activity.
   c. Examination may reveal some local tenderness and occasionally swelling.
   d. X-rays may be negative or reveal a small lucent "dark" line, and in later cases one may see actual periosteal bone production.
   e. Bone scans are helpful if plain films are negative.
   f. Treatment includes rest and limited physical stresses and in time most will heal but may take a prolonged healing time.

3. **Compartment syndromes**
   a. The leg is divided into four compartments that contain specific muscles, nerves, and vessels (see p. 442).
   b. The compartments do not expand, and with either local trauma or exertion the compartment may become tensed secondary to swelling or bleeding.
   c. The patient will complain of pain and later can develop neurological deficits and muscles necrosis if the tight compartment is not relieved.
   d. Exam will reveal a tight, tense compartment to telltale hypesthesia and motor weakness in the foot.
   e. Measurements of compartment pressures are a relatively simple process, with values over 30 mm Hg abnormal.
   f. Treatment includes ice, rest, and close observation for increased swelling and pain, plus any neurological deficit, in which case surgical compartment release is necessary. This may be a surgical emergency in which prolonged observation and inaction can lead to irreversible muscle and nerve damage.

XII. **Ankle and Foot** (See also Chaps. 41 and 42)

A. **Ankle**
1. **Inversion sprains**

a. The most common ankle injury occurs with an inward rolling of the foot.

b. Most injuries are incomplete tears of the anterior talofibular ligament and reveal local tenderness and swelling anterolaterally on the ankle but are stable to anterior drawer and inversion stress testing.

c. X-rays should be done to rule out fractures, and one may see a small avulsion fracture.

d. Treatment includes pressure-wrapping and ice, plus rehabilitation for range of motion and avoiding inversion. Strapping and bracing are helpful for football activities.

e. If the acute injury reveals a positive anterior drawer test, the anterior talofibular ligament is torn and response will be slower. Similarly, if the patient exhibits inversion laxity to examination and stressing, then the calcaneofibular ligament may be torn. A double ligament tear can be treated by cast immobilization or surgical repair, with similar good results in either case. I prefer cast treatment in this situation.

f. Recurrent inversion sprains of a chronic nature lead to lateral laxity and require lateral ligament reconstructive surgery.

2. **Eversion sprains**

a. This injury is less common and involves internal rotation of the leg on the fixed foot, with resultant stresses and injury to the distal tibia and fibula relationship.

b. These can be more serious injuries, with separation of the tibia and fibula and tear of the deltoid ligament.

c. One must rule out displacement or diastasis of the ankle joint and mortice, which would require reduction, casting, or surgical repair. Again, x-ray evaluation is mandatory.

3. **Tendinitis**

a. **Achilles tendinitis**

i. Not uncommon in runners, including football players, with pain along the Achilles tendon.

ii. Examination reveals tenderness and swelling along the course of the Achilles tendon, with sometimes thickening, grating, and crepitation with painful motion.

iii. Treatment includes ultrasound, ice after activity, stretching of the tendon, plus a heel lift and anti-inflammatories. **Never inject a steroid preparation.**

b. **Peroneal subluxation**

i. Relatively rare football injury.

ii. Be suspicious of a lateral ankle injury with anterior pain, and posterior lateral malleolar discomfort too. The peroneal tendon may sublux from posterior to anterior.

iii. Treatment is operative, either acutely to repair the sheath or chronically to deepen the peroneal groove.

4. **Tibial talar spurring**

a. These spurs develop on the anterior lip of the tibia and neck of the talus from repetitive impingement between the tibia and the talus.

b. Exam may reveal restricted dorsiflexion of the foot and local tenderness.

c. X-rays will reveal prominent impingement spurs.

d. Treatment includes anti-inflammatories, rest, and strapping, and if symptoms persist, then surgical removal of the spurs is indicated.

B. **Foot**

1. **Turf toe**

a. A hyperextension injury (dorsiflexion) to the first metatarsophalangeal joint, usually on artificial turf.

     b. Can be temporarily disabling, with swelling, ecchymosis, tenderness, and decreased range of motion.

     c. X-rays are usually negative.

     d. Treatment includes rest, ice, anti-inflammatory medications, and a sole insert to stiffen the shoe forefoot. A single intra-articular corticosteroid injection to the MTP joint can be helpful in difficult cases.

     e. Semirigid metal plates ("turf toe plates") can be placed under the insole of the player's shoe to protect the toe against forced dorsiflexion.

  2. **Plantar fasciitis**

     a. Heel to plantar arch pain that is common in runners, including football players.

     b. Exam reveals some local tenderness in the plantar aspect of the heel or the arch.

     c. X-rays are usually normal, though a traction calcaneal spur may be noted in advanced cases.

     d. Treatment includes plantar stretching, heel cup, soft-molded arch supports, anti-inflammatory medications, and, in resistant cases, corticosteroid injection locally.

  3. **Sesamoiditis**

     a. Plantar pain and tenderness beneath the first metatarsal head.

     b. Acute injury will reveal local swelling and decreased range of motion.

     c. X-rays are important to rule out a fracture, as it is not unusual to see a split or bipartite sesamoid, especially on the medial sesamoid.

     d. To rule out a fracture, a bone scan can be helpful.

     e. Treatment includes metatarsal padding, oral anti-inflammatories, and occasionally surgery.

  4. **Jones fracture**

     a. A fracture of the proximal shaft or diaphysis of the 5th metatarsal, as compared to a fracture of the base of the 5th metatarsal.

     b. This fracture is characteristically slow in healing, with a significant nonunion rate, as compared to a fracture of the base of the 5th metatarsal.

     c. Treatment includes casting with nonweight-bearing status until early healing; then short-leg walking cast until healed—to primary intermedullary screw fixation in the active athlete, which allows for early activity status. If a nonunion occurs, internal fixation and bone grafting are necessary.

XIII. **Prevention:** Because the rate of serious injuries is so high in football (7–9% of football injuries are major), special attention should be paid to preventive strategies.

  A. **Preseason conditioning:** A controllable and predictable factor is off-season conditioning, including weight training and running. Bone, ligaments, and muscles definitely respond to exercise and resistance by gaining size, strength, and power. As a guide, a conditioning program in progressive phases is recommended:

    1. **Phase I** includes establishing a good base of distance running, stretching, and basic weight-lifting. In this phase, one is establishing basic conditioning, and one should not overlift or sprint.

    2. In **Phase II,** one emphasizes higher lifting repetition over poundage, continues basic stretching, and advances in running to ¾ speed workouts. In addition, jumping rope, basketball, and racquetball will improve conditioning and agility.

    3. In **Phase III,** one increases the intensity of workouts to more explosive maneuvers and agility drills. This includes full-speed sprinting and quick starts, plus continued stretching and lifting progressively.

4. The **most useful lifts** include incline and bench press, squats and hip sled, hang cleans, knee extensions and curls, plus neck flexion and extension. In addition, situps and crunches will increase abdominal muscle tone and strength, which are necessary for running. **One needs proper instruction to lift correctly and avoid excessive weights.** For instance, heavy deep squats, in my experience, can lead to injury and need to be done with care and guidance.

B. **Athletic equipment** should be in good condition and fit properly in order to protect. It is important that helmets, pads, etc. be evaluated, repaired, or replaced before each season begins.

1. Coaches and athletic trainers, as well as equipment managers, should know how to evaluate and fit protective equipment.

2. Figures 1 through 5 illustrate basic football protective equipment.

3. **Helmets** should fit snugly so that they do not slide or twist. The front rim should be 2 finger-widths above the eyebrow. The helmet strap should be in good repair and fit firmly. **Face masks** should be high enough to protect the face and low enough to allow a good visual range. They should be secured with rubber or soft plastic attachments that can be cut easily to remove the face mask for emergency treatment.

4. **Athletic mouthpieces** are required for all players. They should be brightly colored to make it obvious when the player is using one. Heat-moulded standard mouthpieces are adequate, but custom-fitted devices are better.

5. **Footwear** has changed, and there appears to be less injury when **multiple-cleated soccer type shoes** are used.
   a. These include shoes with 7–10 cleats for grass and 13–17 shorter cleats for artificial turf.

6. **Prophylactic knee braces** remain controversial after much initial enthusiasm. Most studies have revealed that these braces are not preventing knee ligament injuries. Some information suggests they may lessen the severity of a ligament injury; some indicates there is even an increase in ligament injuries for those wearing the braces. My recommendation is to inform the player and family of these facts, and, if they still desire a brace, to provide it. Again, conditioning and strengthening appear to be more important.

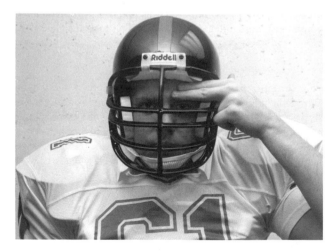

**FIGURE 1.** Helmet with appropriate face mask is standard. Helmet fit is critical, with 2 fingers from the brow to the frontal edge. The back edge should not dig into the neck. The helmet should not slide or turn on the head. A mouthpiece is frequently attached.

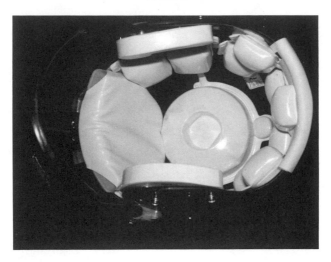

**FIGURE 2.** Interior view of football helmet, demonstrating padding and inflatable air bladders. A hand bulb inflation device should be kept at the sidelines by the equipment manager, athletic trainer, or coach during all practice and competitions.

    C. **Protective rule changes** have decreased injuries. Most notable have been rules **penalizing:**
      1. Spearing
      2. Head-butting
      3. Leg-whipping
      4. Blocking below the waist outside the line of scrimmage.
    D. **Nutritional concerns**
      1. **Proper diet** contributes to improved athletic performance, too. Increased intake of carbohydrates, moderate use of protein, and decreased fat in the diet are the recognized approach for good health. Often, large lean football players will be

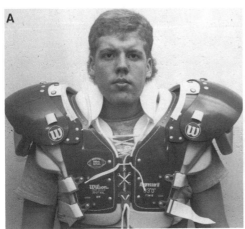
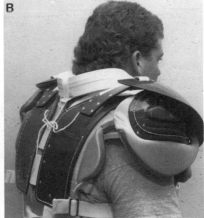

**FIGURE 3A, B.** Shoulder pads (lineman). The inner pad should cover the shoulder tip, while the outer pad cups the deltoid. The clavicle should be covered and the neck should not be constricted. A collar roll is attached to the shoulder pads shown. Quarterbacks typically use a smaller, somewhat less protective model, which allows more shoulder mobility for passing.

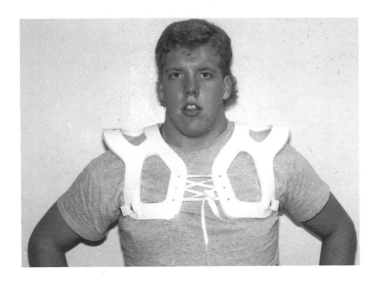

**FIGURE 4.** Acromioclavicular (AC) pad ("spider"). The AC pad is worn underneath shoulder pads in an athlete who has sustained a previous AC joint sprain or separation. When the shoulder pads are applied over the AC pad, they are elevated off of the AC joint.

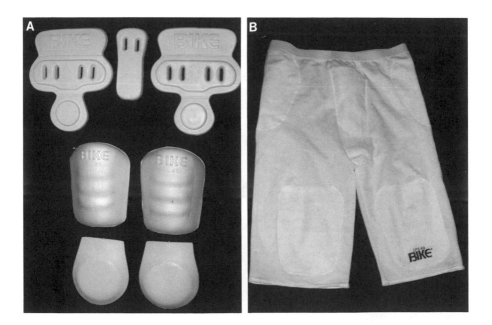

**FIGURE 5.** *A*, Lower extremity pads, including hip, coccyx, anterior thigh, and knee pads. *B*, Girdle worn by football players to hold the hip, coccyx, and thigh pads. The knee pads are held in place by the football pants.

unable to maintain optimal playing weight during the season without a marked increase in carbohydrates and a moderate increase in dietary fats. Multiple snacks may be necessary between meals to supply the $\geq$ 5000 kcal daily requirements of these athletes.

2. **Fluids** should never be restricted, especially during the warmer times of the season. Cool water is quite adequate during games and practice. Salt loss can be replaced by salting foods at mealtimes during the season. Salt tablets are not necessary and are not recommended.
3. **Drugs, stimulants, and anabolic steroids** are only mentioned to condemn their use because of associated and often devastating side-effects, and because using them is cheating.

E. **Medical coverage on the field**
   1. **Ideally, a physician knowledgeable in sports medicine and emergency care should be present for every game and practice session.**
   2. **Certified athletic trainers** should supplement the care of the physician. If a physician is not available, a certified athletic trainer should be present.
      a. Universities, colleges and high schools should budget for the athletic trainer's services.
   3. All coaches should currently be certified in American Red Cross Advanced First Aid and Cardiopulmonary Resuscitation or the equivalent.

XIX. **Summary.** American football, as played primarily in the U.S. and with some variation in Canada, is both a "contact and collision sport." Young men participate in football at most levels of school and college, in professional teams, and play touch or nontackle football in organized leagues for pure recreation. Touch football may involve less pure contact, but any collegiate intramural program will reveal a significant injury incidence. The availability of a team physician and/or certified athletic trainer on the field is encouraged for diagnosis, treatment, and, when indicated, referral of football injuries. Any school or district with such professional help available is a better, safer program.

Football, especially at the high school level, is basically a positive experience, since it is a team- and goal-oriented sport that requires personal and physical sacrifices by the players, yet with some risks. It is imperative to provide these athletes with proper care and protection from team physicians and trainers.

## REFERENCES

1. Mueller FO, Blyth CS, Cantu RC: Catastrophic spine injuries in football. Phys Sportsmed 17(10):51–53, 1989.
2. Olson CO: Prevention of Football Injuries: Protecting the Health of the Student Athlete. Philadelphia, Lea & Febiger, 1971.
3. Dick RW: Football: 1989–1990 NCAA Surveillance System. Mission, KS, National Collegiate Athletic Association, 1990.
4. Dick RW: NCAA Football Injury Surveillance System (Fall) for Academic Year 1989–1990; Injury Exposure Summary as of 1/12/90. Mission, KS, National Collegiate Athletic Association, 1990.
5. Thompson N, Halpern B, Curl WW, et al: High school football injuries: Evaluation. Am J Sports Med 15:117–124, 1987.
6. Torg JS, Vegso JJ, O'Neil MJ, et al: The epidemiologic, pathologic, biomechanical, and cinematographic analysis of football-induced cervical spine trauma. Am J Sports Med 18:50–57, 1990.
7. Yost FH: Football for Player and Spectator. Ann Arbor, MI, University Publishing Company, 1905.
8. Halpern B, et al: High school football injuries: Defining the risk factors. Am J Sports Med 15:316–320, 1987.
9. Lackland DJ, et al: The utilization of athletic trainer-team physician services and high school football injuries. Athletic Training 20(Spring):20–23, 1985.

# Chapter 45: Volleyball

DENISE FANDEL, MS, ATC
MORRIS B. MELLION, MD

I. **Introduction and General Concerns**

  A. Origin: Volleyball was invented in 1895 in Holyoke, Massachusetts, as a recreational sport of modest intensity.

  B. **Power volleyball** is an increasingly popular competitive men's and women's sport that requires:

    1. Explosive movement

    2. Quickness and agility

      a. Frequent changes in direction and intensity

    3. Rapid reaction time

      a. Ball may travel at 75 mph

    4. Total body control

    5. Aerobic and anaerobic fitness

    6. Mental toughness.

  C. Volleyball is a contact sport in which the player may be injured due to contact with:

    1. The ball

    2. The floor

    3. Other players

    4. The nets and supporting apparatus.

  D. Certain aspects of volleyball **predispose the athlete to specific types of overuse injuries.**

    1. **The underhand passing position** of volleyball stresses the patellofemoral joint.

    2. Jumping and landing with **recurrent intense deceleration forces** further stress the patellofemoral joint as well as the patella tendon and its origin and insertion into the tibial tubercle.

    3. **The hitting motion of volleyball in serving and spiking (hitting)** subject the shoulder to several overuse injuries.

    4. Repetitive, intense **hyperextension of the lumbosacral spine in hitting and blocking** subject the low back to injury.

  E. Highly competitive volleyball players tended to be **lean and angular.** Height is a marked advantage for the hitting and blocking on the front line (Fig. 1). Agility and quickness are critical for defense.

    1. Similar characteristics as front court and back court basketball players.

    2. Volleyball requires both **strength and endurance.**

    3. **Weight management** may be a problem for some athletes.

II. **Volleyball Injuries**

  A. **General patterns**

    1. Overuse injuries are more frequent than trauma.

      a. Of traumatic injuries, highest number due to contact with floor.

        i. Especially sprains and strains occurring with body rotation over or around a planted foot.

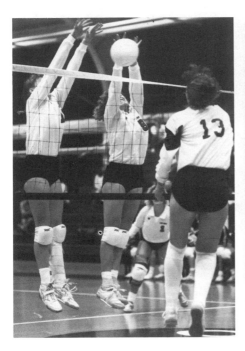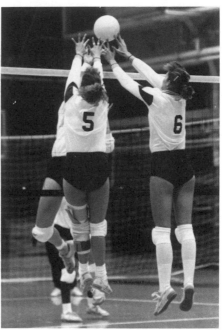

**FIGURE 1** *(left).*    Height is a marked advantage for hitting and blocking on the front line.

**FIGURE 2** *(right).*    Finger injuries are common in volleyball from contact with the ball.

    2. College freshman and sophomores are injured more frequently than juniors and seniors.
      a. Higher conditioning and skill level appear to be protective.
    3. Injuries in college volleyball generally result in players missing 1–6 days per injury.
  B. **Traumatic injuries**
    1. Contact with the ball (Fig. 2)
      a. Finger injuries (see Chapt. 36)
        i. "Jammed fingers" (tenosynovitis).
        ii. Mallet finger and boutonniere deformity from poor blocking technique.
        iii. Hyperextension injuries from poor setting technique.
          (a) Flexor tendon strain and volar plate injuries.
        iv. Finger tip contusions.
      b. **Hands, wrists, and forearms**
        i. **Contusions** from recurrent ball trauma.
          (a) Frequent in inexperienced players but occur at all levels.
          (b) Occasionally severe.
        ii. **Traumatic aneurysms** have been reported in small arteries of the hand.
      c. **Facial injuries.**
    2. **Contact with the floor produces a wide variety** of trauma (Fig. 3), but certain injuries are relatively common.
      a. **Shoulder**
        i. Acute rotator cuff strains (traumatic tendinitis) occur in digging and diving motions.
          (a) There may be an underlying overuse problem that is "asymptomatic" or "subclinical" prior to trauma in some cases.

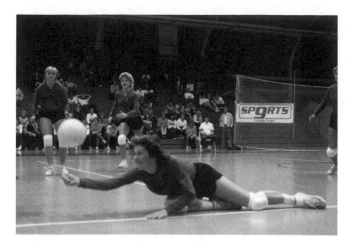

**FIGURE 3.** Contact with the floor produces a wide variety of traumatic injuries.

        ii. Contusions
        iii. Acromioclavicular separations
        iv. Glenohumeral dislocations.
    b. **Knee**
        i. **Prepatellar bursitis** ("housemaid's knee")
          (a) Prevent by using knee pad.
        ii. Ligament sprains
        iii. Mensical tears.
    c. **Ankle**
        i. **Sprains**
        ii. **Strains**
          (a) Achilles
          (b) Medial head of gastrocnemius
          (c) Peroneals and posterior tibial.
    d. **Foot**
        i. **Metatarsal arch**
    e. **Elbow**
        i. Olecranon bursitis
    f. **Hand**
        i. Sprain of the thumb ulnar collateral ligament ("gamekeeper's thumb").
          (a) Floor contact
          (b) Poor blocking technique
             (i) "Check-rein" taping may be useful in caring for this injury.
    g. **Skin**
        i. Abrasions
  3. **Contact with other players**
    a. Occurs when more than one player digging or diving for the ball
    b. Jumping and landing on other player's foot during hitting and blocking.
  4. **Contact with net and support apparatus.**
C. **Overuse**
  1. **Knee**—most common site
    a. **Problems of the extensor mechanism due to jumping** (see also Chap 40).

**TABLE 1.** The Relationship Between Frequency of Practices and Games and the Incidence of Knee Extensor Mechanism Overuse Injuries in Competitive Volleyball Players (Adapted from Ferretti A, et al: Jumper's knee: An epidemiological study of volleyball players. Phys Sportsmed 12(10):97–106, 1984.)

| Weekly Practices/Games | Players Affected |
|:---:|:---:|
| 2 | 3.2% |
| 3 | 14.6% |
| 4 | 29.1% |
| >4 | 41.8% |

  i. **Mechanism:** Landing with quadricep mechanism contracted and allowing it to absorb an intense load while the muscle is lengthened. Microtrauma results at the quadriceps tendon, the patellofemoral interface, the patellar origin of the patellar tendon, and the insertion of the patella at the tibial tubercle.
 ii. Predisposing factors
   (a) Intrinsic (anatomic) factors. See Chap. 40.
   (b) Extrinsic factors
      (i) Incidence varies directly with number of practices/games per week (Table 1).
        • Increase in volume and intensity of participation adds to risk
      (ii) Hard playing surfaces raise incidence, and shock-absorbing surface lowers risk (Table 2).
iii. Common syndromes
   (a) "Jumper's knee"—patellar tendinitis (The term "jumper's knee" is also occasionally used to include all extensor mechanism problems in the jumping sports.)
      (i) Most common extensor mechanism problem in the jumping sports.
      (ii) Somehow related to weakness of ankle dorsiflexor muscles, but mechanism is not clear.
      (iii) Very high incidence of patella alta.
   (b) Patellofemoral pain
   (c) Quadriceps tendinitis
   (d) Osgood-Schlatter's disease
      (i) Pubertal and peripubertal athletes.
 iv. Other knee overuse
   (a) Semimembranosis tendinitis.
2. **Ankle/foot**
   a. Achilles tendinitis
   b. Plantar fasciitis.

**TABLE 2.** The Relationship Between Playing Surface and the Incidence of Knee Extensor Mechanism Overuse Injuries in Competitive Volleyball Players. (Adapted from Ferretti A, et al: Jumper's knee: An epidemiological study of volleyball players. Phys Sportsmed 12(10):97–106, 1984.)

| Playing Surface | Players Affected | |
|:---|:---:|:---:|
| Cement | 24/64 | (37.5%) |
| Linoleum | 55/237 | (23.2%) |
| Wood parquet | 3/64 | ( 4.7%) |
| Other surfaces | 11/42 | (26.2%) |

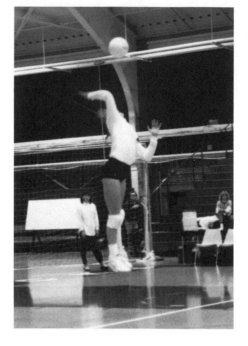

**FIGURE 4.** Repetitive overhead hitting, blocking, and serving can cause impingement and overuse syndromes.

3. **Shoulder**
   a. **Etiology:** Repetitive overhead hitting, blocking, serving, and setting (Fig. 4).
   b. **Rotator cuff tendinitis and impingement syndromes** include:
      i. Rotator cuff tears—acute and chronic
      ii. Supraspinatus tendinitis
      iii. Biceps tendinitis
      iv. Subdeltoid bursitis
      v. Glenoid labrum avulsion.
   c. **Predisposing factors**
      i. Poor technique
      ii. Lack of sport specific conditioning
         (a) Strength (Fig. 5)
         (b) Flexibility
         (c) Endurance.
      iii. Improper or inadequate warm-up.
4. **Lumbosacral spine**
   a. **Etiological factors**
      i. Flexed hip posture of underhand passing position stresses lumbosacral spine (Fig. 6).
      ii. Forced hyperextension of low back in hitting, blocking, and setting stresses the pars interarticularis of the lower lumbar vertebrae.
   b. **Common syndromes** (see Chap. 38)
      i. Low back strain
      ii. Spondylolysis/spondylolisthesis
      iii. Sacroiliac joint sprain/contracture.
5. Shin splints and stress fractures (see Chap. 41)
   a. Etiology
      i. Recurrent impact from jumping

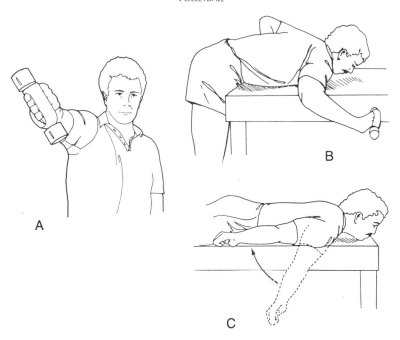

**FIGURE 5.** Shoulder strengthening exercises particularly useful in rehabilitating and preventing rotator-cuff injuries in volleyball players: *A,* The supraspinatus muscle is strengthened by internally rotating and abducting the humerus. *B,* Strengthening exercise for the posterior portion of the deltoid muscle and the rotator cuff. *C,* By elevating the arm in an externally rotated position (with the thumb pointed outward), the athlete exercises the external rotators of the shoulder and the stabilizers of scapula.

    ii. Common anatomical factors
      (a) Hyperpronating feet
      (b) Genu varum (bow legs).
    iii. Inadequate sport-specific conditioning
      (a) Inadequate flexibility
      (b) Imbalance between anterior and posterior musculature.
    iv. Increase in intensity or duration of participation.
  b. **Common stress fracture sites in volleyball**
    i. Metatarsals
    ii. Tibia
    iii. Fibula.
  c. **Bracing**
    i. Some athletes may be able to participate with shin splints or mild stress fractures of the tibia or fibula after ≥ 10 days rest by using an Aircast leg brace.
D. **Preventative strategies: special prehabilitation and rehabilitation**
  1. **Year-round conditioning**
    a. Sport specific
    b. Strength, endurance, flexibility, agility, reaction time
    c. **Avoid plyometrics in athletes until a high level of strength, endurance and flexibility have been attained.**
  2. Employ a **gradual progression of skill** training.
    a. Allow the athlete time to build body awareness while learning new skill.
    b. Chart the total number of foot contacts per training session to plan gradual increase in intensity.

    c. Do not allow plyometric training until the athlete can lift a minimum of two times their body weight in the hip sled/squat.

3. **Diving and digging drills**

    a. Special tumbling drills to prepare player to dive and dig for the ball without injury.

4. **Proprioception training**

    a. Body position awareness is vital to lower extremity landings and to the diving and digging movements in volleyball.

    b. Proprioception drills can reduce injuries

        i. Lower extremity drills

            (a) Jumping rope

            (b) Balance board

            (c) Footwork drills (See Box).

        ii. Diving and digging drills have a proprioceptive component.

---

## FOOTSPEED DRILLS

This drills will be done 3 times a week. If done correctly and intensively, you will help yourself and your team by:

1. Increasing your footspeed
2. Increasing your quickness
3. Improving your coordination
4. Improving and increasing your lower leg strength.

The entire drill will take only 12 minutes a day.

**Materials**

1. A piece of chalk or carpet
2. A flat, firm surface
3. A timing device.

Choose an area where you can lay out a figure such as the one below:

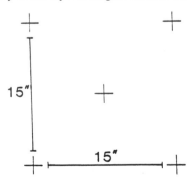

Set 1. Double Foot—Clockwise 4 corner
Set 2. Double Foot—Counterclockwise 4 corner
Set 3. Double Foot—Left clockwise triangle
Set 4. Double Foot—Counterclockwise left triangle
Set 5. Double Foot—Clockwise right triangle
Set 6. Double Foot—Forward triangle
Set 7. Double Foot—Backward triangle

The goal of these drills is to do one more rep each time you do drills. Each set lasts 30 seconds. Rest 45 seconds between sets. Record the number of attempts.

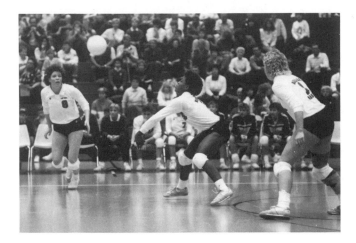

**FIGURE 6.** The flexed hip posture of the underhand passing position stresses the lumbosacral spine.

III. **Sport Specific Facilities and Protective Equipment**
  A. **Playing surface**
     1. Softer, more shock-absorbent surface reduces incidence of injuries (see Table 2).
        a. Suspended wooden (parquet) floor is currently best.
     2. Sweat on floor should be wiped up.
        a. At higher competition levels, rules are being tightened to prevent abuse of time-out to wipe the floor.
  B. **Padded apparatus**
     1. Net supports and cables.
     2. Officials' stand.
  C. **Uniforms**
     1. Padded hip briefs.
     2. Knee pads.
  D. **Footwear**
     1. Court shoes required.
        a. Special volleyball shoes available.
     2. High-tops may provide added ankle support if the lacing on the upper part of the shoe is tied separately from the lacing over the foot.
        a. This arrangement provides a looser tension over the foot and more support from higher tension over the ankle and lower leg.

IV. **Taping and Bracing**

  A. **General policy regarding taping and bracing:**
     1. Ankles are a common site of injury in volleyball. Lace-up style braces are preferred, even over adhesive taping.
     2. Knees can require patellofemoral joint supports, but generally there is not a need for ligamentous braces.
        a. Palumbo brace (neoprene style).
  B. **Specific taping**
     1. **Fingers**
        a. Buddy tape for PIP and DIP joint injuries caused most commonly by blocking.
     2. **Thumb**

a. Gamekeeper's thumb—use check-rein tape or modified figure-of-eight tape to prevent hyperextension.

    i. Occurs from contact with the floor and improper blocking skills (blocking with the thumbs facing forward toward the opponent).

V. **Rules to Protect the Athlete**

A. No hard materials on extremities.

    1. Braces must have all hard exposed surfaces padded and all metal covered.

B. No penetration completely over the centerline.

C. Wiping the floor

    1. Collegiate and interscholastic level of play—players allowed to wipe floor. At Olympic level, players must carry wiping cloth and cannot delay the game to wipe perspiration off the floor.

VI. **Other Sport-specific Concerns**

A. Dehydration.

*SUGGESTED READINGS*

1. Black JE, Alten SR: How I manage infrapatellar tendinitis. Phys Sportsmed 12(10):86–92, 1984.
2. Ferretti A, Puddu G, Mariani PP, Massimo N: Jumper's knee: An epidemiological study of volleyball players. Phys Sportsmed 12(10):97–103, 1984.
3. Ferretti A: Epidemiology of jumper's knee. Sports Med 3:289–295, 1986.
4. Lund PM: Marathon volleyball: Changes after 61 hours of play. Br J Sports Med 19(4):228–229, 1985.
5. Yi ZR, Lian HY, Peng WK, Nan ZY: A biomechanical study of suprascapular nerve injuries in volleyball. Intl Series on Biomechanics, Vol. 6B. Champaign, IL, Human Kinetics, 1987, pp 951–954.

# Chapter 46: Soccer

GIANCARLO PUDDU, MD
IGNAZIO CARUSO, MD
GUGLIELMO CERULLO, MD
VITTORIO FRANCO, MD
W. MICHAEL WALSH, MD

I. **Soccer and Special Sports Medicine Concerns**

A. **Introduction**

1. **Historical aspect**

a. The Japanese "kemani" of the 7th century B.C., Greek "episkiros" of the 4th century B.C., and the Roman "harpostum" of the 1st century B.C. represent first games resembling modern soccer.

b. In Florence during 16th century A.D. (Medici dynasty), a game was played that was very much like the soccer of today.

c. Most of the rules of modern soccer were defined on October 26, 1863, by the Football Association of England.

2. **Current participation**

a. Soccer has propagated to become the most popular sport in the world, with about 40,000,000 participants in all countries.

b. In Italy (55,000,000 population), soccer is the national sport; 2,000,000 players are registered with the Soccer Federation.

c. Popularity in U.S. has been slow to grow, with only 40,000 participants 20 years ago; today, 2,000,000 people play soccer in the U.S.

d. U.S. high school participation climbed to 196,000 boys and 85,000 girls in 1985–1986.[32]

e. More than 1,000,000 players under age 19 are registered with the U.S. Soccer Federation.[32]

3. **Epidemiology**

a. **Injury rates**

i. Injury rates in NCAA soccer are 8.05 per 1,000 athlete exposures for women, and 7.78 per 1,000 athlete exposures for men.[7] These rates are comparable to American football, but the level of severity is lower.

ii. Older soccer players are injured more frequently, with 15 to 30 times as many injuries in senior and professional players compared to youth participants.[12]

iii. Severe soccer injuries occur infrequently but are more common among older participants.[12]

iv. No matter what the age, injury incidence increases as the intensity of play increases.[12]

v. Outdoor soccer is reported to produce more injuries than indoor soccer among professional athletes.[12]

b. **Youth soccer**

i. Youth soccer may have one-fifth to one-half the injury rate of American football.[12]

    ii. Some indication that tall but muscularly weak boys (ages 6–17) may be more susceptible than peers.[3]

    iii. Some indication that females in youth soccer may sustain as many as twice the number of injuries as male counterparts.[12]

    iv. In youth programs, goalkeepers may be more likely to be injured; otherwise, no influence of position played on likelihood of injury.[12]

    v. Among youth participants, indoor soccer is reported to produce 4–6 times as many injuries as outdoor soccer.[11]

  c. **Anatomical considerations**

    i. The lower extremity is injured more frequently, with knee and ankle accounting for about 20% of all injuries in all age groups.[12]

    ii. Head and upper extremity injuries occur more commonly in youth, whereas hip and thigh injuries are seen more commonly in older athletes.[12]

    iii. Knee and ankle ligament sprains make up one-third of soccer injuries across all age groups; muscle strains occur more commonly in older participants; contusions represent more severe injury in young participants.[12]

    iv. Congenital knee joint laxity, past history of ankle sprain, poor flexibility, and incomplete rehabilitation from previous injury are significant factors in producing soccer injury.[12]

  d. **Other predisposing conditions**

    i. Inadequate equipment, poor field conditions, and rule violations are also associated with injuries.[12]

B. **Special attributes and abilities of soccer players**

  1. European soccer coaches believe that successful soccer players are characterized by specific physical attributes (power, endurance, and, above all, speed), outstanding technical ability, and most of all, an understanding of tactics.

  2. During a game, the running required is a series of repeated bouts of brief duration (generally between 6 and 15 seconds), recurring regularly (on average once a minute).

  3. Equally as important as performing well during bursts of activity, the player must recover sufficiently between bursts.

  4. Tests we propose to evaluate the soccer player include:

    a. Cooper's 12-minute run to determine aerobic capacity.

    b. Kovac's test, requiring a continuous activity of medium duration (2 to 2½ minutes), including running, dribbling, and shooting.

    c. Comucci's test, which involves 5 repetitions of a 50-meter run (10 meters in one direction, 10 meters in the opposite direction, 15 meters in the opposite direction, and 15 meters in the opposite direction). Each 50 meters should take 10 seconds.

  5. In collegiate soccer players, no significant differences in flexibility or strength have been found between the dominant and the nondominant leg.[1]

  6. Compared to players under 16 years of age, Canadian players under 18 years have shown greater absolute lean body mass and greater isokinetic leg extension, force, and explosive lower extremity strength.[14]

C. **Injury prevention—general concerns**

  1. Factors in preventing soccer injuries can be divided into three groups:

    a. **Technical factors:** type of training, preventive exercises, taping and bracing, shoes and other equipment.

    b. **Hygienic and dietetic factors:** lifestyle, rest and sleep, food habits.

    c. **Individual factors:** age, predisposition, psychological status, other health problems.

2. Many of these factors are the same as in other sports, but two deserve emphasis in soccer players: **training** and **diet.**

    a. Typical **training** of an Italian professional soccer player is divided into **three phases.**

        i. **First phase** (preseason training) lasts 20–25 days, usually in the mountains. This phase is divided into **two stages. First stage** is endurance exercise and general agility, followed by strengthening exercises, and finally stretching. After 5–6 days of acclimatization, **2nd stage** is composed of technical activities (e.g., playing soccer basketball, or soccer tennis).

        ii. **Second phase** generally lasts 2 weeks, composed of interval training, speed exercises, individual technique work, 2-times-per-week acrobatic and agility exercises.

        iii. **Third phase** lasts all season. Speed and specific resistance exercises are emphasized (circuit training, uphill running).

    b. **Diet:** Depending on the part of the season, the player has different energy needs.

        i. **Preseason training,** especially in hot climates, requires significant amounts of starches, fruits, vegetables, and, of course, water. Energy requirements are between 2,900 and 3,200 kcal/day (55% carbohydrates, 26% fats, 19% proteins).

        ii. **During the season,** energy requirements are between 3,000 and 3,500 kcal/day (55% carbohydrates, 28% fats, and 17% proteins). May be divided into three meals plus one lighter meal following afternoon training session. On a game day, carbohydrates may be increased.

3. Controlled warm-up and stretching program is important in injury prevention.[1,12]

4. Complete rehabilitation from previous injury should be assured.[12,32]

5. Women soccer players may be more susceptible to traumatic injuries during the premenstrual and menstrual periods compared to the rest of the menstrual cycle. Especially true for players with definite premenstrual symptoms.[19]

II. **Specific Injuries:** The typical distribution for soccer injuries is shown in Figure 1. Table 1 shows soccer injuries according to mechanism of injury.

  A. **Head injuries**

    1. **Pattern of injury**

      a. Head injuries in soccer account for 5%–10% of injuries.

      b. Fatal head injuries have occurred on rare occasions.[9]

      c. Symptoms may include headache, neck pain, dizziness, irritability, insomnia, impaired hearing, impaired memory.[28]

      d. EEG studies have shown neuronal damage that may be more pronounced among younger (professional) players.[13,30]

        i. Younger player may be more susceptible: the skull may be less skeletally mature and player may have poorer heading technique.[30]

    2. **Mechanism of injury**

      a. Mechanisms of injury include heading the ball improperly; making head-to-head contact; forcefully kicked ball striking a player's head.[9]

      b. Most head injuries occur while the player is heading a soccer ball, with a cumulative effect over the course of the individual's playing career.

        i. Plastic-coated soccer ball weighs from 396–453 gm (13.86–18.85 oz), and the speed can reach 60–120 km/hr (37.2–74.4 miles/hr).

        ii. Professional soccer participants head the ball 5 times/game on average, adding up to over 5,000 impacts in a 15-year career. Impact may be as forceful as 200 kp.[28]

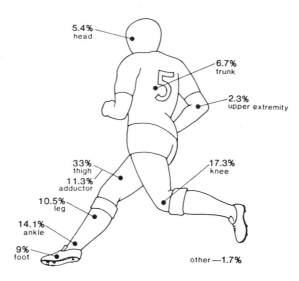

**FIGURE 1.**   Frequency of injury according to body part.

   iii. Computer modelling techniques have shown greater injury risk from angular head acceleration than linear head acceleration, with apparent increased risk from lateral head impacts compared to frontal impacts.[25]

  c. Goalkeepers may experience head injury when they strike the goal post, playing surface, or another player.[9]

3. **Prevention**

  a. The modern soccer ball is currently plastic-coated to prevent water saturation, the extra weight of which is responsible for more head injuries.[9]

  b. In children, there is a greater risk of injury that can be reduced by using only smaller-sized soccer balls.[25]

B. **Eye injuries**

1. **Pattern of injury**

  a. Overall incidence of eye injury is low, but a series of 24 injuries from soccer ball impact has been reported.[5]

  b. When compared with hockey and racquet sports, soccer eye injuries were less serious, with low likelihood of permanent visual acuity loss.[5]

2. **Mechanism of injury**

  a. A study of 13 children and adolescents who sustained soccer trauma to the eye showed cause by ball contact (6), a kick (3), and head butt (1); in 3 cases, cause was unknown.[32]

**TABLE 1.**   Mechanisms of Injury in Soccer

| Mechanism of Injury | During Match | During Training | Total |
|---------------------|:------------:|:---------------:|:-----:|
| Fall                | 23%          | 6%              | 29%   |
| Contact             | 39%          | 9%              | 48%   |
| Bruise              | 11%          | 2%              | 13%   |
| Twisting            | 3%           | 2%              | 5%    |
| Heading             | 2%           | 0%              | 2%    |
| Other               | 1%           | 2%              | 3%    |
| TOTAL               | 79%          | 21%             | 100%  |

3. **Prevention**
   a. Protective eyewear is strongly recommended for soccer activity.[5]
   b. Additional preventive techniques include education of coaching staff, parents, and officials; proper conditioning to reduce fatigue; mastery of basic skills; strict enforcement of rules.[22]

C. **Maxillofacial and dental**
   1. **Pattern of injury**
      a. In a Norwegian study, 20% of soccer injuries were to the teeth,[21] whereas a Finnish report showed 6.4% of total soccer injuries to affect maxillofacial and dental regions.[23] 80.8% of those affected teeth or alveolar process, whereas 11.2% were fractures of lower or middle third of facial skeleton, including a relatively high incidence of nasal fractures.[23] Uncomplicated crown fracture of maxillary incisors was most common dental injury.[21]
      b. Majority of dental injuries occurred among male players, with relative frequency higher than in women.[21]
      c. Players over age 20 are more susceptible to dental and maxillofacial injuries,[23] with prevalence of dental injuries highest in the top competitive divisions.[21] Goalkeepers appeared to be most susceptible to dental injuries.[21]
      d. In Finnish study, 40% of patients needed prosthetic treatment, and over 30% required endodontic treatment.[23]
      e. Lacerations of the forehead and scalp may occur in association with injuries to underlying tissues, including facial fractures.
   2. **Mechanism of injury**
      a. Maxillofacial and dental injuries more likely to occur during games than during practices.[23]
      b. Most frequent cause was contact with another player.[23]
      c. Injuries commonly occur when two players try to head the ball simultaneously.
   3. **Prevention**
      a. **Mouth guards** to protect against injury.

D. **Spine**
   1. **Pattern of injury**
      a. Frequency and degree of degenerative cervical spine changes may be significantly higher in soccer players.[29]
      b. Central cord syndrome after heading a ball, subluxation, fracture of cervical spine, and cervical disc herniation have all been reported in association with soccer.[29]
      c. Nonradiating low back pain affects almost 5% of soccer players, especially in older age groups.
   2. **Mechanism of injury**
      a. Cervical spine commonly injured by heading soccer ball.
      b. Like other low back problems in sports, lumbar pain in soccer can occur for a variety of reasons.

E. **Internal organs:** A variety of internal injuries common to any contact sport have been reported in soccer, including pneumomediastinum[6] and pancreatic rupture.[10]

F. **Groin pain (pubalgia):** Groin pain is extremely common in soccer players. Can be caused by inflammation due to overuse, or ruptures (partial or total) of muscle-tendon unit. Additionally, there are many nonmuscular causes for groin pain in soccer players, including bursitis, hernia, pain from abdominal organs and genitalia, and various nerve entrapments.

1. **Adductor tendinitis and tenoperiostitis**
   a. **Pattern**
      i. Muscles that adduct the thigh (adductor longus, adductor magnus, adductor brevis, gracilis, and the pectineus) may be involved.
      ii. Onset usually insidious.
      iii. **Symptoms:** Pain located at proximal attachment of these muscles. May radiate toward the mid-medial thigh. Characterized by pain when sprinting, pivoting, or shooting; increased with fatigue; more pronounced immediately after play, and the following day, stiffness with pain on getting in and out of chair or car.[15]
      iv. Tenderness may be elicited by direct palpation or by adduction of the thigh against resistance.
      v. **X-rays** may show various stages of bony changes, including osteolysis, erosions, arthrosis of symphysis, and calcification at the muscular attachments to the pubis.[27]
      vi. Differential diagnosis includes orthopedic conditions of hip, sacrum, or lower back, as well as other conditions listed in Section II.F.4. (below).
   b. **Mechanism of injury**
      i. Overloading of these muscles caused by sideways kicks typical of soccer.
      ii. Generally due to poor warm-ups, intensive training, or sometimes hard playing surfaces.
   c. **Prevention**
      i. Incidence of groin strain may be reduced by controlled warm-up and stretching program.[1]
      ii. Thorough flexibility exercises for adductor muscles.
   d. **Prehabilitation/rehabilitation**
      i. Athlete should stop as soon as groin pain is felt.
      ii. Rest and anti-inflammatory drugs are usually prescribed.
      iii. Physical therapy consisting of stationary bicycling, stretching the adductors, isometric and isotonic low-resistance exercises.
      iv. One or two local steroid injections may be tried.
      v. Operative intervention recommended for resistant adductor tendinitis is a simple subcutaneous adductor tenotomy.[15]
2. **Abdominal muscle injuries**
   a. **Pattern of injury**
      i. Rectus abdominis usually involved, occasionally oblique and transverse abdominal muscles.
   b. **Specific injuries**
      i. Rectus abdominis strain
         (a) Rectus abdominis lesion causes pain with sprinting and sudden changes of direction; pain after sports or daily activities; often, pain on coughing.[15]
         (b) Usually tenderness at the rectus insertion on the pubis. Pain elicited by contraction of the abdominal muscles, as when athlete, while lying flat, lifts head and both legs off ground simultaneously.
         (c) **Mechanism of injury:** Usually overuse inflammation rather than distinct tear.
         (d) **Treatment:** Flexibility exercises for rectus abdominis, nonsteroidal anti-inflammatory medication, physical modalities, and steroid injection may be useful.

(e) Surgical treatment recommended for resistant rectus abdominis tendonopathy is a rectus abdominis tenotomy combined with a fasciaplasty.[15]

 ii. **"Perforating nerve syndrome"**

  (a) **Symptoms:** spontaneous or provoked pain located along the lateral edge of the rectus abdominis, 4–5 cm from the groin arch.

  (b) **Etiology:** entrapment of distal branch of the iliohypogastric nerve by the aponeurosis of the rectus abdominis.

  (c) Surgical treatment for perforating nerve syndrome is surgical release of the entrapped nerve.

3. **Iliopsoas injury**

 a. **Pattern of injury**

  i. Less common source of groin pain in soccer players is injury to iliopsoas muscle.[20]

  ii. Usually no direct trauma, with pain appearing only while playing.[20]

  iii. Pain pattern is different from that of other causes of groin pain: pain located in lower abdominal quadrant, frequently with radiation to groin.

   (a) Pain is lateral to rectus abdominis and above inguinal ligament, aggravated by forced flexion of the hip, as in kicking.[20]

  iv. **Examination:** Pain is provoked by pressure over iliopsoas with active flexion of thigh against resistance.[20]

 c. **Prehabilitation/rehabilitation**

  i. May be treated by rest, medication, and appropriate flexibility exercises.

  ii. If weakness occurs, will need restrengthening exercises.

  iii. May be treated best by injection directly into iliopsoas muscle.[20]

4. **Nonmuscular causes**

 a. **Pattern of injury**

  i. Other orthopedic causes include symphysitis pubis.

  ii. Nonorthopedic causes include inguinal hernia and genitourinary conditions, such as posterior urethritis, prostatitis, epididymitis, or chronic varicocele or hydrocele.[27]

  iii. Pain may radiate in different directions: along adductors to scrotum, testicles, and perineum; laterally to hip; to pelvis and sacrum; in rare cases, into bladder.[27]

  iv. Herniography may be extremely helpful in diagnosing a hernia in cases of obscure groin pain, including those athletes with normal physical examination; also helpful in selecting those that need repair.[16]

  v. Many patients with chronic groin pain will show multiple positive studies, all of which may be related to the symptoms.[8] These problems are often a diagnostic dilemma.

  vi. Rectus abdominis muscles may also be involved in "perforating nerve syndrome."

G. **Thigh injuries**

1. **Pattern of injury**

 a. An injury from a direct blow may occur to the quadriceps, whereas strains occur commonly to both the quadriceps and hamstrings.

 b. **Symptoms:** acute intense pain in injured area; tenderness of the involved muscle; localized hematoma and swelling after a few hours; in more complete rupture, a palpable defect in the muscle.

2. **Mechanism of injury:** Direct trauma against the contracted quadriceps during play; sudden and vigorous contraction of quadriceps or hamstrings.

3. **Prehabilitation/rehabilitation:** Ice, compression, rest; nonweight-bearing with crutches. Rehabilitation: rehabilitative exercises, including stretching and strengthening, can usually start after about 72 hours following the injury.

H. **Knee injuries** (See also Chap. 40)

 1. **Pattern of injury**

   a. Most common knee injury in soccer is ligamentous injury. This injury follows the same pattern seen when knee is injured in other sports that demand twisting, pivoting, cutting.

   b. Meniscus injuries in soccer are usually combined with ligamentous lesions. Since soccer player needs an entirely stable knee, it is usually fruitless to treat only meniscal disorder and not ligamentous laxity.

 2. **Mechanism of injury**

   a. Valgus external rotation of tibia on femur occurs with impact against lateral side of knee, or when two players simultaneously kick the ball with inside of foot.

     i. Can produce tears of the medial collateral ligament, medial capsular ligament, or, in severe cases, anterior cruciate ligament.

   b. Varus internal rotation of the tibia is a very frequent mechanism in soccer, usually because of sudden change of direction while player is running. May be caused by shoe cleats becoming stuck in turf. Usually produces tear of anterior cruciate ligament.

   c. Hyperextension injury is not infrequent. May be from kicking or an impact on the anterior knee, as when a goalkeeper runs into an attacker with the ball.

I. **Achilles tendinitis**

 1. **Pattern of injury:** Condition may be acute or chronic. Since chronic condition is extremely difficult to treat, it is important for the athlete to address the problem in its earliest stage.

 2. **Mechanism of injury:** Inflammation of the Achilles tendon can occur as a result of prolonged and repeated running on a hard, uneven playing surface.

 3. **Prevention:** Warm-up and stretching exercises. Effort should be given to maintaining playing surface in good condition.

J. **Ankle injuries**

 1. **Pattern of injury**

   a. Ankle injury is the most common joint injury in soccer.

   b. Ankle injuries in soccer players should never be neglected, since the ankle may well be the most important joint used in this sport. The ankle is used not only in running, but also in controlling and kicking the ball. Players may say, "I feel the ball with my foot."

   c. Ligament sprain is the most common type of ankle injury.

   d. Osteochondral fractures of the talus occur not infrequently in soccer players.

 2. **Specific injuries**

   a. Ankle sprain

     i. Usually inversion injuries

   b. **"Footballer's ankle"** is a very common cause of anterior ankle pain in soccer players over age 30.

     i. **Symptoms** include anterior tenderness of the ankle, anterior ankle pain while running and kicking, and mild loss of motion of the ankle.

     ii. **X-rays** reveal anterior osteophytes on tibia and talus.

     iii. **Mechanism:** Footballer's ankle is due to repeated overloading of the ankle, producing traction osteophytes of the anterior capsular attachment to both talus and tibia. Hyperextension or hyperflexion of the ankle can cause minor avulsion or compression fractures of the osteophytes.

    iv. **Treatment** for footballer's ankle may include:

        (a) Rehabilitation through bicycling, swimming, and stretching exercises; however, anterior osteophytes may preclude normal methods of Achilles tendon stretching.

        (b) Steroid injection may be attempted.

        (c) Surgical excision of osteophytes often required.

  c. **Meniscoid lesion:** a mass of hyalinized soft tissue located in anterior portion of ankle joint between fibula and talus.

    i. May give **symptoms** of pain, swelling, and pseudo-locking episodes.

    ii. **Mechanism:** Meniscoid lesions are usually the result of repeated inversion sprains.[17]

    iii. **Treatment:** Meniscoid lesions may be treated by physical therapy, taping, and anti-inflammatory medication. Persistent symptoms treated by arthroscopic debridement of the fibrous tissue (see Chap. 41).

  d. **Osteochondral fractures of the talus**

    i. Specific **symptom** may be locking of the ankle.

    ii. **Diagnosis** can be very difficult. Special studies such as tomography may be necessary to demonstrate fracture.

3. **Prevention**

  a. Ankle taping, especially of previously injured ankles, can be an effective preventive technique.

  b. Thorough warm-up, including heel cord flexibility program, may help prevent injuries.

  c. Proper footwear and playing surfaces also can be important in prevention of ankle injuries.

4. **Prehabilitation/rehabilitation**

  a. Rehabilitation of soccer ankle injuries can be handled as described elsewhere in this handbook (Chap. 30).

  b. Total rehabilitation of previous ankle injury is critically important in preventing future ankle sprains.

III. **Sport-specific Facilities and Protective Equipment**

  A. **Facilities:** Soccer requires little in the way of specific facilities. A playing field 65–70 meters wide by 110–120 meters long is required, along with a ball of 68–71 cm in circumference and 396–455 g in weight.

  B. **Footwear** is especially important:

    1. The shoe represents the means by which the player touches the ball. Therefore, it must have qualities of softness and toughness at the same time: a soft shoe lets the foot "feel" the ball, while toughness allows violent shots on goal.

    2. The traditional soccer shoe has 6 aluminum cleats. In recent years in the U.S., molded rubber soles with multiple (15 or more) cleats measuring no more than 1.25 by 1.25 cm each, are more common. These are especially useful on artificial surfaces, whether indoors or outdoors.

    3. Because shoes must allow maximum mobility of the foot, they do not provide significant support for the ankle, exposing it to twisting injuries. In addition, the soccer shoe has little to no heel elevation, increasing the likelihood of Achilles tendon or calcaneal problems.

  C. Male players should use protective cup supporter.

  D. All players should use shin guards. Compliance with wearing shin guards may be highly variable, and those worn may be inadequate.[12] Shin guards that cover full length of tibia and malleoli may provide increased protection.[12] Shin guards may be extremely efficient in dispersing forces, even of the magnitude that might cause tibial fractures.[31]

E. **Goalkeeper** may use padding for elbows, flanks, and knees, and a pair of special gloves to facilitate catching the ball. The goalkeeper may also wear a cap to shade eyes from strong sunlight.

F. Protective eyewear has been suggested, especially for children and adolescents.[22]

## IV. Specific Taping and Bracing

A. International rules prohibit wearing any article that could be dangerous for other players, including braces with hard prominent parts.

B. Ankle taping is especially prevalent because of the frequency of ankle joint injuries. A program to prevent soccer injuries, including ankle taping for players with a history of previous sprain or clinical ankle instabilities, has been shown to be effective.[12]

## V. Rules to Protect the Athlete

A. Rules to protect the athlete are several, but they can be summed up in one phrase: the player is not allowed to touch an opponent except for shoulder-to-shoulder contact. Violations, depending on their severity, are punished by a penalty kick, admonition (indicated by a yellow card), or expulsion (red card).

B. Tight officiating of games with no toleration of unsportsmanlike conduct has been suggested as a method of preventing eye injury.[22]

C. As many as 30% of traumatic injuries may be due to foul play, according to one study.[12] The player committing the foul is more likely to be the injured player.[12]

## VI. Sport-specific Special Concerns of the Team Physician

A. As shown above, most soccer injuries are musculoskeletal, so the team physician must be well versed in orthopedic evaluation and treatment. However, he/she must also be prepared for cardiovascular, ophthalmologic, maxillofacial, and neurologic problems.

B. Like all physicians caring for athletes in contact sports, the soccer team physician must be able to assess quickly the player's ability to return to competition.

C. Awareness of factors surrounding soccer head injuries is especially important, since soccer is one of very few sports in which players purposely sustain repeated blows to the head.

D. Soccer injury studies have shown the following to be associated with injury:[12]
  1. Pathologic knee ligament laxity
  2. Previous ankle injury
  3. Muscle weakness
     a. Persistent muscular weakness of the leg following previous injury
     b. Decreased musculotendinous flexibility
     c. Inadequate muscular rehabilitation
  4. Inadequate equipment
  5. Poor field conditions
  6. Foul play.

E. A peak in injury rates during the first 5 minutes of the 2nd half has been shown,[4] suggesting that an additional warm-up period before the start of the 2nd half would be beneficial.

# REFERENCES

1. Agre JC, Baxter TL: Musculoskeletal profile of male collegiate soccer players. Arch Phys Med Rehabil 68:147–150, 1987.
2. Antao NA: Myositis of the hip in a professional soccer player. Am J Sports Med 16:82–83, 1988.
3. Backous DD, Friedl KE, Smith NJ, et al: Soccer injuries and their relation to physical maturity. Am J Dis Child 142:839–842, 1988.
4. Berger-Vachon C, Gabard G, Moyen B: Soccer accidents in the French Rhône-Alpes Soccer Association. Sports Med 3:69–77, 1986.
5. Burke MJ, Sanitato JJ, Vinger PF, et al: Soccer-ball induced eye injuries. JAMA 249:2682–2685, 1983.
6. Doyle M, Given F: Pneumomediastinum as a complication of athletic activity. Two case reports. Ir J Med Sci 156:272–273, 1987.
7. Duda M: NCAA study: Football injury rate dips again. Phys Sportsmed 17(4):28, 1989.
8. Ekberg O, Persson NH, Abrahamsson P-A, et al: Longstanding groin pain in athletes. A multidisciplinary approach. Sports Med 6:56–61, 1988.
9. Fields KB: Head injuries in soccer. Phys Sportsmed 17(1):69–73, 1989.
10. Harrison JD, Branicki FJ, Makin GS: Pancreatic injury in association football. Injury 16:232, 1985.
11. Hoff GL, Martin TA: Outdoor and indoor soccer: Injuries among youth players. Am J Sports Med 14:231–233, 1986.
12. Keller CS, Noyes FR, Buncher CR: The medical aspects of soccer injury epidemiology. Am J Sports Med 15(suppl):S105–S112, 1987.
13. Kròss R, Öhler K, Barolin GS: Cerebral trauma due to heading—Computerized EEG analysis in football players. Z EEG-EMG 14:209–212, 1983.
14. Leatt P, Shephard RJ, Plyley MJ: Specific muscular development in under-18 soccer players. J Sports Sci 5:165–175, 1987.
15. Martens MA, Hansen L, Mulier JC: Adductor tendinitis and musculus rectus abdominis tendopathy. Am J Sports Med 15:353–356, 1987.
16. McCarroll JR, Ritter MA, Schrader J, Carlson S: The "isolated" posterior cruciate ligament injury. Phys Sportsmed 11(2):146–152, 1983.
17. McCarroll JR, Schrader JW, Shelbourne KD, et al: Meniscoid lesions of the ankle in soccer players. Am J Sports Med 15:255–257, 1987.
18. McCarroll JR, Meaney C, Sieber JM: Profile of youth soccer injuries. Phys Sportsmed 12(2):113–117, 1984.
19. Møller-Nielsen J, Hammar M: Women's soccer injuries in relation to the menstrual cycle and oral contraceptive use. Med Sci Sports Exerc 21:126–129, 1989.
20. Mozes M, Papa MZ, Zweig A, et al: Iliopsoas injury in soccer players. Br J Sports Med 19:168–170, 1985.
21. Nysether S: Dental injuries among Norwegian soccer players. Community Dent Oral Epidemiol 15:141–143, 1987.
22. Orlando RG: Soccer-related eye injuries in children and adolescents. Phys Sportsmed 16(11):103–106, 1988.
23. Sane J, Ylipaavalniemi P: Maxillofacial and dental soccer injuries in Finland. Br J Oral Maxillofacial Surg 25:383–390, 1987.
24. Schmidt-Olsen S, Bünemann LKH, Lade V, Brassoe JOK: Soccer injuries of youth. Br J Sports Med 19:161–164, 1985.
25. Schneider K, Zernicke RF: Computer simulation of head impact: Estimation of head-injury risk during soccer heading. Int J Sport Biomech 4:358–371, 1988.
26. Smedberg SGG, Broome AEA, Gullmo A, Roos H: Herniography in athletes with groin pain. Am J Surg 149:378–382, 1985.
27. Smodlaka VN: Groin pain in soccer players. Phys Sportsmed 8(8):57–61, 1980.
28. Smodlaka VN: Medical aspects of heading the ball in soccer. Phys Sportsmed 12(2):127–131, 1984.
29. Tysvaer AT: Cervical disc herniation in a football player. Br J Sports Med 19(1):43–44, 1985.
30. Tysvaer AT, Storli O-V: Soccer injuries to the brain. A neurological and electroencephalographic study of active football players. Am J Sports Med 17:573–578, 1989.
31. Van Laack W: Experimental studies of the effectiveness of various shin guards in association football. Z Orthop 123:951–956, 1985.
32. Ward A: Soccer: Safe kicks for kids. Phys Sportsmed 15(8):151–156, 1987.

# Chapter 47: Basketball

MICHAEL A. SITORIUS, MD
MARK KWIKKEL, ATC

I. **Introduction**

  A. Basketball was invented by James Naismith in 1891 in Springfield, Massachusetts as a recreational, noncontact sport. Since the early 1960s, with increasing interest and participation and increasing athlete size and athletic skills, the injuries associated with the sport have rapidly increased. **Basketball is now a contact sport.**

    1. Ranked 13th in number of participants ($>$ 25 million).

    2. Greater than 1 million treated injuries annually.

  B. **Competitive basketball** (male/female) requires:

    1. Size (height/weight)

    2. Quickness

    3. Agility

    4. Repetitive explosive movement

    5. Conditioning—physical and mental

    6. Excellent hand-eye coordination and reactions

    7. Speed

    8. Strength.

  C. **Mechanisms of injury:** Contact with:

    1. Other players

    2. Ball

    3. Floor

    4. Backboard, rim, net

    5. Objects surrounding floor

      a. Fixed, e.g., bleachers, walls

      b. Loose, e.g., towels, warm-up suits, chairs, tables, electronic cables, backboard and supports.

  D. **Anatomic distribution of injuries**

    1. Upper extremity (most frequent)

      a. Wrist

      b. Hand

      c. Finger.

    2. Lower extremity

      a. Ankle

      b. Knee

      c. Hip.

    3. Spine

    4. Facial.

  E. **Common types of injury**

    1. Strain

    2. Sprain

    3. Contusion

    4. Inflammatory conditions

      a. Tendinitis

      b. Bursitis

      c. Synovitis

      d. Myositis.

5. Overuse
   a. Secondary to running, jumping, quick acceleration/deceleration
6. Fractures/dislocations
7. Lacerations.

## II. Specific Problems—By Anatomic Location

### A. Head

1. Lacerations—scalp and forehead are the most common sites.
2. Contusions
3. The mechanism is striking court-site equipment, backboard, or another player.
   a. Example: player is undercut while rebounding or shooting a lay-up.
4. **Prevention is key.**
   a. Adequate padding to backboard and support.
   b. Removal of nonessential court-side loose objects.
   c. Adequate distance from court of "essential" court-side objects (scorer's table, benches, chairs).

### B. Face

1. **Lacerations**
   a. Eyebrows and chin are common locations.
   b. Usually secondary to contact with another player's elbow or head.
   c. Treatment:
      i. Suture
      ii. Steri-Strip.
   d. Usually does not limit return to immediate participation.
2. **Nasal fractures**
   a. Due to contact with another player's elbow.
      i. Ball strike is a less common cause.
   b. Displaced vs nondisplaced
      i. Clinical exam—check for obstruction and nasal or septal hematoma.
      ii. X-ray study may or may not be indicated.
   c. Treatment
      i. Ice
      ii. NSAIDs
      iii. Reduction if malaligned or if nasal passages are obstructed.
      iv. Face mask to allow return to participation—multiple types of face masks are available.
   d. Complications
      i. Bleeding
      ii. Cosmetic—malalignment
      iii. Obstruction of nasal passages (nasal septal hematoma).
   e. Risk of reinjury is great.
3. **Eye**
   a. **Corneal abrasion**
      i. Due to trauma from finger/fingernail, glasses shattering (rare), or contact lenses.
      ii. Symptoms—pain, blurred vision.
      iii. Diagnosis
         (a) Physical exam
         (b) Visual acuity testing
         (c) Fluorescein staining of eye.

        iv. Treatment
           (a) Eye patch for 24–48 hours.
              (i) Most resolve spontaneously.
           (b) Re-examine after 24 hours.
           (c) Antibiotic ointment—prophylactic initially.
           (d) Analgesic eye drops only for examination.
           (e) Prevention
              (i) Eye goggles
              (ii) Trimmed fingernails.

    b. **Blunt trauma**
       i. Mechanisms: Being struck by ball or body parts.
      ii. Potentially serious, though uncommon.
     iii. Thorough ophthalmologic exam (i.e., slit lamp and fundoscopic, etc.) necessary if visual acuity decreased or severe pain is present.
      iv. Check extraocular movements looking for an orbital blow-out fracture.
       v. Treatment depends on recognizing the disorder.

  4. **Dental/oropharyngeal**
    a. **Teeth**
       i. Fracture
          (a) Management is dependent on symptoms.
          (b) Dental referral is often necessary.
      ii. Avulsion—see Chap. 33.
     iii. **Prevention: mouth guard.**
    b. **Soft tissue**
       i. Lacerations—cheeks, tongue
      ii. Contusions.

C. **Neck**
  1. **Abrasions**—increasingly common
    a. Due to jewelry
    b. Prevent by removing jewelry.
  2. **Strains/sprains—rare**
  3. **Fracture**—cervical spine fracture is rare.
    a. Mechanism: striking floor or court-side equipment with hyperflexed cervical spine.
    b. Be prepared—have proper equipment available
       i. Spine board
      ii. Neck collar (Philadelphia collar)
     iii. Resuscitation equipment.

D. **Upper extremity**
  1. **Fingers**
    a. Most common upper extremity injury.
    b. Sprain—collateral ligaments of interphalangeal joints
       i. Common, most are uncomplicated.
      ii. Proximal interphalangeal joint most common site of injury.
     iii. Treatment—ice, "buddy taping."
      iv. Distal interphalangeal injury
         (a) Due to forced flexion of joint by ball hitting end of finger.
         (b) May result in digital extensor tendon avulsion/fracture
           (i) Mallet finger deformity
         (c) Diagnosis by exam, x-ray studies.
         (d) Treatment—dorsal stack finger splint, 2–4 weeks.
    c. Fractures—rare.

       d. Dislocations—rare
          i. Usually safe to reduce on site.
          ii. X-ray post-reduction.
          iii. Splint in flexion 7–10 days.

  2. **Thumb**
       a. Ulnar collateral ligament sprain most common.
       b. Mechanism—forced abduction due to contact with:
          i. Ball-mild (grade 1).
          ii. Other player, floor—potentially more severe.
       c. Diagnosis
          i. Exam—stress test is valuable.
          ii. X-rays to include stress views.
       d. Treatment
          i. Definite endpoint on exam (x-ray, stress test $< 45°$): immobilization with thumb spica cast for 2–3 weeks, then taping.
          ii. No definite endpoint to exam (x-ray, stress test $> 45°$): surgical referral.

  3. **Wrist**
       a. Sprain
          i. Mechanism—a fall on an outstretched hand.
          ii. Diagnosis—clinical exam, x-ray study.
          iii. Treatment—ice, NSAID, splint.
       b. Fracture
          i. Relatively uncommon
          ii. Sport specific
          iii. Scaphoid bone is primary area of concern.

  4. **Elbow**—rare
       a. Due to direct trauma—falls.
       b. Olecranon bursitis is most common.
       c. Fracture/dislocation rare.

E. **Chest**
  1. **Contusions**—common
       a. Mechanism—contact with bony prominence of another player, i.e., elbow, knee.
       b. Treatment—ice, NSAID
          i. Female—add compression and good supporting bra.
       c. Complications rare.

  2. **"Rebound rib"—stress-induced first rib fracture**
       a. Proposed mechanism is a sudden, violent contraction of the anterior scalene muscle.
       b. Symptom: Poorly defined shoulder pain.
       c. Diagnosis
          i. Physical exam
          ii. X-ray.
       d. Treatment—conservative
          i. Sling 4–6 weeks
          ii. Analgesics
          iii. Complications are rare.

F. **Back**
  1. Strain
       a. Common
       b. Secondary to:
          i. Jumping and twisting with outstretched arms.

          (a) Increases stress forces of compression, flexion, and lateral rotation on the lumbar discs.

        ii. Height of athlete results in increased leverage.

        iii. Inappropriate resistance training—"rebounder" machine.

    c. Risk increased by:

        i. Poor conditioning and stretching

        ii. Improper mechanics

        iii. Overuse

        iv. Incomplete rehabilitation of previous injury.

    d. Treatment

        i. Rest

        ii. Ice for acute injury

        iii. Heat for chronic injury

        iv. Muscle stimulation or transcutaneous electrical nerve stimulation (TENS) for chronic injury

        v. Stretching and rehabilitation exercises for low back disorder (flexion, extension, etc.)

        vi. NSAIDs

    e. Prevention

        i. Stretching and rehabilitation exercises continually.

        ii. Remove offending mechanism ("rebounder") if possible.

2. Lumbar disc

    a. Common symptoms—pain, limited range of motion.

    b. Diagnosis

        i. Clinical exam

        ii. MRI of lumbar spine.

    c. Treatment

        i. Conserative

          (a) Rest

          (b) Ice/heat

          (c) Rehabilitation exercises, stretching

          (d) NSAIDs

        ii. Surgery

          (a) Indicated if patient doesn't respond to conservative treatment, if disc disease is documented.

          (b) Persistent neurologic deficit.

3. Spondylolysis

    a. Fracture of pars interarticularis.

    b. Suspect in adolescent with "low back pain."

    c. L5 most common.

    d. Pain on hyperextension.

    e. Diagnosis

        i. Oblique spine x-rays help confirm diagnosis.

        ii. Bone scan

          (a) Indicated if x-rays not conclusive.

    f. Treatment

        i. Rest

        ii. Stretching—increase flexibility and muscle strengthening.

        iii. Casting or anterior-opening Boston brace

          (a) Semirigid orthosis

          (b) Lessens loading on spine by preventing hyperextension.

4. Scoliosis
   a. Noted with screening exam
      i. Shoulder, pelvic alignment are noted.
      ii. Check leg length.
   b. Scoliosis x-ray studies to define extent.
   c. Mild abnormality—rare cause of disqualification.
   d. Severe abnormality
      i. Needs treatment (bracing, casting, etc.).
      ii. Disqualification until further evaluation by orthopedic consultant.
5. Contusion
   a. Common
   b. Secondary to collision with another player—direct trauma.
   c. Treatment
      i. Rest
      ii. Ice
      iii. Compression.

G. **Hip**
   1. Greater trochanter bursitis
      a. Uncommon
      b. Secondary to diving for loose balls.
      c. Often repetitive injury
         i. Inflammation and pain initially
         ii. Bursa later may fill with fluid.
      d. Treatment
         i. Rest
         ii. Ice
         iii. Padding over area of repetitive trauma
         iv. NSAIDs
         v. Corticosteroid injection.
   2. Strains
      a. Adductor muscle group strains are the most common.
         i. Occasionally difficult to distinguish from inguinal hernia.
      b. Treatment
         i. Rest
         ii. Ice
         iii. Stretching to limit pain (continued once healed)
         iv. Time.

H. **Upper leg**
   1. Strains—common
      a. Location
         i. Quadriceps—middle area of rectus femoris
         ii. Groin—upper portion of adductor longus/magnus
         iii. Hamstrings—lower or middle biceps femoris.
      b. Mechanism: Excessive tension on contracted muscle.
      c. Diagnosis
         i. Pain
         ii. Decreased ROM
         iii. Palpable defect in muscle in severe strains
         iv. X-ray: soft tissue swelling is possible.
      d. Treatment
         i. RICE (rest, ice, compression, elevation)

   ii. Stretching as tolerated—important to prevent muscle contracture. Continue long-term.

 2. Contusion—commmon, often severe
  a. Mechanism secondary to collision with another player "taking a charge."
  b. Quadriceps—common site
  c. Treatment
   i. Immediate, aggressive icing
   ii. Rest; crutches in moderate to severe cases
   iii. Compression
   iv. Avoid NSAIDs—may increase hemorrhaging secondary to coagulation system effects of NSAIDs.
  d. Myositis ossificans is a possible long-term consequence.

## I. Knee

 1. Less common site than in other contact sports (i.e., football, soccer), but second in frequency to ankle injuries in basketball players.
 2. Type
  a. Ligament
  b. Meniscal
  c. Patellofemoral pain syndrome
  d. Patellar dislocation
  e. Plica syndrome.
 3. Ligament
  a. Strain, tear
  b. Mechanisms in basketball:
   i. Deceleration—valgus and external rotation injury most common.
    (a) Medial collateral ligament
    (b) Anterior cruciate ligament
    (c) Lateral collateral ligament
    (d) Posterior cruciate ligament.
   ii. Hyperextension second most common.
   iii. Also direct blow to knee with resultant abnormal valgus, varus, or rotational forces.
  c. Diagnosis, treatment, and rehabilitation, see Chap. 40.
 4. Mensical tear
  a. Common
  b. Mechanism
   i. Direct valgus/varus stress
   ii. Hyperextension
   iii. Repetitive trauma.
  c. Diagnosis, treatment, and rehabilitation, see Chap. 40.
 5. Patellofemoral pain syndrome
  a. Common
  b. Results from constant acceleration, deceleration, and jumping.
  c. Pain is primary complaint.
  d. Treatment
   i. Conservative
    (a) Rest
    (b) Ice
    (c) Resistance exercises in extension
    (d) NSAIDs
    (e) Patellar restraining brace.
   ii. Arthroscopy if refractory to conservative treatment.

      (a) Confirm diagnosis.

      (b) Positive or negative lateral release.

      (c) Intensive rehabilitation postoperatively.

6. Patellar dislocation
   a. Mechanism
      i. Laterally directed force to patella—knee-to-knee contact, knee striking fixed object.
      ii. Medial retinaculum—stretched or torn.
   b. Treatment
      i. Reduction after x-rays to rule out fracture (many self-reduce).
      ii. Immobilization in extension up to 6 weeks.
         (a) First dislocation may warrant immobilization up to 6 weeks in an attempt to prevent recurrences.
         (b) Immobilize recurrent dislocations until pain and swelling are well controlled.
      iii. Quadriceps strengthening exercises
      iv. Patellar restraining brace
      v. Surgery occasionally warranted with major tear of medial quadriceps tendon.
   c. Recurrence is common.
7. Patellar tendonitis—"jumper's knee"
   a. Common
   b. Functional overload injury of knee extension mechanism.
   c. Symptoms—dull aching pain in the inferior aspect of patella and proximal patella tendon.
   d. Patella alta is a common predisposing condition.
   e. Treatment
      i. Rest
      ii. Ice
      iii. NSAIDs
      iv. Quadriceps strengthening exercises in extension
      v. Ankle dorsiflexion exercises
      vi. Stretching of biceps femoris—flexibility is cornerstone of therapy.
      vii. Neoprene knee sleeve
      viii. Phonophoresis or iontophoresis
      ix. No steroid injection—increased risk of tendon rupture reported.
   f. Rupture of tendon
      i. Rare
      ii. Risk increased with chronic pain, increasing age of participant.
      iii. Often a complications of previous corticosteroid injections.
   g. Prevention
      i. Decrease jumping drills.
      ii. Increase quadriceps strength.
      iii. Biceps femoris and quadriceps stretching can help prevent.

J. **Shin/calf injuries**
   1. Rare
   2. Contusion—secondary to blunt trauma
      a. RICE
      b. NSAIDs
      c. Rule out acute compartment syndrome.
   3. "Shin splints"
      a. Syndrome of pain inner distal two-thirds of tibia.

        b. Initially pain after running.

        c. Pain

            i. Dull

            ii. Located posterior medial border of tibia.

        d. Treatment

            i. Rest

            ii. Ice

            iii. NSAIDs

            iv. Heal cord and hamstring stretching.

        e. Consider other etiologies, i.e., stress fracture tibia/fibula, muscle and tendon tears, facial tears with muscle herniation, compartment syndromes.

**K. Ankle**

    1. Is the most common site of basketball injury.

    2. Sprain—lateral ligaments most common.

        a. Mechanism: inversion stress from:

            i. Landing on another player's foot

            ii. Sudden directional change

            iii. Inadequately rehabilitated previous injury

            iv. Weak ankles, history of previous injury.

        b. Ligaments involved:

            i. Anterior talofibular

              (a) Prevents anterior displacement.

            ii. Calcaneofibular

              (a) Largest ligament in complex

              (b) Resists inversion.

            iii. Posterior talofibular

              (a) Strongest ligament of complex

              (b) Resists anterior and medial displacement.

        c. Diagnosis—see Chap. 41.

            i. Physical exam, include anterior drawer testing.

            ii. X-rays—stress films are helpful (anterior drawer, talar tilt).

            iii. May need local anesthetic to examine adequately.

        d. Treatment

            i. Grade 1—RICE, immobilization with taping, rehabilitation.

            ii. Grade 2—RICE plus crutches, rehabilitation.

            iii. Grade 3—rare in basketball

              (a) Surgical treatment occasionally required.

        e. Prevention

            i. Strengthening ankle dorsiflexors, plantar flexors, invertors, and evertors (tilt board; resistance exercises).

            ii. Taping

            iii. Braces—helpful for chronic sprain.

            iv. Shoes—high top; leather or canvas (Nylon stretches).

    3. Medial ligaments

        a. Deep/superficial deltoid ligament.

        b. Less common (15% of ankle injuries).

        c. Treatment is similar as for lateral compartment sprain.

        d. Deep deltoid sprains frequently warrant surgery.

            i. Diagnosis made on mortise x-ray view if medial clear space is increased.

    4. Fracture—consider; rule out with x-rays.

    5. Achilles tendon rupture

        a. Achilles tendon initiates jumping motion.

      b. More common in recreational athletes over 30 years old.

      c. Sudden "pop," pain with forced plantar flexion.

      d. Contributing factors

         i. Chronic injury

        ii. Chronic inflammation (Achilles tendonitis)

       iii. Previous corticosteroid injection.

      e. Diagnosis

         i. Palpable musculotendinous defect

        ii. Positive Thompson's test.

      f. Treatment

         i. Acute

          (a) RICE

          (b) Referral for surgery

            (i) Elite athlete

            (ii) Younger athlete

            (iii) Tear at attachment.

          (c) Conservative—rest, casting, rehabilitation

            (i) Recreational athlete

            (ii) Older athlete.

          (d) Rehabilitation—1 year to return to high level of competition.

L. **Foot**—Foot injuries are more common in basketball than in many other sports.

  1. Fracture of base of 5th metatarsal

    a. Secondary to forced inversion and plantar flexion.

    b. Avulsion of the peroneus brevis from its insertion.

    c. Diagnosis

      i. Pain over base of 5th metatarsal

     ii. X-ray.

    d. Treatment conservative

      i. Rest

     ii. Ice

     iii. NSAIDs

     iv. Hard-soled shoe

     v. Improved biomechanics.

  2. Jones fracture—base of 5th metatarsal.

    a. May be a stress fracture or may appear to be a traumatic fracture in an area of pre-existing stress.

    b. Involves the proximal part of the diaphysis distal to tuberosity.

    c. Due to vertical and mediolateral forces concentrated over 5th metatarsal.

    d. Bone scan if suspicion high and normal x-rays.

    e. More frequent in young athletes.

    f. Incidence highest in early training period.

    g. Often very disabling.

    h. Treatment

      i. Conservative

        (a) Immobilization, nonweight-bearing for 6–8 weeks.

        (b) Rehabilitation gradual after healing on x-ray and no symptoms.

     ii. Surgery—may allow earlier return to competition.

        (a) Consider for competitive, elite athlete.

        (b) Delayed union greather than 12 weeks.

        (c) Non-union

        (d) Recreational athlete with persistent symptoms limiting daily activity.

(e) Type

    (i) Intramedullary screw

    (ii) Bone grafting.

3. Tarsal navicular stress fracture

  a. Uncommon in all athletes—most frequently occurs in basketball players.

  b. Pain

    i. Insidious onset

    ii. Dorsum of foot

    iii. Medial longitudinal arch.

  c. Aggravated with activity.

  d. Bone scan often necessary.

  e. Treatment

    i. Cast immobilization for 6–8 weeks

    ii. Nonweight-bearing

    iii. Rehabilitation of lower leg when pain-free.

4. Metatarsal stress fracture

  a. Common—increasing incidence.

    i. Year-round commitment

    ii. Increased intensity of practice.

  b. Often secondary to sudden increase in running/jogging (early training).

  c. Identified in every bone in foot; metatarsals more common.

  d. Diagnosis

    i. Plain x-rays

    ii. Bone scan may identify earlier.

  e. Treatment:

    i. Rest

    ii. NSAIDs

    iii. Moderate training regimen.

5. Arch sprains

  a. Involve plantar fascia, intrinsic muscles of foot, ligaments of midfoot.

  b. Pes planus predisposing factor.

  c. Improper jumping mechanics.

  d. Treatment

    i. RICE

    ii. Taping

    iii. Orthotics.

6. Plantar fasciitis

  a. Overuse is a major contributor.

  b. Occurs in origin of plantar fascia from calcaneus.

  c. Associated with decreased flexibility of biceps femoris and Achilles tendon.

  d. Treatment

    i. Heat

    ii. NSAIDs

    iii. Stretching exercises—increased flexibility

    iv. Tuli's heel cups

    v. Corticosteroid injection

    vi. Orthotics.

7. Skin—most common injury to foot.

  a. Blisters

    i. Occur early in the season.

    ii. Due to constant start and stop, pivoting.

      iii. Treatment
        (a) Proper shoe fit
        (b) Two pairs of socks worn—laundered daily.
        (c) Moleskin applied to affected area.
    b. Calluses—trim frequently.
    c. Corns—local theapy with salicylic acid plaster or excision.

III. **General**

    A. Sprains are the most common injury in basketball.
       1. Prevention is the key.
         a. Conditioning
           i. Strength and power should be increased to prevent joint injury—muscle lends dynamic stability to passive protection of ligaments.
       2. Flexibility
         a. Warm-up stretching is important.
         b. Maintain good flexibility year-round.
       3. Preseason moderation of frequency and duration of practice.
       4. Once injured—long-term plan for rehabilitation to decrease recurrence rate.
    B. Male and female basketball players
       1. Experience same types of injuries:
         a. Sprains
         b. Contusions
         c. Strains
         d. Muscle cramps
         e. Tendonitis.
       2. Female
         a. More sprains—prevent with greater emphasis on conditioning.
         b. More contusions—may be related to increased capillary fragility related to both endogenous and exogenous birth control pills hormone.

## *RECOMMENDED READING*

1. Apple DF: Basketball injuries: An overview. Phys Sportsmed 16(12):64–74, 1988.
2. Basset FH: Basketball. In Schneider RC, et al (eds): Sports Injuries: Mechanisms, Prevention and Treatment. Baltimore, Williams & Wilkins, 1985, pp 79–89.
3. Henry JH, Lareau B, Neigut D: The injury rate in professional athletes. Am J Sports Med 10:16–18, 1982.
4. Kavanaugh JH, Brown TD, Mann RV: The Jones fracture revisited. J Bone Joint Surg 60A:776–781, 1978.
5. Mellion MB: Overuse syndromes in athletes. In Mellion MB (ed): Office Management of Sports Injuries & Athletic Problems. Philadelphia, Hanley & Belfus, 1988, pp 289–309.
6. Saccjetti AD, Beswick DR, Morse SD: Rebound rib: Stress-induced first rib fracture. Ann Emerg Med 12(3):177–179, 1983.
7. Torg JS, Baldwin FC, Zelko RR, et al: Fracture of the base of the fifth metatarsal distal to the tuberosity. J Bone Joint Surg 66A:209–214, 1984.
8. Yost JH, Ellfeldf HJ: Basketball injuries. In Nicholas JA, Hershman EB (eds): The Lower Extremity and Spine in Sports Medicine. St. Louis, CV Mosby, 1986, pp 1440–1466.
9. Zelisko JA, Noble HB, Ponter M: Comparison of men's and women's professional basketball injuries. Am J Sports Med 10:297–299, 1982.

# Chapter 48: Wrestling

TIMOTHY F. KELLY, MA, ATC

I. **Introduction and General Sports Medicine Concerns**

Wrestling is one of the oldest forms of sport known to man. References to this ancient sport date back as far as 2160 B.C.[2] **Greco-Roman** and **international freestyle** are two of the most popular styles practiced today. Both styles are Olympic sports.

Wrestling enjoys strong participation at all levels of competition. Organized youth programs at YMCAs and Boys Clubs provide younger competitors the opportunity to enjoy wrestling. Junior high, high school, AAU, and collegiate programs all offer older competitors the opportunity to compete. The formation of wrestling clubs has also become a popular way for successful ex-collegians to train for International and Olympic competition.

A working knowledge of the sport of wrestling is necessary in order to treat the injured wrestler effectively. Physicians working with these athletes should be aware of the high incidence of injury associated with competitive wrestling. Weight-cutting practices and their health consequences remain a constant source of criticism of the sport.

A. **Wrestling styles**
   1. **Greco-Roman** wrestling was developed in the 19th century by the French and is typified by upper-body throws in which one wrestler takes his opponent to the mat. It is a more restrictive style of wrestling in which wrestlers are prohibited from actively using their legs or grabbing their opponent below the waist in order to execute a throw to the mat. Points are awarded for the degree of skill a wrestler displays in throwing his opponent to the mat. A fall is awarded when one wrestler throws his opponent to the mat in a manner by which both shoulders touch the mat simultaneously.
   2. **International freestyle** wrestling is the most popular wrestling style in the world. Unlike Greco-Roman, the legs play an integral part in the execution of many maneuvers in freestyle wrestling. Holds below the waist are permissible as are trips and throws. Participants wrestle two 3-minute periods with 1 minute of rest between periods. Points are awarded for take-downs, reversals, and the exposure of the opponent's back to the mat. Pins are awarded when a wrestler holds his opponent to the mat for a 1 second count.
   3. **Intercollegiate freestyle** wrestling is almost exclusive to high school and collegiate programs in the U.S. It varies only slightly from international freestyle in that wrestlers are awarded additional points for controlling or "riding" their opponent and for escaping from their opponent's control. Refer to Table 1 for weight-class divisions.
B. **Mechanisms of injury** in wrestling have been classified into six different categories. The first five were identified by Snook[20]:
   1. **Direct blows** may occur during takedowns, clashing of heads, or from an errant elbow and usually result in contusions or lacerations.
   2. **Friction** occurs with constant contact with the mat and/or the opponent and may result in abrasions, skin infections, and bursitis.

**TABLE 1.** Weight Classifications in Wrestling

### International Greco-Roman and freestyle wrestling

| | |
|---|---|
| 1. 48 kg or 105.5 lb | 6. 74 kg or 163.0 lb |
| 2. 52 kg or 114.5 lb | 7. 82 kg or 180.5 lb |
| 3. 57 kg or 125.5 lb | 8. 90 kg or 198.0 lb |
| 4. 62 kg or 136.5 lb | 9. 100 kg or 220.0 lb |
| 5. 68 kg or 149.5 lb | 10. 130 kg or 286.0 lb |

### Intercollegiate freestyle

| | |
|---|---|
| 1. 118 lb | 6. 158 lb |
| 2. 126 lb | 7. 167 lb |
| 3. 134 lb | 8. 177 lbs |
| 4. 142 lb | 9. 190 lb |
| 5. 150 lb | 10. Hwt (177 to 275 lb) |

### Interscholastic freestyle

| | |
|---|---|
| 1. 103 lb (88 lb minimum) | 7. 140 lb |
| 2. 112 lbs (97 lb minimum) | 8. 145 lb |
| 3. 119 lb | 9. 152 lb |
| 4. 125 lb | 10. 160 lb |
| 5. 130 lb | 11. 171 lb |
| 6. 135 lb | 12. 189 lb |
| | 13. 275 lb (188 to 275 lb) |

### USA Kids Division—Three age group classifications

| (9–10) | | (11–12) | | (13–14) | |
|---|---|---|---|---|---|
| 50 lb | 85 lb | 60 lb | 105 lb | 70 lb | 115 lb |
| 55 lb | 90 lb | 65 lb | 110 lb | 75 lb | 120 lb |
| 60 lb | 95 lb | 70 lb | 120 lb | 80 lb | 125 lb |
| 65 lb | 100 lb | 75 lb | 130 lb | 85 lb | 130 lb |
| 70 lb | 110 lb | 80 lb | 140 lb | 90 lb | 135 lb |
| 75 lb | 120 lb | 85 lb | 150 lb | 95 lb | 145 lb |
| 80 lb | 130 lb | 90 lb | 165 lb | 100 lb | 155 lb |
| | Hwt | 95 lb | Hwt | 105 lb | 165 lb |
| | | 100 lb | | 110 lb | 175 lb |
| | | | | | Hwt |

3. **Falls** can occur during takedowns, trips, or throws and can be exacerbated by the weight of the opponent landing upon the bottom wrestler. There exists a potential for serious injury with any type of fall.

4. **Twisting and leverage** mechanisms are common with the holds and maneuvers in wrestling and may lead to strains and sprains.

5. **Self-induced injuries** are uncommon and are usually caused by the wrestler's own exertion, such as a back strain when attempting to lift a resisting opponent.

6. **Insidious** mechanisms may be observed in wrestlers with significant injuries. Many wrestlers may be unable to remember the exact mechanism or the onset of their injuries. Some of these injuries are likely to be attributed to overuse.

II. Wrestling Injuries

  A. **Patterns of injury**

    1. Because of the combative nature of wrestling and the heavy body contact, the incidence of injury is relatively high and has been compared to that of football,[16] soccer, lacrosse, and ice hockey.[19] However, the occurrence of serious injuries appears low.

    2. More injuries occur during practice than during competition because of the far greater time spent practicing;[4,16,20] however, matches carry a much higher risk of injury.[16,25]

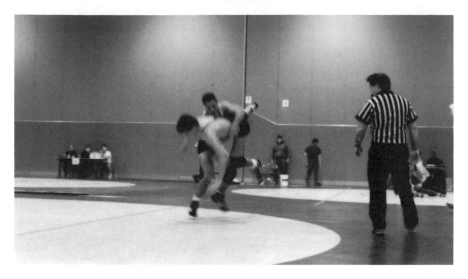

**FIGURE 1.** The takedown process places the wrestler at high risk for injury.

3. The **knee** is the most frequently injured anatomic site,[3,18,25] although injuries are distributed over the entire body.[3,16,17]
4. **Ligament sprains and musculotendinous strains** are the most common injuries in wrestling.[16,17]
5. Younger wrestlers are injured less seriously and less often than older, more competitive wrestlers.[9,17]
   a. Wrestling appears to be a relatively safe sport for preadolescent boys.[6]
6. The **takedown process,** in which one wrestler takes his opponent to the mat, places wrestler's at high risk for injury. During a takedown, one wrestler is usually caught off-guard and is taken to the mat in a manner over which he has very little control (Fig. 1).
7. **Reinjuries** are often noted in wrestlers who attempt to return to activity before complete healing and rehabilitation has occurred.[16,25]

B. **Specific injuries**
1. **Head and face injuries**
   a. **Lacerations** occur frequently during wrestling and are usually the result of a direct blow, as in the clash of heads or an errant elbow. Lacerations are noted around the orbit, scalp, zygomatic arch, and lower mentum.
      i. **Treatment**
         (a) Application of Steri-Strips may provide a temporary closure of the wound and allow continued participation. Supportive dressings are usually warranted.
      ii. **Precautions:**
         (a) Lacerations should be cleaned and dressed daily and monitored closely for signs of infection.
         (b) Consideration should be given to the use of relatively heavy Nylon (4.0–5.0) sutures, which may be deemed more appropriate when wrestlers continue to actively participate.
         (c) Cosmetic suturing should be avoided. If needed, wrestlers may opt for cosmetic revision at the end of the wrestling season.
   b. **Epistaxis** may occur with incidental contact to the nose. A direct blow or contact to the nose, as seen with a cross-face maneuver, can injure the highly

vascular nasal septum. Epistaxis may present with mild to profuse bleeding from one or both nares.

  i. **Treatment**

   (a) Mild epistaxis may resolve spontaneously with little intervention.

   (b) Persistent cases of epistaxis should be treated with **direct pressure** over the affected nares while the head is tilted slightly forward, reducing the chance of blood traveling down the oropharynx. Ice application may prove beneficial.

   (c) A **pledget or "nose plug"** treated with petroleum jelly may be inserted or gently screwed into the affected nostril.

     (i) Pledgets soaked with vasoconstrictors, such as 1% phenylephrine or 4% cocaine, have been used for many years, but these substances are banned at many levels of competition.

  ii. **Precautions:**

   (a) Allowing the end of the nose plug to slightly protrude from the naris will facilitate easy removal upon completion of activity.

   (b) Athletes should be instructed not to blow their noses following significant bouts of epistaxis.

   (c) If the above treatment fails to achieve hemostasis, proper referral to a medical facility for nasal packing may be indicated.

   (d) **Recurrent bouts** of nasal epistaxis may be treated with nasal cauterization:

     (i) Chemically with silver nitrate sticks.

     (ii) Electrocautery under local anesthesia.

 c. **Nasal fractures** may occur following a blow to the nose.

  i. **Treatment:** Wrestlers can often return to activity by wearing a protective face guard that adequately protects the nose.

 d. **"Cauliflower ear"**

  i. **Etiology**

   (a) Continuous friction and/or direct trauma to the auricle produces bleeding into the soft tissue of the ear.

   (b) Failure to wear headgear while wrestling.

  ii. **Diagnosis**

   (a) Localized perichondral swelling with disappearance of the normal convexities of the auricle, mild discomfort, and disfigurement.

   (b) Differential diagnosis

     (i) Cellulitis

     (ii) Perichondritis.

  iii. **Treatment**

   (a) Immediate aspiration with 25–27 gauge needle. Multiple incisions may be necessary to drain the ear completely. Aseptic practices should be rigidly followed.

   (b) Compression dressing following aspiration to prevent reaccumulation of blood and serum.

   (c) Methods of ear compression include:

     (i) Strips of gauze soaked in flexible collodion may be layered from the anterior to posterior aspect of the ear, which, upon drying, form a small cast around the ear.

     (ii) A commercial silicone that is easily molded to the contours of the ear has also been utilized.[5]

     (iii) A fluffy, gauze, mastoid dressing can also be used.

iv. **Precautions**

    (a) The ear canal should not be blocked or obstructed following application of the compressive dressing, as it is imperative that the athlete be able to equalize ear pressure.

    (b) Monitor daily for signs of infection.

    (c) Potentially disfiguring if left untreated.

e. **Concussions** may occur with a hard fall or heavy contact to the head. Proper evaluation and treatment are essential.

2. **Neck injuries** occur infrequently due to enforcement of the rules prohibiting slams and certain types of throws.

  a. Common neck injuries observed in wrestlers include:

    i. Sprains/strains

    ii. Degenerative disc changes

    iii. Neurogenic pain syndromes

    iv. Cervical spondylosis

    v. Facet syndrome.

  b. **Etiology**

    i. **"Bulling"** or spearing with the head held in slight hyperextension while attempting a takedown or blocking a takedown is common in wrestling. This technique is associated with the greatest number of neck injuries.[24]

    ii. **Stretch and pinch** mechanisms are commonly noted during the takedown process, when the head and neck are forced laterally while the shoulder is depressed.

    iii. **Forced extension and axial compression** can be observed when one wrestler is taken directly to the mat in a manner by which the head is the first part of the wrestler to strike the mat.

    iv. **Combinations** of neck motion.

  c. **Treatment**

    i. **Prevention**

      (a) Rule enforcement

      (b) Preseason x-ray examination of individuals with prior history of neck injury.

      (c) Preseason neck strength conditioning program.

3. **Chest and trunk injuries** common to wrestling include:

  a. **Rib and costochondral injuries**

    i. **Etiology**

      (a) **Direct blows** can be observed when one wrestler lands on his opponent's arm or leg following the takedown maneuver.

      (b) **Forced compression** injuries may occur when one wrestler falls forcefully on top of his prone or supine opponent following a takedown.

      (c) **Torsional strain** is common to various wrestling maneuvers and can result in muscle strains and costochondral separations.

      (d) **Exertional** injuries can be noted when one wrestler may expend enormous effort in performing a maneuver against the resistance of his opponent.

    ii. **Diagnosis**

      (a) Labored breathing, point tenderness, mild to severe, debilitating pain mostly associated with motion.

      (b) X-ray examination.

    iii. **Treatment**

      (a) Any injury involving the ribs is usually quite painful and **self-regulating** to the participation of the wrestler.

(b) **Rest and anti-inflammatory medication**

(c) Local **Corticosteroid injection** may be beneficial in highly competitive wrestlers.

(d) **Padding and taping** for practice are advisable when symptoms have subsided. A commercial rib belt may offer additional support.

  iv. **Precautions**

(a) Careful evaluation of injury before moving athlete with suspected rib injury.

(b) Pneumothorax, hemothorax.

  b. **Muscle strains** may result from sudden torsional movements or rigorous exertion common to many wrestling maneuvers. The oblique and rectus abdominis muscles may become involved.

  c. **Contusions** are also common.

4. **Back injuries** occur infrequently in wrestling. Most injuries are observed during the takedown process.[24]

  a. Back injuries observed in wrestlers include:

    i. Sprain

    ii. Strain

    iii. Spondylolysis/spondylolisthesis

    iv. Sciatica

    v. Sacroiliac sprain.

  b. **Etiology**

    i. May occur when wrestlers "spar" for position, placing the back in **mild hyperextension.**

    ii. **Torsional mechanisms**

    iii. **Extension against resistance,** as when a wrestler attempts to lift an opponent.

    iv. **Hyperflexion mechanisms** have been reported in various rolling maneuvers.

  c. **Treatment** (general)

    i. Rest/modified activity

    ii. Reduction of pain and spasm

    iii. Patient education

    iv. Stretching and conditioning programs

    v. Strengthening exercises.

5. **Shoulder injuries** occur frequently in wrestlers, usually when one wrestler is taken to the mat and lands forcibly on the tip of the shoulder. This mechanism usually results in a sprain of the AC joint. Occasionally, a wrestler may subluxate or completely dislocate his shoulder. This is not surprising, because the glenohumeral joint is subjected to considerable strain when used as a lever arm, and extreme ranges in motion are often applied during competitive wrestling.

  a. Common shoulder injuries include:

    i. Dislocation

    ii. Subluxation

    iii. Acromioclavicular strain

    iv. Sternoclavicular sprain

    v. Capsule strain.

6. **Elbow injuries** may result when a wrestler "posts" or completely extends his elbow to break his fall when landing on the mat following a takedown. This maneuver may lead to hyperextension or a fracture-dislocation injury. Wrestlers should be instructed to flex the elbow slightly when it is to be used

in this manner. Hyperextension taping is effective in preventing full extension of the elbow.

  a. Common elbow injuries include:
     i. Fracture
     ii. Hyperextension
     iii. Olecranon bursitis
     iv. Epicondylitis.

7. **Hand and wrist injuries** occur occasionally. Finger sprains can be buddy-taped to allow functional use during practice or competition. Finger dislocations can be properly splinted and padded to allow further competition.

  a. Frequent hand and finger injuries include:
     i. Sprain
     ii. Dislocation
     iii. Subluxation.

8. **Thumb injuries** can be debilitating to the wrestler. Most injuries of the thumb involve the ulnar collateral ligament, which is injured when the thumb is forcefully abducted. This represents a serious injury if the wrestler lacks strong opposition of the thumb, which is needed to grasp and hold an opponent. Surgery and a thumb spica cast may be required for serious injuries.

9. **Knee injuries** account for a large portion of all injuries sustained in wrestling.[3,11,18,25] Severe strain is often placed on the knee during certain wrestling maneuvers.

  a. Common knee injuries in wrestling include:
     i. Meniscal tears
     ii. Sprains
     iii. Strains
     iv. Subluxation/dislocation
     v. Bursitis.

  b. **Meniscal injuries** are common in wrestling. Wrestlers appear to injure the **lateral menisci** more frequently than do athletes in any other sport.[25] The takedown is a highly vulnerable period for a meniscal injury. The lead leg used during takedowns and defensive maneuvers appears to be injured more frequently.

     i. **Etiology.** Athough the exact pathomechanics of meniscal injuries are not always identified, Wroble et al.[25] have cited the following mechanisms:
       (a) **Indirect forces**
       (b) **Torsion**
       (c) **Shearing/hyperflexion**
       (d) **Insidious/overuse.**

     ii. **Diagnosis**
       (a) May present atypically in wrestlers.
       (b) Lateral rather than medial meniscal injuries occur.
       (c) Minimal symptoms, other than complaint of "locking," are present.
       (d) Many wrestlers may attempt to "wrestle through" meniscal injuries.

  c. **Sprains and strains** are the most common knee injuries.[25]
     i. Incidence of **ACL** and other catastrophic knee injuries is low.[25]
     ii. **Indirect force** accounts for most of these injuries.
     iii. The **takedown** is associated with the most injuries.
     iv. **Leg wrestling** may carry a higher potential for MCL and LCL injuries. Some wrestlers ride their opponents, almost exclusively using their legs to control their opponents (Fig. 2).

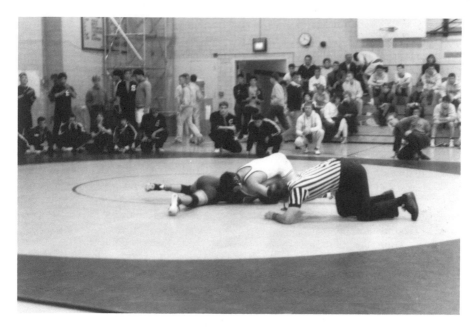

**FIGURE 2.** Extreme torsional forces on the back of a wrestler being pinned.

 d. **Patellar subluxation/dislocation** injuries are sometimes observed in younger wrestlers.
  i. Wrestlers sustaining these injuries may benefit from wearing a specialized neoprene sleeve designed to enclose and stabilize the patella.
 e. **Prepatellar bursitis** is a frequent knee problem in wrestlers.[13] The lead leg used during takedowns is most often afflicted. Recurrences are not uncommon.
  i. **Etiology**
   (a) Single traumatic event
   (b) Repeated bouts of irritation or trauma.
  ii. **Diagnosis**
   (a) History of trauma or irritation
   (b) Superficial patellar swelling
   (c) May have NROM, except with extreme flexion.
  iii. **Treatment**
   (a) Immediate aspiration (culture and Gram stain) of all cases
   (b) Compressive wrap
   (c) Nonsteroidal anti-inflammatory agents
   (d) 1 week of immobilization in recurrent cases
   (e) Steroid injections produce variable results.
   (f) Repeated bouts of inflammation in the competitive wrestler may necessitate a bursectomy.
   (g) Knee pads should be worn while wrestling.
 f. **Septic bursitis** may also afflict wrestlers.
  i. **Etiology**
   (a) *Staphylococcus aureus* is usually the invading organism.
  ii. **Diagnosis**
   (a) Often **asymptomatic.**

      (b) May show local signs of infection, including erythema, warmth, and fever.

      (c) Culture and sensitivity of bursal aspirate.

      (d) Laboratory tests (bursal glucose values, WBC count, Gram stain, and lactic acid tests) are not always reliable in distinguishing traumatic from septic bursitis.

   iii. **Treatment**

      (a) Same treatment as above

      (b) **Penicillinase-resistant penicillin** is the drug of choice until sensitivity tests are available.

10. **Ankle injuries** occur infrequently in wrestlers. A sprain may occur when a wrestler's foot "sticks" in the mat while performing a maneuver. Sprains can be adequately taped for participation following a proper rehabilitation program. Ankle injuries include sprain, fracture, and overuse injury.

C. **Treatment on the mat**

  1. **Time constraints**

    a. Injury time allotment is outlined in Table 2.

    b. Physician/trainer must work quickly yet thoroughly in evaluating and treating the injured wrestler during the injury time-out.

  2. **Epistaxis**

    a. The treatment of epistaxis during a match does not count toward the allotted injury time.

  3. **Rules regarding treatment**

    a. Taping an injured area (fingers, ankle, etc.) is permissible during an injury time-out.

      i. Taping that substantially reduces the normal motion of a joint is prohibited.

    b. The use of braces or mechanical devices that do not permit normal range of motion of a joint or that prevent an opponent from applying a hold are prohibited.

    c. The use of medications during a match to relieve a preexisting condition such as asthma or diabetes is strictly prohibited.

  4. **Return to wrestling**

    a. At the end of the allotted injury time, a decision about whether the athlete can continue participation must be rendered to the referee.

**TABLE 2.** Major Differences in Rules for Interscholastic and Intercollegiate Wrestling

| Parameter | High School | | Collegiate |
|---|---|---|---|
| **Length of Matches** | Period 1 | 2 min | 3 min |
| | Period 2 | 2 min | 2 min |
| | Period 3 | 2 min | 2 min |
| **Number of matches/day** | 5 full matches | | No limit |
| **Time between matches** | 45 min | | 1 hr |
| **Weigh-ins** | 1½ hr before meet | | 5 hr before meet |
| **Injury time allowed** | 1½ min | | 2 min |
| **Dehydrating equipment** | Sauna, plastic suits, and other dehydrating devices are strictly prohibited. | | No similar rule |
| **Certification** | Wrestlers are required to certify the weight at which they intend to wrestle the majority of the season. | | No similar rule |

    b. The referee has the authority to end the match when, in his opinion, a wrestler may be in danger of further injury if he continues to wrestle.

    c. Coaches, trainers, and parents cannot override the referee's decision.

    d. The attending physician may prohibit an injured wrestler from returning to participation. The physician may, after careful examination, deem the wrestler fit to continue wrestling.

    e. The referee may override the physician's *opinion* to allow an injured wrestler to continue participation.

    f. The decision of the attending physician that a wrestler cannot continue participation may not be overruled by anyone, including the referee.

D. **Common skin conditions** (see Chap. 28)

  1. **Pyodermic infections**

    a. Staphylococcus

    b. Streptococcus.

  2. **Viral infections**

    a. Herpes gladiatorum

    b. Herpes zoster

    c. Molluscum contagiosum.

  3. **Fungal infections**

    a. Tinea pedis

    b. Tinea cruris

    c. Tinea corporis.

  4. **Infestations**

    a. Scabies.

  5. **General treatment strategies**

    a. **Proper hygiene**

      i. Frequent showering

      ii. Daily laundering of wrestling gear

      iii. Fingernails cut short and cleaned daily.

    b. **Mat cleaning** done after every practice with an appropriate antiseptic solution.

      i. Antibacterial

      ii. Antiviral

      iii. Antifungal.

    c. **Medication** must be taken as directed.

    d. **Isolation** of infected wrestler(s) for 7–10 days with staphylococcal or streptococcal infections.

    e. **Proper wound care**

      i. Mat burns and other open wounds should be meticulously cleaned and monitored daily for infection.

    f. **Visual inspection** of wrestlers at weigh-ins for contagious skin conditions. **Disqualification** if skin condition is present.

III. **Prevention Strategies**

A. **Medical supervision**

  1. **Physician** present at all meets and tournaments.

  2. **Athletic trainer** or another qualified person at all practices.

  3. An **emergency plan** including initial triage, first aid, communication, and transportation.

  4. An accurate system of **record keeping** in which injuries are thoroughly documented.

B. **Coaching**

  1. Wrestlers should be made aware of illegal holds and potentially dangerous maneuvers and learn proper defenses against them.

C. **Conditioning and strength programs**
   1. Should be aimed at developing:
      a. Muscular endurance          d. Flexibility
      b. Muscular strength           e. Ideal wrestling weight.
      c. Aerobic fitness
D. **Proper warm-up/cool-down**
   1. Jogging
   2. Stretching
   3. Rehearsal of wrestling skills.
E. **Officiating**
   1. It is vital that the referee anticipate and position himself so he may whistle or stop a potentially dangerous or illegal hold before an injury is allowed to occur (Figs. 3 and 4).

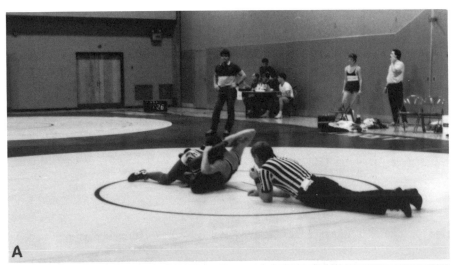

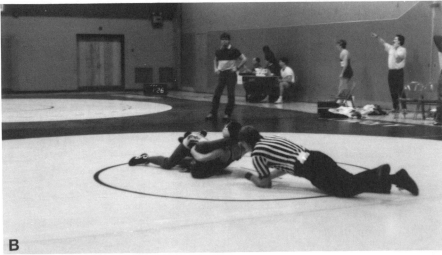

**FIGURE 3.**   *A,* High torquing forces are applied to the shoulder of the wrestler on the left in what is known as the "guillotine maneuver." *B,* The official is in position to interrupt the match and bring the wrestler's back to the referee's position if the hold becomes potentially dangerous.

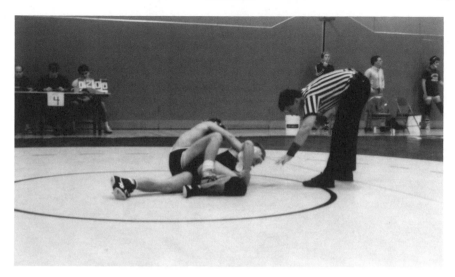

**FIGURE 4.** The left foot of the wrestler on top is trapped in a position that may lead to injury. The official is evaluating whether it is a potentially dangerous hold.

    F.  **Equipment** (shoes, elbow and knee pads, headgear, etc.)
        1.  Properly fitted
        2.  High quality
        3.  Protective features.

IV.  **Special Aspects of Prehabilitation and Rehabilitation**

    A.  **Prehabilitation**
        1.  **Strength assessment**
        2.  **Cardiovascular assessment**
        3.  **Flexibility assessment:** Wrestling demands extensive joint mobility for optimal performance. Emphasis should be placed on the following areas: heel cords, hamstrings, quads, adductors, abductors, low back, and shoulders.
        4.  **Maturation assessment:** The evaluation of preadolescent wrestlers may be necessary for proper matching younger competitors. Proper matching is important in reducing injuries as well as ensuring satisfaction in younger wrestlers.
        5.  **Previous injury assessment**—evaluation and rehabilitation of preexisting injuries.

    B.  **Rehabilitation**
        1.  **Compliance:** Collegiate wrestlers are often noncompliant athletes who must be carefully monitored throughout the rehabilitation process.
        2.  **Coach:** The coach can provide the impetus to stimulate compliance by the wrestlers. The coach can demand that a wrestler adhere to the physician's or trainer's recommendations.
        3.  **Weight control:** Wrestlers must stay within a reasonable reach of their wrestling weight during the rehabilitation process.

V.  **Wrestling Facilities and Protective Equipment**

    A.  **Facilities**
        1.  **Wrestling mats**—constructed from Ensolite foam, which has a outer vinyl coating that permits easy cleaning. The mat exhibits properties of controlled compression and controlled recovery, which provide shock absorption for the heavy impact that occurs in takedowns and throwing maneuvers.

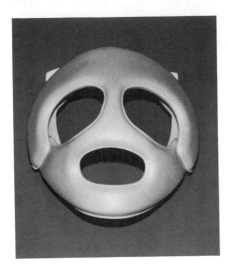

**FIGURE 5.**   Face guard attached to the wrestler's headgear to protect facial injuries.

2. **Wrestling room:** Dimensions should be at least 50 sq. ft. per wrestler to minimize the chance of injury from collisions with other wrestlers.[15] Walls and pillars in the wrestling room should be padded at least 5 feet high.
B. **Equipment**
   1. **Faceguard:** Wrestlers with facial sutures or nasal fractures may benefit from wearing a protective faceguard (Fig. 5).
   2. **Mouthguard:** All wrestlers, especially younger wrestlers with orthodontic braces, should wear mouthpieces.
   3. **Knee and elbow pads** provide protection of previously injured areas. Pads of neoprene construction are currently popular.
   4. **Footwear:** Soles are of a gum-rubber composition that allows ankle and foot mobility while maintaining adequate traction with the mat. These shoes should never be used for running as they provide no shock-absorbing qualities.
   5. **Athletic supporter**—provides protection of the testicles.
   6. **Headgear:** The use of properly fitted headgear is essential for the protection of the ears during wrestling (Fig. 6).

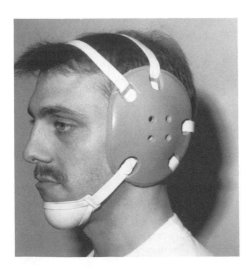

**FIGURE 6.**   Protective headgear designed to prevent ear injuries.

VI. **Rules to Protect Wrestlers**

  A. **Governing bodies**

    1. Members of the National Collegiate Athletic Association (NCAA) Rules Committee and the National Federation of State High School Associations (NFSHSA) have established their own individual sets of wrestling rules.

    2. International wrestling rules and regulations are set by the Federation Internationale des Luttes Amateurs (FILA).

  B. **Specific rules**

    1. Most rules are the same or very similar; however, subtle differences do exist between interscholastic and collegiate wrestling. For specific differences, see Table 2.

    2. To ensure safety, the referee may temporarily halt a match for illegal holds, unnecessary roughness, or potentially dangerous situations.

      a. **Illegal holds** are maneuvers that inflict pain and are dangerous to the receiving wrestler, such as holds that cover the mouth, throat, and eyes. The offending wrestler is penalized.

      b. **Potentially dangerous** situations are those in which a hold or maneuver may place a wrestler in danger of injury. These moves usually force a joint beyond its normal mobility. The referee can break these holds before an injury is allowed to occur. No penalty is assessed, as these are usually unintentional.

      c. **Unnecessary roughness** may be assessed when one wrestler uses more force or aggressiveness than is necessary, such as a forceful trip or an aggressive cross-face. A penalty is assessed.

VII. **Special Concerns of the Team Physician**

  A. **"Making weight"**

    1. **Certification of scholastic wrestlers**

      a. Each state is allowed to regulate the certification process by which wrestlers seek to qualify (make weight) for a given weight classification at which they desire to compete for the majority of the wrestling season.

      b. Predetermined dates are set by which the wrestler must make the requirements of the weight classification.

      c. A wrestler may not wrestle below his certification weight but may wrestle at a higher weight class.

      d. If a wrestler fails to make weight for a meet, he may become eligible to compete in the next higher weight classification.

      e. Recertification at a lower weight classification should be strongly discouraged.

      f. Physicians are urged to become actively involved in the certification process.

      g. Certification weight should be based not only on visual assessment and current weight, but also on body composition assessment.

    2. **Weight-cutting practices**

      a. Why wrestlers cut weight

        i. Wrestlers seek to gain an advantage over their opponents by reducing body weight and body fat to a minimal level in order to compete in the lowest possible weight classification over a supposedly smaller and weaker opponent.

        ii. There may be two good wrestlers at one weight, which means one wrestler may not compete unless he moves to another weight classification.

        iii. Most wrestlers believe they can make weight for a lower weight class with no loss in performance.[23] This belief is often unsound.

    b. Methods of weight cutting
       i. Thermal methods
         (a) Plastic or rubber suits
         (b) Saunas or steam rooms
         (c) Excessive exercise.
       ii. Nutritional method
         (a) Diet restriction
         (b) Fluid restriction.
       iii. Other less common methods
         (a) Excessive spitting
         (b) Self-induced vomiting
         (c) Diuretics
         (d) Laxatives

**3. The process of making weight**

    a. The actual process of making weight is usually undertaken 2 or 3 days prior to the official weigh-in when wrestlers begin to restrict their food and water intake while continuing to exercise and wrestle at rigorous levels.

    b. Several hours before the official weigh-in, wrestlers unable to meet the weight requirement may attempt acute dehydration to lose the necessary weight in order to qualify for their weight classification.

    c. Wrestlers may lose up to 10% of their body weight or more following these methods.

    d. Following the weigh-in, wrestlers frequently attempt to rehydrate themselves by consuming large quantities of fluids. Research has shown that a 5-hour rehydration period does not allow the body enough time to rehydrate,[8,26,27] and that most high school and collegiate wrestlers are competing in a dehydrated state.[10,26]

    e. This weight-cutting process is then repeated many times throughout a wrestling season.

    f. Fellow wrestlers and coaches are most frequently consulted for information concerning making weight; physicians and parents are rarely consulted about these problems.[23]

**4. Health consequences associated with making weight**

    a. **Thermal injuries**
       i. Heat cramps
       ii. Heat exhaustion
       iii. Heat stroke.

    b. **Renal and cardiac disturbances**[1]
       i. Lower plasma and blood volumes
       ii. Decreased cardiac output
       iii. Decreased renal blood flow and urine output.
       iv. Electrolyte problems
       v. Possible renal damage.

    c. **Other disturbances**
       i. Learning ability is reduced.[21]
       ii. Anxiety may occur during the weight-cutting process.[12]
       iii. Depression[12]
       iv. Eating disorders
         (a) Bulimia nervosa
         (b) Anorexia nervosa.

    d. **Decrements in physical performance**[7]
       i. 2% loss of body weight impairs thermoregulatory system.
       ii. 3% loss reduces muscular endurance time.

      iii. 4–6% loss results in reduced muscular strength, reduced endurance time, and heat cramps.

      iv. > 6% loss can lead to heat cramps, exhaustion, stroke, coma, and death.

   e. **Long-term studies needed** to examine dehydration in wrestlers.

      i. Delayed renal damage may present during the middle decades of the wrestler's life.[22]

      ii. Possible stunting of growth and maturation in younger wrestlers.

**B. Preventive strategies against weight abuses**

   1. **Education**

   2. **Nutritional guidance**

   3. **Preseason conditioning programs**

   4. **Weight monitoring**—a daily record of each wrestler's weight before and after each practice.

   5. **Body composition assessment:** Following the preseason conditioning program, an assessment of body composition should be undertaken by qualified personnel.

     a. A 5% level of body fat should be considered the minimal percentage at which a wrestler can safely compete.[22]

     b. Most wrestlers completing a 4–6 week preseason conditioning program will be close to their actual wrestling weight.

     c. Any wrestler seeking to reduce weight further must get prior approval from the physician, so that an appropriate weight reduction plan can be set up.

     d. Caloric intake and expenditure should be monitored closely.

     e. Wrestlers should be discouraged from losing more than 2–3 lbs. per week.

   6. **Method of body composition**

     a. Opplinger and Tipton regression equation designed specifically for wrestlers (Table 3).[14]

     b. This equation uses various anthropometric measurements to compute minimal wrestling weight. The use of a anthropometer or similar body caliper device is required for measurements.

     c. Coaches, trainers, and physicians can easily use this equation for assessment of body composition.

**TABLE 3.** Opplinger and Tipton Regression Equation for Prediction of a Minimal Wrestling Weight in Scholastic Wrestlers

| **Opplinger and Tipton Model** (r. 962) | | |
|---|---|---|
| (0.49)* (current weight in lb) | = | _____ |
| (1.65)* (height in inches) | = | _____ |
| (1.81)* (chest diameter) | = | _____ |
| (6.70)* (right wrist diameter) | = | _____ |
| (1.35)* (chest depth) | = | _____ |
| | Sum total − 156.56 = Minimal wrestling weight | |

\* All measurements in centimeters unless otherwise noted.
From Opplinger RA, Tipton CM: Iowa wrestling study: Cross validation of the Tcheng-Tipton minimal weight prediction formulas for high school wrestlers. Med Sci Sports 20:310–316, 1988, with permission.

## REFERENCES

1. American College of Sports Medicine: Position Stand on Weight Loss in Wrestlers. Madison, WI, American College of Sports Medicine, 1976.
2. Boring WJ: Science and Skills of Wrestling. St. Louis, CV Mosby, 1975.
3. Estwanik JJ, Bergfeld J, Canty T: Report of injuries sustained during the United States Olympic wrestling trials. Am J Sports Med 6:335–340, 1978.

4. Estwanik JJ, Bergfeld JA, Collins HR, Hall R: Injuries in interscholastic wrestling. Phys Sportsmed 8:111–121, 1980.
5. Gross CG: Treating "cauliflower ear" with silicone mold. Am J Sports Med 6:4–5, 1978.
6. Hartmann PM: Injuries in preadolescent wrestlers. Phys Sportsmed 6:79–82, 1978.
7. Hecker AL, Wheeler KB: Impact of hydration and energy intake on performance. In Kaverman D (ed): Schering Symposium. Athletic Training Winter 1984, pp 260–264.
8. Herbert WG, Ribisl PM: Effects of dehydration upon physical working capacity of wrestlers under competitive conditions. Res Q 43:416–422, 1972.
9. Hinkamp JF: High school athletic injuries. Ill Med J 148:127–129, 1975.
10. Hursh LM: Food and water restriction in the wrestler. JAMA 241:915–916, 1979.
11. Lok V, Yuceturk G: Injuries in wrestling. J Sports Med 2:324–328, 1974.
12. Morgan WP: Psychological effect of weight reduction in the college wrestler. Med Sci Sports 2:24–27, 1970.
13. Mysnyk MC, Wroble RR, Foster DT, Albright JP: Prepatellar bursitis in wrestlers. Am J Sports Med 14:46–54, 1986.
14. Opplinger RA, Tipton CM: Iowa wrestling study: Cross validation of the Tcheng-Tipton minimal weight prediction formulas for high school wrestlers. Med Sci Sports 20:310–316, 1988.
15. Rasch PG, Kroll W: What Research Tells the Coach about Wrestling. Washington, D.C., American Association for Health, Physical Education and Recreation, 1964.
16. Requa R, Garrick JG: Injuries in interscholastic wrestling. Phys Sportsmed 9:51, 1981.
17. Strauss RH, Lanese RR: Injuries among wrestlers in school and college tournaments. JAMA 248:2016–2019, 1982.
18. Snook GA: Injuries in intercollegiate wrestling. Am J Sports Med 10:142–144, 1982.
19. Snook GA: The injury problem in wrestling. Am J Sports Med 9:184–188, 1976.
20. Snook GA: Wrestling. In Schneider RC (ed): Sports Injuries: Mechanisms, Prevention, and Treatment. Baltimore, Williams & Wilkins, 1985, pp 129–138.
21. Taylor HL, Herschel A, Mickelson O, et al: Some effects of acute starvation with hard work on body weight, body fluids, and metabolism. J Appl Physiol 6:613–623, 1954.
22. Tipton CM: Physiological problems associated with the "making of weight." Am J Sports Med 8:449–450, 1980.
23. Tipton CM, Tcheng TK: Iowa wrestling study: Weight loss in high school students. JAMA 214:1269–1274, 1970.
24. Wroble RR, Albright JP: Neck and low back injuries in wrestling. Clin Sports Med 2:295–324, 1986.
25. Wroble RR, Mysnyk MC, Foster DT, Albright JP: Patterns of knee injuries in wrestling: A six year study. Am J Sports Med 14:55–66, 1986.
26. Zambraski EJ, Tipton CM, Tcheng TK, et al: Iowa wrestling study: Changes in the urinary profiles of wrestlers prior to and after competition. Med Sci Sports 7:217–220, 1975.
27. Zambraski EJ, Foster DT, Gross PM, Tipton CM: Iowa wrestling study: Weight loss and urinary profiles of collegiate wrestlers. Med Sci Sports 8:105–108, 1976.

## RECOMMENDED READING

28. Carson RF: Championship Wrestling. New York, AS Barnes and Co., 1974.
29. Gable D, Peterson JA: Conditioning for Wrestling: The Iowa Way. West Point, NY, Leisure Press, 1980.
30. Gibney R: Safety in Individual and Dual Sports. Sports Safety Monographs 4. Washington, D.C., American School and Community Safety Association, American Alliance for Health, Physical Education, and Recreation 12:43–46, 1977.
31. Katch FI, McArdle WD: Nutrition, Weight Control and Exercise. Boston, Houghton-Mifflin, 1977.
32. Porter PS, Baughman RD: Epidemiology of herpes simplex among wrestlers. JAMA 194:998–1000, 1965.
33. Rasch PG, Kroll W: What Research Tells the Coach about Wrestling. Washington, D.C., American Association for Health, Physical Education and Recreation, 1964.
34. Reek CC: A national study of incidence of accidents in high school wrestling. Res Q 10:72–73, 1939.
35. Round Table: Weight reduction in wrestling. Phys Sportsmed 9:79–96, 1981.
36. Tcheng TK, Tipton CM: Iowa wrestling study: Anthropometric measurements and the prediction of a "minimal" body weight for high school wrestlers. Med Sci Sports 5:1–10, 1973.
37. Tipton CM, Tcheng TK: Iowa wrestling study: Weight loss in high school students. JAMA 214:1269–1274, 1970.
38. Wheeler CE, Cabaniss WH: Epidemic cutaneous herpes simplex in wrestlers (herpes gladiatorum). JAMA 194:993–997, 1965.

# Chapter 49: Swimming and Diving

RICHARD W. HAMMER, MD

## I. General

A. **Perspective:** Both swimming and diving are popular recreational water activities as well as competitive sports.[1]

B. **Scope:** All ages from water babies to elderly persons swim; divers are usually not as young or as old.[2]

C. **Focus:** Competitive events begin in water sports around age 8 (sometimes earlier) and extend through college. Masters programs involve all ages beyond 25. This chapter will not discuss water polo or water skiing, although they share many similar problems.

D. Sports medicine concerns vary by age of swimmer or diver and stroke or dive involved. Most concerns focus on practice and training; more time is spent in these situations. Safety programs should be introduced early to protect the athlete. Swimming is a sprint, middle distance, and endurance activity, diving more a spatial orientation sport.

## II. Traumatic and Overuse Injuries

A. **Shoulder**
1. **Generally develops during training.** Related to overuse but sometimes develops during a change in stroke as a child matures, from change in coaches, from adjustment of stroke to increase speed/power, or from using improper stroke technique.[3]
2. **As fatigue develops, stroke changes, and in the process pain develops and/or stroke efficiency decreases.**
3. Anatomy of shoulder is shown in Figure 1.[4] Biceps tendon, rotator cuff, and impingement of shoulder and related muscles are often involved.
4. **Muscles**
   a. Subscapularis
   b. Supraspinatus
   c. Infraspinatus
   d. Teres minor
      i. Detection of these small muscle injuries depends on attention to the location of each and knowledge of function.
   e. Deltoid muscle—injury to a particular segment can be identified. Differentiate from subacromial bursitis or rotator cuff injury.
5. **Ligaments**
   a. Coracoacromial ligament
   b. Acromioclavicular ligament. More often injured during direct trauma applied to shoulder.
   c. Coracoclavicular ligament—rarely involved in swimming.
6. **Tendons**
   a. Biceps—most common tendon of shoulder to be involved in overuse injury.
   b. Deltoid—need to differentiate from subdeltoid bursitis.

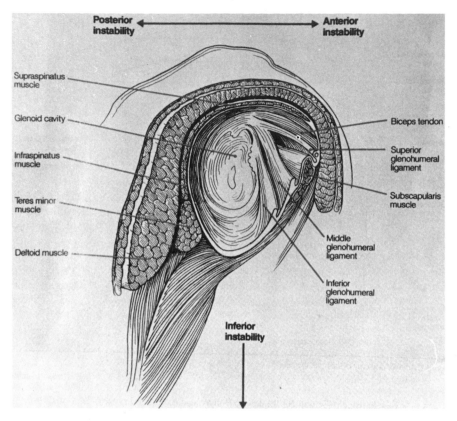

**FIGURE 1.** Anatomy of the shoulder showing parts that may be involved in overuse shoulder injuries. (From McMaster WC: Painful shoulder in swimmers: A diagnostic challenge. Phys Sportsmed 14(12):108–122, 1986, with permission.)

7. **Bursae**
   a. Subacromial
   b. Subdeltoid. May become inflamed and/or swollen and limit motion through mechanical obstruction and/or from pain.
8. **Shoulder joint**
   a. Dislocation, subluxation
   b. Synovitis
   c. Capsulitis.
9. **Other problems affecting shoulder:**
   a. Neck
      i. Arthritis
      ii. Disc problems
      iii. Tumors, cord problems.
   b. Miscellaneous
      i. Congenital problems
      ii. Thoracic outlet syndrome
      iii. Upper chest problems encroaching on shoulder or brachial plexus.
10. **History and physical examination, and other evaluations**
    a. Obtain **history** of:
       i. Mechanism of injury (Figs. 2 and 3)

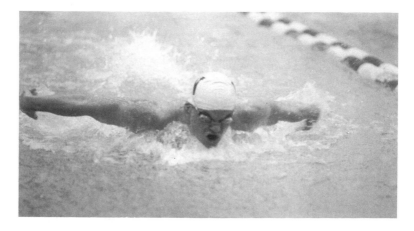

**FIGURE 2.**   Butterfly stroke is one of the overuse mechanisms resulting in shoulder injuries. (Photograph courtesy of Sports Information Office, University of Nebraska-Lincoln.)

      ii. Prior injuries
     iii. Current medications.
  b. **Observe shoulder in relaxed position.**
      i. Notice depressions.
       (a) Torn ligaments
       (b) Acromioclavicular separations.
     ii. Notice swellings.
       (a) Capsulitis
       (b) Bursitis.

**FIGURE 3.**   Backstroke is an example of overuse injury to the shoulder as well as to the back. (Photograph courtesy of the Sports Information Office, University of Nebraska-Lincoln.)

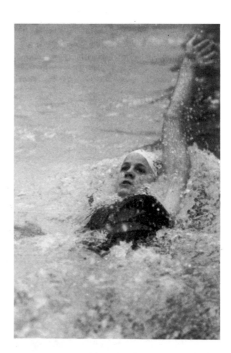

   c. **Observe abnormal movements.**
      i. Torn muscle
      ii. Contused muscles
      iii. Inability to raise shoulder laterally.
        (a) Injury to deltoid
        (b) Acromioclavicular separation.
      iv. Painful flexion of elbow—biceps tendonitis.
   d. **Palpation** (point tenderness aids in localizing injury)
      i. Acromioclavicular joint
      ii. Joint capsule area
      iii. Biceps tendon.
   e. **Measure loss of strength**
      i. Estimate by appearance.
      ii. Measure upper arm circumference.
      iii. Specific strength measured by machines with digital readouts.
   f. **Neurologic evaluation**
      i. Reflexes—biceps tendon.
      ii. Sensory, pain perception—brachial plexus, local nerve.
   g. **Laboratory evaluations** as complement to above:
      i. Uric acid—gout, pseudogout.
      ii. RA factor, ANA, HLA—rheumatoid arthritis, other collagen vascular diseases.
      iii. Serum iron—hemochromatosis.
      iv. Serum copper—liver problems (Wilson's disease).
   h. **Other confirming evaluations:**
      i. **Electromyography**—muscular damage or diseases and nerve damage.
      ii. **Arthrography**—cuff deficits, damage to muscular capsular component of joint.
      iii. **Magnetic resonance imaging**—may be done with or without enhancement, best for soft tissue visualization.
      iv. **Ultrasound**—helps to see cuff structures.
   i. **Special treatments.** Use principles already outlined in Chap. 34 for "sore shoulder":
      i. Work with swimmer and coach to **adjust workout and/or stroke.**
      ii. Give shoulder **adequate rest,** avoiding continuing injury in other activities.
      iii. Insure **adequate warm-up; ice after workout.**
      iv. **Complete rest of shoulder** if above does not help.

B. **Back**
  1. **General:**
    a. **Most back problems for swimmers and divers are in lower back and sacral areas.**
    b. Back injuries occur from constant pounding, from turns at the end of the pool, or from striking water at the end of a dive.
    c. Severe injuries may result from improper technique, diving into shallow water, diving onto another swimmer/diver, falling on deck.
  2. **Specific injuries:**
    a. Myofascial strain
    b. Fracture of vertebra
    c. Ligament strain
    d. Disc syndromes—lumbar, cervical.

3. Other problems
    a. Defective atlantooccipital formation
        i. Particularly in Down's syndrome.
    b. Arthritis
        i. Marie-Strümpell's disease
        ii. Rehumatoid
        iii. Gout.
    c. Scheuermann's disease
    d. Spondylolysis, spondylosis—steppe defect
    e. Bursitis—most common in the lumbosacral area.
    f. Congenital problems, developmental:
        i. Scoliosis
        ii. Other problems require special examinations to determine possible participation in handicapped programs.

4. **Evaluations:**
    a. Obtain history.
        i. Mechanism of injury
        ii. Past injuries
        iii. Past treatments.
    b. Physical exam:
        i. Observe for deformities of spine.
        ii. Observe movement of patient.
        iii. Notice swellings or discolorations.
    c. Palpation: feel for depressions, swellings or protrusions.
    d. Neurological exam
        i. Check knee and ankle reflexes.
        ii. Check sensation, vibration, and pain perception.
        e. Radiology
        i. Spine x-rays with oblique views for baseline, definitive diagnosis.
        ii. Magnetic resonance imaging—particularly for discs.
        iii. CT scan
        iv. Myelogram.

5. **Limitations of participation**
    a. Defective atlantooccipital structure:
        i. Avoid diving.
        ii. Start races in water.
        iii. Avoid water polo.
    b. Arthritis, gout:
        i. Depends on stage, symptoms, and degree of control.
    c. Disc syndromes:
        i. Avoid diving.
        ii. Avoid flip turns and grab starts.
            (a) Lap swimming without flip turns may be prescribed as therapy in some patients.
    d. Scoliosis
        i. Adaptation depends on degree of involvement.
        ii. May lead to bracing and/or surgery.
        iii. Some swimmers/divers remove braces during competition and do well.

C. **Head**
    1. Lacerations
        a. Most common to divers in the water sports. Most famous recent occurrence was in the 1988 Summer Olympics to diver Greg Louganis.

      b. Could also occur when head hits wall of the pool, most likely in back-stroke.

  2. Contusions

      a. From striking head against wall on turns or finishes.

      b. On diving board.

      c. Observe for further neurological deficits.

      d. May have headache for several days.

  3. Cervical spine injuries

      a. May occur in diving—either in a specific dive or from chronic trauma to cervical spine.

      b. May occur when diving into shallow water or onto another participant.

  4. Treatment

      a. Lacerations—appropriate wound care.

      b. Contusions, concussions—ice if needed, observation counseling.

      c. Cervical spine—immobilization until definitive diagnosis is made and appropriate care is initiated.

**D. Knee**

  1. The knee may be involved as in other sports (see Chap. 40).

  **2. In swimmers, the major problem occurs in breaststrokers:[5]**

      a. Another overuse/abuse problem: "breaststroker's knee."

      b. One form occurs in medial aspect of knee:

         i. Tibial collateral ligament

        ii. Medial retinaculum

       iii. Gracilis tendon

       iv. Also extensor mechanism malalignment may be a form of "breaststrok-er's" knee (see Chap. 40).

      c. Occurs when overtraining or adjusting stroke—a valgus stress with external rotation.

      d. Treatment varies

         i. Proper warm-ups, stretching

        ii. Ice after use

       iii. Aspirin or nonsteroidal anti-inflammatory drugs

       iv. Complete rest

       v. Physical therapy.

**E. Groin injuries**

  1. May be involved, as in other sports.

  2. In swimmers, more likely to occur in breaststrokers.

      a. Can be an overuse problem or sudden stress on iliopsoas muscle.

      b. Can occur when not properly warmed up.

      c. Swimmer has trouble flexing hip. Can palpate tenderness in groin area.

      d. The iliopsoas is a muscle used in all strokes, so complete rest from swimming, along with analgesics and physical therapy may be needed.

**F. Miscellaneous**

  **1. Swimmer's ear[6,7]**

      a. Swollen inflamed external ear canal (Fig. 4).

      b. Responds to combination antibiotic-corticosteroid drops or acetic acid with or without steroid drops.

         i. If swelling is severe, use wick to help to get drops to inflamed area.

      c. May require oral antibiotics as well as local and/or oral analgesics.

      d. May need long-term prophylaxis after each swim with 2% vinegar (acetic acid), 70% alcohol, or 3% boric acid in isopropyl alcohol or aluminate sulfate-calcium acetate solution.

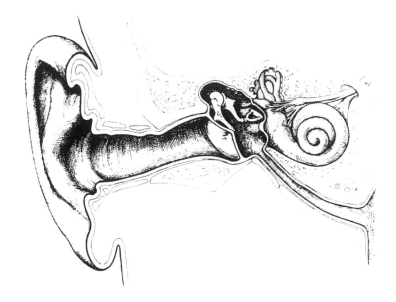

**FIGURE 4.** Anatomy of the ear. (With permission of the artist. ©Jane Hurd, 1981.)

    e. Ear plugs
        i. Commercial ones not usually helpful.
        ii. May require professionally produced plugs from an audiologist or oto-laryngologist.
    f. With adequate treatment and response, the athlete may be able to continue to participate in the water.
    g. Perforated drum—occurs when the diver lands improperly with side of head hitting water first.
        i. Occurs also with severe otitis media.
        ii. Needs proper protection before resuming water activity.
2. **Conjunctivitis**
    a. If infectious, treat appropriately.
    b. May be from chlorine irritation.
        i. Use of goggles may help.
        ii. Give trial of ophthalmic cromolyn sodium (also used in allergic conjunctivitis).
        iii. May respond to over-the-counter eye drops or may require steroid ophthalmic preparations after viral infection is ruled out.
3. **Athlete's foot**
    a. Restrict from pool or showers where patient may expose others.
    b. Treat with antifungal topically; if severe, may also need oral medication.
    c. Advise shower clogs for protection and prevention.
4. **Warts**
    a. Use quick method to get athlete back into action: liquid nitrogen or hyfrecation.
    b. Advise shower clogs for prevention.
    c. If topical methods are used, restrict from pool and shower areas until healed.

5. **Lacerations**
   a. May occur from sharp edges of starting blocks, exposed bolts on deck or block, or from glass on pool decks.
   b. Repair appropriately, using adherent strips or sutures.
   c. Avoid water unless wound is properly protected (note—Greg Louganis was able to complete another dive after repair and won another gold medal a week later).
6. **Ankle**
   a. Most likely overuse occurs from flutter kick and involves the extensor retinaculum of the ankle.
   b. Adjust stroke, stretching, ice, anti-inflammatory medication.
   c. May require rest, physical therapy.

III. **Other Problems in Swimmers and Divers.** Unless otherwise noted, treat as in other sports.

A. **Skin rashes**—possibly due to water, chemicals in the water, or rubdown materials. Visit with coach and respond according to findings; otherwise treat as other athletes.

B. **Fractures**—more often in divers. If injury occurs during practice or competition, it is usually from striking the diving platform while performing a dive, particularly the fingers, wrist, and nose. **In some instances the person may continue to swim/dive if fiberglass cast is used.**

C. **Pneumonia**—same as other athletes.

D. **Asthma**—Athlete may need to take pre-exercise medication to prevent exercise-induced asthma.[9]

E. **Gastroenteritis**—If epidemic among users of the pool, ask pool manager to have pool tested (may be bacterial such as Shigella, Cholera, or others, or viral such as Rotavirus or parasitic-like Giardia.[10,11]

F. **Sunburn, sunstroke, heat exhaustion**—rare, but could happen in long meets under just the right circumstances. Encourage adequate fluid intake as prevention; also, sun-blocker application. Water sports competitors get many hours of sun exposure but rarely use any sun blocker protection except early in the season.[12]

G. **Hypothermia**—more likely in long-distance swimmers but could also occur in early morning hours of meet/practice. Observe for alertness, coordination, skin color, shivering.

H. **Nutrition**
   1. Swimmers, divers tend to be low to medium body fat percentage.[13]
   2. **Otherwise, trained and fit long-distance swimmers may need extra body fat for buoyancy and insulation.**[14]
   3. "Pregame" meals are a problem for all or partial day meets. **Most important to stay hydrated, avoid "quick" energy sources such as sugars just prior to an event.**[15]

I. **Menstruation**[16]
   1. Rarely causes absence from the pool.
   2. Early intense competition/practice may delay menarche.
   3. If a problem involves menstruation, also inquire about other problems, including anorexia, thyroid, pregnancy, or personal problems as possible causes.[17]

J. **Surfing injuries**
   1. Also a popular water sport with some injuries peculiar to it.[18]
   2. Lacerations—75% to lower extremity.
   3. Soft tissue injury
      a. Sprains, strains, dislocations
      b. Primarily to knee, lower back, shoulder, ankle, and neck, in descending order of frequency.

4. Fractures—uncommon
   a. Primarily nose, feet, arms, ribs, and teeth.
5. Cause—surfer's own board
   a. 80–90%: fins, tails, or rails of board.

K. **Drowning**
   1. Same problem as with other persons using water for sport, recreation, or commerce.
   2. May occur following inhalation of water and secondary laryngospasm.
   3. May result from "diving reflex" in swimmer who hyperventilates, enters water, and while swimming stays at bottom of pool.[19]

IV. **Warm-up, Cool-down, and Stretching**

A. A controversial area[20,21]
B. Swimmers have traditionally **"stretched"** each other prior to competition, often involving movements not used in swimming/diving.
C. Some authorities prefer more general warm-up activities, putting joints through full range of swimming motion. Avoid over-stretching as a harmful activity, possibly leading to some loss of strength.
D. **Warm-up**—length of time varies among swimmers. Start of warm-up is on deck to loosen muscle and start heart activity, then move to water for a time to get body ready for competition, then wear warm-up suits while waiting for one's event. If meet is long, swimmer may need to repeat these phases at appropriate times to be ready for the event.
E. **Rubdowns**—also traditional, best in hands of practicing therapists. Avoid overrelaxing and avoid abnormal absorption of amounts of chemicals from substances applied to skin.
F. **"Swim down"**—valuable for swimmer to gradually cool down after event, usually done in an adjoining pool to avoid tightening muscles after event.

V. **Sport-specific Facilities and Protective Equipment**

A. **Pool configuration,** markings, blocks, and lane lines are specified by the governing body under which the swimmer competes. Diving boards and pool configuration are similarly regulated for divers.
B. **Protective equipment**
   1. Swimmers may use goggles.
   2. Rubdown oil allowed unless judged excessive or not permitted by the pool operator.
   3. Long distance swimmers use lard or similar substance for insulation in some events.
   4. Swimming caps may be used to reduce friction with water.
   5. For additional speed, swimmers may "shave" body and/or head hair.
C. **Sport-specific taping and bracing**
   1. None is specific for swimming. Water negates most efforts at taping.
   2. In some instances, temporary taping may be useful in sprains or simple fractures of digits.
   3. With orthopedist's approval, swimmer/diver may compete with certain fractures, especially if covered with fiberglass cast.

VI. **Rules to Protect the Athlete**

A. **Age group divisions, male and female**
   1. Standards set for 8-year-old as lowest age group.
   2. Age divisions go up by 2-year increments for more equal competition.

    3. Swimmers younger than 8 compete, but more for recreation and learning fundamentals.

    4. Masters swimmers also divided by age groups.

B. **Coach certification: U.S. Swimming (USS)**

    1. Safety certified.

    2. CPR certified.

    3. Registered USS members.

    4. Standard set for individuals to belong to coaches organizations; levels of proficiency outlined.

    5. Other aquatic programs may follow implementation of the USS program and/ or establish their own programs for protection of participants (some already have).

C. **Safety advisors**—U.S. swimming members—to coordinate safety aspects.

    1. National chairperson

    2. Local sport committee chairperson

    3. Local swim/diving club safety person.

D. **Specified warm-ups**

    1. Designated lanes for a club, sprints.

    2. Diving monitor to signal water clear.

    3. No diving by divers or swimmers unless supervised.

E. **Water depth**

    1. Starting only in water of specified depth or deeper.

    2. Diving only in water of specified depth or deeper.

F. No jumping into the pool when a race is in progress and, then, only with the referee's approval.

G. No interference allowed during diving/swimming competition.

H. Specifications listed for starting block surfaces, composition, and structure of diving boards and towers; also, pool size and depth, wall surfaces, lighting, and electrical cords/apparatus.

I. Certified officials when possible.

J. Clearing pool before each event starts.

K. Giving each diver time between the announcement of a dive and its execution.

L. Competition between those of similar abilities. Time standards used to separate abilities within an age group.

M. In long-distance swimming, officials in boats following swimmers can order swimmer out of water if hypothermia is suspected.

N. Swimming officials should be alert to possibility of troubled swimmers with exercise-induced asthma, laryngospasm, or "diving reflex."

O. Referees have authority to stop a meet when lightning or other severe weather threatens.

P. Referees have authority to adjust, postpone, or cancel meets if conditions of the meet jeopardize the safety of the swimmers/divers.

Q. Note—complete rules of the national governing bodies for swimming and diving may be obtained from U.S. Swimming and U.S. Diving (see reference). Other organizations may have their own rules (NCAA, high school, YMCA, for example) or follow USS/USD rules (copies available to members). There may be a modest charge.

VII. **Sport-specific Special Concern of the Team Physician**

    A. Swimmer's shoulder

    B. Swimmer's ear

    C. Breaststroker's knee

D. Nutrition and hydration when dealing with long meets and multiple events per day.

E. Water as the medium in which sport takes place.

F. Temperature problems ranging from hypothermia to heat stroke.

G. Stretching activities specific to swimming/diving.

H. All of above items are discussed within body of chapter.

## REFERENCES

*1. United States Swimming's Sports Medicine Informational Series: Training Concepts for the Age-Group Swimmer (#4), 1985.

*2. Burd B: Infant swimming classes: Immersed in controversy. Phys Sportsmed 14(3):238–244, 1986.

*3. United States Swimming's Sports Medicine Informational Series: Swimmer's Shoulder and Rehabilitation (#7), 1985.

4. McMaster WC: Painful shoulder in swimmers: A diagnostic challenge. Phys Sportsmed 14(12):108–122, 1986.

5. Rory S, Irvin R: Sports Medicine. Englewood Cliffs, Prentice-Hall, 1983, pp 452–453.

6. Eichel BS: How I manage external otitis in competitive swimmers. Phys Sportsmed 14(8):108–116, 1986.

*7. United States Swimming's Sports Medicine Informational Series: Swimmer's Ear (#8), 1985.

*8. United States Swimming's Sports Medicine Informational Series: Eat to Compete (#2), 1987.

*9. United States Swimming's Sports Medicine Informational Series: Exercise Induced Asthma and the Competitive Swimmer (#3), 1987.

10. Makintubee S, Millonee J, Istie G: Shigellosis outbreak associated with swimming. Am J Public Health 72:166–168, 1987.

*11. United States Swimming's Sports Medicine Informational Series: Diarrhea (#6), 1987.

12. Davidson TM, Wolfe DP: Sunscreens, skin cancer and your patient. Phys Sportsmed 14(8):65–79, 1986.

13. Ross Laboratories: Nutrition and Hydration in Swimming: How They Can Affect Your Performance. Columbus, OH, Ross Laboratories, Dec 1986.

*14. United States Swimming's Sports Medicine Informational Series: Nutrition and Competition (#1), 1985.

*15. United States Swimming's Sports Medicine Informational Series: Travel and Competition (#5), 1985.

*16. United States Swimming's Sports Medicine Informational Series: Training Considerations for the Female Athlete (#3), 1985.

17. Dummer GM, Rosen LW, Heusner WW, et al: Pathogenic weight control behaviors in competitive swimmers. Phys Sportsmed 15(5):75–86, 1987.

18. Renneker M: Surfing: The sport and life style. Phys Sportsmed 15(10):156–162, 1987.

19. Higgins P, Simenski J, Pearson R: Near drowning—lap swimming (letter). N Engl J Med 315:1551–1553, 1986.

20. Levine M, Lombardo J, McNeeley J, Anderson T: An analysis of individual stretching programs of intercollegiate athletes. Phys Sportsmed 15(3):130–138, 1987.

*21. United States Swimming's Sports Medicine Informational Series: Strength Training for Age Group and Senior Swimmers, 1985.

---

* Copies of the referenced USS Series may be obtained from: Dr. John Troup, U.S. Swimming, 1750 E. Boulder, Colorado Springs, CO 80909-5770.

Copies of the complete series may also be obtained from the same source. Swimming rule books can be obtained by writing U.S. Swimming at the above address. Diving rules from U.S. Diving, Pan American Plaza, 201 S. Capitol Avenue -Suite 430, Indianapolis, IN 46225.

# Chapter 50: Baseball and Softball

T. A. BLACKBURN, Jr., RPT, ATC

I. **Overview**
   A. Extremely popular sports—large number of participants at many levels.
      1. Professional
      2. Amateur
      3. Recreational.
   B. Classified as "limited contact impact" sports.
   C. Common types of injuries
      1. High speed collisions do occur:
         a. Between players
         b. With fences and equipment
         c. Ball striking player
         d. Bat striking player.
      2. Running injuries
      3. Throwing injuries.

II. **Biomechanical and Pathomechanical Considerations in Baseball and Softball**

   A. **Biomechanics of overhand throwing.** Efficient throwing depends on a coordinated **transfer of momentum** (momentum = mass × velocity) from larger, slower body segments to segments of smaller mass that can move faster, thus imparting a **high velocity** to the ball (up to 100 mph) at ball release.
      1. **Wind-up phase\***—variable among pitchers; **establishes the rhythm** (Fig. 1A).
         a. Initiates with a downward swing of the arms, which are then raised overhead **(gathered position).**
         b. Weight shifts forward on the right foot and then back to the left foot during the arm swing.
         c. Rotation of the shoulders and hips occurs as the arms go overhead and the body shifts from facing the batter to being perpendicular to the line of throw.
         d. The right foot must move from its perpendicular position on top of the rubber, to a position parallel to the rubber and just in front of it.
         e. Pitcher must maintain balance as the stretched left leg goes into the air, with hip and knee flexed at approximately chest-high level.
         f. Spine flexes with leftward rotation.
         g. **Wind-up phase ends when the hands come apart from the gathered position.**
         h. Wind-up lets pitcher hid the ball.
         i. Lasts anywhere from 0.5 to 1.3 seconds.
         j. Sequence is as follows: initiation/pivot foot/"gather."
         k. **Wind-up from the stretch**
            i. Used when runner is on base
            ii. Eliminates the first half of the wind-up
            iii. Pitcher may lose some rhythm

---

\* Description of phases assumes right-handed pitcher.

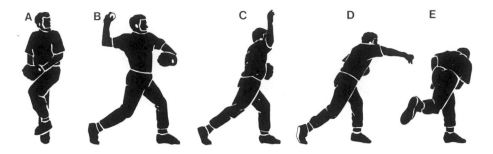

**FIGURE 1.** Phases of the overhand throw: *A,* Windup. *B,* Cocking: late phase before maximum external rotation. *C,* Late acceleration, near ball release. *D,* Deceleration. *E,* Follow-through.

1. **Balk**
    i. The thrower turns his shoulders to look at the man on base, but throws the ball to the plate.
2. **Cocking phase** (Fig. 1B)
    a. Begins at hands apart.
    b. Ends when the right arm is at its most extreme external rotation.
    c. **Early cocking**
        i. Stride leg extends forward as hips begin to derotate or "open up." Center of gravity moves forward caused by the push leg (takes approximately 0.5 second).
        ii. Right arm moves into external rotation and horizontal abduction.
            (a) Rotator cuff stabilizes humeral head and externally rotates humerus.
            (b) Scapulothoracic muscles retract the scapula.
            (c) Deltoid pulls humerus into horizontal abduction.
        iii. Anterior chest muscles and humeral internal rotators are put on stretch.
            (a) Pectoralis major and minor
            (b) Latissimus dorsi
            (c) Subscapularis
            (d) Teres major.
    d. **Late cocking**
        i. Stance leg pushes center of gravity forward.
        ii. Stride leg plants with foot parallel to line to plate and just left of center. Quadriceps, hamstrings, and hip extensors decelerate the body from rotation and forward motion. **This allows the momentum transfer to begin its progression proximally through the body to the arm.**
        iii. Shoulder reaches maximum amount of external rotation/horizontal abduction, **"winding" the glenohumeral joint capsule like a spring** (Fig. 2).
        iv. Glenohumeral joint is at 90° of abduction and 25–30° of horizontal abduction. The wrist is supinated. Spine is hyperextended and elbow is flexed to approximately 90°.
3. **Acceleration phase** (Fig. 1C)
    a. Begins when the ball moves forward.
    b. Ends when ball is released.
    c. **High constant forces** are developed through momentum transfer from the trunk to the arm as the glenohumeral capsule is "un-wound."

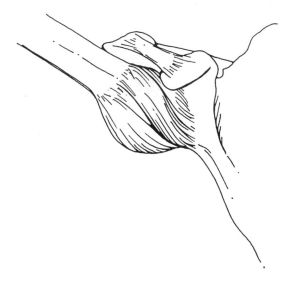

**FIGURE 2.** "Winding" of anterior capsule with external rotation and horizontal abduction during cocking phase.

d. Occurs in approximately 0.1 second.
e. Burst of muscle action occurs.
   i. Latissimus
   ii. Pectoralis major and minor
   iii. Serratus anterior
   iv. Triceps.
f. Two distinct motions occur at the shoulder during the acceleration phase:
   i. Horizontal adduction (40 msec)
   ii. Internal rotation (40 msec); occurs at an angular velocity of 6,000° per second.
g. Triceps extends elbow from 90° of flexion to 25° of extension, at approximately 7,000° per second. Valgus stress occurs across the elbow (Fig. 3), stressing the medial ligaments, flexor muscle mass, radiohumeral joint, and the olecranon fossa.
h. Pathomechanics during acceleration
   i. **Mid-shaft spiral humeral fractures**—infrequent

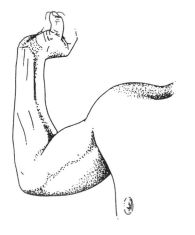

**FIGURE 3.** Valgus stress on the elbow during acceleration.

    ii. **Muscle strains**—attempt to control high forces and protect anterior capsule.

      (a) Pectoralis major

      (b) Latissimus dorsi

      (c) Subscapularis

      (d) Biceps.

    iii. **Glenohumeral joint laxity**

      (a) **Extreme external rotation and horizontal abduction** of the glenohumeral joint stretches anterior capsule and can cause anterior subluxation.

      (b) **High force production of acceleration muscles** pulls humeral head forward and can cause anterior subluxation.

      (c) **"Opening" up too soon"** can aggravate this type of problem.

    iv. **Superior glenoid labrum lesion**

      (a) **Laxity of anterior capsule** allows humeral head to sublux anteriorly and abrade the labrum, causing breakdown.

      (b) **"Labrum grinding factor"** created by **internal rotation and horizontal abduction of the humeral head** may cause abrasion (grinding) of the labrum even in a stable shoulder.

4. **Release arc**

  a. Hand is moving at speed of pitch at release.

  b. Ball must be released at **critical point** to be accurate.

  c. Muscles about shoulder are relatively quiet by EMG measurements at release.

  d. Stride leg continues to decelerate trunk momentum.

  e. **Variations in release**

    i. **"Bull whip" release**

      (a) **Causes**

        (i) Pitcher locks stride leg in recurvatum rather than allowing leg to flex.

        (ii) This decelerates forward momentum to create trunk rotation and extra "whipping" motion through rest of body to arm.

      (b) **Results of "bull whip release"**

        (i) Impact forces transmitted through lower extremity and pelvis.

        (ii) Increased derotation forces at pelvis.

        (iii) Increased stress on shoulder during acceleration.

        (iv) May lead to injury.

    ii. **"Opening up too soon"**

      (a) **Causes**

        (i) Squaring shoulders to batter too soon before release.

        (ii) Hips are derotated too quickly.

        (iii) Stride is too short.

        (iv) Stride leg is too far left of mid-line.

        (v) Hip and knee of stride leg are not flexed adequately during late cocking.

        (vi) Rushing a pitch.

      (b) **Results of "opening up too soon"**

        (i) Arm lags behind body at release.

        (ii) Increased stress on anterior shoulder and medial elbow during acceleration.

        (iii) Elbow drops toward side attempting to locate proper release point.

        (iv) Increased injury potential.

    iii. **"Opening up too late"**
      (a) **Causes**
        (i) Squaring shoulders to batter too late.
        (ii) Stride leg is too far right of mid-line.
        (iii) Hips are derotated too slowly.
      (b) **Results of "opening up too late"**
        (i) Arm is ahead of body at release.
        (ii) Body loses momentum.
        (iii) Decreases effectiveness.
        (iv) Relatively few injuries result.

5. **Deceleration** (Fig. 1D)
  a. Begins at ball release.
  b. Ends after strongest contraction phase of the rotator cuff muscles.
  c. Strong but variable forces on posterior rotator cuff.
  d. Posterior rotator cuff must slow the 6,000–9,000°/sec internal rotation and horizontal abduction motion of the humerus.
  e. Stride leg aids in deceleration.
  f. Biceps decelerates elbow extension and supports the anterior shoulder.
  g. **Scapulothoracic muscles are very important during this phase for stabilizing the scapula, controlling scapula protraction, and providing a stable base** for the rotator cuff to decelerate the arm.
  h. **Pathomechanics during deceleration**
    i. **Muscle strains**
      (a) **Posterior rotator cuff**
        (i) High deceleration forces required of these small muscles cause breakdown in the tendons of the rotator cuff near their humeral attachment.
        (ii) Pain causes the thrower to decrease speed because deceleration from higher speed cannot be tolerated.
      (b) **Biceps**
        (i) Biceps **controls deceleration of the elbow** via forces on its origin at the glenoid fossa and attachments to the glenoid labrum. The biceps tendon may also become inflamed.
        (ii) A **weak rotator cuff** forces the biceps tendon to work harder during deceleration, causing more irritation to the biceps tendon and usually a rotator cuff problem as well.
    ii. **Glenoid labrum**
      (a) May tear or degenerate because of these forces, especially if rotator cuff or biceps is weak.

6. **Follow-through** (Fig. 1E)
  a. Begins following strongest contraction phase of the rotator cuff muscles.
  b. Ends when trailing leg contacts ground.
  c. Completes dissipation of the momentum of throwing motion.
  d. Puts body in a position to field batted balls.

7. **Types of deliveries:** All show glenohumeral joint to be at about 90° of abduction. The degree of **body lean** affects the way the delivery appears.
  a. **Overhead**
    i. Similar to outfielder's throw.
    ii. Better use of body.
    iii. Mechanically allows for higher velocity with less prime mover exercise, and gives a much longer lever arm.

        iv. Curve ball is much more deceptive because of the angle of delivery.

        v. More **control problems** with this type of pitch.

    b. **Three-quarters**

        i. Shorter lever arm—prime movers do more work.

        ii. Flatter trajectory, so curve ball is not so deceptive.

        iii. Pitcher usually has **better control.**

    c. **Sidearm**

        i. Increased elbow valgus stress and anterior shoulder stress.

        ii. More "drag"—relies on whipping motion.

        iii. Pitch is very flat so it is easier to hit.

        iv. Associated with more injuries.

  8. **Pathomechanics of overhand throwing**

    a. Most throwing injuries occur over a period of time and are termed **overuse injuries.**

    b. **Any factor** (sprained ankle, patellar tendinitis, low back dysfunction, shoulder pain, coaching, etc.) **that changes the form, rhythm, coordination, and timing** of a pitcher can **cause injury to the throwing arm.**

B. **Biomechanics of underhand pitching: Very little research** has been done on the underhand fast pitch motion. **Very few career-ending injuries** occur with this type of pitch, possibly explaining the lack of research. The **rotator cuff is not loaded** as it is in the overhand pitch, and **extreme external rotation is avoided.**

  1. **Phases**

    a. **Wind-up and cocking**

        i. Stride leg moves forward, while stance leg pushes the body forward.

        ii. Glenohumeral joint moves in an arc of flexion, abduction, and then extension.

        iii. Radius and form of arc will vary with the pitcher's style.

    b. **Acceleration:** Begins with forward motion of the ball.

        i. Shoulder flexors, depressors, and horizontal adductors provide for speed of arm into the forward-flexed position. The muscles involved are:

          (a) Pectoralis major and minor

          (b) Subscapularis

          (c) Deltoid.

        ii. At the elbow and shoulder, the biceps contracts to propel the ball forward.

    c. **Release:** Occurs in front of the body.

    d. **Deceleration:** Forces here are much **less stressful,** and the position of the arm allows **larger muscles** to absorb the shock:

        i. Triceps

        ii. Latissimus dorsi

        iii. Posterior rotator cuff

        iv. Teres major

        v. Posterior deltoid.

    e. **Follow-through:** Puts body in position to field ball.

C. **Biomechanics of sliding:** Sliding allows the base runner to reach a base (other than running from the batter's box to first base) at the fastest possible speed without going past the base, and allows the runner to be as small a target as possible to prevent being tagged.

  1. **Types**

    a. **Feet first:** The runner slides in on either the right or left side, according to preference. Right-sided slide is described here. For left-sided slide, right and left designations are reversed.

      i. Right-sided slide has the runner flexing right knee as much as 90°, with the left leg extended.

     ii. The feet-first slide is timed to allow the left foot to touch the base first. Sliding forces are usually absorbed over the entire right thigh.

    iii. Variations:

       (a) **"Pop-up slide"**

         (i) Runner's weight never transfers entirely to the thigh, but stays at the leading edge of the right **flexed shin and knee.**

        (ii) This allows runner to quickly assume a standing and running position.

       (b) **"Hook slide"**

         (i) Runner attempts to slide away from the area of the base or plate where he thinks the thrown ball will arrive, thus trying to avoid the tag.

        (ii) Runner is usually outside of the direct path to the base but must still make contact with his left foot as he slides by the base and decelerates.

    iv. **Injuries**

       (a) Abrasions

       (b) Cleat laceration to areas of ankle and shin may occur to the opposing player as he tries to make the tag.

       (c) Fractures, dislocations, and sprains of the foot, ankle, and leg as lower extremities contact base and possibly the opposing player.

       (d) Ball may strike the player.

  b. **Head first**

      i. Many feel that this technique is a bit **faster** than the feet-first slide.

     ii. Landing occurs on the chest, with head up and arms outstretched.

    iii. An even **smaller target** is available for the tag.

    iv. **Injuries**

       (a) Abrasions

       (b) **Head and neck** are much **more exposed** to injury from collision and from being hit by the ball.

       (c) **Hands and fingers** are at greater risk of injury by cleats and collisions.

## III. Common injuries in baseball and softball

  A. **Lacerations and abrasions**

    1. **Etiology**

      a. Sliding

      b. Spikes

      c. Field/stadium disrepair

      d. Collisions.

    2. **Evaluation and treatment**

      a. As provided in Chap. 28.

      b. Protect area during participation until healed.

    3. **Complications**

      a. Infections

      b. Loss of playing time.

  B. **Ankle and foot injuries**

    1. **Types**

      a. Various fractures

      b. Medial and lateral sprains

      c. Contusions

      d. Great toe dysfunction in pitchers.

  2. **Etiology**

      a. Sliding

      b. Running

      c. Ball impact

      d. Bases

      e. Pitching from mound.

C. **Contusions/myositis ossificans**

  1. **Etiology**

      a. Collision between players

      b. Ball striking a player

      c. Collision with other objects.

D. **Muscle strains**

  1. **Etiology**

      a. Inadequate conditioning

         i. Strength

         ii. Flexibility

         iii. Endurance.

      b. Inadequate warm-up and maintenance of warm-up.

      c. Overuse.

E. **Knee injuries:** Various knee ligament, meniscal, and patellofemoral problems occur, as in other running and contact sports.

  1. **Etiology**

      a. Usual causes as in other running and contact sports.

      b. Impact with baseball environment (bases, sprinklers, fences, grandstand, etc.).

      c. Cleats and spikes allow for more foot fixation and increased risk of knee injury.

F. Lumbosacral dysfunction

  1. **Etiology**

      a. Injury rate not unusually high vs. other sports.

      b. Pitching—sacroiliac joint and lumbar facets stressed

         i. Rotational component of pitching act

         ii. Height of pitching mound

         iii. Landing forces on front leg.

G. **Head and face injuries**

  1. Injury potential is high.

      a. Swinging bats

      b. Thrown and batted balls.

IV. **Management of Throwing Arm Injuries**

A. **Introduction**

  1. Rather than simply treating symptoms, a **careful clinical and biomechanical evaluation** of the athlete will help the examiner define the nature and cause of the injury. As presented in Chap. 30, basic treatment principles, modalities, rest, and rehabilitation are called for. Emphasis should be placed on the total athlete. Cardiovascular fitness, lower body strength and flexibility, trunk strength and flexibility, as well as reconditioning of the throwing arm, are essential to successful treatment and rehabilitation. The following sections will focus on major injuries to the throwing arm that don't resolve with a few days of care.

**TABLE 1.**  Interval Throwing Program

Each phase consists of several throwing sessions. The athlete should work up to the parameters within each phase. Generally, the athlete throws daily. However, if soreness or stiffness develops after a throwing session and persists, then the next session should be reduced or skipped. Progression to the subsequent phase is based on achieving the phase goals without any symptoms.

Session sequence:
— Warm up (break sweat, stretch, "soft-toss" 10–15′ until loose, work to long-toss distance)
— Long-toss interval
— Short-toss interval
— Rest 10–30 minutes
— Repeat warm up
— Long-toss interval
— Short-toss interval
— Cool down (stretch, ice, monitor symptoms)

| Phase | Long-toss interval | | Short-toss interval | | Speed/Pitch type/Surface |
|---|---|---|---|---|---|
| | Distance | # throws* | Distance | # throws* | |
| 1 | 90′ | 25 | 30′ | 50 | ½, straight, flat |
| 2 | 120′ | 25 | 60′ | 50 | ½, straight, flat |
| 3 | 150′ | 25 | 60′ | 50 | ¾, straight, flat |
| 4 | 180′ | 25 | 60′ | 50 | ¾, straight, mound |
| 5 | 210′ | 25 | 60′ | 50 | ½–¾, breaking, mound |
| 6 | 240′ | 25 | 60+′ | 50 | ¾–full, all, mound |
| 7 | Work to game situations; number of pitches in game situation should be increased as able; monitor mechanics and accuracy (85% of pitches should be strikes). | | | | |

\* In each phase, prescribed number of throws should be completed within a 5-minute time period.

2. **Interval throwing program**
    a. Provides a **gradual** increase in throwing intensity at a controlled pace based on symptoms.
    b. See Table 1 for details.
B. **Rotator cuff injuries:** Can vary from a mild case of tendinitis to partial or full-thickness tears.
    1. **Etiology**
        a. Overuse
        b. Change in mechanics
        c. Weakness in rotator cuff.
    2. **Symptoms**
        a. Pain when trying to pitch intensely, generally in the early phase of deceleration.
            i. May or may not have pain at rest or night.
            ii. May have trouble even warming up when problem becomes severe.
        b. Often the injury pattern falls into one of injury, rest and return to full play; then reinjury, rest, return to full play, and so on. It may take the athlete 6 to 12 months before medical help is sought and a good diagnosis is made.
    3. **Examination** (see Chap. 34)
        a. **Weakness (and sometimes pain)** to manual muscle testing:
            i. Supraspinatus (Jobe's test)
            ii. External rotation at 90° abduction
            iii. Abduction at 90°
            iv. External rotation at 0° abduction.
        b. **Impingement test(s)** positive.
        c. Pain on palpation of rotator cuff.
        d. External rotation and abduction demonstrate increase in pain.
        e. Biceps tendon and coracoid process may be tender to palpation.
        f. Slow-motion analysis of video tape of throwing to identify **mechanical flaws.**

4. **Differential diagnosis**
   a. Biceps tendinitis
   b. Glenoid labrum tear
   c. Subdeltoid bursitis.
5. **Treatment**
   a. Rest: anywhere from 1 to 6 weeks, depending on severity.
   b. Modalities
      i. Ice
      ii. Ultrasound
      iii. High-voltage electrical stimulation
      iv. Phonophoresis
      v. Iontophoresis
      vi. Anti-inflammatory medication.
   c. Therapeutic exercise program is based on physical exam.
      i. Strength
      ii. Flexibility
   d. Surgery—**only after exhaustive conservative care.**
      i. Arthroscopic debridement and evaluation of the rotator cuff as well as the subdeltoid bursa area. Acromioplasty may be needed if impingement is noted.
      ii. **Very difficult to return to competitive level after open surgery, because of scarring.**
   e. Return to throwing (see Table and Chap. 30).
6. **Prognosis:** Tendinitis should clear with proper care. Partial and complete lesions of the rotator cuff may need debridement and then a good rehabilitation and return-to-throwing program. May take a year, even with surgery, for complete return.
C. **Glenoid labrum injuries:** Injury to the anterior superior glenoid labrum **does not result in glenohumeral instability,** as seen in anterior dislocations when the anterior inferior labrum is torn. Occasionally, the posterior superior labrum will be damaged with overuse.
   1. **Etiology**
      a. Falls on outstretched arm
      b. Anterior or posterior instabilities
      c. Rotator cuff weakness
      d. Military and bench-press weight training
      e. Throwing technique changes
      f. Batting
      g. Labrum grinding factor.
   2. **Symptoms**
      a. **Pain during acceleration phase** of throwing:
         i. Unable to move the arm briskly through full range of motion while throwing.
         ii. Once through the painful area (painful arc), it no longer hurts.
      b. Usually no pain at rest or night pain.
      c. No swelling is evident.
      d. Biceps tendinitis may accompany this disorder.
      e. History—either a one-pitch episode or a gradual buildup.
   3. **Examination**
      a. Pain with **over-pressure in horizontal adduction**—over-pressure takes joint into extreme of motion, stressing joint capsule and creating joint compression, which may trap torn labrum and cause discomfort.

    b. **Labrum "clunk" test**—shoulder in external rotation and abduction, forcing an anterior and posterior motion of the humerus in an attempt to catch the torn labrum between the bony segments and creates a "clunk."

        i. May have more pain with forced external rotation at 90° abduction than in a more abducted position.

    c. Palpation of biceps tendon.

  4. **Differential diagnosis**

    a. Rotator cuff tendinitis/tear (often seen in conjunction with one another)

    b. Biceps tendinitis

    c. Abnormal joint laxity.

  5. **Treatment**

    a. Rest: 7–10 days

    b. Therapeutic exercise program

    c. Review mechanics of throwing.

    d. Modalities and medication not much help.

    e. Return to throwing.

    f. **Surgery after failure of exhaustive conservative care**

        i. Arthroscopic debridement of superior labrum

        ii. Tendon of the long head of the biceps may be involved.

  6. **Prognosis:** Conservative treatment may work in the majority of cases. Two to 6 weeks may be required of a rehabilitation program. If arthroscopic debridement is performed, throwing may start in 2–3 weeks, full play by 12 weeks if all goes well.

D. **Anterior glenohumeral joint laxity**

  1. **Etiology**

    a. Repetitive throwing

    b. Poor mechanics

    c. Trauma

    d. Congenital.

  2. **Symptoms**

    a. Extra strain on rotator cuff and biceps tendon as the muscle groups try to stabilize the shoulder.

    b. Glenoid labrum may break down with increased laxity.

    c. Inability to throw hard.

  3. **Examination**

    a. Abduction/external rotation demonstrates laxity.

    b. Labrum "clunk" test.

    c. Rotator cuff may also be symptomatic.

  4. **Differential diagnosis**

    a. Rotator cuff pathology

    b. Labrum tear.

  5. **Treatment**

    a. Rest

    b. Therapeutic exercise program with dynamic stability emphasis

    c. Review of mechanics

    d. Return-to-throwing program

    e. Surgery

        i. Arthroscopic debridement of rotator cuff and labrum

        ii. Open anterior capsule reefing and aggressive postoperative care, so athlete can regain full range of motion and return to throwing.

  6. **Prognosis:** More difficult to return from surgery to full potential.

E. **Valgus extension overload of the elbow:** Injuries to ulnar nerve, wrist flexor mass origin, medial elbow ligaments, radio-capitellum joint, and olecranon fossa.
   1. **Causes**
      a. **Poor mechanics**
         i. "Opening up too soon"
         ii. "Bull whip" release.
      b. Overuse
      c. Occurs during **acceleration phase.**
   2. **Symptoms**
      a. Ulnar nerve
         i. Transient radiating pain is present in early phase.
         ii. In chronic cases, ulnar nerve distribution affected.
      b. Wrist flexors—pain at medial epicondyle at rest and during performance, depending on severity.
      c. Elbow medial compartment laxity—instability during throwing act.
      d. Radiocapitellum joint: Osteochondritis dissecans may develop.
         i. Pain at joint on throwing
         ii. Locking and clicking.
      e. Olecranon fossa degeneration
         i. Pain on medial side of joint
         ii. Spur formation
         iii. Loss of extension in chronic cases.
   3. **Examination**
      a. Ulnar nerve
         i. Positive Tinel sign
         ii. Sensory changes to pin-prick in hypothenar eminence
         iii. Tenderness over ulnar groove
         iv. EMG/NCV changes.
      b. Wrist flexors
         i. Weakness of grip
         ii. Pain/weakness on manual muscle testing of wrist flexors
         iii. Pain to palpation of medial epicondyle area.
      c. Medial compartment laxity
         i. Opening on valgus stress test
         ii. Tenderness over medial collateral ligament.
      d. Radiocapitellum joint
         i. X-ray findings
         ii. Loss of extension.
   4. **Differential diagnosis**
      a. Flexor mass pain and medial ligament pain similar; care must be taken in palpation to discern between the two.
   5. **Treatment**
      a. Acute
         i. Relative rest
         ii. Modalities
         iii. Therapeutic exercise program
         IV. Return-to-throwing program.
      b. Chronic
         i. Arthroscopic surgery for loose body removal, radiocapitellum debridement, and posterior olecranon spur debridement.
            (a) Begin range-of-motion and strengthening program immediately.

           (b) Return-to-throwing program begins at 6 weeks. May take 6 months before full return.
      ii. Open surgery for medial ligament reconstruction and posterior olecranon spur excision.
           (a) 10 days immobilization is recommended.
           (b) Cast brace at 30°–90° until 6 weeks.
           (c) At 6 weeks, begin aggressive range-of-motion and strengthening program.
           (d) Return to throwing begins at 12 weeks postoperative.
           (e) Full play at 6–12 months from surgery.

    6. **Prognosis**
      a. **If this problem is identified early, mechanical problems are corrected,** and the overuse situation is changed, it should clear easily.
      b. **When allowed to progress, it can become quite difficult to manage.** Surgical intervention may allow the athlete to return to play, but **advancement in the sport may not be possible.** That much stress may still cause problems at the elbow.

V. **Prevention of Injuries**

  A. **Proper conditioning**
    1. Off-season programs
      a. Aerobic foundation
      b. General strengthening
      c. Flexibility
      d. Isolated rotator cuff exercises
      e. Throwing program.
    2. In-season program—maintenance program
      a. Running—Sprints especially
      b. Isolated rotator cuff exercises
      c. Flexibility
        i. Hamstrings
        ii. Gastrocnemius
        iii. Quadriceps
        iv. Rectus femoris
        v. Low back.
    3. **Recreational** softball and baseball participants often have a very **poor level of conditioning.**

  B. **Technique training is important—emphasis put on proper mechanics.**
    1. Pitching instruction
    2. Batting
    3. Sliding.

  C. **Overuse**
    1. Have Little League pitcher's schedule based on **pitches thrown** (games and practices), not on innings thrown.
    2. Coaches must pay particular attention to pitchers, no matter at what level.

  D. **Umpires:** Conscientious and quality umpiring will cut down on injuries.

  E. **Playing surfaces**
    1. Warning track should be located between field and fences.
    2. Fence around entire field should be in good repair and padded where appropriate.
    3. Line markings should not be of lime (irritates eyes and skin).
    4. Batter's box and pitcher's mound kept in good repair.

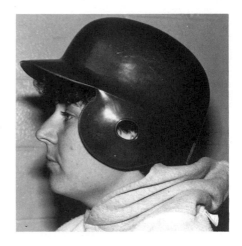

FIGURE 4. Batting helmet.

    5. Smooth infield.
    6. Breakaway bases to decrease sliding injuries.
F. **Equipment**
    1. Batting helmets (Fig. 4)
        a. Jaw protectors
        b. Plastic eye guards
    2. Metal or hard plastic cup inside athletic supporter
    3. Non-metal spikes
    4. Batting gloves
    5. Sliding pads to prevent abrasions ("strawberries")
    6. Ankle and shin protectors
    7. Catcher's and umpire's protective equipment: face mask equipped with throat protector (Fig. 5), chest protector (Fig. 6), shin guards (Fig. 7).

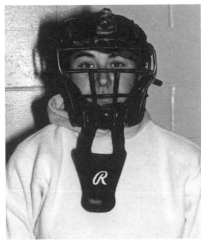

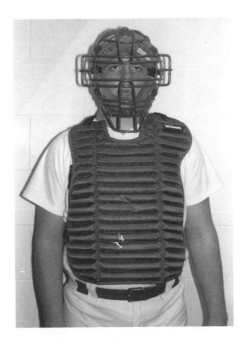

FIGURE 5 *(above).* Face mask with throat protector.

FIGURE 6 *(right).* Face mask with metal extension throat protector and padded chest protector.

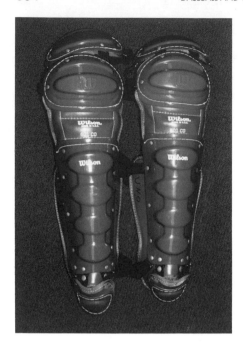

**FIGURE 7.**   Rigid shin guards.

8. Sunglasses
9. Sunscreen
10. During batting practice, screens to protect pitcher, first baseman, and others in the infield from batted balls.
11. Unbreakable aluminum bats may reduce injury potential.
12. Toe guard to prevent pitchers from damaging shoes.

VI. **Other Problems in Baseball and Softball**

A. Oral cancer from chewing tobacco.
B. Blisters on fingertips of pitchers.

# Chapter 51: Track and Field

THOMAS M. HEISER, MD

I. **Introduction**

Events in track and field demand widely diversified skills requiring increased aerobic and/or anaerobic metabolism. The sport is epitomized by the decathlete, who is challenged by a combination of events that test upper body strength in throwing events, jumping ability, sprint speed, and endurance running. Each one of these skills may result in a different type of injury and will be evaluated under the group to which it belongs.

II. **Specific Injuries**

A. **Throwing events** (shot put, discus, javelin throw, hammer throw)
   1. **Training injuries**
      a. **Osteolysis distal clavicle**
         i. History: pain is localized to the acromioclavicular (AC) joint with any activities requiring overhead motion. Pain may have been initiated by an incomplete AC separation, even one seemingly as mild as first degree. Pain also may be brought on by repetitive overhead lifting required in weight training.
         ii. Findings
            (a) Painful arc from 140–180° abduction
            (b) Point tenderness over AC joint
            (c) Radiographic evidence of widening of AC joint.
         iii. Treatment
            (a) Eliminate irritating activities (throwing, lifting above the head).
            (b) Anti-inflammatory medication
            (c) Physical therapy modalities
            (d) Distal clavicle resection.
      b. **Shoulder impingement syndrome**
         i. History: progressive onset of anterior and lateral shoulder pain experienced with repetitive overhead activities or high-velocity overhead activities.
         ii. Findings
            (a) Painful arc from 80–140° abduction and forward flexion
            (b) Positive impingement signs
            (c) Pain with resistance of external rotation (infraspinatus, teres minor) or Jobe's test (resistance with the arm in 80° abduction, 30° forward flexion, and full internal rotation, supraspinatus).
            (d) Tenderness lateral and anterior to acromion
            (e) No detectable instability or signs of labral lesions (clicking or popping with AP stress)
            (f) Radiographic studies usually normal.
         iii. Treatment
            (a) Minimize irritating activities
            (b) Physical therapy modalities directed toward decreasing rotator cuff inflammation

    (c) Anti-inflammatory medication

    (d) Flexibility exercises

    (e) Rotator cuff strengthening exercises at a level not resulting in pain

    (f) Gradual return to throwing activities.

  iv. Prevention

    (a) Well-balanced strengthening program to include strengthening (rhomboids, levator scapulae, trapezius), rotator cuff muscles, paraspinal and abdominal muscles.

    (b) Stretching and proper warm-up before any throwing activity.

c. **Muscle strains**

  i. History: sharp pain within body of a muscle sustained during lifting or throwing activities.

  ii. Findings

    (a) Tenderness in muscle belly with possible palpable defect

    (b) Pain localized to site of injury when muscle contraction is resisted

    (c) Swelling.

  iii. Treatment

    (a) Initial (1–3 days)—ice, stretching, exercise

    (b) Intermediate (3–7 days)—flexibility, strength, endurance

    (c) Advanced—flexibility, strength, endurance, gradual return to throwing.

  iv. Prevention

    (a) Well-balanced strengthening program using isometric, isotonic, and isokinetic exercise; concentric and eccentric strengthening, and proper balance between agonists and antagonists.

    (b) Well-designed stretching and warm-up program before each practice.

d. **Low back strain**

  i. History

    (a) Acute pain experienced during forceful movement while lifting or throwing.

    (b) Chronic recurrent pain experienced during or after lifting or throwing mechanics.

  ii. Findings

    (a) Range-of-motion limitations

    (b) Flexibility

    (c) Radicular signs

    (d) Spasm

    (e) Tenderness.

  iii. Treatment

    (a) Medications as necessary—analgesics, muscle relaxants, anti-inflammatory medication

    (b) Rest

    (c) Modalities

      (i) Ice, electrical stimulation, TENS unit (acute)

      (ii) Soft tissue mobilization and deep stroking massage (intermediate).

    (d) Strengthening

      (i) One-half sit-ups

      (ii) Spine extension exercises

      (iii) Internal and external oblique exercises

      (iv) Lumbar side-bending

      (v) Commercial back machines

(e) Return to throwing or lifting activity
(i) Waist belt for lifting
(ii) Abdominal binder for throwing.
iv. Prevention
(a) Proper lifting techniques
(b) Well-balanced strengthening program for spine flexors, extensors, and rotators.
2. **Throwing injuries**
a. **Shoulder instability syndrome**
i. History: shoulder pain associated with throwing.
ii. Findings
(a) Pain reproduced in shoulder with athlete going through throwing motion.
(b) Impingement signs may be present with arm in position.
(c) Instability in glenohumeral joint when stressed.
iii. Treatment
(a) Modalities
(b) Anti-inflammatory medication
(c) Restore motion and flexibility
(d) Strengthen rotator cuff and scapular stabilizers, with arm in the plane of the scapula and muscles at their normal resting length.
(e) Return to throwing program.
iv. Prevention—see par. II.A.1.b.
b. **Epicondylitis of the elbow**
i. History: gradual onset of pain over medial common flexor tendon origin or lateral common extensor tendon origin.
ii. Findings
(a) Tenderness at site
(b) Pain and weakness with resistance of wrist dorsiflexion or volar flexion.
iii. Treatment
(a) Modalities
(b) Anti-inflammatory medication
(c) Restore pain-free motion.
(d) Flexibility
(e) Restore strength, power, and endurance.
(f) Return to throwing program.
B. **Jumping events**
1. **Muscle strains**
a. History: pain in the muscle belly during or after the performance or jumping activities.
b. Findings
i. Pain to palpation over injured area
ii. Pain with resistance of muscle contraction
iii. Palpable defect, spasm, or knot at site of injury.
c. Treatment
i. Acute
(a) Modalities
(b) Flexibility, exercise
(c) Anti-inflammatory medication.
ii. Intermediate
(a) Modalities

        (b) Flexibility
        (c) Strengthening.
    iii. Advanced
        (a) Flexibility
        (b) Restore strength, power, and endurance
        (c) Progressively challenging jumping activities.
    d. Prevention—see par. II.A.1.c.
2. **Patellar tendinitis**
    a. History: pain experienced at the inferior pole of the patella with jumping activities.
    b. Findings
        i. Tenderness at the inferior pole of the patella.
        ii. Pain with resisted knee extension.
    c. Treatment
        i. Stage I—pain only after sports activity
            (a) Adequate warm-up
            (b) Ice after exercise
            (c) Modalities and anti-inflammatory medications
            (d) Hamstring/quadriceps flexibility and strengthening
            (e) Elastic knee supports.
        ii. Stage II—pain at the beginning of exercise, then disappearing but returning with fatigue.
            (a) Continue Stage I
            (b) Heat modalities before warm-up.
        iii. Stage III—constant pain at rest and during activity.
            (a) Continue Stage II
            (b) Prolonged rest
            (c) Cease jumping activities.
            (d) Restore strength, power, and endurance of lower extremity muscles as pain disappears.
            (e) Progressive return to jumping program.
        iv. Stage IV—complete rupture of the patellar tendon.
            (a) Surgery.
3. **Patellofemoral syndrome**
    a. History: retropatellar pain associated with running or jumping activities. Stages are similar to patellar tendinitis.
    b. Findings
        i. Pain with patellofemoral compression
        ii. Pain with palpation of patellar facets
        iii. Patellofemoral crepitus with active range of motion, especially with axial loading of the foot.
        iv. Patella apprehension
        v. Malaligned extremity
            (a) Femoral anteversion          (c) Squinting patellae
            (b) Genu valgus                  (d) Foot pronation.
        vi. Laterally riding patella with tight retinaculum
        vii. Patella hypomobility
        viii. Vastus medialis oblique (VMO) hypoplasia
    c. Treatment
        i. Modalities
        ii. Medication
        iii. Flexibility

    iv. Restore strength, power, and endurance

    v. VMO reeducation and strengthening

    vi. Support pronated foot with proper footwear and/or orthotics

    vii. Progressive return to jumping activities.

4. **Ligament sprains**

  a. History: acute injury to joint caused by flexion/extension, rotational, or varus/valgus forces when landing.

  b. Findings

    i. Extra-articular ligament

      (a) Point tenderness at site of injury

      (b) Localized swelling proportional to degree of injury

      (c) Degree of instability with stress maneuvers proportional to degree of injury.

    ii. Intra-articular ligament

      (a) Restricted motion

      (b) Effusion

      (c) Degree of instability with stress maneuvers proportional to degree of injury.

  c. Treatment

    i. Acute

      (a) Modalities

      (b) Splinting

      (c) Medication

        (i) Anti-inflammatory medication

        (ii) Analgesics.

      (d) Assisted ambulation

      (e) Discussion related to surgery options.

    ii. Intermediate

      (a) Modalities

      (b) Anti-inflammatory medication

      (c) Progressive weight-bearing

      (d) Range-of-motion activities

      (e) Strengthen thigh and leg muscles within limits of pain.

        (i) Exercise bicycle

        (ii) Electrical stimulation

        (iii) Isometric, isotonic, isokinetic.

    iii. Advanced

      (a) Modalities

      (b) Restore strength, power, and endurance.

      (c) Provide progressive athletic challenges to the joint directed at full return to activity.

5. **Achilles tendinitis**

  a. History: gradual onset of pain associated with workouts localized 1–3 inches proximal to Achilles insertion into os calcis.

  b. Findings

    i. Foot position

      (a) Rigid cavus foot

      (b) Pes planus.

    ii. Localized tenderness

    iii. Localized swelling

    iv. Tight gastrocsoleus complex.

  c. Treatment

    i. Modalities

    ii. Anti-inflammatory medication

    iii. Heel lifts and arch supports

     iv. Stretching of plantar fascia and Achilles

     v. Rest if pain is present with activities of daily living

     vi. Progressive return to usual workouts.

  d. Prevention

     i. Maintain flexibility of gastrocsoleus complex by stretching with flexed and extended knee.

     ii. Proper strength balance between foot dorsi and plantar flexors.

     iii. Comfortable running shoes with slightly elevated heel and well-supported longitudinal arch.

6. **Jumper's ankle**

  a. History: gradual onset of pain at anterior ankle associated with dorsiflexion of the foot at time of take-off and landing when jumping.

  b. Findings

     i. Limited ankle dorsiflexion

     ii. Pain on palpation of anterior ankle

     iii. Palpable spur over talus or anterior tibial plafond

     iv. Radiographic evidence of spur on talus or anterior tibia.

  c. Treatment

     i. Modalities

     ii. Anti-inflammatory medication

     iii. Prophylactic taping

     iv. Surgical excision of spurs.

7. **Plantar fasciitis**

  a. History: onset of pain acutely or subacutely, localized to plantar surface of os calcis.

  b. Findings

     i. Pain and tenderness over plantar-most aspect of os calcis or slightly distal and medial to that point.

     ii. Pain may be reproduced with stretch of plantar fascia.

     iii. Tightness in Achilles' tendon.

  c. Treatment

     i. Modalities

     ii. Anti-inflammatory medication

     iii. Stretching—plantar fascia and gastrocsoleus complex

     iv. Orthotics

       (a) Rigid plastic heel cup

       (b) Custom-molded support of longitudinal arch and first metatarsal.

  d. Prevention

     i. Maintain flexibility of Achilles' tendon.

     ii. Rigid plastic heel cup to maintain heel fat pad thickness to serve as cushion.

     iii. Well-supported longitudinal arch.

8. **Turf toe**

  a. History: pain at MTP joint of great toe associated with push-off phase of running or jumping.

  b. Findings

     i. Diffuse swelling at MTP joint

     ii. Tenderness throughout area of MTP joint

     iii. Restricted plantar flexion and dorsiflexion of great toe.

  c. Treatment

     i. Modalities

     ii. Anti-inflammatory medication

        iii. Taping to reduce joint mobility

        iv. Spring steel or orthoplast forefoot insole to reduce forefoot motion.

C. **Sprint events**

    1. **Muscle strains—lower extremity** (see par. II.B.A.a–c)

        a. Special rehabilitation considerations

            i. Restore flexibility during healing process.

            ii. Strength, power and endurance need to be restored.

                (a) Aerobic and anaerobic training methods

                (b) Isotonically, isometrically, and isokinetically

                (c) Concentrically and eccentrically

                (d) Running progression should be based on progressive challenges in the workout designed to gradually increase speed as tolerated by recovery of the injury, e.g., walk/jog distances; distance jogging; run straight-aways, walk curves, straight-aways to be run, gradually increasing speed to maximum tolerated at 40 to 60 meter mark and decelerating last 40 meters; sprints, gradually increasing distance.

                (e) Faithful stretching and warm-down after practice.

    2. **Tendinitis** (see par. II.B.2.a–c; II.B.5.a–c; II.B.7.a–c)

    3. **Patellofemoral syndrome** (see par. II.B.3.a–c)

D. **Endurance events**

    1. **Stress fractures**

        a. History: resulting from nonviolent stress that is applied in a rhythmic, repeated subthreshold manner.

        b. Findings

            i. Local tenderness

            ii. Possible swelling

            iii. Pain with repetitive impact axial loading

            iv. Radiographs may possibly be positive after minimum of 2 weeks from onset of pain

            v. Bone scan will be positive within days of onset of pain.

        c. Treatment

            i. Nonweight-bearing if pain present with activities of daily living.

            ii. If asymptomatic with walking and running, may resume in 2–4 weeks in atraumatic fashion; i.e., minimal mileage, no hills, no speed work, no hard surfaces, no frequent turns, and at a smooth, easy pace.

            iii. Gradual increase in mileage and pace as allowed by comfort.

            iv. Consider surgery for resistant femoral neck stress fracture or one that appears likely to progress.

        d. Prevention

            i. Avoid abrupt change in workout intensity, especially early in the conditioning period.

    2. **Patellofemoral syndrome** (see II.B.3.a–c)

    3. **Tendinitis**

        a. **Patellar** (see par. II.B.2.a–c)

        b. **Achilles** (see par. II.B.5.a–c)

        c. **Posterior tibialis**

            i. History: gradual onset of pain, posterior and inferior to medial malleolus, present in foot flat phase of stance and toe-off phase of running.

            ii. Findings

                (a) Tenderness localized over course of posterior tibialis tendon around malleolus.

        (b) Mild swelling over course of tendon.

        (c) Pain with resisted inversion/plantar flexion or attempt at single-limb heel rise.

    iii. Treatment

        (a) Modalities

        (b) Anti-inflammatory medication

        (c) Workout modification

        (d) Orthotic support of longitudinal arch to prevent pronation.

    iv. Prevention

        (a) Maintain balance between muscle agonists and antagonists

        (b) Develop endurance strength in addition to absolute strength.

**4. Iliotibial band friction syndrome**

  a. History: pain is localized to lateral aspect of the knee and is worse with running down hills or on banked surfaces.

  b. Findings

    i. Tenderness over lateral epicondyle is present.

    ii. Pain localized to lateral epicondyle as flexed knee is extended to 30°.

    iii. Pain at lateral epicondyle as athlete supports all of his body weight with his knee flexed 30°.

    iv. Tendency toward genu varus.

    v. Hyperpronated foot causing excessive internal tibial rotation.

  c. Treatment

    i. Reduce training, mileage, and avoid running downhill and on banks.

    ii. Modalities

    iii. Anti-inflammatory medication

    iv. Iliotibial band stretching

    v. Support pronated foot.

  d. Prevention

    i. Utilize properly balanced footwear.

    ii. Avoid running frequently on irregular or banked surfaces.

**5. Compartment syndromes**

  a. History: onset of pain is usually gradual over time. Pain consistently present over a certain distance during a run. Pain may persist after running, often into the night. Pain may be accompanied by complaints of weakness or numbness.

  b. Findings

    i. Palpable increase in firmness of size of involved compartment when pain is present.

    ii. Weakness of involved musculature.

    iii. Sensory change of nerves traveling through involved compartment.

    iv. Increased compartment pressures after reproducing pain in treadmill stress test.

  c. Treatment

    i. Subcutaneous fasciotomy.

**6. Periostitis** (shin splints)

  a. Anterior

    i. History: pain or tenderness along the medial or lateral anterior border of the tibia associated with running.

    ii. Findings

        (a) Pain increase with resisted dorsiflexion of passive plantar flexion of the foot.

        (b) Diffuse tenderness over anterior tibial border.

      iii. Treatment
- (a) Anti-inflammatory medication.
- (b) Ice to reduce swelling and inflammation.
- (c) Elastic wrap or tape for compression.
- (d) Rest from running while working on strengthening of dorsiflexors of the ankle.
- (e) Improve flexibility of Achilles and dorsiflexors.
- (f) Return to running by walk/job program.

  b. Posterior
    i. History: posteromedial leg pain in athlete who runs on crowned roads, a track with banked turns, or uneven terrain.
    ii. Findings
- (a) Tenderness along posteromedial border of tibia.
- (b) Foot pronation.

    iii. Treatment
- (a) Anti-inflammatory medication
- (b) Modalities
- (c) Reduce foot pronation
- (d) Run on flat surfaces
- (e) Return to running by walk/job program.

7. **Plantar fasciitis** (see par. II.B.7.)

8. **Metatarsalgia**
  a. History: pain under metatarsal heads associated with repetitive impact from running.
  b. Findings
    i. Tenderness localized to metatarsal heads.
    ii. Callus formation present over prominent metatarsal heads.
  c. Treatment
    i. Custom-molded orthotics for cushioning of metatarsal heads.
    ii. Rocker-bottom modification to orthotic.

9. **Morton's neuroma**
  a. History: pain in the foot localized to the third, or less commonly the second, interspace of the foot. Paresthesias or numbness may be present along the involved digital nerves.
  b. Findings
    i. Tenderness in involved interspace
    ii. Reproduction of symptoms by side-to-side compression of the foot.
  c. Treatment
    i. Properly fitting shoes
    ii. Anti-inflammatory medication
    iii. Orthosis with metatarsal pad to relieve pressure on metatarsal heads.
    iv. Surgery.

10. **Hallux rigidus**
  a. History: gradual onset of aching in the first MTP joint associated with stiffness and enlargement of the joint.
  b. Findings
    i. Limited dorsiflexion and plantar flexion of great toe MTP.
    ii. Palpable hypertrophic changes, especially dorsally, and sometimes associated with skin irritation or bursa formation.
  c. Treatment
    i. Properly fitting shoes
    ii. Stiff-soled shoes

           iii. Anti-inflammatory medication
           iv. Surgery.

11. **Tarsal tunnel syndrome**
    a. History: onset of numbness and paresthesias on the plantar aspect of the foot.
    b. Findings
       i. Positive Tinel's sign
      ii. Tenderness to palpation in the tarsal canal
     iii. Electrodiagnostic evidence of changes in the distal motor latencies in medial and lateral plantar nerves.
    c. Treatment
       i. Modalities
      ii. Anti-inflammatory medication
     iii. Properly fitting shoes with good shock absorption soles
     iv. Surgery.

12. **Athlete's foot**
    a. Itchy, scaly infestation of the foot caused by a fungus.
    b. Treat infections promptly with appropriate medication
    c. Good foot hygiene and use of shower clogs.

III. **Overuse Syndromes in Runners\***
Overuse syndromes can affect any part of the lower extremity and the list of potential injuries is almost limitless. These syndromes are chronic musculoskeletal problems resulting from microtraumatic stress to localized tissues, which leads to inflammation. Usually caused by excess mileage in training, the inflammation develops faster than the body's ability to repair, and eventuates in macroscopic irritation and tissue disruption. These syndromes often affect tissues that are biomechanically critical to running.

   A. **History of injury.** The following information should be obtained in the history-taking process for the present injury:
     1. **Nature of the present injury**
       a. When the injury was noticed
       b. Part injured
       c. Treatment in progress
       d. Recent foot or leg injuries that may have changed gait pattern.
       e. Past medical/orthopedic problems.
       f. Past use of orthotics or other pedal modifications (e.g., for leg-length discrepancy).
     2. **General training practices of the individual**
       a. Weekly mileage
         i. Changes in mileage
          (a) Rate of advancement should not be $\geq 10\%$/week.
        ii. Changes in intensity or pattern of running.
        iii. Excessive mileage. Injury rises over the 30-mile-per-week training threshold.
          (a) $\geq 15\%$/year for males
          (b) $\geq 20\%$/year for females.
       b. Surface
         i. Type of surface (grass, asphalt, clay, etc.) and recent changes from one to another.

---

\* *Note:* Part III is adapted in part from Franz WB: Overuse syndromes in runners. In Mellion MB: Office Management of Sports Injuries & Athletic Problems. Philadelphia, Hanley & Belfus, 1988, with permission.

        ii. Surface grade
          (a) Uphill stresses gastroc-Achilles tendon system.
          (b) Downhill stresses tibial stabilizers or anterior tibialis muscle group.
        iii. Bank of roadway or track
          (a) Pronation of upper foot
          (b) Supination of lower foot.
    c. Nature and extent of running in leisure activities.
    d. Use of lower extremities in activities of daily living.
  3. **Nature of specific training practices**
    a. Interval training—sprints can increase biomechanical strain.
    b. Footwear use
        i. Training footwear
          (a) How often changed?
            (i) Shoes lose 50% of shock absorption capacity in 250–300 miles.
          (b) Wear patterns
          (c) Repaired vs. new footwear
        ii. Racing footwear—should not be used in training because of lack of support and shock absorption.
        iii. Everyday footwear—look for patterns of wear, support characteristics.
    c. Systemic effects of overtraining
        i. Excessive fatigue and stiffness
        ii. "Staleness" and desire for rest
        iii. Deterioration of interest in training.
B. **General treatment approach**
  1. **Classify degree of overuse** (Table 1).
    a. Early stages of overuse (Grades I and II):
        i. Evaluate training program for correctable problems.
        ii. Most athletes will not seek help at this stage.
    b. More advanced overuse (Grades III and IV):
        i. Pain limits competitive performance.
        ii. Training program is interrupted.
        iii. Rest and treatment are necessary.
  2. **Rest**
    a. The more severe the grade of overuse, the more rest is needed.
    b. Usually a decrease in weekly mileage is necessary.

**TABLE 1.** Staging of Overuse Syndromes*

| Grade I | Post-activity soreness<br>Duration of symptoms less than 2 weeks<br>Generalized tenderness |
|---|---|
| Grade II | Pain during end of running and immediately after<br>Duration of symptoms greater than 2 weeks<br>Localized pain, minimal inflammation |
| Grade III | Pain during early training<br>Duration of symptoms greater than 3 weeks<br>Point tenderness, definite objective tissue inflammatory signs<br>(erythema, edema, crepitus) |
| Grade IV | Pain with activities other than training, severity of which<br>prohibits training or competition<br>Grade III symptoms plus—dysfunction of injured structure,<br>muscle atrophy, tissue breakdown |

* From Franz WB: Overuse syndromes in runners. In Mellion MB: Office Management of Sports Injuries and Athletic Problems. Philadelphia, Hanley & Belfus, Inc., 1988, with permission.

    c. Training sessions should be divided into smaller increments, with rest between.

    d. Activities with less biomechanical strain can be substituted for running (e.g., swimming, bicycling).

3. **Cryotherapy and thermotherapy**

    a. Ice applied to inflamed body parts

        i. 20-minute applications or to tolerance, then rewarm and reapply as appropriate.

        ii. Ice is most useful in the acute phase of injury.

           (a) Decreases pain

           (b) Inhibits inflammation.

        iii. Contraindicated with medical conditions that affect sensory nerve supply:

           (a) Diabetes

           (b) Vascular disease

           (c) During use of local anesthetic.

    b. Heat is useful in later rehabilitation of injury.

        i. Increases tissue flexibility and elasticity.

        ii. Allows athlete to stretch more comfortably.

    c. Compression and elevation are used with cryotherapy.

        i. Decreases edema.

        ii. Compression prevents accumulation of inflammatory products in tissue.

        iii. Elevation promotes venous and lymphatic flow.

4. **Pharmacologic treatment**

    a. NSAIDs and salicylates

        i. Useful both acutely and chronically.

        ii. Pain relief initially and during longer term, indicating decrease in inflammation.

    b. Injectable corticosteroids

        i. Indicated after more conservative measures fail.

        ii. Often mixed with local anesthetic.

        iii. Skin surgically prepared.

        iv. Do not inject into tendons.

        v. Watch for systemic effect and infection.

5. **Orthotics for running**

    a. Consider for a specific biomechanical problem related to symptoms.

    b. Usually shoe inserts of plastic or rubber material.

    c. Usual objective is to balance foot in neutral to inhibit pronation and supination.

    d. Initiate slowly, with multiple adjustments during break-in.

    e. Use in symptom-free athlete is contraindicated (may cause symptoms).

6. **Shoes**

    a. Sports-specific shoes have enhanced performance.

    b. Running shoes should have good shock absorption, rigid heel control, good flexibility at midfoot break, provide good traction, and protect the feet.

        i. Soles should be constructed for long wear and shock absorption.

        ii. Wide heal with lift for shock absorption and support of Achilles tendon.

        iii. Curve of sole conforms to foot shape, with greater curve for high arch or cavus foot.

        iv. Snug fit, allowing slight increase in volume during running.

    c. Prescription of footwear is an important component of treatment program for overuse.

    d. Major problem is overworn shoes.

7. **Promote appropriate warm-up and cool-down techniques**
   a. Warm-up long enough to cause sweating and to feel mild exertion. Has several salutary effects:
      i. Enhances oxygen release from hemoglobin
      ii. Increases blood flow
      iii. Decreases blood viscosity
      iv. Enhances muscular contraction
      v. Increases speed of neuromuscular transmission (i.e., improved reaction time)
      vi. Increases tissue elasticity, with decreased viscosity of synovial fluid
      vii. Allows for better gains from subsequent stretching.
   b. Non-ballistic stretching
      i. Follows proper warm-up
      ii. Facilitates enhanced neuromuscular efficiency
      iii. Should be done gently, never past minimal discomfort to the point of pain
      iv. Careful attention to
         (a) Hamstring and gastrocnemius muscle group
         (b) Iliotibial band
   c. If running precedes stretching, warm-up should provide for flexibility.
      i. Alternate 220-yard jog with 20-yard walk for one-half mile
   d. Cool-down
      i. Should be active vs. passive.
         (a) Facilitates removal of lactate from tissue
         (b) Heart rate and respiration decrease to pre-exercise levels
         (c) Additional stretching can be done.

IV. **Sport-specific Facilities and Protective Equipment**

A. **Running shoes**
   1. Wide sole base to prevent running over the side of the shoe.
   2. Tough, flexible, rubber outsole with cushioned heel area to reduce trauma at heel strike.
   3. Firm heel counter with well-padded area to reduce irritation on the Achilles' tendon.
   4. Removable insole to allow for adjustment or replacement, compensating individual arch variations.

B. **Runway approaches**
   1. 85–120 feet in length for pole vault, long and triple jump.
   2. Homogeneous surface of regular consistency to avoid soft spots or uneven edges, preventing unusual stresses on the foot and ankle.

C. **Vaulting boxes**
   1. Construction of cast aluminum or welded steel.
   2. Walls of the box are angled obtusely to avoid contact with the pole.

D. **Vaulting poles**
   1. Fiber glass construction with poles classified by weight and length.
   2. Size and weight of pole to be used depends on size, strength, speed, and skill of athlete.
      a. The athlete should never use a pole with a weight designation lighter than his body weight.
      b. Adjustment of pole can be determined by height of the vault and landing position in the pit, provided the athlete is determined to use proper technique.

   3. The athlete's top hand should always be between 6 and 18 inches from the top of the pole.

   4. The take-off foot should always be in the center of the runway.

  E. **Landing mats for pole vault**

    1. Mat construction is a combination of foam and air cells.

    2. Mats must be held together by a common unit—preferably a tarp with a 2-inch foam pad that breathes and allows the exchange of air in the mats.

    3. Mats should cover an area at least 16½ × 16½ feet and should enclose all sides of the vaulting box except the pole entrance side. Mat depth is generally 26–36 inches. Increased surface area is more important than depth.

## V. Sport-specific Special Concerns of the Team Physician

Track and field is a sport in which the majority of the problems concern injury caused by poor conditioning, overconditioning, or acute strain in the heat of competition. Injuries can be prevented by examining the athlete's general body habitus and foot and leg alignment, and by anticipating problems according to the specific demand of the event.

Thoughtfully designed preseason and in-season training programs can prevent injuries due to "overuse" or stress fractures and similar injuries. Coaches need to be advised that every athlete is different, with variable physical and physiologic responses to conditioning. Each athlete may have an overall limit beyond which further training will have deleterious results. Not every runner will physically be able to tolerate the level of intensity needed in workouts to become a marathon runner, and this is true in other events also.

Recovery from injury requires the athlete reach a near pain-free condition. While the athlete is in the recovery phase of the injury, muscle tone and aerobic fitness can be maintained with a weight-lifting program modified to allow for the disability and with workouts on an exercise bike or in a swimming pool. The athlete should continue to be challenged in some way to maintain enthusiasm and a positive approach to return to activity.

Workouts may then begin as a series of challenges, each of which the athlete must overcome before going on to the next. In this way, muscles, tendons, ligaments, and bones can respond to Wolff's law (form follows function) and develop the necessary strength to survive the demands placed on them.

# Chapter 52: Gymnastics

JERRY WEBER, MS, PT, ATC

## I. General Discussion

A. Participation

The wide popularity of gymnastics as a sport has greatly increased the participation by members of both sexes over the past decade. The benefits of "gymnastic training" for a prospective athlete in the formative years is evidenced by the large number of children's gymnastics clubs and instructional programs. The strenuous requirements of this sport in strength, flexibility, agility, and physical size tend to eliminate most early participants from becoming truly competitive at the high school and most certainly at the college level. A physician who will be working with competitive-level gymnastics must be familiar with the basic requirements of the sport and the different individual events in male and female programs (Table 1).

B. Forces involved

1. Gymnastics events exert tremendous forces on the bodies of the participants.
2. Dismounts may entail great rotational and/or twisting forces from great heights, causing severe injury to the lower body, or, if improperly performed, a fall on the side, back, head, or neck.
3. Forces involved in the swinging apparatus (horizontal bar, rings, uneven bars) exert many times the weight of the body on the shoulders, elbows, and wrists, with the potential for distraction and stress injuries.

C. Medical concerns

1. The physician working with gymnasts must be knowledgeable about potential acute injuries as well as chronic overuse problems.

## II. Overview of Injury Patterns: Body Survey

A. **Head and neck injuries**

1. **Concussion**
   a. **Mechanism:** Striking head on mat or apparatus in a fall or dismount.
   b. **Evaluation:** General neurologic screen; medical observation is recommended for unconsciousness.
   c. **Treatment:** Physician should follow standard head injury guidelines for severity and follow-up.
2. **Cervical subluxation/dislocation/fracture**
   a. **Mechanism:** Fall from apparatus, over- or underrotation on a dismount from apparatus or in a floor tumbling pass, failure to clear the vaulting horse, striking head on end of horse, or being driven into landing mat.
   b. **Evaluation and treatment:** Emergency ABCs, evaluation and life-saving measures instituted.
3. **Neck strain/sprain**—extensor/flexor muscle mass injuries, "whiplash," ligamentous injuries.
   a. **Mechanism:** Fall on head/neck with neck flexed or extended. Injuries to these muscles can occur without contact by use of the head and neck to provide lead momentum in a specific maneuver.

**TABLE 1.** Gymnastic Events for Men and Women

| Men's Events[6] | Women's Events[4] |
|---|---|
| Floor exercise | Vault |
| Pommel horse | Uneven bars |
| Still rings | Balance beam |
| Vault | Floor exercise |
| Parallel bars | |
| Horizontal bar | |

*Note:* The trampoline is no longer a competitive event at the high school, collegiate, or international level.

    b. **Evaluation:** Check neurologic status, active and passive ranges of motion, strength levels, pain levels.

    c. **Treatment:** Ice in acute stage; soft neck collar to provide support if indicated. Encourage early active motion—isometric strengthening. Physical therapy as indicated.

4. **Lacerations** to scalp, forehead, orbit, or chin
    a. **Mechanism:** Lacerations may occur any time the head strikes the hard surface of a mat or in contact with any of the apparatus.
    b. **Evaluation and treatment:** physician's discretion.

5. **Nerve root irritation**
    a. **Mechanism:** Acute episode of neck strain/sprain or insidious onset with pain and/or numbness in a specific neurologic pattern.
    b. **Evaluation:** History of injury in the neck area is important; neurologic exam of involved area.
    c. **Treatment:** Avoidance of irritating activities. Physical therapy includes cervical traction once bony injury eliminated. Appropriate strength maintenance exercises.

B. **Shoulder injuries**
1. **Glenohumeral (GH) dislocation**—acute episode
    a. **Mechanism:** Forced external rotation of the abducted shoulder causing anterior dislocation (most common)—usually from a fall or failure to maintain proper swing on rings or high bar with torsion to arm that maintains grip.
    b. **Evaluation:** History, physical exam of shoulder to evaluate loss of deltoid "roundness." On involved side, palpation of head of humerus in anterior-lateral chest wall. Neurovascular status of distal extremity.
    c. **Treatment:** Reduction of joint if no fracture is suspected. Immobilization with arm at side and hand across abdomen. Ice or medication for pain. X-ray.

2. **Glenohumeral subluxation**
    a. **Mechanism:** Same as dislocation. Athlete may describe shoulder slipping out of joint and back in place.
    b. **Evaluation:** History, physical exam to determine joint stability, apprehension test.
    c. **Treatment:** Immobilization until discomfort is gone then early motion and strengthening, especially of rotator cuff musculature. Repeated episodes of shoulder instability, whether dislocations or subluxations, may effectively eliminate any gymnast from competing in the swing events, either due to pain and failure of the shoulder, or, with repair, the inherent loss of external rotation.

3. **Acromioclavicular (AC) sprain/separation**
    a. **Mechanism:** Fall on the shoulder to mat or apparatus.
    b. **Evaluation:** History and comparative clinical exam to determine appearance, clavicular mobility at the AC joint, and pain. Comparative x-rays with and without distracting weights for degree of separation.

    c. **Treatment**—depends on degree of injury

       i. **First degree:** Ice; return to activity as tolerated by pain and motion.

      ii. **Second degree:** Ice and physical therapy. Immobilization (sling) only if dictated by pain. Work for motion as tolerance allows. May be able to return to certain events earlier than others. Short course of anti-inflammatory medication at discretion of physician.

     iii. **Third degree:** Ice and immobilization. Moist heat therapy at 72 hours. Sling for comfort and stabilization for 10–14 days. NSAIDs. Begin gentle ROM exercises at 2 weeks, followed by resistive motion exercises as tolerated.

4. **Chronic AC inflammation**

    a. **Mechanism:** Irritation of AC joint from constant stress from swing maneuvers and handstand activities. AC joint can become tender to palpation and painful with full AROM activities. Inflammations usually respond well to local physical therapy, rest, or avoidance of irritating activities, and anti-inflammatory medications. Resistant or acutely tender inflammations may respond well to local corticosteroid injection.

5. **Internal derangement**

    a. **Mechanism:** Labrum tears and rotator cuff impingement syndromes are common in gymnasts from stress on the shoulder girdle. Internal derangements may be associated with some degree of glenohumeral instability.

    b. **Evaluation:** Proper evaluation and diagnosis are important to management.

    c. **Treatment:** The majority of these problems respond well to conservative measures such as physical therapy, medication and/or injection therapy, appropriate strengthening activities (rotator cuff), rest and avoidance of sport- and weight-training related activities (e.g., overhead lifts or tricks that compromise stability). The athlete who does not respond to conservative measures may require arthroscopic intervention.

6. **Thoracic outlet syndrome (TOS)**

    a. **Mechanism:** Thoracic outlet syndromes may occur in athletes as a result of repeated overhead rotatory stress.

    b. **Evaluation:** Pain in shoulder and arm with numbness and tingling of hand and swelling or cyanosis of upper extremity with overhead activities suggest thoracic outlet syndrome.

    c. **Treatment:** (see Chap. 34).

C. **Elbow injuries**

1. **Dislocation**

    a. **Mechanism:** Fall on outstretched hand with semiflexed elbow.

    b. **Evaluation:** History, physical exam of bony landmarks. Check neurovascular status distal to injury. Reduction followed by x-ray exam. Obtain x-rays prior to reduction if fracture is suspected.

    c. **Treatment:** Ice and pressure wrap from hand to mid-biceps. Immobilization in posterior 90° elbow splint for 3–6 weeks. **Active** motion in flexion and extension very important. Passive mobilization to be avoided. Early strengthening of elbow extensors encouraged.

2. **Epicondylitis—medial/lateral**

    a. **Mechanism:** Strain of forearm flexor or extensor muscles from varus or valgus stress on the elbow or torsion stress of elbow from specific pivot-like maneuvers in handstand positions.

    b. **Evaluation:** History, active and passive ROM, palpation to determine areas of point tenderness, x-ray to determine possibility of avulsion fractures or hypertrophic bony changes at the epicondyle.

    c. **Treatment:** Physical therapy and strengthening exercises to emphasize resisted supination/pronation. Neoprene elbow sleeve for compression, support, and warmth may be of some benefit to the athlete. Anti-inflammatory medications and/or corticosteroid injection may be indicated.

  3. **Valgus/varus sprains**

    a. **Mechanism:** Falls from or on the apparatus may result in stress to the collateral ligaments, most commonly the medial collateral ligament. This ligament may also be stressed by certain moves on any of the specific events.

    b. **Evaluation:** History, palpation to determine point tenderness, comparative valgus stress test to determine ligament stability.

    c. **Treatment:** Ice, compression, early tolerated motion to maintain full flexion, physical therapy and appropriate strengthening to ensure full return to activity.

  4. **Ulnar neuritis**

    a. **Mechanism:** Insidious overuse problem in which ulnar nerve becomes stretched, contused, or otherwise irritated at the ulnar groove.

    b. **Evaluation:** History—complaints of pain, tingling, numbness down medial forearm to include outside of the hand and fifth finger.

    c. **Treatment:** Avoidance of irritating positions or repetitious elbow movements. Protection from further insult. Physical therapy to relieve swelling. May require surgical intervention in extreme cases.

D. **Forearm injuries**

  1. **Fracture**

    a. **Mechanism:** An injury specific to gymnasts in which the leather grip that the athlete is wearing for horizontal bar "catches" or grabs onto the bar, and, instead of allowing the athlete to complete the "giant swing," holds the hand in position on the bar as the body continues around the circle, causing the forearm to "wrap around" and sustain multiple fractures. This serious injury requires the coach or whoever is present to get the athlete off the apparatus without inflicting further damage to the arm.

    b. **Evaluation and treatment** as appropriate for the fracture(s).

  2. **Forearm splints:** The athlete reports pain and aching in one or both forearms during and after workout. It is caused by an interosseous inflammation, usually of the wrist extensors.

    a. **Mechanism:** Stress to the interosseous region of the forearm from the athlete being in a weight-bearing position on his hands much of the time during floor exercise, vault, and especially the pommel horse and parallel bars.

    b. **Evaluation:** History—usually atraumatic pain with and without palpation and resisted gripping. X-ray to rule out stress fracture to the ulna or radius.

    c. **Treatment:** Ice massage to the area after and during workouts. Anti-inflammatory medication as indicated by level of disability. Pressure wrap or taping of the area for added support.

E. **Wrist:** The wrist is an area of special concern in gymnastics because of the tremendous stress placed on this joint in all events.

  1. **Navicular fracture—acute and stress-induced**

    a. **Mechanism:** Fall on the extended wrist or maneuver in which the weight of the body comes down sharply on one or both wrists. Stress fractures of this bone occur from constant pounding that the wrist undergoes in this sport.

    b. **Evaluation:** Classic signs of navicular fracture are present. Point tenderness over the anatomic snuff box. Painful wrist extension with limitation of wrist extension. History may or may not be specific. X-ray in acute episode may not be positive. If symptoms persist, x-rays must be repeated after 10–14 days.

    c. **Treatment:** Positive navicular signs even in the absence of radiographic evidence should be treated with immobilization until it is proved that there is no fracture present.

2. **Dorsal wrist/hand pain**

    a. **Mechanism:** The insertion of the extensor carpi radialis brevis tendon into the base of the second metacarpal can become raised and point tender due to the resisted wrist extension required in body support in many gymnastic events.

    b. **Evaluation:** Lateral x-ray view of the wrist may reveal an actual avulsion or lifting of the bony surface in extreme cases. The athlete will experience pain in this area while working out as well as after practice.

    c. **Treatment:** Limitation of resisted wrist extension, ice, physical therapy modalities to lessen inflammation, tape for support. Extreme cases of actual avulsion may require immobilization for a limited amount of time.

F. **Hand, fingers, and thumb injuries**

1. **Dislocations:** The most common hand injuries in gymnastics are dislocations of the interphalangeal (IP) joints of the fingers. Metacarpophalangeal (MP) joint dislocations may also occur.

    a. Treatment: Most competitive gymnasts will not tolerate even a 10-day period of immobilization or splinting except for a fracture, but the finger should be splinted in slight flexion during their time out of the gym, with "buddy taping" of the finger for protection during workouts.

2. **Soft tissue injuries, blisters and "rips"**

    a. **Mechanism:** A gymnast's hands are subjected to severe abuse in the sport. Even with the use of leather grips and chalk, the friction between skin and apparatus will at times cause even callused skin to tear away in patches or "rips."

    b. **Treatment:** Soft tissue wounds should be treated to avoid infection. Appropriate protective padding and wrapping should be applied to prevent irritation until the athlete can tolerate friction in the area. Typical blister treatment such as moleskin or second skin to protect the wound site usually will not work on gymnasts' hands and still allow them to practice.

G. **Chest injuries**

1. **Rib injuries**

    a. **Mechanism:** Falls on or from the apparatus can cause rib contusions and/or costochondral sprain/separation injuries. Rib fractures are rare, but, if warranted, x-rays should be performed to rule out this possibility.

    b. **Evaluation:** History, palpation, lateral and AP compression tests to localize injury site and help determine if x-rays are needed.

    c. **Treatment:** Rib binder, medication, activity as tolerated, and appropriate cold or moist heat therapy.

2. **Sternoclavicular (SC) sprain**

    a. **Mechanism:** Acute fall or blow to SC area or overuse injury with insidious onset from "swing" stress or strength moves on rings.

    b. **Evaluation:** History (acute or chronic), palpation and inspection to determine degree of separation if any, x-ray if indicated.

    c. **Treatment:** Local cold/hot applications for swelling and discomfort. Medication as indicated. Rest and progressive return to activities as tolerated.

3. **Sternocostal sprain/separation**

    a. **Mechanism:** Fall through the parallel bars that allows the body to drop below shoulder level while the hands are still holding onto the bars puts distractive force on the pectoral muscles and the ribs at the sternum. This extensive chest injury may incapacitate the athlete for up to 4 weeks.

    b. **Evaluation:** The athlete will present with a very specific history of the above mechanism and extensive chest and possibly shoulder pain and tenderness with associated limitation of ROM.

    c. **Treatment:** Rest, compression binder, medication for discomfort, early return of motions as tolerated, physical therapy and strengthening as indicated.

H. **Lower abdomen, hip, and pelvic injuries**
  1. **Muscle strain**
    a. **Mechanism:** The lower abdominal and hip flexor musculature in both male and female gymnasts is typically very strong from training efforts that require these muscle groups to be strenuously worked at all times. Injuries to this region are not common in the competitive gymnast. Younger gymnasts may strain these muscle groups in training to achieve the higher strength levels.

    b. **Treatment:** Relative rest and therapeutic exercise.

  2. **Contusion to the anterior pelvis**
    a. **Mechanism:** Female gymnasts may incur severe bruises to the anterior superior illiac spine region on uneven bars when swinging down from the high bar to the low bar by slamming the anterior pelvic region into the lower bar. Repeated trauma to this poorly padded area can cause extreme tenderness and bruising.

    b. **Treatment:** Avoidance of the maneuver or padding of anterior bony area. Ice to reduce swelling and decrease tenderness.

I. **Lumbar spine**
Low back pain is a common complaint in both male and female gymnasts. Many gymnasts, especially females, have a pronounced lordotic curve. This abnormal curvature can be attributed to years of back flexion and extension flexibility exercises, "extension walkovers," and abnormal strengthening of the iliopsoas muscles. A gymnast who presents with low back symptoms needs to be examined thoroughly to identify the cause of pain.

  1. **Acute low back pain**
    a. **Mechanism:** Common causes include sudden explosive over-rotation, hard landings on the feet with the knees locked, causing the back to be jammed, or falls to the mats, floor, or apparatus. Pain is associated with spasm of the extensor muscles on one or both sides of the spine, swelling, and loss of normal motion.

    b. **Treatment:** Ice, pain and anti-inflammatory medications, sacral belt for support, physical therapy to include lumbar traction and flexibility and strengthening exercises. The problem resolves in a few days, and the gymnast may return to limited activities. Gymnasts should be cautioned against stressing their backs too soon, and should be observed to be sure that further symptoms do not occur that may warrant other measures.

  2. **Chronic low back pain**
Many gymnasts will have a certain level of chronic back pain because of the nature of their sport. This chronic soreness and pain usually respond to appropriate stretching and physical therapy. When these measures do not control the pain or other symptoms arise, then measures need to be taken to evaluate for more serious conditions.

  3. **Radiculopathy**
    a. **Evaluation:** Unilateral pain down into the buttock and hamstring with associated tingling may be caused by nerve root irritation or sciatic nerve irritation. Pain, tingling, and numbness further down the leg into the foot

may represent specific nerve root irritation and/or a possible disc lesion. Depending on the severity of symptoms, diagnostic measures should include complete clinical exam, x-ray, and CT scan or MRI, if indicated.

   b. **Treatment:** See Chap. 39.

  4. **Spondylolysis and spondylolisthesis**

   a. **Evaluation:** X-rays should always be obtained in an athlete with persistent low back pain. Many gymnasts will have positive radiographic evidence of posterior lamina defects or spondylolisthesis. These may be unilateral or bilateral and typically represent an old injury, especially in a gymnast who has been in the sport since childhood.

   b. **Treatment:** This condition may be fairly benign and may or may not cause symptoms. When spondylolisthesis is present, or anterior slippage of the superior vertebral body occurs, the athlete may have more pronounced symptoms. Depending on the degree of slippage and physical symptoms, the gymnast will have to be advised as to activity level or counselled to quit the sport altogether. The muscle strain and associated muscle spasm often respond favorably to physical therapy.

**J. Knee injuries**

  1. **Mechanism:** Gymnasts are vulnerable to all the various knee injuries common to athletes in all sports that involve running and jumping, but with the added stress, rotation, and twist associated with landing from heights. The majority of knee injuries in gymnasts occur on dismounts or during floor exercise passes that involve tumbling passes. The team physician who is working with gymnasts can expect to see the full complement of knee injuries from infrapatellar tendinitis to anterior cruciate ligament (ACL) tears.

   Note: Gymnasts who have suffered a torn ACL should have full reconstruction of this ligament to prevent further knee deterioration and to allow for eventual return to the sport.

**K. Leg injuries**

  1. **Shin splints**

   a. **Mechanism:** Repeated stress to the lower leg from running, jumping, and dismounts. May be intensified in female gymnasts from beam workouts. Often associated with stress to the medial longitudinal arch, which causes strain on the tibialis posterior muscles.

   b. **Evaluation:** Typical history of shin splint complaints. Pain in anterior shin along interosseous region of tibia and fibula during activities, and deep aching afterward and without activity.

   c. **Treatment:** Ice before, during, and after workouts. Aspirin therapy or other anti-inflammatory medications. Physical therapy in extreme cases to include electrical stimulation, heat, and ultrasound. Anterior shin stretching exercises, lower leg strengthening exercises, and arch supports are indicated in all cases. Typical orthotic type arch supports will not work during workouts, because shoes are not worn; however, they may be of benefit when worn while out of the gym. Proper supportive arch taping should be used during time in the gym.

  2. **Calf strains**

   a. **Mechanism:** Injuries to the triceps surae muscle group do occur in gymnastics during the floor exercise event. The forcible, explosive plantar flexion or "punch" required by the gymnast to be "launched" on tumbling passes or dismounts is stressful and may cause damage, especially to the gastrocnemius group.

   b. **Evaluation:** History, clinical evaluation to determine comparative muscle shape and palpable defects or masses, and strength tests to determine whether the gastrocnemius or soleus muscles are involved.

   c. **Treatment:** Ice with pressure wrap to control effusion. Crutches may be necessary until acute tenderness has subsided. Heel lift may be used if weight-bearing or partial weight-bearing. Gentle early stretching and strengthening exercises depending on severity of the injury.

3. **Strain/rupture of Achilles' tendon**
   a. **Mechanism:** The same mechanism that causes calf muscle strains is responsible for injuries to the Achilles' tendon. Actual ruptures or partial tears of the Achilles' tendon usually occur in older athletes but may occur in high school and college age competitors.
   b. **Evaluation:** History, tenderness will be more distal in the calf to the musculotendinous junction or in the tendon itself. A palpable, visible defect may be present and the ability to actively plantarflex the ankle will be absent or diminished. A common test (Thompson's test) for complete rupture is to squeeze the muscle mass proximal to the injury. In a complete tear the foot will not plantarflex with this passive movement, thus indicating rupture of the Achilles' tendon.
   c. **Treatment:** Ice and compression are the immediate concern. Non-weight bearing crutch walking will be required. The decision as to surgical and non-surgical treatment is up to the experience of the physician.

4. **Fibular stress fracture**
   a. **Mechanism:** Fibular stress fractures in gymnasts are not uncommon owing to the frequency of activity that stresses the lower leg. The possibility of a stress fracture should not be overlooked when treating the athlete for chronic shin splints.
   b. **Evaluation:** Ongoing symptoms that include painful walking outside the gym, extreme isolated point tenderness, or pain with interosseous compression should prompt the physician to order x-ray studies and possibly a bone scan to rule out this possibility.
   c. **Treatment:** Most gymnasts will be able to continue modified workouts with a fibular stress fracture, because they can work the upper body on the various apparati and avoid the dismounts, running, and landings necessary in floor and vault. Once healing has begun the gymnast can slowly return to full activity with support as dictated by tolerance and the physician's discretion.

L. **Ankle injuries**
   1. **Mechanism:** In their competitive careers most gymnasts will fall victim to some type of ankle injury. The ankles absorb a tremendous amount of force when the gymnast lands perfectly, and with a rotational or twisting component involved in many dismounts, the ankle is placed in even more jeopardy. Lateral ankle injuries (inversion-plantar flexion) occur quite often from improper landings, but also from the foot hitting a seam between mats.

      Acute anterior impingement of the tibia against the talus is a special problem in gymnasts caused by landing "short," in which the athlete under-rotates a somersault and lands in a deep squatted position, jamming the anterior ankle. Over a course of time this situation can lead to a chronic inflammatory condition with exostosis of the anterior talar lip. Because of these problems, it is not unusual for many competitive college gymnasts to exhibit early arthritic changes in the ankle that lead to arthroscopic or surgical intervention.
   2. **Evaluation:** History (acute or chronic). Check for effusion, tenderness, and joint laxity. X-rays when indicated to determine extent of bony changes.
   3. **Treatment:** Acute severe sprains need to be treated with pressure and ice. The ankle should be wrapped from the toes to above the ankle to avoid pitting edema of the foot. Extreme injuries may require a bulky dressing or even a cast

for proper healing and weight-bearing. In most cases early motion and strengthening are important to ensure proper return to activity. Management of less severe cases involves physical therapy, strengthening, support, and anti-inflammatory medications as deemed necessary. It is highly recommended that competitive gymnasts protect their ankles with athletic tape or lace-up braces that allow full function while protecting against abnormal range of motion.

M. **Foot injuries:** The same forces that are exerted on the ankle affect the foot structures as well.

1. **Medial longitudinal arch sprain**
   a. **Mechanism:** Pain in the medial aspect of the foot and along the course of the posterior tibialis tendon may or may not be associated with shin splints. Arch pain may be acute or result from chronic overuse syndrome.
   b. **Treatment:** Proper management includes supporting the medial arch with tape and padding. Modification of footwear will not work since no rigid foot support is worn in gymnastics. Appropriate physical therapy to control pain and swelling along with rest or modification of activity are also important.

2. **Heel bruising**
   a. **Mechanism:** In working dismounts from a somersault, athletes may over-rotate the maneuver, which will cause them to land with full weight on their heels. This can cause significant injury to the heel pad of one or both feet.
   b. **Evaluation:** History. Physical exam reveals diffuse or specific point tenderness, localized heel pad swelling, and perhaps ecchymosis.
   c. **Treatment:** Ice massage, padding for comfort, or solid plastic heel cup. Avoidance of reinjury is important to avoid chronic problems. Physical therapy after 3–4 days to include moist heat, ultrasound, and electrical stimulation. Heel taping or heel cup draws natural padding of heel fat pad together.

III. **Traumatic and Overuse Injury:** Traumatic injuries in gymnastics, although many times quite serious, may be easier to deal with for everybody concerned than chronic overuse conditions. Typically, the acute injury has a specific onset with predictable diagnosis and prognosis. Ground rules can be laid out in a specific manner in black and white. On the other hand, overuse syndromes can be hard to document, with symptoms coming and going until the athlete finally mentions them and usually wants something done immediately. Many gymnasts attempt to work through most injury situations, and often will be successful, so that by the time the resistant injury is reported, it will have become a full-blown chronic problem with a frustrating and lengthy return to activity. It is important that the team physician allow the athlete to remain as active as possible without compromising treatment of the injury in question.

IV. **Injury Prevention: Prevention of gymnastics injuries is directly related to organization and supervision in the gym itself. Proper coaching and spotting techniques** are vital in preventing many serious injuries. **Recognition of the gymnast's abilities** by the coach is important to make sure that the athlete is not attempting maneuvers before going through the proper learning sequence. **Strengthening and flexibility training** along with proper warm-up are also essential in assuring lower incidence of injury.

V. **Special Aspects of Prehabilitation and Rehabilitation:** At the competitive level it is important that the athlete be allowed to continue working on flexibility, strength, and cardiovascular conditioning as permitted. Skill training can also continue within limits with lower extremity injuries, such as allowing modified swinging skill on apparatus, even though wearing a brace or even a short leg cast. Other activities that may be permitted include swimming and cycling.

VI. **Sport-specific Facilities and Protective Equipment:** Properly maintained and safe gymnastics apparatus are important in preventing injuries. The use of tumbling pits and spotting belts where possible can decrease the incidence of injuries while the athlete is learning tumbling sequences, dismounts and vaults. Properly fitted, well-maintained hand grips are necessary in preventing injury. It is up to the gymnast and coach to recognize and correct any possible problems before they occur.

VII. **Sports-specific Taping and Bracing:** It is highly recommended that ankle taping and/ or bracing be routine for competitive gymnasts. Support at the wrist with various wraps, straps, compression sleeves, and athletic tapes is the norm for gymnasts. Every gymnast will develop his or her own method of wrist support that may be different for each event or hand grip combination. Taping the ankle to prevent extremes of dorsiflexion may help to prevent problems in landing short and anterior ankle impingement.

VIII. **Special Concerns of the Gymnastic Team Physician**

A. **Compliance:** Compliance with physician's request and orders may be a problem with some athletes, and gymnasts are no different. Coaches, parents, teammates, and the athletes themselves at times may resist orders for rest or modification of activities to allow an injury to heal. It is important that the physician discuss specific problems directly with not only the athlete but also the parents and coach to ensure that the entire story gets back to them to avoid this problem.

B. **Burnout:** Gymnasts may begin their sport career as early as 4 or 5 years of age and continue past college working out 5–6 days a week every week of the year. Even a highly successful young gymnast can develop signs of burnout and may continue in the sport only to please the coach or parents. **Injury and illness can be a way for the athlete to find a way out of the dilemma.** When this problem is suspected, it may be up to the physician to approach this problem and bring it out into the open for discussion by all concerned.

C. **Eating Disorders:** For gymnasts at any level to be successful, many have to control their body weight. If gymnasts are overweight, their sport can be much more difficult for them and may even lead to stress injuries. In an effort to control weight, both male and female gymnasts, but especially females, may develop eating disorders such as anorexia nervosa and bulimia, which can lead to serious physical and mental health problems and, if identified, should be dealt with by the physician for proper referral.

# Chapter 53: Bicycling

MORRIS B. MELLION, MD
JEFFREY W. HILL, MD

I. **Bicycling and Bicycle Racing**

A. **Introduction and general concerns.** Stimulated by four American bicycle racing gold medals in the 1984 Olympics and Greg Le Mond's victory in the 1986 and 1989 Tour de France, bicycling has experienced an explosive increase in popularity in the United States. Most notable has been the rapidly increasing interest in serious and competitive bicycling. Racing, touring, and off-road riding are among the fastest growing sports in the country. The growth of the various forms of bicycling as sports warrants increased physician understanding of how to prevent, evaluate, and manage the wide variety of traumatic and overuse injuries commonly experienced by the cyclist. **To treat bicyclists effectively, physicians need to know the basic design and function of the bicycle, the relationship of proper and improper bicycle "fit" to injuries, and the potential of the various forms of serious riding and racing for injury.**

1. **Road racing** is a term used to describe both all forms of bicycle racing on the open road and a specific event.

   a. The **time trial** is a race against the clock in which riders start at intervals of generally 1 minute.

      i. A short race, generally 9–50 miles (15–80 km)

      ii. Intense test of physical and mental strength

      iii. **Relatively trauma-free** because of distance between riders

      iv. **Variation: team time trial**–four cyclists per team riding in a pace line.

   b. The **criterium** is a fast race of many laps around a short course beginning with a mass start.

      i. Distance usually 15–65 miles (24–104 km).

      ii. **Many fast racers in a pack** making tight turns at close range.

         (a) **Many spills** occur.

         (b) **Skill and experience are paramount.**

   c. **The road race event** is a one-day race over a long stretch of open road beginning with a mass start.

      i. Distance generally > 40 miles (64 km); > 100 miles (160 km) typical for high-level riders.

      ii. **Grueling endurance event. Medical concerns include trauma, overuse, dehydration and heat illness, nutritional problems, and, hypothermia in cooler weather.**

   d. A **stage race** is a set of various road-race events on consecutive days.

      i. Generally scored both as individual stages and as a collective single race.

      ii. Two short stages may be held on a single day.

   e. **"Ultra races"** are multiday distance races that generally continue through the night.

      i. Examples: Race across American ("RAAM") and Paris-Brest-Paris Race.

      ii. **Medical concerns: extreme fatigue and sleep deprivation, fluids and nutrition, hyperthermia and hypothermia, overuse and trauma.**

2. **Track racing** includes a variety of individual and team events in which **specialized bicycles, generally without brakes** are ridden on steeply banked indoor and outdoor tracks.
   a. **Medical concerns: Trauma** related to riding at close quarters through tight turns on a relatively narrow track.
      i. There are relatively few velodromes in the United States, and several have relatively rough, poor-quality surfaces.
3. **Triathalon** is an endurance competition consisting of swimming, bicycling, and running portions in immediate succession.
   a. **Medical concerns: hyperthermia and hypothermia, dehydration and nutrition, overuse and trauma.**
4. **All-terrain bicycle (ATB) racing** involves heavier, lower-geared bicycles with wide balloon tires and upright handlebars in competition in rough or hilly terrain. These bicycles are also very popular for recreational riding in similar terrain, as well as on the open road and in urban areas. They are usually ridden without toe clips
   a. **Medical concerns: overuse on flat or uphill terrain and trauma on the downhills.**
5. **Cyclo-cross** is an off-road race in which the competitor who covers the greatest distance in laps around a 1–2 mile course of rough terrain in a set amount of time wins. The type of bicycle used varies with the course. The racer may have to carry the bicycle around or over obstacles.
   a. **Medical concerns: trauma and overuse.**
B. **Bicycle touring** is open-road riding for recreation.
   1. **Light touring:** Riding with only a handlebar bag or seat bag.
      a. May be supported by vehicles often called **"sag wagons,"** especially for multi-day trips.
   2. **Loaded touring:** Carrying large amounts of luggage in panniers (saddle bags) attached to racks mounted adjacent to the front and rear tires.
   3. **Medical concerns: overuse and trauma, thermoregulation, dehydration, and sun exposure.**

## II. The Bicycle

A. **Anatomy and terminology of the modern bicycle**
   1. Bicycle consists of a **frame** ("frameset") with various **components**, such as handlebars, brakes, and wheels, attached (Fig. 1).
      a. The frame is shaped like a diamond lying on its side (Fig. 2).
         i. Racing bicycles have more upright geometry with steeper angles to the diamond.
            (a) Stiffer frame that is more responsive in the turns.
         ii. Touring bicycles have somewhat flatter geometry.
            (a) More shock absorption with some sacrifice in cornering.
         iii. All terrain bicycles have somewhat flatter geometry.
            (a) Absorb shock of rough surface with greater sacrifice in cornering.
B. **Proper fit of the bicycle to the rider** is critical for prevention and treatment of overuse injuries in cyclists.
   1. The most efficient, accurate method to fit a bicycle for a racer or serious rider is with **a set of measuring devices known as a Fit Kit.** This service is generally provided for a fee by bicycle mechanics at shops that cater to racers.
      a. Riders using cleated shoes or step-in pedals may have their cleat adjustment checked and set using the rotational adjustment device (RAD) associated with the Fit Kit.

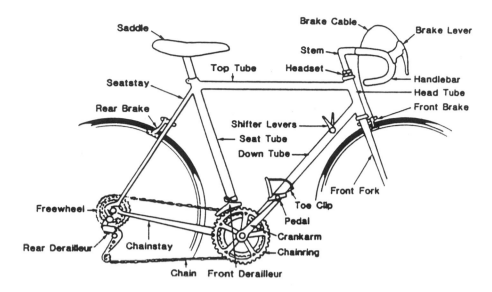

**FIGURE 1.** Anatomy and terminology of a modern bicycle. (From Hill JW, Mellion MB: Bicycling injuries: Prevention, diagnosis and treatment. In Mellion MB (ed): Office Management of Sports Injuries and Athletic Problems. Philadelphia, Hanley & Belfus, 1988, pp 257-269, with permission.)

    2. Frame size selection and the five basic fit adjustments may be made by estimates using these guidelines:
        a. **Frame size:** With the rider straddling the frame, there should be 1–2 inch clearance between the crotch and the top tube (Fig. 3).
        b. **Seat height:** several scientific and quasi-scientific methods exist:
            i. **Inseam method:** With rider wearing cycling shoes, measure inseam (floor to crotch) and multiply by 1.09 to obtain seat height (Fig. 4).

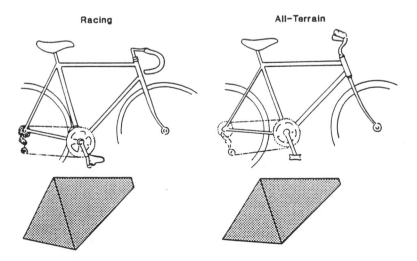

**FIGURE 2.** The bicycle frame is shaped like a diamond lying on its side. Racing bicycles have more upright geometry with steeper angles to the diamond. All terrain bicycles have somewhat flatter geometry with more shallow angles. Touring bicycles are generally in between.

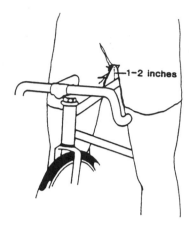

**FIGURE 3.**   Proper frame size. Allow 1–2 inches between the crotch and the top frame tube. (From Hill JW, Mellion MB: Bicycling injuries: Prevention, diagnosis and treatment. In Mellion MB (ed): Office Management of Sports Injuries and Athletic Problems. Philadelphia, Hanley & Belfus, 1988, pp 257–269, with permission.)

    ii. **Bone length method:** With the rider standing upright, back flat against a wall and legs spread 6 inches, measure upper leg length from greater trochanter to lateral femoral condyle and lower leg length from lateral femoral condyle to tip of lateral malleolus. Seat height equals the sum of upper and lower leg length multiplied by 0.96 (Fig. 5).

    iii. **Estimation from leg length:** With the bicycle positioned next to a wall or vehicle for support, the rider sits with the pedals in the 6 and 12 o'clock positions with the heels on the pedals. The seat should be raised or lowered until the leg on the 6 o'clock pedal is barely straight (Fig. 6).

    iv. **"Rocking in the saddle" method:** Raise the seat to the point at which the rider must rock from side to side in order to pedal; then lower it until the rocking disappears.

       (a) Roughest estimate, although many coaches swear by it.

       (b) Not as reliable in less experienced cyclists who may pedal in toe-down position.

    v. **All seat height formulas are estimates.** Adjustments of ¼ inch at a time, usually upward, may be made after a trial of several rides.

  c. **Fore and aft saddle position:** The bicycle saddle is built on a pair of rails that are connected to the seatpost and allow approximately 1½ inch adjustment range. With the rider in the saddle and the pedals at the 3 and 9 o'clock positions, the seat should be adjusted so that a plumb line dropped from the tibial tubercle would intercept the axle of the forward pedal (Fig. 7).

  d. **Saddle angle:** A carpenter's level placed along the longitudinal axis of the saddle should indicate that the saddle is level or slightly angled with the front end up.

  e. **Reach:** Handlebar reach is the distance from the saddle to the transverse part of the handlebars. A rough estimate of proper reach may be obtained by placing the elbow at the front of the seat with the fingers fully extended (Fig. 8).

    i. More accurate determinations of reach may be made using trunk measurements with the Fit Kit, or according to formulas in the bicycle literature.

    ii. The reach is adjusted by replacing the stem, with one having more or less extension (Fig. 9).

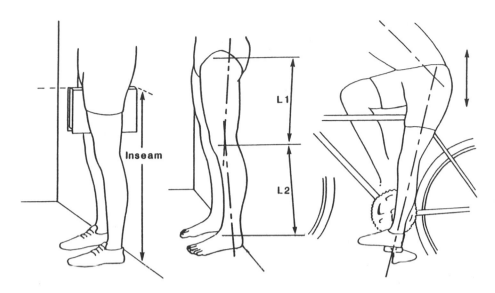

FIGURE 4 *(left)*.  Seat height by inseam method. With rider wearing cycling shoes measure inseam (floor to crotch) and multiply by 1.09 to obtain seat height.

FIGURE 5 *(center)*.  Seat height by bone length method. With the rider standing upright, back flat against a wall and legs spread 6 inches, measure upper leg length from greater trochanter to lateral femoral condyle and lower leg length from lateral femoral condyle to tip of lateral malleolus. Seat height equals the sum of upper and lower leg length multiplied by 0.96.

FIGURE 6 *(right)*.  Seat height estimation from leg length. With the bicycle positioned next to a wall or vehicle for support, the rider sits with the pedals in the 6 and 12 o'clock positions with the heels on the pedals. The seat should be raised or lowered until the leg on the 6 o'clock pedal is barely straight.

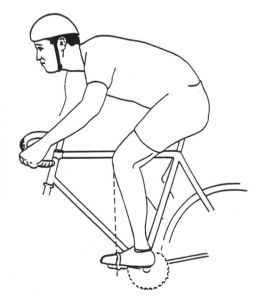

FIGURE 7.  Fore and aft saddle position. The bicycle saddle is built on a pair of rails which are connected to the seatpost and allow approximately 1½" adjustment range. With the rider in the saddle and the pedals at the 3 and 9 o'clock positions, the seat should be adjusted so that a plumb line dropped from the tibial tubercle would intercept the axle of the forward pedal.

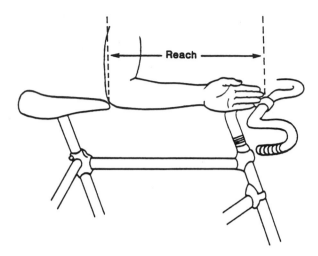

**FIGURE 8.** Handlebar reach is the distance from the saddle to the transverse part of the handlebars. A rough estimate of proper reach may be obtained by placing the elbow at the front of the seat with the fingers fully extended.

   f. **Handlebar height:** The handlebar height should always be at or lower than seat height.
    i. For racing, it should always be lower than seat height.
     (a) How low depends on individual characteristics of the rider and specific type of race.
  C. **Pedalling and gearing.** Riding with too much pedal resistance at too low a cadence (pedal revolutions per minute) is second only to improper bicycle fit as a cause of overuse problems in cyclists.
   1. **General principles.** The human body functions most effectively and safely in a narrow range of pedal resistance to effort.
    a. **Sources of resistance to bicycle movement:**
     i. **Inertia of bicycle and rider**

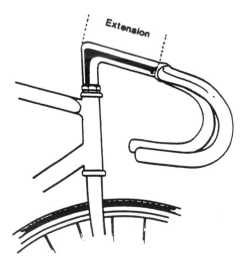

**FIGURE 9.** Extension is the horizontal length of the handlebar stem. The reach is adjusted by replacing the stem with one having more or less extension. (From Hill JW, Mellion MB: Bicycling injuries: Prevention, diagnosis and treatment. In Mellion MB (ed): Office Management of Sports Injuries and Athletic Problems. Philadelphia, Hanley & Belfus, 1988, pp 257–269, with permission.)

ii. **Uphill grade** (gravity)

iii. **Wind**

iv. **Friction of air.** Approximately 90% of the energy expended riding 20 mph on a calm day is used to overcome the friction of the bicycle and the rider against the still air.

v. **Rolling resistance** of tires on road surface

vi. **Fatigue.** Strength, force, and efficiency are all reduced in fatigued muscles.

b. **Gearing:** A method of overcoming resistance that allows the cyclist to pedal comfortably with a relatively constant pedal resistance at a generally constant pedal resistance at a generally uniform cadence by shifting through a range of 10–21 "speeds" or gears (Fig. 10).

i. **Chainwheels** are the relatively large front gears attached to the "crank," or axle, around which the rider pedals.

(a) **Large chainwheel** and **small chainwheel** used on virtually all road bicycles and ATBs.

(b) **"Granny":** A very small chainwheel used for hill climbing on touring bikes and ATBs.

iii. The **freewheel** is a cluster of 5–8 gears ("cogs") mounted to the right of the rear wheel on the same axle.

iii. A **chain** composed of evenly spaced links connects one of the chainwheels to one of the freewheel cogs to drive the rear wheel of the bicycle. Since the gear teeth must be evenly spaced and uniform size in order to mesh with the links of the chain, the size of the gears may be expressed by the number of teeth they have.

(a) The front derailleur shifts the chain from one chainwheel to another.

(b) The rear derailleur shifts the chain from one cog of the freewheel to another.

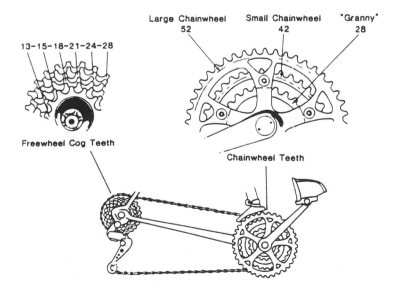

**FIGURE 10.** Modern bicycle gearing. This example is from a touring bicycle with 3 chainwheels on the crank and 6 cogs on the freewheel. (From Hill JW, Mellion MB: Bicycling injuries: Prevention, diagnosis and treatment. In Mellion MB (ed): Office Management of Sports Injuries and Athletic Problems. Philadelphia, Hanley & Belfus, 1988, pp 257–269, with permission.)

  iv. **Gear ratio** is the ratio of the size of the chainwheel in use to that of the freewheel cog in use:

$$\text{Gear Ratio} = \frac{\text{\# of teeth on chainwheel}}{\text{\# of teeth on freewheel cog}}$$

    (a) Higher gear ratios result in higher pedal resistance in given riding conditions.

     (i) Riding safely with higher gear ratios requires strength, endurance, and better technique.

    (b) Lower gear ratios result in lower pedal resistance and may permit pedalling, or "spinning," at a higher cadence.

  v. Generally, racers and other serious bicyclists in the United States multiply the gear ratio by the diameter of the rear wheel to obtain a ratio known as **gear number** or **gear inches:**

    (a) **Gear number** (gear inches) = Gear ratio × rear wheel diameter, expressed in inches

    (b) Table 1A indicates the ranges of gear ratios generally available on road and all terrain bicycles, and Table 1B describes the uses of these gear ratios.

 2. **Optimal cadence** (= pedal revolutions per minute) varies with the type of riding and the skill, strength, and endurance of the athlete.

  a. **May be expressed in terms of several variables:**

   i. **Gross efficiency** (= work performed/energy cost):

    (a) 60–80 rpm optimal

    (b) Falls off sharply > 100 rpm.

   ii. **Heart rate**

    (a) 80 rpm optimal peak

    (b) 60–100 rpm optimal range.

**TABLE 1.** Ranges of Gear Ratios (A) and Uses of Gear Ratios (B)

A.

| Examples | Gear Ratio $= \dfrac{\text{\# of teeth on chainwheel}}{\text{\# of teeth on freewheel cog}}$ | Gear Inches = gear ratio × wheel dia. |
|---|---|---|
| Very high gear | $\dfrac{52}{13} = 4$ | 4 × 27 = 108 |
| Lower gear | $\dfrac{52}{26} = 2$ | 2 × 27 = 54 |
| Very low gear | $\dfrac{28}{28} = 1$ | 1 × 27 = 27 |

B.

| Gear Inches | Use |
|---|---|
| 27–35 (or lower) | Very low gears. Used for climbing steep hills. Also used for touring hilly terrain with a heavily loaded bicycle. |
| 36–44 | Low gears. Used for climbing hills or riding into a severe headwind. |
| 45–60 | Slightly low gears. Used for gentle hills or mild headwind. |
| 61–85 | Standard gears. Used for riding on level ground. Effort may be maintained for a long time. |
| 86–108 | High gears. Used for high speed riding. Used when riding downhill or riding with a tailwind. |
| > 108 | Special gearing, not available on most bicycles. Used by competitive racers. |

   iii. **Perceived exertion**
    (a) 80 rpm optimal peak
    (b) 60–100 rpm optimal range.
   iv. **Lactate concentration**
    (a) 80 rpm optimal peak
    (b) 60–100+ rpm optimal range
    (c) At 110–120 rpm lactate rises steeply.
   v. **Generation of power for effective racing**
    (a) 90–110 rpm optimal range
    (b) Short bursts at higher rpm.
  b. **Racers must often sacrifice efficiency for speed.**
  c. **Relatively high cadence/low resistance pedalling reduces the incidence of overuse injuries.**
   i. **Racers and serious cyclists should begin their seasons with 500–1000 miles of this kind of riding.**

III. **Bicycle Injuries**

 A. **General injury data**
  1. $>$ 500,000 bicycle injury visits/year to U.S. emergency rooms.
  2. **Approximately half of hospital admissions from cycling accidents involved motor vehicles.**
   a. **Most often, the vehicle driver fails to see the bicyclist.**
    i. Especially in low-light dawn and dusk hours and at night.
  3. **Road surface damage and obstacles often involved:**
   a. Road cracks and potholes
   b. Damaged shoulders
   c. Trash on road
   d. Gravel on surface (often left from previous winter's snow control)
   e. Railroad crossings
   f. Sewer openings and rain drainage grates
   g. Cattle guards
   h. Curbs.

 B. **Traumatic injuries**
  1. **Head injuries**
   a. Account for most of deaths
   b. Generally preventable
   c. Victims rarely wearing helmets.
  2. **Face injuries**
   a. Most often abrasions and contusions
   b. Good helmet offers partial protection.
  3. **Musculoskeletal injuries**
   a. Contusions, sprains, and fractures
   b. Common sites:
    i. Hand
    ii. Wrist and lower arm
    iii. Shoulder
    iv. Ankle and lower leg.
  4. **Abominal and genital injuries**
   a. From handlebar trauma when stopping short.
  5. **Skin injuries**
   a. Lacerations
   b. Abrasions: **"road rash"**

        i. Grading system similar to burns
           (a) 1st degree: superficial
           (b) 2nd degree: partial thickness
           (c) 3rd degree: full thickness.
        ii. Treatment:
           (a) 1st, 2nd, and small 3rd degree
              (i) DuoDerm hydroactive dressings
              (ii) Silvadene cream, t.i.d.
           (b) Larger 3rd degree
              (i) Silvadene cream, t.i.d.
              (ii) Wet-to-dry soaks.
           (c) Tetanus prophylaxis.

6. **Spoke injuries**
    a. Loose spokes must be tightened or removed.
    b. If a spoke must be removed, loosen the two adjacent spokes. Ride slowly home or to assistance until the wheel is either replaced or fixed.
    c. Spoke injuries often caused by getting a finger, foot, or piece of clothing caught in the wheel while riding.
        i. Almost always avoidable.

C. **Strategies to prevent trauma**
  1. **Use proper protective clothing and safety equipment** (see IV. below).
  2. **Maintain bicycle in top mechanical condition.**
    a. **Check brakes frequently.**
        i. Ensure that there is no lubricant on the brake pad surface or on the adjacent braking surface of the wheel.
           (a) May clean wheel braking surface with acetone if necessary.
    b. **Check tires and tubes frequently;** repair or replace if even slightly damaged.
    c. **Perform a preride check routinely.**
        i. Check quick-release levers on wheels whenever getting on bicycle.
  3. **Anticipate the errors of others.**
    a. Assume that the other riders or vehicle drivers do not see you.
    b. Watch the eyes of motor vehicle drivers.
  4. **Riding strategies**
    a. Control speed.
        i. Reduce speed when brakes are wet.
    b. Anticipate obstacles and road damage.
    c. Practice with extra clothing in a protected area.
        i. Diverting around obstacles
        ii. Jumping over obstacles
        iii. Braking technique
        iv. Forced turns and tight downhill turns.

D. **Overuse injuries**
  1. **Neck and backache**
    a. Common problem; up to 60% of riders.
    b. Upper left trapezius and levator scapula muscles also common sites.
        i. Due to muscle tension from watching for overtaking traffic, either by turning head or by looking through helmet mirror.
    c. Mechanism of injury
        i. Increased load on arms and shoulders to support rider.
        ii. Increased handlebar "reach" causing hyperextension of neck and exaggerated flexion of low back.
           (a) Accentuated by drop handlebars.

    d. Management
      i. Mechanical
        (a) Raise handlebars.
        (b) Use stem with shorter extension.
        (c) Move seat forward.
        (d) Use handlebars with less drop.
        (e) Ride with "unlocked" elbows.
        (f) Change hand position frequently.
        (g) Change mirror placement.
        (h) Switch to upright handlebar.
      ii. Medical
        (a) Strength and flexibility exercises
          (i) Neck, back, and shoulders
        (b) Ice massage
        (c) Nonsteroidal anti-inflammatory drug
        (d) Skeletal muscle relaxants
          (i) Not benzodiazepines.
    e. Evaluate treatment failures for:
      i. Degenerative disc disease
        (a) Radiculopathy
      ii. Degenerative arthritis.
 2. **Handlebar problems**
    a. **Ulnar neuropathy** ("cyclist's palsy"; "handlebar palsy")
      i. Gradual onset of numbness, tingling, and/or weakness in the ring and little fingers
        (a) Generally occurs after several days of long or intensive rides.
      ii. Duration: several days to months.
      iii. Etiology
        (a) Ulnar nerve compression at the wrist
          (i) In or near Guyon's canal
        (b) Hyperextension of wrists causing nerve traction.
      iv. Management
        (a) Mechanical
          (i) Wear padded gloves.
          (ii) Add handle bar padding.
          (iii) Decrease length, intensity of rides.
          (iv) Change hand position frequently.
          (v) Avoid hand positions with marked wrist hyperextension.
        (b) Medical
          (i) Generally resolves spontaneously
          (ii) Rarely, surgical decompression.
    b. **Carpal tunnel syndrome**
      i. Rarely result of handle bar trauma alone
      ii. Management similar to ulnar neuropathy.
 3. **Saddle problems**
    a. Ischial tuberosity soreness
      i. Tenderness associated with infrequent riding
        (a) Occurs at beginning of riding season.
      ii. Generally self-limited.
    b. **Skin problems**
      i. Chafing
        (a) Management

        (i) Mechanical
- Padded riding shorts
- Adjust seat position and height.
- Saddle pad
- Change saddle to different shape or padded saddle.

       (ii) Medical
- Talcum powder: effective only for short rides.
- Lubricating ointments, e.g., Cramer's Skin Lube or Mueller's lubricant.
- Anusol or Anusol HC creams
- Nonfluorinated corticosteroid creams
- Shave perineum prophylactically to prevent irritation caused by traction on hairs.

ii. Furuncles, folliculitis
  (a) Management
    (i) Warm soaks
    (ii) Incision and drainage
    (iii) Antibiotics
- May involve coliforms in this area.

c. **Pudendal neuropathy**
  i. Numbness, tingling in scrotum, penile shaft.
  ii. Etiology: compression of dorsal branch of pudendal nerve between bike seat and pubic symphysis.
  iii. Management
    (a) Mechanical
      (i) Adjust saddle angle to horizontal or only slightly upward in the front.
      (ii) Change saddle width.
      (iii) Wear padded cycling shorts.
      (iv) Add saddle padding.

d. **Traumatic urethritis**
  i. Varies from silent hematuria to marked dysuria with hematuria and pyuria.
    (a) Predisposes outflow tract to obstruction and infection.
  ii. Easily mistaken for benign prostatic hypertrophy.
  iii. Management
    (a) Similar to pudendal neuropathy.

e. **Vulva trauma**
  i. Superficial abrasions
  ii. Lacerations
  iii. Contusions
  iv. Hematomas
  v. Management:
    (a) Similar to pudendal neuropathy.

f. **Torsion of testes**
  i. Described in association with bicycling
  ii. No definite cause and effect relationship

g. **Male impotence**
  i. Inability to attain an erection documented in cyclists after repeated or multi-day rides.
  ii. Incidence low.
  iii. Treatment:
    (a) Stop riding until symptoms resolve.

(b) Bicycle adjustments
(i) Fit kit recommended
(ii) Padded shorts and seat.

4. **Hip problems**
   a. Trochanteric bursitis
      i. Mechanisms
         (a) Repetitive sliding of fascia lata over greater trochanter.
         (b) Generally occurs when rocking from side to side while pedalling because seat is too high.
      ii. Management
         (a) Mechanical
            (i) Lower seat height
            (ii) Change frame size if too large to adjust.
         (b) Medical
            (i) Iliotibial band stretching
            (ii) Ice massage
            (iii) Nonsteroidal anti-inflammatory drugs
            (iv) Occasional local steroid injection into bursa.
   b. **Iliopsoas tendinitis**
      i. Pain in medial, proximal aspect of thigh
      ii. Management
         (a) Mechanical
            (i) Same as trochanteric bursitis
         (b) Medical
            (i) Stretching
            (ii) Ice massage
            (iii) Rest
            (iv) Nonsteroidal anti-inflammatory drugs.

5. **"Biker's knee"** = extensor mechanism malalignment syndrome = patellofemoral pain syndrome.
   a. Tracking problem of the kneecap in the intercondylar groove of the femur
   b. Mechanism of injury
      i. Commonly, seat is too low or too far forward.
      ii. Improper foot position; kneecap should be pointing straight forward when riding.
         (a) May be due to improper cleat adjustment.
      iii. Hyperpronating feet with rear foot valgus.
      iv. Riding at relatively low cadence with high pedal resistance.
   c. Management
      i. Mechanical
         (a) Modify bicycle position.
            (i) Raise seat height.
               • Increments as small as 5–6 mm may make a difference.
               • Move seat back.
         (b) Adjust cleat alignment in racing shoes (consider RAD, par. II.B. above)
            (i) Consider newer cleats that allow several degrees of rotatory motion.
         (c) Correct for hyperpronating feet.
            (i) Orthotics placed in shoes.
            (ii) 1/8–3/16 inch medial wedge glued to sole of shoe.
            (iii) Special pedals.

(d) Modify technique.
  (i) Ride at high RPM with low resistance.
    • May necessitate changing freewheel.
  (ii) Decrease intensity and duration of training rides.

6. **Foot and ankle problems**
  a. **Paresthesias**
    i. Common when riding long distance; self-limited
    ii. Etiology
      (a) Tight shoe straps and clips
      (b) Increased pedal pressure.
    iii. Management
      (a) Mechanical
        (i) Loosen toe straps; proper toe clip size.
        (ii) Ride at higher cadence with lower pedal resistance.
        (iii) Switch to newer "step-in" shoe-pedal combination.
  b. **Metatarsalgia**
    i. Etiology
      (a) Poor foot position
      (b) Improperly placed shoe cleats
      (c) Poor gearing and cadence.
    ii. Management
      (a) Mechanical
        (i) Adjust toe clip size
        (ii) Proper cleat adjustment
        (iii) Metatarsal pad
        (iv) Ride at higher cadence with lower pedal resistance.
  c. **Achilles tendinitis**
    i. Etiology: low saddle height causes pronounced ankle dorsiflexion during pedal rotation.
    ii. Management
      (a) Mechanical
        (i) Raise seat height.
        (ii) Adjust pedalling technique.
      (b) Medical
        (i) Heel cord stretching
        (ii) Ice massage
        (iii) NSAID therapy
        (iv) **Avoid local corticosteroid injections.**
  d. **Plantar fasciitis**
    i. Pain in sole at origin of plantar fascia on anterior calcaneus
    ii. Management
      (a) Mechanical: same as Achilles tendinitis.
      (b) Medical
        (i) Head cord stretching
        (ii) Ice massage
        (iii) NSAID therapy
        (iv) Iontophoresis
        (v) Corticosteroid injection

7. Other common problems
  a. **Dehydration**
    i. Rapid sweat evaporation causes rider to underestimate fluid needs.
    ii. Thirst inadequate guide.

iii. Management/prevention
    (a) Conscious hydration several days prior to event should be undertaken.
    (b) Keep two bottles of fluid on bicycle.
        (i) Note well: **Standard bicycle water bottles hold only 20 oz, and large bicycle bottles hold 27 oz.**
    (c) Adequate hydration if passing clear urine every 1–2 hours.

b. **Sunburn**
    i. Common problem relating to exposure time
    ii. Common areas
        (a) Arms
        (b) Thighs
        (c) Lips.
    iii. Prudent use of sunscreen advised.
        (a) Caveat: May cause some impairment of evaporation.

## IV. Safety Equipment and Protective Clothing

A. **The bicycle helmet is generally very effective in preventing serious head injuries because of the relatively low speed at impact in bicycle compared with motorcycle injuries.**
    1. **Required**
        a. All U.S. Cycling Federation sanctioned events
        b. All Triathalon Federation USA competitions
        c. Most local club and charity races and rides.
    2. **Mechanism of action: High-density, expanded polystyrene (EPS) or polyurethane foam crushes to absorb the shock of a severe impact. More resilient materials may produce a recoil that may add to the trauma.**
    3. **Three types**
        a. **"Hard shell" helmet** consists of a hard shell that spreads the shock over a wider area and a crushable foam liner to absorb the shock.
            i. Advantage: proven safety record in actual use.
            ii. Disadvantage: slightly bulkier and heavier.
        b. **"No shell" helmet** generally consists only of a single, molded, EPS layer with a Lycra cover.
            i. Advantages: light and attractive
            ii. Disadvantages: tested in laboratory but limited experience in actual crashes. Some experts fear that the EPS layer may crack on impact.
        c. **"Mini shell" helmet** is similar to "no shell" helmet, but it has a thin, smooth, hard outer shell layer.
            i. Advantages:
                (a) Light and attractive
                (b) Smooth hard surface glides on pavement causing a more glancing impact and, consequently, less head trauma.
            ii. Disadvantage: very little actual experience yet.
    4. **Standards**
        a. **American National Standards Institute (ANSI) Z90.4 standard**
            i. Minimum required for racing.
        b. **Snell Memorial Foundation standard**
            i. More stringent
                (a) Higher test impact
                (b) Will probably become even more stringent in the near future

5. Other important features:
   a. Good retention system (straps and buckle).
   b. Aerodynamically designed to reduce drag.
   c. Airflow entrained to avoid thermal stress.
B. **Mirrors** allow cyclist to observe overtaking vehicles without turning head.
   1. Various models mount on:
      a. Helmet
      b. Eyeglasses (sunglasses)
      c. Handlebars.
C. **Protective eyewear**
   1. Protects rider from:
      a. Radiation of sun
      b. Flying objects such as bugs, dust, stones
      c. Irritants such as wind, rain, cold air, and allergens.
   2. Wraparound or semi-wraparound preferred
      a. Goggles for extreme conditions.
   3. Polycarbonate or other unbreakable material.
D. **Cycling gloves**
   1. Functions
      a. Cushion hands from road shock.
      b. Provide good handlebar grip.
      c. Prevent blisters.
      d. Protect hands in a fall.
      e. Some have terry backing to wipe sweat from face.
      f. Winter gloves protect from cold injury.
   2. Palms are padded with shock-absorbent elastopolymer or neoprene.
   3. Summer gloves: fingerless, leather palms, mesh or lightweight fabric backing.
   4. Winter gloves: full fingers and insulation.
E. **Handlebar tape and padding**
   1. Most racers use colorful, lightweight tape to enhance handlebar grip.
   2. Padded handlebar tape and slip-on foam rubber pads may be used for greater shock absorption.
F. **Saddle pads and padded saddles** may provide extra shock absorption.
   1. Saddle pads
      a. Elastopolymer in closed-cell neoprene cover
      b. May reduce pedalling power slightly.
   2. Padded saddles
      a. Elastopolymer or other high-tech material incorporated into the saddle itself.
G. **Reflectors**
   1. **Bicycle reflectors**
      a. Generally removed by racers to reduce drag.
      b. Wheel-mounted reflectors should be removed for riding at high speed or in windy conditions because they may cause the bicycle to vibrate and become unsteady.
      c. Important for night and urban riding.
   2. **Reflective tape**
      a. Most important on back of shoes
      b. On helmet
      c. On wheels.
   3. Reflective clothing.

H. **Lights**
1. Halogen headlights
2. Flashing light or strobe behind rider.
I. **Protective Clothing**
1. **Bright tight cycling clothing**
a. **"Advertises" presence of cyclist to other riders and motor vehicle drivers.**
b. Special materials keep cyclists cool in hot weather and warm in cold windy weather.
c. Reduces drag.
2. **Cycling shorts** protect inner thighs, groin, and buttocks from chafing and pressure trauma.
a. Seamless crotch pad
i. Traditionally, natural chamois, that requires lubricating with lanolin.
ii. Newer synthetic padding only needs washing.
J. **Bicycle shoes**
1. **Stiff midsole distributes pedalling forces over entire foot.**
a. **Helps prevent foot and ankle overuse syndromes.**
2. **Racing shoes connect to pedals with slotted cleats and toe clips or with step-in cleats.**
a. Designed to transmit force to the pedal throughout the full revolution.
b. Roomy toe box necessary to prevent toe trauma.
c. Tight lacing or firm Velcro fastener high up on arch to anchor foot in proper position and prevent toe trauma.
d. **Cleat adjustment critical for smooth pedalling and overuse prevention.**
i. **Rotational adjustment device (RAD) is most accurate adjustment system (see par. II.B.1.a. above)**
e. Racers with biomechanical foot problems may require:
i. Orthotics in shoes
ii. Canted shims between shoe and cleat
iii. Adjustable pedals (Biopedal).
3. **Touring shoes** resemble court shoes with roomy toe box still small enough to fit in toe clips.
a. More freedom of movement than racing shoes.
i. Less overuse problems
ii. Less force transmitted to pedals.

V. **Rules to Protect the Cyclist**

A. Helmet requirements
B. Gearing limitations by age of racer (U.S. Cycling Federation)
C. Pre-race equipment checks by officials
D. Requirement for water and aid stations at races
E. Riding conduct rules

## RECOMMENDED READING

1. Bicycling Magazine: Overcoming cycling ailments. Emmaus, PA, Rodale Press, 1984.
2. Burke ER: Safety standards for bicycle helmets. Phys Sportsmed 16(1):148–153, 1985.
3. Burke ER (ed): Science of Cycling. Champaign, IL, Human Kinetics Publishers, 1986.
4. Burke ER, Newsom MM (eds): Medical and Scientific Aspects of Cycling. Champaign, IL, Human Kinetics Books, 1988.
5. Dickson TB: Preventing overuse cycling injuries. Phys Sportsmed 13(10):116–123, 1985.
6. Grisolfi CV, Rohlf DP, Navarude SN, et al: Effects of wearing a helmet on thermal balance while cycling in the heat. Phys Sportsmed 16(1):139–146, 1988.

7. Hill JW, Mellion MB. Bicycling injuries: Prevention, diagnosis and treatment. In Mellion MB (ed): Office Management of Sports Injuries and Athletic Problems. Philadelphia, Hanley & Belfus, 1988, pp 257–269.
8. Mayer RJ: Helping your patients avoid bicycling injuries. I. What injuries to anticipate this summer. J Musculoskel Med 2:31–40, 1985.
9. Mayer RJ: Helping your patients avoid bicycling injuries. II. How to choose, adjust, and use a bicycle properly. J Musculoskel Med 2:31–38, 1985.
10. Powell B: Correction and prevention of bicycle saddle problems. Phys Sportsmed 10(10):60–67, 1982.
11. Van der Plas R: The Bicycle Racing Guide. San Francisco, Bicycle Books, 1986.

# Chapter 54: Golf

## MARK AMUNDSON, MS, PT, ATC

I. **Golf and Special Sports Medicine Concerns**

The history of golf is hard to pinpoint. A variety of stick and ball games were played in Northern Europe as early as the 12th Century. Golf, as we know it, made rapid developments in Scotland during the 19th Century, and championship golf was inaugurated in 1860. The National Sporting Goods Association estimates that 18.5 million Americans golf at least twice a year. Because of the vast number of golfers in the U.S. and other countries, injuries are inevitable, and the primary care physician will need skills in the care of these injuries.

II. **Overuse and Traumatic Injuries Related to the Golf Swing**

A. **Lumbar strain/sprain**
   1. Definition
      a. An injury, either acute or chronic, involving the muscles and/or ligaments of the low back region.
   2. Evaluation
      a. History of violent muscular contraction against resistance.
      b. History of overstretching.
      c. History of overuse or repeated positioning.
      d. Pain upon palpation of the lumbar musculature.
      e. Pain with movement of the lumbar spine.
      f. Pain with resistance to movement of the lumbar spine.
      g. Pain with prolonged sitting or standing.
      h. Pain in the buttocks and hip region.
      i. Lack of neurologic signs or symptoms.
      j. Loss of function.
      k. History of stress and tension.
   3. Mechanisms
      a. Low back strain/sprain during the takeaway phase of the swing results from the hyperrotation of the lumbar spine.
      b. Low back strain/sprain during the impact phase of the swing results from the uncoiling of the lumbar spine and from the jarring force of contact with the ground.
      c. Low back strain/sprain during the follow-through phase of the swing results from the hyperextension and rotation of the lumbar spine (reverse "C" position).
   4. Frequency
      a. In a study of professional golfers, injuries to the low back accounted for 23.7% of the total.[7]
   5. Treatment
      a. Flexibility exercises for the low back, hip, and hamstring muscles.
      b. Strengthening exercises for the low back, abdominal, and hip muscles.
      c. Physical therapy procedures
      d. Proper posture and lifting techniques.

6. Prevention
  a. Proper swing mechanics are essential.
  b. Proper conditioning (see sec. V, "Conditioning").
  c. Education in proper posture and daily living techniques for the low back.
  d. Lumbar support during activity.

B. **Impingement syndrome of shoulder**
  1. Definition
    a. An overuse injury resulting in the impingement (squeezing) of the soft tissue structures of the shoulder between the coracoacromial arch and the greater tuberosity of the humerus.
  2. Evaluation
    a. History of repeated use of the arm for internal and external rotation activities.
    b. History of repeated use of the arm for overhead activities.
    c. Pain with abduction of arm, especially from 80–130° of motion (**painful arc syndrome**).
    d. Pain with resisted movement of internal or external rotation.
    e. Pain when lying on involved arm.
    f. Pain when sleeping and difficult to get into comfortable position.
    g. Tenderness over anterior/lateral aspect of the shoulder, just distal to the tip of the acromion.
  3. Mechanisms
    a. **Right shoulder impingement** results from abduction of the shoulder during the take-away phase of the swing.
    b. **Left shoulder impingement** results from hyperabduction of the shoulder during the follow-through phase of the swing.
  4. Frequency
    a. In a study of professional golfers, left shoulder injuries accounted for 6.9% and right shoulder injuries 2.5% of the total.[7]
  5. Treatment
    a. Flexibility exercises for the rotator cuff, latissimus dorsi, and pectoral muscles.
    b. Strengthening exercises for the rotator cuff, latissimus dorsi and pectoral muscles.
    c. Physical therapy procedures
    d. Decompression surgery.
  6. Prevention
    a. Proper swing mechanics
    b. Proper conditioning (see sec. V, "Conditioning").

C. **Medial epicondylitis (golfer's elbow)**
  1. Definition
    a. An overuse injury of the medial aspect of the elbow involving the epicondyle of the humerus, the wrist and finger flexor muscles, and the pronator muscles.
  2. Evaluation
    a. History of sudden overload to contractile units of the medial elbow.
    b. Tenderness over medial epicondyle of humerus.
    c. Pain with flexion of wrist or fingers.
    d. Pain with resistance to flexion of wrist or fingers.
    e. Loss of function or palpable gap in muscle.
    f. History of chronic use of wrist flexors or pronators.
  3. Mechanisms
    a. Right medial epicondylitis in right-handed golfer due to extension of the right elbow during the impact phase of the swing while the right wrist remains dorsiflexed.

  b. Left medial epicondylitis in right-handed golfer due to supination of the left forearm during the follow-through phase of the swing.

 4. Frequency

  a. In a study of injuries to professional golfers, elbow injuries accounted for 6.6% of the total.[7]

 5. Treatment

  a. Flexibility exercises for wrist and finger flexor muscles and pronator muscles.

  b. Strengthening exercises for wrist and finger flexor muscles and pronator muscles.

  c. Physical therapy procedures.

 6. Prevention

  a. Proper swing mechanics

  b. Proper conditioning (see sec. V, "Conditioning")

  c. Wear a "tennis elbow" band around proximal forearm.

D. **Lateral epicondylitis**

 1. Definition

  a. An overuse injury involving the lateral epicondyle of the humerus, the wrist and finger extensor muscles, and the supinator muscles.

 2. Evaluation

  a. History of sudden overload to the wrist or finger extensors or the supinators.

  b. Tenderness over the lateral epicondyle of the humerus.

  c. Pain with use of the wrist or finger extensors, or supinators.

  d. Pain with resistance to the finger or wrist extensors or the supinator muscles.

  e. Loss of function of wrist or finger extension or palpable gap in the muscle.

  f. History of chronic overuse of the wrist or finger extensors or supinators.

 3. Mechanisms

  a. **Left lateral epicondylitis** in right-handed golfer due to forceful contraction of the left elbow extensors during the impact phase of the swing.

  b. **Right lateral epicondylitis** in right-handed golfer due to pronation of forearm during the follow-through phase of the swing.

 4. Frequency

  a. In a study of professional golfers, elbow injuries accounted for 6.6% of the total.[7]

 5. Treatment

  a. Flexibility exercises for the wrist and finger extensors and supinator muscles.

  b. Strengthening exercises for the wrist and finger extensors and supinator muscles.

  c. Physical therapy procedures.

 6. Prevention

  a. Proper swing mechanics

  b. Proper conditioning (see sec. V, "Conditioning").

  c. Wear a "tennis elbow" band around proximal forearm.

E. **Wrist tendinitis**

 1. Definition

  a. An overuse injury resulting in inflammation and irritation of the tendons of the wrist flexors and extensors, and the tendons of the finger flexors and extensors.

 2. Evaluation

  a. History of violent contraction against resistance.

  b. History of overstretching or chronic overuse.

  c. Pain with wrist motion.

  d. Pain with movement against resistance.

  e. Palpable or audible click in the wrist.

  f. Tenderness in the wrist.

  g. Loss of function.

 3. Mechanisms

  a. **Left wrist tendinitis** in right-handed golfer due to repeated radial deviation of the wrist during the take-away phase of the swing.

  b. **Right wrist tendinitis** in right-handed golfer due to repeated dorsiflexion of the wrist during the take-away phase of the swing.

  c. **Left wrist tendinitis** in the right-handed golfer due to forceful contact with the ball and ground during the impact phase of the swing.

 4. Frequency

  a. In a study of professional golfers, right wrist injuries accounted for 3.1% and left wrist injuries 23.9% of the total (all types of wrist injuries together).[7]

 5. Treatment

  a. Physical therapy procedures.

 6. Prevention

  a. Proper swing mechanics

  b. Tape or wrap wrist or wear wrist brace.

F. **Carpal fractures**

 1. Definition

  a. Any fracture of one or more carpal bones due to the golf swing.

 2. Evaluation

  a. History of direct blow or fall on wrist or hand.

  b. History of forceful hyperextension of wrist.

  c. Acute pain in the wrist.

  d. Pain with palpation of involved area.

  e. Pain with movement of wrist.

  f. Swelling in the wrist area.

  g. Positive roentgenogram.

 3. Mechanism

  a. **Hamate fracture** of the left wrist in a right-handed golfer due to the force of the wrist and hand being thrust into the ball during the impact phase of the swing.

  b. **Scaphoid (navicular) fracture** of the right wrist in a right-handed golfer due to the compressive force of hitting the ground during the impact phase of the swing.

 4. Frequency

  a. No specific frequency was noted for carpal fractures.

 5. Treatment

  a. Cast for 4–6 weeks; if a navicular fracture, casting may possibly take 6 months. May also require surgical intervention.

  b. Post-cast

   i. Restoration of normal range of motion

   ii. Strengthening exercises for all muscles of the forearm.

   iii. Physical therapy procedures.

 6. Prevention

  a. Proper swing mechanics.

G. **Degenerative arthritis of the MCP joint of the thumb**

 1. Definition

  a. A degenerative process occurring at the MCP joint of the thumb due to repetitive stress from the golf swing.

 2. Evaluation

  a. History of jamming injury to thumb.

  b. History of repeated stress to MCP joint.

  c. Pain with use of thumb.
  d. Pain with pressure of MCP joint.
  e. Swelling of MCP joint.
  f. Loss of function and stiffness of MCP joint.
  g. Crepitation with passive motion.
3. Mechanisms
  a. **Left MCP degenerative arthritis** in right-handed golfer due to repeated hyperabduction of the thumb during the take-away phase of the swing.
4. Frequency
  a. In a study of professional golfers, injuries to the left thumb (right-handed golfers) accounted for 3.3% of the total.[7]
5. Treatment
  a. Physical therapy procedures
  b. Arthroscopic debridement of joint.
6. Prevention
  a. Proper swing mechanics
  b. Proper sized grips
  c. Range of motion exercises for joint
  d. Splint or taping for support.

## III. Treatment of Overuse Injuries

### A. Physical therapy procedures
1. Complete rest of the injured area for a period of 3–10 days. This may require the involved joints to be restricted in a sling or splint.
2. Ice packs or ice massage for 20–30 min, 3–4 times/day for the first 3–5 days.
3. Heat packs or warm whirlpool for 15–20 min, 1–2 times/day after the initial 3–5 days of cold therapy.
4. Anti-inflammatory medication for 7–14 days.
5. Ultrasound with the use of 10% hydrocortisone cream as the medium (phono-phoresis) for 8–10 min 1–2 times/day for 8–10 days.
6. Iontophoresis: Transportation of dexamethasone sodium phosphate (4%, 1 ml) and lidocaine (4%, 2 ml) ions through the skin with the use of electrical stimulation (4 mA). Treatment is for 20 min on an every-other-day basis for a total of 3–5 treatments.
7. Cortisone injection
8. Appropriate supportive device (such as lumbosacral corset or neoprene elbow sleeve).

## IV. Other Golf-related Problems

A. **Ocular trauma** in golf is rare. It has been reported that chemical injuries to the eye have taken place when persons have cut into a liquid-center golf ball and been squirted in the eye with the chemical. A player may be struck in the eye with a golf ball in flight or by a club while someone is swinging it.[2]

B. **Head injuries** have been reported in golf when a person is struck in the head with a golf ball or club. A study done in England showed that of 52 head injuries that occurred in sport and were serious enough to be reported to a regional neurologic center, 14 (27%) were golf-related.[5]

C. **Skin cancer** has been reported to be more prevalent among golfers than non-golfers, and has been reported to occur at a younger age in golfers than non-golfers. In a study of women professional and amateur golfers, the professionals received five times as much sun as the amateurs, and five professional players had developed basal cell carcinomas at an average age of 25.5 years.[3]

D. **Psychomotor difficulties,** known as the "yipps," have been reported by great players such as Ben Hogan, Bobby Jones, and Sam Snead. The "yipps" attack golfers on short putts and totally disable the player from hitting the putt properly. Most often the player either strikes the ball with a sudden forceful jerk or stubs the putter on the ground before ever hitting the ball. No successful treatment has ever been found for the "yipps," and this disability has been the undoing of many great golfers.[6]

E. **Oculophysical disability** occurs when a golfer who suffers from refractive errors such as astigmatism or muscle imbalance has difficulty with the short game in golf. The long game appears to rely heavily on physical action rather than oculophysical coordination, whereas the short game relies heavily on oculophysical coordination. Thus, some persons will have problems with chipping and putting owing to eye dysfunction.[6]

F. **Sudden death** does occur in golf. It is rare, but some of the causes that have been reported include cardiac events, lightning, and heat stroke. Accidents such as a shaft of the club being broken around a tree and plunging into the body have also been reported.[6]

V. **Conditioning Program for Golf**

A. **Flexibility exercises**

All flexibility exercises should be repeated 5–10 times on each side of the body and each repetition should be held for 10–20 sec. Each stretch should be gradual in nature with no bouncing.

1. **Neck**
   a. Turn head to look over each shoulder, bend chin to chest and look to ceiling, tilt ear toward shoulder without elevating the shoulder.

2. **Shoulder**
   a. Lie on back with arm out to side at 90° and elbow bent to 90°; let arm rotate backward.
   b. Pull arm across chest and under chin without rotating torso.
   c. Reach arm overhead with elbow bent completely; place behind head and pull with other hand.

3. **Forearm**
   a. Extend elbow completely while flexing wrist and fingers as far as possible.
   b. Extend elbow completely while extending wrist and fingers as far as possible.

4. **Chest**
   a. Stand in a corner; place forearm of each arm on wall and lean into corner.
   b. Grasp hands behind back, pull arms up backward.

5. **Trunk**
   a. Clasp hands above head and lean body sideways.
   b. Lie on back with arms at shoulder level and flat on ground, roll onto one hip while keeping back flat, pull the top leg toward chest while keeping bottom leg straight.

6. **Low back and hip**
   a. Lie on back, pull one knee to chest.
   b. Lie on back, pull both knees toward chest.
   c. Lie on back, keep one leg straight while pulling other leg to waist and then across chest.

7. **Hamstring**
   a. Sit with both legs out straight, knees flat on floor, and toes pointed toward ceiling. Bend forward at hips, keeping the back straight.
   b. Stand with knees bent and touch toes, keep touching toes while straightening knees.

8. **Calf**
   a. Stand facing wall, keep knees straight, heels flat, and toes straight ahead, lean into wall by bending arms.

    b. Stand facing wall, bend knees, keep heels flat, and toes straight ahead, lean into wall.

B. **Muscle strengthening exercises**

Strengthening exercises should be done with light weights in order to increase strength gradually. The exercises should be done with both sides of the body, and the weights should be gradually increased over a period of time. Initially a person should do 1–2 sets of 10 repetitions and increase to 2–3 sets of 10 repetitions.

  1. **Neck**
    a. Start with head in neutral position, place hand against forehead, and try to bend head down. Resist with hand so no movement takes place. Hold contraction for 3–5 sec. Repeat for extension, lateral side bending, and rotation each direction.

  2. **Rotator cuff**
    a. Hang arm by side with elbow straight, turn hand inward as far as possible, then raise arm up at 45°. Rotate arm so the hand is pointing toward the ceiling.
    b. Lie on side, rest top arm on body, bend elbow to 90°. Rotate arm so hand turns up toward ceiling.
    c. Lie on side, place bottom arm under the body, bend elbow to 90°, and rest hand on floor. Rotate arm so hand turns up toward stomach.

  3. **Latissimus dorsi**
    a. Lie on stomach with arm by side, lift arm up backward as far as possible.
    b. Sit in chair with arm rests, place hands on arm rests and push down so the body is lifted off the chair.
    c. Stand with arms above head, grasp pulleys or rubber tubing, and pull down and back as far as possible.

  4. **Forearm**
    a. Sit with forearm resting on table and wrist hanging over edge with palm up; bend wrist up as far as possible.
    b. Sit with forearm resting on table and wrist hanging over edge with palm down; bend wrist up as far as possible.
    c. Sit with forearm resting on table and wrist hanging over edge with palm up; rotate forearm so palm faces down.
    d. Sit with forearm resting on table and wrist hanging over edge with palm down; rotate forearm so palm faces up.
    e. Stand with arm hanging by side, bend wrist laterally toward thumb side.
    f. Stand with arm by side and bend wrist laterally toward little finger.

  5. **Chest**
    a. Lie on back with arms out to side at 90° at shoulder; raise arms toward the midline until hands touch.

  6. **Abdominal muscles**
    a. Lie on back on floor, knees bent and feet flat on floor, place arms by side or across chest, raise torso off floor until shoulder blades come off floor.

  7. **Back**
    a. Lie on stomach with arms by side, raise one leg up backwards, keeping knee straight.
    b. Get on hands and knees, raise one arm and opposite leg up backwards to level of body.

  8. **Hip**
    a. Lie on side with top leg straight and bottom knee bent for stability; raise top leg up sideways as far as possible.
    b. Lie on stomach with one leg hanging over edge of table; lift the leg up backwards as far as possible keeping the knee straight.

### C. Cardiovascular exercise

1. Cardiovascular fitness is an integral component of a person's overall fitness. Golfer's need cardiovascular fitness in order to walk 18 holes or more and not become fatigued.
2. There are many different modes for developing cardiovascular endurance. Biking, swimming, walking, and jogging are a few of the more common. Initially a person should exercise for 10–15 min 3 times/week and then gradually build up to 20–30 min 3 times/week of aerobic exercise at an intensity level of 70–80% of their target heart rate.

## VI. Equipment and Technique

### A. Equipment

1. Length of club
   a. The length of the shaft is determined by the length of the golfer's arm and the distance of the finger tips from the ground.
2. Grip size
   a. The grip size is an individual preference. A standard size is when the fingertip of the long finger of the left hand just touches the palm of the left hand when the club is gripped properly.
3. Shaft flexibility
   a. The proper shaft flexibility differs for each individual. Usually the shaft flexibility is determined by the direction that the golfer consistently hits the ball.
4. Swing weight of club
   a. The swing weight of the club is also individual for each golfer. The size of the individual as well as the direction of the normal shot help determine the proper swing weight.

### B. Technique

1. The proper technique for the golf swing is a complex issue and goes beyond the scope of this chapter. Proper technique is one way of preventing the many overuse injuries that have been described. The best advice for developing proper technique is to take lessons from a PGA Golf Professional.

## VII. Special Rules for Protection

### A. Rule 6-8a

1. Rule 6-8a states that when a golfer believes he is in danger from lightning, the golfer may discontinue play of his own accord.

## REFERENCES

1. Duda M: Golf injuries: They really do happen. Phys Sportsmed 15(7):191–196, 1987.
2. Farley KG: Ocular trauma resulting from the explosive rupture of a liquid center golf ball. J Am Optom Assoc 56:310–314, 1985.
3. Hanke WC, Zollinger TW, O'Brian JJ, Bianco L: Skin cancer in professional and amateur female golfers. Phys Sportsmed 13(8):51–52, 61–63, 66–68, 1985.
4. Jobe FW, Moynes DR: 30 Exercises for Better Golf. Inglewood, Champion Press, 1986.
5. Lindsay KW, McLatchie G, Jennett B: Serious head injury in sport. Br Med J 281:789–791, 1980.
6. McCarroll JR: Golf. In Schneider RC, et al: Sports Injuries: Mechanism, Prevention, and Treatment. Baltimore, Williams & Wilkins, 1985, pp 290–294.
7. McCarroll JR, Gioe TJ: Professional golfers and the price they pay. Phys Sportsmed 10(7):64–70, 1982.
8. Roberts J: Injuries, handicaps, mashies, and cleeks. Phys Sportsmed 6:121–123, 1978.
9. Stover CN, Wiren G, Topaz SR: The modern golf swing and stress syndromes. Phys Sportsmed 4:42–47, 1976.
10. Vaupel GL, Andrews JR: Diagnostic and operative arthroscopy of the thumb metacarpophalangeal joint. Am J Sports Med 13:139–141, 1985.

# Chapter 55: Skiing

## Part I: Alpine (Downhill) Skiing

JOHN A. FEAGIN, JR, MD
J. RICHARD STEADMAN, MD

I. **General Introduction and Medical Coverage**

A. **The responsibility of the ski team physician** is a privileged one. Alpine ski racing requires special equipment, facilities, training, and climate that set it apart in many ways from other sports. Despite these differences, some fundamentals remain: the special bond between physician and athlete, the privileged relationship between physician and trainer, and the coach/physician interaction. This chapter will emphasize the general knowledge and responsibilities requisite for the "Ski Team Doctor" and the specific responsibilities for the Alpine and Nordic team physicians.

   Alpine skiing is one of the fastest growing sports in the world. It is estimated that there are one hundred million skiers, and more youth and affluence suggest that growth will continue.

   As the worldwide base of recreational skiers expands, it is understandable that more and more opportunities have become available for the exceptional skier: the secondary school team, the regional team, the national team, and finally Olympic and World Cup competition for the "elite" skier.

B. **"On the mountain" responsibilities**
   1. **Skiing ability.** The ski team physician should ski well enough to attend practices and competition on the ski mountain itself.
      a. **On the mountain experience is necessary to:**
         i. Supervise preparations for event coverage.
         ii. Develop preventive strategies.
         iii. Ensure proper first aid and evacuation procedures.
         iv. Develop rapport with athletes and coaches.
      b. **Ski patrol training helpful:**
         i. Physician as trainee
         ii. Physician as trainer
   2. **Radio communication**
      a. **Mandatory for event coverage**
         i. With coach/team
         ii. With ski patrol and mountain manager.
      b. Radio communication with coach and team is highly recommended both at home and away.
   3. **Event coverage at home**
      a. **Coordination with:**
         i. **Mountain manager and/or ski area manager**
            (a) General planning and logistics
            (b) Grooming and condition of course.
         ii. **Ski patrol leader**
            (a) Personnel, supplies, and equipment on hill
            (b) Ski traffic patterns and crowd control

        (c) Evacuation plan
             (i) Physician availability on hill and at base
        (d) Spectator medical support.
    iii. **Support medical personnel**
        (a) Assign duties to assisting physicians, trainers, and medical support personnel.
        (b) Coordinate availability of medical facility at mountain and/or local hospital.
             (i) Coordinate ambulance availability if appropriate.
    iv. **Medical support personnel and/or coaches from attending teams**
    v. **Personal equipment**
        (a) Ski equipment well maintained
        (b) Warm clothing for "standing and waiting" by race course
        (c) "Fanny pack" or backpack with emergency supplies.

## II. Preparation of the Athlete

  A. **General:** The Alpine competitive skier is one of the most fit and well-proportioned of athletes. The $VO_2$max, leg strength, agility, and endurance are at peak. Upper-body strength is usually excellent. How is this fitness acquired? Through selection and years of dedication and training. Most competitive skiers were on skis by age 5, they have competed locally and regionally, and they have traveled extensively to seek competition and/or conditions conducive to training.

      "Dry-land" training is essential to competition and is usually conducted with coaching supervision. Dry-land training consists of 3–4 months of strength training (particularly quadriceps work), endurance and interval training, roller skiing, bicycling, running, and agility drills. Most skiers are nutrition-conscious, and body fat is low. Training or competition may occupy 10 or 11 months of the year.

  B. **Clothing and equipment**
    1. **Layered clothing** is essential, particularly for warm-up and warm-down.
    2. **Lightness and airfoil characteristics** are important for competition.
    3. **Reliable bindings,** with multimode adjustable toe and heel releases, are essential.
    4. **Quality skis** that will not delaminate under the stress of binding loads.
    5. **Goggles** must be well ventilated and must protect the eyes from ultraviolet radiation as well as injury.
      a. **Lenses should be color-adjusted** to provide optimum visibility, given changing conditions.
    6. For the slalom skier, **pads** are helpful in protecting against injury from slalom poles.
      a. Padded gloves and uniforms
      b. Additional arm pads.
    7. **Helmets** are required for the downhill.
      a. Use in practice and competition.
    8. **Break-away poles** for slalom and giant slalom
      a. Must have optimum strength and flexibility.
  C. **Cardiovascular and pulmonary systems**
    1. Alpine competitive skiing requires **high levels of aerobic and anaerobic conditioning** (see sec. III, Physiology).
  D. **Musculoskeletal strength, endurance, agility**
    1. **Must be gained preseason and maintained in season. "Peaking"** is important and sometimes must be obtained 2–3 times per season.

2. **Overtraining** is difficult to evaluate and recognize—an increasing pulse rate is sometimes helpful in diagnosis. Overtraining seems to occur more often in women athletes (see Chap. 21).
3. **Agility** can be taught.
   a. Simple drills are available in the coaching manuals, and in addition to these, soccer, water-skiing, and plyometrics are components of an agility program.
   b. The "SAID" principle (Specific Adaptation to Individual Demands) must be recognized so that some of the conditioning, both aerobic and anaerobic, is attained "on slope."

III. **Physiology**

A. **General:** The pioneer and pace-setter in the physiology of downhill skiing was Bengt Saltin (1965). His work laid the foundation and challenge for those who would follow and has placed our training programs on a physiologic basis.

B. **Cardiovascular**
1. The competitive Alpine skier is characterized by a **significantly increased VO₂max,** an **increased stroke volume,** and an **increased blood volume.**
2. The **lactic acid threshold** is increased with training.
3. **Fluid loss occurs rapidly at high altitude and low humidity,** and if not replaced promptly, will result in decreased performance. Water or hypotonic sugar/salt solutions are preferable.

C. **Musculoskeletal system**
1. Leg strength, both static and dynamic, is remarkable.
   a. Best measured at low torque velocity, i.e., 30°/sec.
2. Upper body strength is excellent.
3. Abdominal and truncal muscles work hard in skiing and must be included in the training process.
4. Muscle fiber type tends to show a preponderance of slow-twitch fibers, but generalizations are inconclusive. Muscle biopsies show increased mitochondria with enhanced peripheral $O_2$ utilization as a response to training.
5. Body fat for men averages 8%, for women 17%.

D. **Specific training recommendations**
1. **Strength training** should be static and dynamic. It should be concentric and eccentric.
   a. The vastus lateralis, biceps femoris, and tibialis anticus should be emphasized.
   b. Back muscles and abdominal rectus, as well as gluteus maximus and hamstring, are key to performance.
2. **Specific exercises** shown to be helpful are: uphill lateral jumping, dynamic tuck training, backward walking, downhill running (in moderation), roller skiing (which approximates running in muscle demand), and bicycling.
3. **Nutrition** during competition should consist of high carbohydrate intake. Nutritional supplementation is optional, but most athletes perceive the need and partake of vitamin supplementation. Body fat should be measured on a regular basis.

IV. **Injury: incidence and epidemiology**

A. **General:** The injury rate for recreational skiers is 3–5 injuries/1,000 skier days. No comparable statistic is known for competitive skiers. It is common knowledge, however, that fractures and knee injuries in competitive skiers are frequent.
1. Most fractures are binding-related, but bindings must be "screwed down" to prevent prerelease. There is a fine line between safety and prerelease.
2. **Speed** often determines injury severity, and the downhill skier will approach 100 kilometers an hour.

   3. **Muscle strength and endurance are known to decrease incidence** and should be emphasized.
B. **Axial injuries**
   1. **Spine injury** does happen and paralysis can result. The cervical and thoracolumbar junctions are at particular risk.
      a. **A "downed" skier should not be moved without palpating the spine and checking neurologically.**
   2. **Concussion** is not uncommon and will impair performance and safety.
   3. Check for **pelvic injuries.**
C. **Appendicular injuries**
   1. Knee ligament injuries are the most common injuries sustained by competitive skiers.
      a. The **medial collateral ligament (MCL)** is the most frequently injured ligament.
         i. Common mechanism: catching inside edge of the ski leads to forceful external rotation and valgus loading of the tibia relative to the femur.
         ii. Surgery is seldom required.
      b. The **anterior cruciate ligament (ACL)** is the second most frequently injured knee ligament.
         i. Common presentation in skiers:
            (a) Skier feels a "pop" or tear at time of injury.
            (b) Sense of "giving way" or instability.
            (c) Effusion within 24 hours.
         ii. **Etiology:** The stiff ski boot has deflected the stress from the ankle and lower tibia to the knee.
         iii. **Mechanisms**
            (a) **"Anterior drawer" mechanism:** Several situations occur in which momentum pulls the skier's lower leg and boot forward while the body falls backward, thus producing a large "anterior drawer" stress.
               (i) Skier lands leaning backward off-balance coming off a jump. Ski shoots forward as skier falls back, and lower leg is forced forward by its own momentum in the direction of an anterior drawer test.
               (ii) Same forces produced when skier catches an inside edge of a ski with body weight too far back on the skis.
               (iii) Same forces produced when racer leans backward near the finish line to pick up extra speed, and catches inside edge.
            (b) **Hyperextension-external rotation mechanism:** Skier catches tip of ski in snow or skis into a bump or obstacle in such a way that the involved knee hyperextends and the femur externally rotates on the relatively fixed tibia.
         iv. Anterior cruciate ligament injuries are serious and warrant early orthopedic consultation.
   2. **Fractures** to the ankle mortise, tibia, and femur are relatively common.
   3. **Shoulder injuries** are relatively common in upper level skiers due to the impact of high-speed falls.
      a. **Shoulder dislocations** are usually anterior and/or inferior.
         i. They may be difficult to reduce because of bony impingement (Hill-Sachs defect), and are often associated with fractures of the greater tuberosity.
         ii. All shoulder dislocations should be x-rayed.

      b. **Acromioclavicular separations** are common when skier lands on tip of shoulder on hard-packed snow or ice.

   4. **Sprains of the thumb ulnar collateral ligaments** are common ("skier's thumb," "gamekeeper's thumb").

      a. Caused by catching thumb on ski pole straps or on hard-packed snow surface in a fall.

      b. Surgical repair of Grade III sprains.

      c. Thumb spica cast for Grades I and II sprains.

   5. **Collisions with fixed objects** occur too frequently. The course should be surveyed repeatedly for safety by skier, coach, and physician.

  D. **Weather-related injuries**

   1. Cold (see also Chap. 12)

      a. Frostbite of the nose, ears, and cheeks is common.

         i. If caught early, in frost-nip stage, massage will usually restore circulation and reverse damage.

      b. Skiers should check each other for frostbite, and the physician should be alerted to the risk.

      c. The wind-chill factor should be known to the physician, who should add this to the skier's speed.

      d. Hypothermia may be a problem if frostbite injury is severe and evacuation delayed.

   2. **Sun**

      a. **Ultraviolet** rays can be intense with altitude and reflected light.

      b. The eyes need protection, and **ordinary glasses may not be enough, since 10% of ultraviolet light may enter from the top and sides.**

      c. **Maximum protection sunscreen** should be liberally used on exposed parts.

         i. Formerly frostbitten areas are particularly vulnerable to ultraviolet damage.

      d. **Herpes labialis** is common and should be treated preventively with protective screens.

      e. Carelessness in protecting the skin leads to an increased incidence of basal cell carcinoma in later life.

      f. **Visibility** is critical to racers. Snow, fogging, flat light, and glare all impair performance and jeopardize safety.

## V. **Injury: Diagnosis and Treatment**

  A. **General**

   1. "Common injuries occur commonly"—expect knee sprain, ACL tear, fractured tibia or ankle, fractured femur, fractured pelvis, dislocated shoulder, ulnar collateral ligament tears, and the occasional concussion.

   2. **Palpation** is the essence of on-the-slope diagnosis. Palpate the entire spine first, then the pelvis and hip joints, then long bones for tenderness and deformity.

   3. **Splint all fractures and joint injuries on site.** When in doubt, use a backboard/cervical collar.

   4. Coordinate evacuation to a definitive treatment center appropriate to the injury. **Whenever possible, stay with the patient until definitive care is arranged.**

   5. **Do not allow evacuation until preliminary diagnosis by history and manual examination is accomplished, and all long-bone fractures are splinted.**

      a. Protect against hypothermia.

  B. **Axial**

   1. **Check cervical and thoracolumbar spines thoroughly by palpation.**

      a. **Splint/backboard if any tenderness, or doubt.**

    2. Neurologic evaluation for major muscle group function and sensation.

       a. Bowel and bladder checks are usually impractical "on slope."

    3. Be alert to rule out rib fracture/pneumothorax.

  C. **Appendicular**

    1. **Palpation** is the key to diagnosis. Crepitation, pain, and tenderness are diagnostic of fracture until proven otherwise by x-ray. When in doubt, x-ray.

    2. **Watch for any dislocation and vascular compromise.** Reduce immediately if this occurs.

    3. **Splint, splint, splint.**

VII. **Injury Prevention**

  A. **Axial**

    1. **Most skull and spine trauma is the result of either high-velocity fall and/or collision with an object.**

    2. **The course should be clear, well marked, and access-controlled.**

    3. **Visibility** should be adequate.

    4. Racers should have a voice in the decision to race if course or weather conditions are marginal.

    5. **Course grooming equipment should be stowed.**

    6. **Helmets** should be requisite for the downhill.

    7. Helmet and goggles should fit well.

  B. **Appendicular**

    1. **Bindings should be checked at least daily by the racer.**

       a. **Self-release should be possible.**

       b. Modern bindings have done a great deal to decrease fractures of the lower extremity. Stiffer, higher boots, however, transfer the strain to the knee ligament. The hope lies in a boot that will allow forward-rearward flexion without sacrificing lateral support. Present binding technology seems to have reached a plateau, but the latest and best should be available and should be adjusted by a competent ski mechanic.

    2. Ski clothing should be streamlined and should fit well to avoid catching on gates or objects encountered in a fall.

## RECOMMENDED READING

1. Johnson RJ (ed): Skiing injuries. Clin Sports Med 1(2), 1982.
2. Karlsson J, et al: The Physiology of Alpine Skiing. U.S. Ski Coaches Association, P.O. Box 1747, Park City, Utah 84060, 1978.
3. Mote CD, Johnson RJ (eds): Skiing Trauma and Safety. Philadelphia, American Society for Testing and Materials, May 1987.
4. Sharkey BJ: Training for Cross-country Ski Racing. Champaign, IL, Human Kinetics Publishers, 1984.
5. U.S. Alpine Ski Training Manual, U.S. Ski Coaches Association, P.O. Box 1747, Park City, UT 84060.

# Part II: Nordic Skiing, Cross Country, Combined, and Special Jumping

## WILLIAM G. CLANCY, JR, MD

I. **General Introduction and Medical Coverage**

The three Nordic sports are less familiar to North Americans than to the European sporting population. Indeed, a major ski-jumping competition such as the Holmenkollen in Oslo, Norway, or the Intersport Springer Tournee in Garmisch, West Germany, will attract over 100,000 fans for a day's events. In Europe, world-champion ski jumpers such as Switzerland's Walter Steiner and Finland's present world and Olympic champion Matti Nykanen are held in almost the same esteem as the world Alpine ski champions. The Nordic cross-country champions are held in only slightly less adulation. These three Nordic competitive events have been held for over a century in all of Western and Eastern Europe, both at the grass roots level and at the world and Olympic levels. This has been in great contrast to the few competitions held in North America. Fortunately, there has been a vast increase in North America in the number of competitive events in cross-country ski racing over the past 5 years. The tremendous interest in cross-country skiing as a recreational sport has led to the development of numerous competitions for the recreational, master, and elite athlete. Unfortunately, the numbers involved in Nordic combine and special jumping are still extremely small.

A. **Medical coverage**
   1. **Special concerns**
      a. **Cross-country**
         i. Long courses: 10–50 km (6.2–31 miles)
            (a) Trails through forest require appropriate paramedical personnel positioned throughout race course.
            (b) Radio communication is necessary.
         ii. Threat of hypothermia
            (a) Low temperature
            (b) Wind-chill effect
               (i) Increased by effect of long, high-speed, downhill runs.
         iii. Dehydration
         iv. Glycogen depletion.
      b. **Ski jumping**
         i. Possibility of high-impact injuries exists.
            (a) Head and neck
            (b) Trunk and limbs.
         ii. Fortunately injury incidence is low.
   2. **Skiing ability of team physician**
      a. Less of a concern than in Alpine skiing, but team physician should be competent to ski to any site being covered.
   3. **Event coverage**
      a. Team physician often responsible for more basic organization and provision of personnel than in Alpine skiing.
         i. Can seek help from:
            (a) Nearby Nordic centers
            (b) Ski clubs

(c) Ski patrols—Alpine or Nordic
(d) State or national park service or forest service
(e) Mountain rescue organizations
(f) Other community organizations.

   b. **Requirements**
      i. Adequate trained personnel to cover course
      ii. Adequate first aid, rescue, and evacuation equipment
      iii. Radio communication
      iv. Appropriate medical transportation to evacuate any medical emergency
      v. Liaison with hospital or local health care facility
   c. **Important sites for medical/paramedical coverage**
      i. Cross country race finish line
      ii. Bottom of ski jump.

## II. Preparation of the Athlete

### A. General

1. **Cross-country racing** is the most demanding of all endurance sports, as documented by $VO_2max$ testing. With the introduction of the skating technique, agility as well as increased upper body strength become more important. Unlike cross-country and distance runners, who usually run only one race a week, the cross-country skier will frequently compete in several races in a weekend. The elite racer at a major competition may race 15 km, then 1 or 2 days later race a 30 km or 50 km race and a day later race 10 km on a 4 × 10 km team relay, with all races being held in subfreezing conditions. It takes approximately 10 years of year-round arduous training and conditioning to achieve this level of effort.

   a. Since cross-country skiers incorporate a good deal of road running during their **dry-land training,** they will frequently develop similar overuse injuries as does the long distance runner (see Chap. 29 and 51). The incidence of these injuries is probably less in skiers than in runners because their dry-land training is intermixed with a great deal of bicycling and roller skiing.

2. **The ski jumper** must focus his training to develop power, quickness, and agility as well as the ability to ride the air. A great deal of time must be spent on developing the ability to gather all body parts into the correct position at the exact spot where take-off should be initiated. The skier may be coming out of the compression portion of the inrun at speeds of up to 50–60 miles an hour. Head, shoulders, arms, and back, knee, and ankle flexion positions must be adjusted in that short interval to the take-off, and cannot be too early or too late. Once the skier is airborne, the ideal aerodynamic position must be held until the landing point.

   a. Special jumping is not so much an endurance sport as it is an explosive sport. Summer dry-land training is aimed at developing a good endurance base with running and bicycling, but is more pointed in developing lower leg strength, speed and agility. Dry-land conditioning consists of upper- and lower-body weight training, agility drills, and plyometrics. Additionally, a great deal of practice time is spent on actual ski jumps that have specialized plastic inruns or have a frost rail inrun. There are several in North America and many in Europe. Wind-tunnel testing for the ideal body position is also utilized during dry-land training.

3. The **Nordic combined athlete** must spend his dry-land training working on both aspects, a most difficult task.

### B. Clothing and equipment

1. **Cross-country skiers**
   a. The **competitive suit** must be aerodynamic as well as lightweight, allowing free, uninhibited movement.
   b. **Gloves** must be flexible and warm.
   c. The **skis** will vary, depending on whether the race is the traditional diagonal technique, or a freestyle or skating technique.
   d. The **poles** must be quite strong, as breakage will lead to a disastrous race finish.
   e. **Sunglasses or windshields** are a must in snowy conditions.
2. **Ski jumpers**
   a. **Layered clothing** is essential when waiting during the long periods between jumps.
   b. The **jumpsuit** is a specially tested aerodynamic suit that must be tested and approved by the FIS (Federation Internationale de Sport) and has the same specifications for all jumpers.
   c. The **jumping ski** must also meet FIS regulations but may vary in length.
   d. The **bindings** are, unfortunately, a single mode cable release that has limited safety value during a fall.
   e. **Goggles** must be well ventilated and the lenses must be color-adjusted to provide optimum visibility given changing conditions.
   f. A **helmet** is mandatory and must be properly fitted.

C. **Cardiovascular system**
   1. Nordic cross-country ski racers are quite similar to long-distance runners both in body composition and cardiovascular make-up. **The elite cross-country skier tends to have a slightly higher $VO_2$max than the distance runner.** This may be due to the fact that, in addition to their leg muscles, cross-country skiers must also use all of their upper body musculature when poling.
   2. Improvement of cardiovascular parameters is far more important in the cross-country skier than in the ski jumper, as cross-country skiing is the most demanding endurance (aerobic) sport. Dry-land training is designed to develop and maximize the cardiovascular system's ability to deliver oxygen to the working muscle groups. The muscle cell must be stimulated to develop its oxidative respiratory system to the highest efficiency, keeping lactic acid production as low as possible. Combinations of long-distance running and interval training programs utilizing bicycling, running, and roller skiing are intermixed to achieve this goal, as well as focused weight training.

D. **Musculoskeletal system**
   1. Cross-country: Upper- and lower-body muscle training must be designed to improve two distinct needs in the cross-country skier:
      a. **Muscular strength** must be increased to produce stronger upper-body poling action, as well as lower-body strength, to climb or skate up steep hills.
      b. **Muscle endurance** must be developed to maintain speed in long races.
   2. The jumper must focus his training to the development of strength and power. The development of strength alone is not sufficient, as the jumper must recruit all the muscle fibers within a very short time period and then explode them (power).
      a. **Strength training** programs will involve the back, hip, thigh, knee, and lower leg muscles.
      b. **Power training** involves the back extensor group, the hip extensors, knee extensors, and the ankle plantar flexor groups.

III. **Injury**

A. **Cross-country skiing**
   1. **General:** The injury rate for the competitive cross-country skier on snow has not

been reported; however, injuries in these skiers are considered to be quite uncommon. The injury rate for recreational skiers is only 0.1 per 1,000 skier days. Most injuries occur during the dry-land training and are generally overuse/overload in nature, as seen in the long distance runner (see Chap. 51).

2. **Axial**
   a. **Low back pain** is relatively common in the skier, occurs most often during the ski season, and is associated more often with the diagonal technique than with the skating technique.
      i. Treatment
         (a) Work on technique
         (b) Rehabilitative exercise and stretching.

3. **Appendicular**
   a. **Dry-land training:** Lower extremity overuse injuries: patellofemoral stress syndrome, shin splints, compartment syndromes, Achilles tendinitis, and stress fractures of the tibia, fibular, and metatarsals.
   b. **Training on snow and competition**
      i. Lower extremity problems are uncommon, probably due to the change from impact loading to gliding.
      ii. Upper extremity overuse problems common due to poling:
         (a) Rotator cuff tendinitis
         (b) Flexor-pronator tendinitis
         (c) Sprain of elbow medial collateral ligaments.

3. Weather-related injuries (see Chap. 12)

B. **Ski jumping**
   1. **General:** The injury rates for ski jumping are far less than one would expect, and similar to those of Alpine racing. A 5-year study on ski-jumping injuries sustained at the Lake Place U.S. Olympic Training Center revealed that the injury rate ranged from 1.2 per 1,000 skier days in World Cup competition to 4.3 per 1,000 skier days for non-World Cup competitions.
      a. Dry-land training injuries are associated more with weight training overload than with impact endurance training.
         i. The more common injuries involve low back pain, patellofemoral pain, and patellar tendinitis.
      b. On snow, jumping injuries are essentially the same as those seen in the Alpine racer.
   2. **Specific Injuries:** See Part I of this chapter, "Alpine Skiing."
   3. **Injury prevention**
      a. **Ski-jumping safety is determined by the competition judges who are responsible for making sure that the ski-jump inrun, landing hill, and outrun are in proper condition.** These judges must also determine whether the **wind and visibility conditions are adequate** for safe competition.
      b. The skier must make sure that the **ski bindings are properly set** so that the ski will not come off in flight, but are set loosely enough to release if a fall ensues.

## *RECOMMENDED READING*

1. Wright JR, Hixon EG, Rand JJ: Injury patterns in Nordic ski jumpers. Am J Sports Med 14:393–397, 1986.
2. Clancy WG Jr, McConkey JP: Nordic and Alpine skiing. In Schneider RC, Kennedy JC, Plant ML (eds): Sports Injuries: Mechanisms, Prevention, and Treatment. Baltimore, Williams & Wilkins, 1984, pp 247–270.
3. Clancy WG Jr: Cross country ski injuries. Clin Sports Med 1(2):333–338, 1982.

# Chapter 56: Tennis

TERRY L. NICOLA, MD, MS

I. **Tennis-specific Conditioning and Body Mechanics**

A. **A combined endurance and strength sport**

1. A typical match requires **300 to 500 bursts of effort,** necessitating strength and efficiency of form for each burst, without fatiguing during the final games and points.

2. **Aerobic performance level:** Averages 60–70% of the predicted maximum heart rate during a singles match, 40% for a doubles match.

3. Given the high demands of lower extremity endurance for repeated bursts of running, a focus on lower extremity conditioning is recommended.

   a. Stationary bicycling at 90 rpm with 1-min high-intensity bursts alternated with 4-min light pedalling may simulate the intensity of tennis play.

   b. 30-min sessions, three times per week, are a necessary minimum for a conditioning effect.

   c. The desired result is a consistent level of performance for an entire match.

4. Specificity of strength and coordination training necessitates that athletes play tennis to be good at tennis.

   a. A progressive resistance strengthening program to key muscle groups (e.g., the rotator cuff) serves to increase the body's tolerance for progressive tennis drills and match play.

      i. Prepare needed muscles for each tennis stroke.

      ii. Balance conditioning of agonist and antagonist muscles for skeletal joint stability.

B. **Tennis form evaluation of specific components for injury prevention**

1. **General concepts**

   a. **Service stroke phases**

      i. **Wind-up phase:** lower extremity preparation with hips, knees, and ankles flexed for recoil, abdominal muscles set.

      ii. **Cocking phase:** ball toss and recoil of service arm, shoulder muscles on maximum stretch.

      iii. **Acceleration phase:** energy release from lower extremity drive, abdominal flexion, and finally upper extremity swing and ball contact.

      iv. **Deceleration phase** of the service arm: primarily from the shoulder and upper trunk.

   b. **Backhand and forehand stroke phases**

      i. **Preparation phase:** trunk rotation, running or jumping to planned set point with "stop" foot planted, racquet drawn back.

      ii. **Acceleration phase:** lower extremity and trunk lean into the stroke, motion of arm-racquet lever primarily from shoulder, finally racquet contact with the ball.

      iii. **Deceleration phase:** lower extremity and trunk rotation toward the net.

   c. **Return strokes at the net**

      i. Quick lower extremity and trunk movements are similar to those described above in par. I.B.1.b., abbreviated by short punch strokes.

2. **Back and trunk motion**
   a. **The primary concern is lower back (lumbar spine) hyperextension during service and overhead strokes.** This stress can be minimized by tossing the ball slightly ahead of the service line and launching into the service driving from the lower extremities, with less back and neck hyperextension.
   b. Thoracic spine flexibility for rotation is necessary for the ground strokes.
   c. There may be excessive back motion in an attempt to compensate for shoulder and lower extremity inflexibility.
3. **Shoulder motion**
   a. **Primary concern is loading of the shoulder structures during service and overhead strokes.**
      i. From wind-up to cocking phases, the combined glenohumeral and scapular motion is responsible for 90° abduction, another 30° by thoracic lateral tilt (Fig. 1).
      ii. The abducted glenohumeral joint also externally rotates up to 120°, which may overstretch the anterior joint capsule.
4. **Elbow and wrist motion**
   a. These components are a relatively fixed part of the arm-racquet lever, responsible for reach and conduction of energy generated by motion of the lower extremities, trunk, and shoulder.
   b. **Error in form is generally due to unwanted wrist-snapping motion during the backhand stroke.** Wrist motion should not occur except in the service stroke during acceleration phase of wrist flexion.
   c. **Grip mechanism** involves the wrist extension muscles as stabilizers for the wrist and finger flexor tendons as they cross the wrist.
      i. The grip should be as relaxed as possible to minimize stress on the above wrist muscles and their origin at the elbow epicondyles (see par. II.B.).
      ii. The racquet handle should have a "sticky" grip.
      iii. **Correct handle circumference:** the handle circumference should be equal to the distance from the tip of the ring finger to the proximal palmar crease, measured along the radial border of the ring finger.
5. **Hip, knee, and ankle motion**
   a. The lower extremity stresses seen in sprinting events are present in pursuits that are part of a tennis volley. Stresses on quadriceps, hamstrings, patella, and calf muscles are **similar to the stresses of sprinting.**
   b. **Lower extremity set and preparation** for each stroke involves predominantly a partial squat (hip flexion, knee flexion, and ankle dorsiflexion) to drive into the stroke with spring from the legs rather than compensatory back and arm motion.
   c. The triceps surae muscles (posterior calf) are stressed during ankle and foot push-off in service strokes and jumps when hip and knee are fully extended (see par. II.B.6.a.i.).
C. **Equipment and force transmission**
   1. **Upper extremity injuries are closely associated with the forces transmitted from the racquet to the upper extremity and trunk.** The ball may reach speeds of over 100 mph. In cases of poor control or recent upper-body injuries:
      a. Reduce string tension by 3–5 lb from that recommended by the manufacturer.
      b. Use natural gut strings.
      c. The weight of the racquet is a factor, especially the racquet head, situated at the distal end of the lever formed by arm and racquet. Consider larger ceramic composite racquets, which are lighter and dissipate energy well.

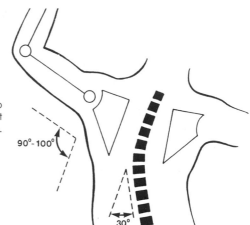

**FIGURE 1.** This view of the service wind-up illustrates the addition of 30° lateral thoracic tilt to the 90°–100° of scapulohumeral abduction.

d. Check for fitted grip.

e. Use only new tennis balls.

2. **Footwear:** Important for shock absorption and dissipation of ground reaction forces.

a. A stable shoe must have a **good heel counter** and **snug fit** with a flexible forefoot to allow a base of support for rapid directional changes on the court. **Such side-side stability may not be seen in other sport shoes such as running shoes.**

b. A lighter tennis shoe may be used for clay courts.

c. Shoes and orthotic devices should be considered in someone who has already corrected for errors in tennis form or conditioning.

3. **Court surfaces may be clay, composition, hard court, grass, or carpet.**

a. In rehabilitation of tennis injuries, carpet, composition, and clay are more forgiving to the lower extremities.

b. Slower ball velocity on clay court is more forgiving to the upper extremities.

## II. **Traumatic and overuse injuries**

A. Severe disruptive injuries such as tendon ruptures, completed stress fractures, and adolescent physeal plate injuries will present as sudden loss of motion and strength, with pain increasing in severity on repeated attempts to keep playing.

B. The predominant mode of tennis injury is **overuse** stress to bone, ligament, muscle, tendon, and nerve.

1. **Lateral tennis elbow**

a. Pain at the lateral elbow: an estimated 50% of all tennis players will suffer injury to the extensor carpi radialis brevis (ECRB) at the common wrist extensor tendon origin at the lateral epicondyle. Risk factors are as follows:

   i. Age of player (> 30 years old)

   ii. Improper grip size

   iii. Use of a metal racquet

   iv. Duration of average practice (greater than 2 hours per day)

   v. Tight strings

   vi. Incorrect backhand technique including snapping wrist

   (a) Both technique errors cause contraction and pull of the ECRB on the lateral epicondyle.

   (b) Symptoms can be elicited by wrist extension or tight grip.

(c) Passive wrist flexion range, with elbow extended and forearm pronated, may be restricted.

2. **Medial tennis elbow**
   a. Pain at the medial elbow is generally attributed to strain at the common flexor tendon origin at the medial epicondyle.
   b. This injury, common to elite or highly ranked recreational players, is due to repeated wrist flexion overload during the service, or to a powerful forehand top spin (pronation stress).
   c. Diagnosis: Local tenderness is present over the medial epicondyle, with pain on active wrist flexion and passive, supinated, elbow-extended wrist extension.

3. **Other concomitant elbow injuries**
   a. Other rare disorders found with classic elbow injuries include **triceps tendinitis** (posterior tennis elbow), **medial collateral ligament injury** elicited by valgus stress to the elbow, and **osteochondral articular loose bodies.**
   b. **Concomitant neurologic injury** may include ulnar nerve (cubital tunnel), median nerve (pronator teres syndrome, carpal tunnel syndrome), or radial nerve entrapment (radial tunnel syndrome).
   c. Occasional anterior elbow compartment pain with flexion contracture can represent **elbow synovitis** from service overuse (biceps in acceleration phase), and is responsive to rest and flexibility exercises.
   d. A large forearm on the dominant side will represent adaptation to sport-specific demands as long as flexibility is not lost.

4. **Shoulder injuries (tennis shoulder)**
   a. **Adaptive changes to the dominant shoulder (King Kong arm)** include a drooped and hypertrophied shoulder girdle with chronic overstretch to the trapezius, levator scapulae, and rhomboid muscles. There may also be a reversible upper thoracic scoliosis.
   b. **Overuse of the rotator cuff muscles** (supraspinatus, infraspinatus, teres minor, subscapularis) leads to glenohumeral joint instability. Combined with scapular droop, joint instability may subject the cuff muscles to impingement under the coracoacromial arch during service and overhead strokes.
      i. Injury may also occur to other subacromial structures such as the subacromial bursa and biceps long-head tendon.
      ii. In younger athletes, overuse to these muscles is possible without actual impingement.
   c. The athlete typically presents with subacromial pain and pain referred to the lateral arm.
   d. The athlete will report **the involved arm "feels dead" during tennis play.**
   e. Passive shoulder abduction–internal rotation by the examiner or simulation of service motion will reproduce symptoms.
   f. Tenderness in the bicipital groove may be present.
   g. Rotator cuff muscles may not be weak on exam in early injury.
   h. **Neurologic exam** should look for axillary nerve traction injury with deltoid muscle weakness and lateral shoulder hypesthesia. Winged scapula from weakness of the serratus anterior due to traction injury to the long thoracic nerve may be missed. This nerve, as it arises from the C5, 6, 7 nerve roots, is susceptible to traction from shoulder depression during the service stroke or chronic tennis shoulder droop.

5. **Wrist and hand injuries**
   a. **Relatively uncommon in tennis,** these injuries relate to **repetitive direct trauma from the racquet handle.** Examples include fracture to the hook of

the hamate or injury to the digital nerve from pressure over the MCP heads. Focal tenderness, numbness, and dysesthesias in wrist or hand should raise suspicion of local trauma. Racquet grip should be evaluated and adjusted for fit and padding after the injury has resolved.

6. **Lower extremity injuries**
   a. **Rupture of the medial head of the gastrocnemius muscle (tennis leg)**
      i. May occur due to repetitive push-off from service and jumping overload to a knee-extended, ankle-plantarflexed leg (see Chap. 39).
   b. **Achilles tendinitis** and rupture
      i. May follow a similar mechanism of injury, with strain or rupture at the tendon component of the triceps surae mechanism (see Chap. 41).
   c. **Patella and quadriceps tendinitis**
      i. May be associated with aggressive side-to-side and vertical jumps.
      ii. Patellofemoral loads are also high during deep knee bends in preparation for ground-stroke returns (see Chap. 40).
   d. **Plantar fasciitis**
      i. Believed due to repetitive forefoot push-off during volleys. As the long arch of the foot depresses, traction occurs to the fascia at its origin on the medial tubercle of the os calcis, with heel pain and tenderness over the area.
      ii. The majority of injuries are shoe-related with poor heel fit (necessitating addition of a heel cup) or inadequate arch to support a cavus foot.
      iii. A hyperflexible (pronating) foot should be evaluated for heel fit and a medial heel counter addition to the midsole.
   e. **Lateral ankle sprains**
      i. See Chap. 41.
      ii. Inadequate heel counter and worn outsole should be suspected causes.
      iii. This injury is more likely to occur on hard than clay court. The clay court allows foot slippage; fixed foot inversion stress is possible on hard courts.

7. **Back injuries**
   a. **Cervical and interscapular pain**
      i. In association with drooped or protracted shoulder posture, there may be compensatory cervical hypertension. Findings may include cervical paraspinal tenderness, decreased cervical motion, tender and fatigued scapular support muscles (levator scapulae, trapezius, and rhomboid), constricted flexibility of pectoralis minor muscle (with protracted shoulder posture).
      ii. There may be an upper thoracic scoliosis and King Kong arm.
      iii. The overuse pattern is associated with the downward motion (acceleration and deceleration phases) of the service and overhead strokes.
      iv. Cervical symptoms may be aggravated by service ball toss too far behind the baseline, causing excessive cervical hyperextension (Fig. 2). See Table 1 for secondary sequelae.
   b. **Injuries to the lumbosacral spine**
      i. Such injuries may be due to a similar **service-related back hyperextension mechanism,** as discussed for the cervical spine.
      ii. The majority of injuries are referable to the facet joints of the lower lumbar segments, less commonly the discs.
      iii. The low back may be stressed from compensatory rotation when thoracic spine rotation is constricted by poor flexibility.
      iv. Combined lumbar lateral rotation/extension on exam may worsen facet joint symptoms.

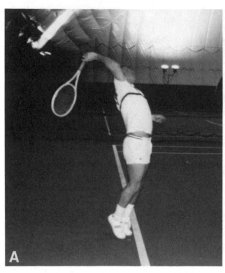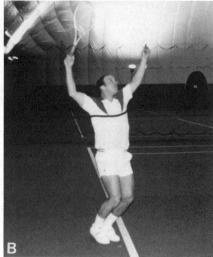

**FIGURE 2.** *A,* Back and neck hyperextension should be avoided during the service motion. *B,* Service ball toss in front of the service line will ensure the hyperextension is avoided.

     v. If sitting is worse than standing, suspect disc injury.

     vi. Secondary L5 or S1 root impingement may be present.

     vii. Examine for lower extremity signs of neuropathy.

  c. **Abdominal wall strain**

     i. Muscles involved include rectus abdominis and internal and external oblique muscles. If symptoms are more toward the groin, think of iliopsoas strain.

     ii. Diagnosis can be **confirmed by hook-lying sit-ups.** Crossed elbow to opposite knee sit-up will be specific for oblique muscle injury (Fig. 3).

     iii. Other differential diagnoses for abdominal symptoms are listed in Table 2.

8. **Eye injuries**

  a. Given tennis ball velocities greater than 100 mph, sport goggles are recommended. For tennis, the safety of open vs. closed goggles needs further research (see Chap. 32).

9. **Tennis and the adolescent athlete**

  a. **Poor flexibility is a concern.** The bones may grow faster than the muscles and tendons. Aggressive flexibility program for tight muscles in the back and extremities is essential.

  b. **Growth plate (physis) injuries** may include:

     i. Slipped capital femoral epiphysis

     ii. Supraspinatus traction to the apophysis at the humerus lesser tuberosity

     iii. Osgood-Schlatter disease

     iv. Sever's disease

     v. Humeral medial epicondyle apophysitis (adolescent medial tennis elbow).

**TABLE 1.** Sequelae Secondary to Cervical Hyperextension

Facet joint injury
Brachial plexus traction injuries
Thoracic outlet syndrome (ulnar nerve)

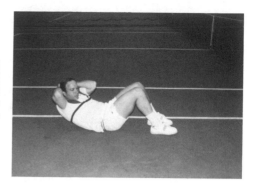

**FIGURE 3.** Sit-ups with hips and knees flexed in a "hook-lying" position will avoid unwanted use of hip flexors and emphasize abdominal muscle groups, preferably opposite elbow to opposite knee to focus on abdominal oblique muscles.

III. **Rehabilitation**

    A. **Acute injuries**

        a. See general guidelines in Chap. 30.

        b. No return to formal tennis training and competition should be allowed until strengthening, flexibility, and equipment modification have arrested symptoms.

        c. Initiate tennis-specific drills to the recovering body part prior to formal participation in training and competition.

        d. Aerobic fitness through cross-training should be maintained, with protection of the injured body part.

    B. **Protection, strength, and flexibility**

        1. **Shoulder**

            a. **Protect the injury** by avoidance of daily overhead activities, and sports such as pitching, volleyball, and the crawl or butterfly swimming strokes. Refractory symptoms may require a part-time sling.

            b. **Active range-of-motion program** of glenohumeral joint: internal and external rotation with the shoulder positioned at 0°; progress gradually to 90° shoulder-abducted position for these exercises.

            c. **Muscles of particular concern**

                i. Rotator cuff and serratus anterior muscles for all strokes.

                ii. Latissmus dorsi and deltoid muscles for overhead and backhand strokes.

                iii. Trapezius and rhomboid muscles to counter effects of shoulder droop.

            d. **Shoulder flexibility** program for the anterior capsule should be modified if the anterior capsule is already chronically stretched (see Chap. 34).

            e. In general, **full scapulohumeral rhythm** must be returned before return to formal training and competition.

        2. **Elbow**

            a. **Protect the injury** by avoiding use of manual tools that require a firm grasp (hammer, screwdriver) or heavy household utensils.

                i. A cock-up wrist splint will protect daily overuse of wrist flexors and extensors during early healing period.

**TABLE 2.** Differential Diagnosis for Nonmuscular Abdominal Pain

| | |
|---|---|
| Acute abdominal process | Inguinal hernia |
| Epididymitis | Testicular torsion |
| Herniated disc | Osteitis pubis |
| Stress fracture | Entrapped intercostal nerve |

ii. Forearm counterforce band ("tennis elbow splint") may be used when athlete resumes tennis-related drills and practice or for mild (inconsistent symptoms) tennis elbow.

iii. If injury is complicated by elbow swelling, medial-lateral instability, or articular lesion, an elbow flexion splint may be necessary.

b. **Progressive resistance program** should include ordered sequence of isometric to isotonic strengthening of grip and wrist flexion and extension. Pronation-supination and flexion-extension of elbow may be added as symptoms allow.

c. **Stretching**

i. Wrist flexor tendon injury (medial tennis elbow): wrist extension stretch with forearm supinated, elbow extended.

ii. Wrist extensor tendon injury (lateral tennis elbow): wrist flexion stretch with forearm pronated, elbow extended.

3. **Functional skills rehabilitation for the upper extremity**

a. Start with **"anchored racquet" exercises,** with racquet secured by rubberized tubing to a wall post or door. The athlete should simulate backhand, forehand, and overhead strokes against this elastic resistance (Fig. 4).

i. Any post-injury incoordination patterns can be corrected at this time.

ii. Backhand simulation is most important for lateral tennis elbow.

iii. Overhead stroke simulation is most important for shoulder injuries and medial tennis elbow.

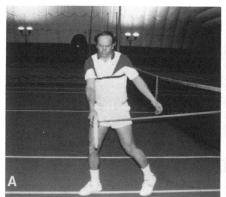
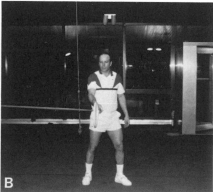
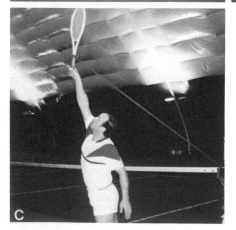

**FIGURE 4.** *A–C,* Tennis strokes such as the backhand may be practiced during later phases of injury rehabilitation by "anchoring" of the racquet with elastic tubing to any fixed handle, knob, or pole.

b. Overhead stroke-related injuries can progress from anchored racquet exercises as tolerated to **"windmill" simulation of service** without racquet, then with racquet. There is no contact made with a tennis ball during these full-service simulations—hence, the term "windmill."

c. The asymptomatic athlete then can begin ball contact service, starting with high-arc service lobs from behind baseline, progressing to full-speed service.

d. **Lateral tennis elbow** should follow a similar pattern of easy, high-arc backhand strokes, progressing to full-speed, short-arc strokes. Backboard volleying drills may provide high-level endurance and provide a test for the stroke.

e. **Refractory lateral tennis elbow may require learning a two-handed backhand technique.**

4. **Back**

a. Rehabilitation by a medical team skilled in back disorders is essential, given that the spine is multiarthrodial, has multiple motor functions and flexibility patterns, and protects the spinal cord.

b. See Chaps. 31 and 38 for protection of the acutely injured spine and basic rehabilitation program, and avoidance of aggravating daily activities and sports.

c. Functional drills outlined in this chapter for the upper and lower extremities should be tolerated without back symptoms prior to formal training and competition.

d. **Back hyperextension should be avoided** during the service stroke (see par. I.B.7.).

5. **Lower extremity**

a. Refer to Chaps. 42 and 51 for fundamental rehabilitation of sprinters' injuries.

b. When full strengthening and flexibility are attained, and endurance is intact for a 3-mile jog, the rehabilitation program may progress to a **plyometric and sprint agility program** prior to sports participation.

  i. An average 2-hour match will include approximately 30 min of actual play, each point 10 sec in duration, with over 20 sec of rest.

  ii. Sprinting and side-to-side jumping plyometric drills should gradually approach these parameters.

c. **The athlete should display full range of motion at the hip, knee, and ankle needed during jumps, service, and low ground strokes.**

d. Initial entry into tennis volleying

  i. For ankle injury: should include ankle taping, air splint, or similar mediolateral stabilizer for ankle injury.

  ii. For knee injury: rarely requires bracing other than simple neoprene patellar knee sleeve.

C. **Proprioceptive neuromuscular facilitation (PNF)**

1. Methods proposed to enhance flexibility and motor coordination via sensorimotor pathways:

a. **Contract-relax stretching** is a form of PNF in which contraction of a given muscle group allows for greater post-contraction passive stretch.

b. PNF may describe the hands-on technique by which trained therapists place inhibitory and facilitatory resistance to key muscle groups and limbs to alter incorrect movement patterns learned during the post-injury period.

  i. In tennis this PNF technique may consist of slowly simulated strokes, with a therapist manually controlling a given body part, such as the shoulder or back. One example would be a therapist facilitating better abduction and elevation of the scapula during a service stroke.

c. **Non–therapist-mediated forms of motor awareness enhancement**
   i. The use of **plyometric techniques,** in which lower extremity muscles are put through a horizontal or vertical jump drill to augment responsive power output and decrease reaction time.
   ii. For the upper extremity, one might lightly weight a tennis racquet with a 1-lb racquet necklace during simulated volleying drills.
   iii. **Injury prevention and effects on performance by these techniques are uncertain.** If done incorrectly, they may increase the risk of overload injury.

IV. **Facilities**

A. Tennis court surfaces (see par. I.C.3. and Chap. 9).
B. **Year-round facilities** allow for continued endurance base to be maintained during the off-season by indoor tennis and tennis drills, bicycling for lower-extremity conditioning, swimming for upper-extremity conditioning, and rowing for back conditioning.
C. **Tennis camps**
   1. For those athletes seeking off-season coaching or who do not have access to a coach, there are many quality tennis camps available and publicized in the major tennis magazines.

V. **Team safety and sportsmanship**

A. **Practice session injuries**
   1. **Racquet and ball missile injuries can be avoided** by clearly defined rules regarding boundaries on tennis courts where players are warming up or volleying in close parallel files. In doubles matches, team partners should have a clear strategy or strict playing zone agreement.
B. **Unsportsmanlike aggression**
   1. A direct tennis ball return to the face of an opponent should be considered unsportsmanlike aggression until decided otherwise.
   2. Overhead return should have a planned trajectory, specifically *away* from an opponent's face.
   3. No player should return a volley at an opponent's feet unless control is adequate to miss other parts of an opponent's body. The player should also be held accountable for the safety of his opponent in such risky shots.
   4. Any throwing of a racquet during a match should be considered unsafe and prohibited, preferably with a penalty rule included. Of course, throwing the racquet vertically in the air after victory is jut plain fun!

## *RECOMMENDED READING*

1. Lehman RC (ed): Racquet sports: Injury treatment and prevention. Clin Sports Med 7(2):April 1988.
2. Saal JA (ed): Rehabilitation of Sports Injuries. Phys Med Rehabil State Art Rev 1(4):597–638, Philadelphia, Hanley & Belfus, 1987.
3. Ryu RKN, McCornmick J, Jobe FW, et al: An electromyographic analysis of shoulder function in tennis players. Am J Sports Med 16:481, 1988.
4. Snijders CJ, Volkers ACW, Mechelse K, et al: Provocation of epicondylalgia lateralis (tennis elbow) by power grip or pinching. Med Sci Sports 19:518, 1987.
5. Wadsworth TG: Tennis elbow: Conservative, surgical, and manipulative treatment. Br Med J 294:621, 1987.
6. Grabiner MD, Groppel JL, Campbell KR: Resultant tennis ball velocity as a function of off-center impact and grip firmness. Med Sci Sports Exerc 15:541, 1983:
7. Elliott BC: Tennis: The influence of grip tightness or reaction impulse and rebound velocity. Med Sci Sports Exerc 14:348, 1982.
8. Kuprian W, et al: Physical Therapy for Sports. Philadelphia, W.B. Saunders, 1982.
9. Murakami Y: Stress fracture of the metacarpal in an adolescent tennis player. Am J Sports Med 16:419, 1988.
10. Rettig AC, Beltz HF: Stress fracture in the humcrus in an adolescent tennis tournament player. Am J Sports Med 13:55, 1985.

# Chapter 57: Dance Injuries

## JAMES G. GARRICK, MD

I. **General Considerations**
  A. **Ballet**
   1. **Training**
     a. **The successful begin young.**
        i. **Novices in late teens prone to more problems.**
           (a) Unique problems among college dance students.
        ii. Training may begin as early as age 5 (weekly).
        iii. Serious training (daily) begins early teens.
        iv. Generally professional status must be attained by late teens.
         v. Professionals may dance into 40s and 50s.
           (a) Ballet activities often continue into adulthood for the "recreational" dancer.
     b. **Training highly structured**
        i. **Practitioner MUST know what goes on in classes.**
        ii. Classes are precisely structured around a gradual warm-up (at the barre) with increasing speed and range of motion, concluding with actual "steps" and jumps carried out around and across the classroom.
        iii. Classes are taken daily, even during the performing season.
           (a) Performance season days include classes, rehearsals, and performances.
     c. Year-round
        i. May perform only a few months.
        ii. Classes continue virtually every day, throughout the entire year.
   2. **Sex differences**
     a. The majority of dancers are female.
        i. Professional companies have nearly equal numbers of males and females.
     b. **Male dancers often begin later (teens).**
        i. Many with previous athletic experience (and injuries).
     c. Male/female differences
        i. Female dancers dance en pointe (on their toes).
           (a) Usually begin pointe work at age 12.
           (b) Going en pointe depends on training and strength, not musculoskeletal maturity.
        ii. Males dance on metatarsal heads (MTP joint dorsiflexion 90°).
        iii. Males responsible for lifting (partnering).
           (a) Lifting begins mid- to late teens.
           (b) Boys frequently ill-prepared with respect to upper body strength.
   3. **Psychology**
     a. **Pyramid system**
        i. Hundreds of thousands of little girls take ballet lessons.
        ii. Only hundreds achieve professional status.
        iii. Competition continues within professional companies.
           (a) Corps de ballet
           (b) Soloist
           (c) Principal dancer.

b. **Advancement based on subjective judgments.**
   i. Students must audition (compete) for entry into professional schools.
   ii. Body type (dancer unable to alter).
   iii. Weight
       (a) Among the most weight-conscious of all athletes.
       (b) Anorexia nervosa and bulimia nervosa more common than in perhaps any other activity.
c. **Teenage dancers often separated from parents.**
   i. Live where training is appropriate.
   ii. Only adult input/supervision may come from teachers.
d. Education usually ceases with high school.
   i. Some do not complete high school.
e. Experience with medical care often bad.
   i. Practitioners do not understand demands of continuous training.
   ii. Treatment of injuries often superficial and expedient.
       (a) Most injuries are of overuse variety, and cause must be found to prevent recurrence.

B. **Modern: From the artistic standpoint modern dance differs appreciably from ballet. From a medical standpoint the differences seem largely related to the factors presented below:**
   1. Generally, modern dance is:
      a. Performed barefoot.
      b. Does not emphasize external rotation of the hips.
      c. Involves more movements requiring hyperflexion of the knees.
      d. Involves more abrupt movements.
   2. There are greater differences among the characteristics and demands of the various forms of modern dance than in ballet.
   3. Most modern dancers (like all dancers) have some background in ballet.
   4. Modern dance training usually begins later than ballet, often in the late teens and 20s.
   5. Modern dance companies are usually smaller than ballet companies and thus are less likely to have structured medical care systems.

C. **Jazz**
   1. Among teenagers, jazz may be the most popular dance form.
   2. Weight restrictions are not as demanding as in ballet.
   3. Choreography does not demand external rotation of the hips as in ballet but generally requires better than average hip motion (splits and high kicks).

II. **Medical Problems**

A. **Menstrual abnormalities**
   1. Both primary and secondary amenorrhea are common.
   2. Delayed onset of menses is the rule rather than the exception in the serious dance student.
B. Contagious diseases spread rapidly within a dance company or school because of daily, close contact of participants.
C. Smoking appears to be more common in the dance (ballet) community than in the general population.
D. **Nutritional disorders are common in the dance community.**
   1. Bulimia and anorexia nervosa occur more frequently in the dance community than in the general population.
   2. Found mainly in teenagers but can occur at any age.
   3. May enhance the problems associated with injuries (demineralization, slowed healing, worsened side effects with medications).

III. **Injuries:** While virtually any acute or overuse injury can be seen among dancers, **some injuries are so closely related to the specific demands of dance** (ballet in most instances) that their diagnosis and treatment merit special consideration.

A. **Types**
1. **Acute**
   a. **Few are unique to ballet.**
   b. Generally same as seen with any running/jumping sport.
   c. Occasional "environmental" injuries are seen.
      i. Falls from sets
      ii. Objects falling on dancers.
2. **Overuse**
   a. Vast majority of injuries are from overuse.
   b. **Frequently related to turn-out (external rotation of hips) or lack thereof.**
   c. Related to activity variances:
      i. Following layoffs
      ii. New demands from new chorcography
      iii. Increased activity during performance season.
   d. Most difficult to treat.
      i. Not totally disabling
      ii. Gradual onset and thus presented for treatment late in course.

B. **Diagnosis**
1. **Must be precise.**
   a. Often related to the very specific demands of dance technique (knowing the demands makes treatment easier).
   b. If vague, cause will not be found and reinjury will occur.
2. **Must be immediate.**
   a. Little time available for reflection (dancer is de-training while waiting).
3. Must be explained to dancer (and often teacher or artistic director).

C. **Treatment**
1. **Maintenance of conditioning (strength, flexibility, and endurance) is of paramount importance.**
2. Programs must allow continuation of as much training as possible.
   a. Must understand classwork and training in order to manipulate activities during treatment.
3. Dancer must understand goals and rationale of treatment.
   a. Must actively participate in program.
   b. Muscular rehabilitation (strength, endurance, and flexibility) is involved in the management of **every** injury.
4. Program must be taught so dancer can carry it out on his/her own (away from medical facility)
5. Frequent demands for expedient treatment (i.e., corticosteroid injection, etc.) must be tempered with long-term goals.
6. Side effects of medications must be considered.
   a. Muscle relaxants—loss of timing and coordination.
   b. NSAIDs—food intake is irregular.

D. **Trunk and thoracic spine**
1. **Parathoracic strains—often actually involve the scapular stabilizing muscles** (rhomboids, trapezius, and levator).
   a. **Cause—often related to lifting partner.**
      i. Not uncommon to see males lacking in upper body strength.
   b. Treatment is symptomatic and should include an upper body conditioning program.

2. **Scoliosis** has been reported to be more common in female ballet dancers than in the general population.
  a. May be related to a combination of delayed onset of menses and dietary anomalies.

E. **Lumbar spine**
  1. **Spondylolysis**
    a. **Cause**
      i. May be prompted by lordosis secondary to inadequate external rotation of hips.
        (a) External rotation of the hips is increased by slight hip flexion.
        (b) In order to maintain an upright posture, increased lordosis is used to compensate for hip flexion.
      ii. Condition may be more common in dancers than in general population.
    b. **Diagnosis**
      i. Midline pain with hyperextension
        (a) Arabesque position in ballet.
      ii. Oblique x-rays to reveal defect.
      iii. Bone scan to reveal maturity of lesion.
    c. **Treatment**
      i. Pain-free activity is the keystone for management.
      ii. Brace is necessary for pain-free activities of daily living.
      iii. Abdominal strengthening exercises are helpful.
      iv. Gradual resumption of dance activities
        (a) Jumping and partnering resumed last.

F. **Hips**
  1. **Overuse**
    a. **Piriformis syndrome**
      i. Cause: inadequate external rotation of hips or weak external rotators.
      ii. Diagnosis
        (a) Deep posterior hip (gluteal) pain.
        (b) Pain when arising from a low chair or car seat.
        (c) May be sciatic radiation.
        (d) Pain on exam with increased internal rotation or external rotation against resistance.
      iii. Treatment
        (a) Stretching and strengthening of external rotators of hip.
    b. **Degenerative joint disease**
      i. Cause: possibly long-term dance activities with repetitive microtrauma.
      ii. Diagnosis
        (a) May be seen in younger age groups than usually expected.
        (b) Anterior hip pain: activity-related.
        (c) Limitation of motion
          (i) Rotation, pure flexion, and abduction.
        (d) Weakness of musculature
      iii. Treatment
        (a) Strengthen hip musculature
        (b) Surgical treatment usually means an end to dancing.

G. **Thigh**
  1. **Overuse**
    a. **Sartorius tendinitis**
      i. Cause: overuse as an external rotator of hip (weight-bearing or nonweight-bearing leg).

      ii. Diagnosis
         (a) Tenderness at origin
         (b) Pain with resisted hip flexion, external rotation, and abduction.
      iii. Treatment
         (a) NSAIDs
         (b) Physical therapy local modalities for symptoms
         (c) Stretching and strengthening exercises.

## H. Knee

### 1. Acute

#### a. Sprains

      i. **ACL injuries** do occur in ballet
         (a) Treatment: Surgical management is not necessarily indicated, as a substantial number of dancers are known to be performing with an absent ACL and no appreciable disability. Any surgical complication, even in small limitation of knee extension, is career-halting for a ballet dancer.

#### b. Meniscal injuries

      i. Definitive diagnosis should be established early, as prolonged watchful waiting results in deterioration of conditioning. Early use of MRI or arthroscopy is often indicated. Meniscus repairs should not be mindlessly performed, because the period of immobilization may in itself be career-threatening.

### 2. Overuse

#### a. Patellofemoral dysfunction is very common.

      i. Cause
         (a) Inadequate quadriceps (vastus medialis) strength for demands of dancing.
         (b) External rotation of leg to compensate for inadequate hip external rotation (increase of Q angle).
         (c) Inadequate rehabilitation of prior knee injury.
      ii. Diagnosis
         (a) Activity-related, retro- or peripatellar pain
            (i) More often in region of medial retinaculum.
         (b) Occasional effusion if seen late in course.
         (c) Decreased tone or bulk of vastus medialis.
         (d) X-ray changes and crepitation are usually of confirmatory value only.
      iii. Treatment
         (a) Relative rest
         (b) Avoidance of deep squats (grand plié)
         (c) Physical therapy modalities if effusion present.
         (d) NSAIDs
         (e) Quadriceps isometrics (full extension)
         (f) Electrical muscular stimulation for vastus medialis if exercises are painful or ineffective.
         (g) Neoprene sleeve with lateral pad
         (h) Surgical intervention should be considered only as a last resort and then only if the alternative is to stop dancing.

#### b. Patellar tendinitis

      i. Cause: may be repetitive jumping; relative quadriceps inflexibility (tight quadriceps not uncommon in ballet dancers).
      ii. Diagnosis
         (a) Activity-related infrapatellar pain
         (b) Focal tenderness at origin of tendon fibers at inferior pole of patella
         (c) Rarely swelling or x-ray changes.

          iii. Treatment

             (a) Relative rest (jumping)

             (b) NSAIDs

             (c) Ice

             (d) Quadriceps stretching and strengthening

             (e) Neoprene sleeve with lateral pad

             (f) Steroid injections not indicated.

## I. **Leg**

### 1. **Acute**

#### a. **Achilles' tendon rupture**

    i. Cause often previous episode(s) of Achilles' tendinitis.

    ii. Males predominate.

    iii. Diagnosis

       (a) Sudden, often loud, snap in distal calf.

       (b) Dancer describes being struck in calf.

       (c) Defect in tendon.

       (d) Positive Thompson test.

    iv. Treatment

       (a) Surgical treatment favored by most, but closed management has been effective in dancers.

### 2. **Overuse**

#### a. **Achilles tendinitis**

    i. Cause:

       (a) Usually overuse but may be minor sprain.

       (b) May be mechanical from pressure.

          (i) Ribbons on toe shoes tied too tightly.

          (ii) Footware used with character roles (e.g., cowboy boots).

    ii. Diagnosis

       (a) Achilles' tendon pain with activities

       (b) Pain with passive dorsiflexion

       (c) Pain with (or inability to) arise on toes (relevé)

       (d) Swelling

       (e) Crepitation (uncommon).

    iii. Treatment

       (a) Physical therapy modalities

       (b) Relative rest (may have to avoid all dancing temporarily and use heel lift in shoes for daily activities).

       (c) Stretching and strengthening are helpful.

       (d) Gradual return to dancing with avoidance of all pain.

       (e) Steroid injections not appropriate.

    iv. **Cautions**

       (a) Posterior ankle impingement often misdiagnosed as Achilles' tendinitis.

       (b) May enhance likelihood of rupture of Achilles' tendon.

#### b. **Stress fractures**—may involve distal tibia or fibula or (more uncommon) anterior border of mid-shaft of tibia with transverse fracture line through anterior cortex on x-ray (the "dreaded black line" of Hamilton).

    i. Cause: usually change in activity.

    ii. Diagnosis

       (a) Activity-related, localized pain at site of fracture.

       (b) Focal tenderness.

       (c) X-rays may not reveal if seen early in course.

       (d) Bone scan.

iii. Treatment
 (a) Rest to the point of **pain-free activities of daily living** for 7–10 consecutive days.
 (b) Gradual resumption of dancing activities—must remain pain-free.
 (c) Stress fracture of anterior border of mid-tibia must be treated with extreme caution, as this lesion has a propensity to go on to overt fracture. Surgical drilling of the fracture site hastens safe return to dancing activities.

J. **Ankle**
1. **Acute**
 a. **Sprains—usually lateral (inversion)**
  i. Treatment
   (a) With grade III sprains, some advocate surgical repair because instability in plantarflexed position (de riguer in ballet) is so disabling.
   (b) We prefer active, aggressive rehabilitation.
   (c) Cast immobilization results in needless time loss.
  ii. **Cautions**
   (a) **Peroneal tendon dislocations are often mistaken for lateral ankle sprains.**
    (i) Tenderness localized to posterior distal fibula.
    (ii) Ecchymosis may be extensive along course of peroneal tendons.
    (iii) Flake of bone off lateral malleolus (x-ray).
    (iv) Should be managed surgically when acute.
   (b) **Avulsion fracture of base of the fifth metatarsal styloid.**
    (i) Similar mechanism of injury
    (ii) Pain and tenderness at base of fifth metatarsal
    (iii) May usually be treated as ankle sprain.
 b. **Ankle impingement**
  i. **Posterior**
   (a) Cause: impingement of posterior process of talus or os trigonum.
   (b) Diagnosis
    (i) Posterior ankle pain with plantar flexion.
    (ii) Pain reproduced with active or passive plantar flexion.
    (iii) Presence of large posterior process of talus or os trigonum on x-ray.
   (c) Treatment
    (i) First (few) episodes
     • NSAIDs
     • Physical therapy modalities for swelling
     • Contrast baths
     • Ankle strengthening (invertors and evertors).
    (ii) Recurrent episodes
     • Surgical removal of posterior process of talus or os trigonum.
  ii. **Anterior**
   (a) Cause: usually osteophytes of anterior tibia and/or anterior articular margin of dome of talus.
   (b) Diagnosis
    (i) Anterior ankle pain with extreme of dorsiflexion
    (ii) X-rays reveal impingement of osteophytes.
   (c) Treatment
    (i) First episodes (as above)
    (ii) Recurrent episodes—surgical excision of osteophytes.

K. **Foot**
   1. **Acute**
      a. **Spiral fracture of shaft of fifth metatarsal (dancer's fracture)**
         i. Cause: inversion injury while on toes.
         ii. Diagnosis by x-ray.
         iii. Treatment—short period of immobilization followed by protection with taping and attenuated dance activities.
   2. **Overuse**
      a. **Stress fractures**
         i. Cause: usually activity changes.
            (a) May involve **metatarsal shaft** (metatarsals 2–4).
            (b) May involve base of second metatarsal.
               (i) A "ballet-specific" injury often resulting in long-term disability.
               (ii) Usually requires bone scan for diagnosis.
               (iii) Uncommon.
            (c) **Sesamoids**
               (i) Utilize bone scan to assist in differentiating from bipartite sesamoid or sesamoiditis.
         ii. Diagnosis
            (a) Activity-related pain, often well-localized.
            (b) Tenderness (focal) at fracture site.
            (c) X-rays (many not reveal if seen early).
            (d) Bone scan.
         iii. Treatment
            (a) Activity attenuation until activities of daily living are pain-free for at least 7 consecutive days (longer for base of second metatarsal).
            (b) Gradual resumption of dance activities—must remain pain-free.
      b. **Degenerative joint disease of first MTP joint**
         i. Cause: more often seen in male dancers, because their positions require more frequent dorsiflexion of this joint.
            (a) Pain at dorsum of MTP joint with hyperdorsiflexion (worsened with weight-bearing in this position).
            (b) Loss of dorsiflexion at MTP joint.
            (c) Tenderness at dorsum of joint.
            (d) X-rays reveal osteophyte at articular margin of dorsum of metatarsal head.
         iii. Treatment
            (a) Early—NSAIDs, contrast baths, taping to restrict motion of toe (which also compromises dancing).
            (b) Late—surgical excision of osteophytes.
      c. **Morton's neuroma**
         i. Cause
            (a) May be related to constrictive footwear.
            (b) Usually at 3–4 interspace.
         ii. Diagnosis
            (a) Weight-bearing, activity-related pain.
            (b) Often "shock-like" sensation in involved toes.
            (c) Usually relief with removal of footwear.
         i. Can be seen with barefoot dancing (rare).
         iii. Treatment
            (a) Metatarsal pad placed just proximal to metatarsal heads.
            (b) Local injections of corticosteroid (3 or fewer).
            (c) Surgical excision (probably successful in no more than 80% of cases).

# INDEX

Entries in **boldface type** indicate complete chapters.